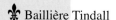 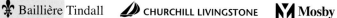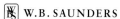

Manual of
Hypertension

Commissioning Editor: Michael Houston
Project Manager: Kim Howell
Designer: Sarah Russell
Illustrators: Robin Dean, Tim Loughead and Marion Tasker

Manual of
Hypertension

Edited by

Giuseppe Mancia MD
Professor of Medicine
University of Milan-Bicocca
Ospedale San Gerardo
Monza (Milan), Italy

John Chalmers AC FAA PhD MD (Hon) FRACP FRCP (Hon)
Professor of Medicine
Institute for International Health
University of Sydney
Newtown, NSW, Australia

Stevo Julius MD ScD
Professor of Medicine and Physiology and
Frederick G. H. Huetwell Professor of Hypertension
University of Michigan Health System
Ann Arbor, MI, USA

Takao Saruta MD PhD
Professor of Internal Medicine
Keio University
Tokyo, Japan

Michael A. Weber MD
Professor of Medicine
State University of New York
Downstate College of Medicine
Brooklyn, NY, USA

Alberto U. Ferrari MD
Associate Professor of Medicine
Centro di Fisiologia Clinica e Ipertensione
University of Milan-Bicocca
Milan, Italy

Ian B. Wilkinson MA BM BCh MRCP
Lecturer in Clinical Pharmacology and Honorary Consultant Physician
Addenbrooke's Hospital
University of Cambridge
Cambridge, UK

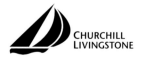
CHURCHILL
LIVINGSTONE

LONDON   EDINBURGH   NEW YORK   PHILADELPHIA   ST LOUIS   SYDNEY   TORONTO   2002

CHURCHILL LIVINGSTONE
An imprint of Harcourt Publishers Limited

© Harcourt Publishers Limited 2002

 is a registered trademark of Harcourt Publishers Limited

The right of G. Mancia, J. Chalmers, S. Julius, T. Saruta, M. Weber, A. Ferrari and
I. Wilkinson to be identified as editors of this work has been asserted by them in
accordance with the Copyright, Designs and Patents Act 1988

First published 2002

ISBN 0 443 06195 5

British Library Cataloguing in Publication Data
A catalogue record for this book is available from the British Library

Library of Congress Cataloging in Publication Data
A catalog record for this book is available from the Library of Congress

Note
Medical knowledge is constantly changing. As new information becomes available,
changes in treatment, procedures, equipment and the use of drugs become necessary. The
editors/authors/contributors and the publishers have taken care to ensure that the
information given in this text is accurate and up to date. However, readers are strongly
advised to confirm that the information, especially with regard to drug usage, complies
with the latest legislation and standards of practice.

Existing UK nomenclature is changing to the system of Recommended International
Nonpropriety Names (rINNs). Until the UK names are no longer in use, these more
familiar names are used in this book in preference to rINNs, details of which may be
obtained from the British National Formulary.

The
publisher's
policy is to use
**paper manufactured
from sustainable forests**

Printed in China by RDC Group Limited

Contents

Contents

Contents

Section 9

Changing aspects of hypertension

Contributors

Ettore Ambrosioni
Professor of Medicine
Dipartimento di Medicine e Biotechnologia
Applicate 'D. Campanacci'
University of Bologna
Bologna
Italy

Stephen E. Bakir MD
Fellow in Interventional Cardiology
Emory University
Atlanta, GA
USA

M. Barenbrock
c/o K. H. Rahn MD
Professor of Medicine
Chairman, Department of Medicine D
University of Münster
Münster
Germany

Lawrence J. Beilin MB BS (London) MD MA FRCP
(England) FRACP
Professor of Medicine
University Department of Medicine
Royal Perth Hospital
Perth, WA
Australia

Mark A. Brown MB BS FRACP MD
Professor of Medicine and Senior Staff
Nephrologist
St George Hospital and University of NSW
Kogarah
Sydney, NSW
Australia

Hans R. Brunner MD
Professor of Medicine
Chief, Division of Hypertension and Vascular
Medicine
University Hospital
Lausanne
Switzerland

Valerie Burke MD FRACP
Senior Research Officer
University Department of Medicine
Royal Perth Hospital
Perth, WA
Australia

Michel Burnier MD
Associate Professor of Medicine
Division of Hypertension and Vascular
Medicine
CHUV
Lausanne
Switzerland

Edoardo Casiglia MD
Researcher
Department of Clinical and Experimental
Medicine
University of Padua
Padua
Italy

John Chalmers AC FAA PhD MD (Hon) FRACP
FRCP (Hon)
Professor of Medicine
Institute for International Health
University of Sydney
Newtown, NSW
Australia

Paula Chattington MB ChB MRCP
Consultant Endocrinologist
Warrington Hospital
Warrington
UK

Denis L. Clement MD PhD
Emeritus Professor of Cardiovascular Diseases
Department of Cardiology–Angiology
University Hospital
Ghent
Belgium

Mark E. Cooper MB BS PhD FRACP
Professor of Medicine
University of Melbourne
Austin and Repatriation Medical Centre
West Heidelberg, VIC
Australia

Francesco V. Costa
Professor of Medicine
Dipartimento di Medicine e Biotechnologia
Applicate 'D. Campanacci'
University of Bologna
Bologna
Italy

J. M. Cruikshank BM BCH DM (Oxon) FRCP
Independent Cardiovascular Consultant
Suffolk
UK

Gregory K. Davis MB ChB MD FRCOG FRANZCOG
Staff Specialist
Department of Women's Health
St George Hospital
Kogarah
Sydney, NSW
Australia

Alan Y. Deng PhD
Chief of Molecular Genetics and
Associate Professor of Medicine
Research Centre
Centre hospitalier de l'Université de Montréal
Montréal, QC
Canada

Henry L. Elliott MD FRCP
Senior Lecturer in Medicine and Therapeutics
University of Glasgow
Department of Medicine and Therapeutics
Western Infirmary, Glasgow
UK

Murray Epstein MD FACP
Professor of Medicine
Nephrology Section
University of Miami School of Medicine
Miami, FL
USA

Murray Esler MBBS PhD
Professor of Medicine
Monash University
Associate Director, Baker Medical Research
Institute
Melbourne, VIC
Australia

Robert Fagard MD PhD
Professor of Medicine
University of Leuven
UZ Gasthuisberg
IG – Hypertensie
Leuven
Belgium

Bonita Falkner MD
Professor of Medicine and Pediatrics
Division of Nephrology
Thomas Jefferson University
Philadelphia, PA
USA

Alberto U. Ferrari MD
Associate Professor of Medicine
Centro di Fisiologia Clinica e Ipertensione
University of Milan-Bicocca
Milan
Italy

Guido Grassi MD
Associate Professor of Medicine
Clinica Medica
University of Milan-Bicocca
Ospedale San Gerardo
Monza (Milan)
Italy

Shawn A. Gregory BS MD
Chief Medical Resident and Instructor of Medicine
University of Alabama at Birmingham
Birmingham, AL
USA

Tomasz Grodzicki MD PhD
Professor of Medicine
Department of Internal Medicine and Gerontology
Jagiellonian University Medical College
Kracow
Poland

Pavel Hamet MD PhD FRCPC
Professor of Medicine
Director of Research, Research Centre
Centre hospitalier de l'Université de Montréal
Montréal, QC
Canada

Lennart Hansson MD
Professor of Medicine
Clinical Hypertension Research
Department of Public Health
University of Uppsala
Uppsala
Sweden

G. L. R. Jennings MBBS MRCP FRACP MD FRCP
Director, Cardiovascular Medicine
The Alfred Hospital
Deputy Director, Baker Medical Research Institute
Melbourne, VIC
Australia

Stevo Julius MD ScD
Professor of Medicine and Physiology and Frederick G. H. Huetwell Professor of Hypertension
Department of Internal Medicine, Division of Hypertension
University of Michigan Health System
Ann Arbor, MI
USA

William B. Kannel MD MPH
Professor of Medicine and Public Health
Boston University School of Medicine/ Framlington Health Study
Framlington, MA
USA

Kazuomi Kario
c/o Thomas G. Pickering MD DPhil
Professor of Medicine
Cardiovascular Institute
Mount Sinai Medical Center
New York, NY
USA

Abraham A. Kroon MD PhD
Assistant Professor of Medicine
University Hospital Maastricht
Maastricht
The Netherlands

Peter W. de Leeuw MD PhD
Professor of Medicine
University Hospital Maastricht
Maastricht
The Netherlands

Professor Jean-Michel Mallion
Cardiologie et Hypertension Artérielle
Centre Hospitalier Universitaire de Grenoble
Grenoble
France

Giuseppe Mancia MD
Professor of Medicine
Clinica Medica
University of Milan-Bicocca
Ospedale San Gerardo
Monza (Milan)
Italy

Barry J. Materson MD MBA
Professor of Medicine
University of Miami
Miami, FL
USA

Peter A. Meredith BSc PhD
Reader in Clinical Pharmacology
Glasgow University
Department of Medicine and Therapeutics
Western Infirmary
Glasgow
UK

Franz H. Messerli MD
Ochsner Clinic and Alton Ochsner Medical
Foundation
Professor of Medicine
Tulane University School of Medicine
New Orleans, LA
USA

Albert Mimran
Professor of Internal Medicine
Hôpital Lapeyronie/Centre Hospitalier
Universitaire
Montpellier
France

Alessandra Monari MD
Research Assistant
Department of Clinical and Experimental
Medicine
Policlinico Universitario
Padua
Italy

Professor Alberto Morganti
Full Professor of Internal Medicine
Centro di Fisiologia Clinica e Ipertensione
University of Milan
Department of Internal Medicine
Ospedale Maggiore
IRCCS
Milan
Italy

Georges Mourad MD
Professor of Nephrology and Transplantation
Head, Department of Nephrology
Hôpital Lapeyronie
Montpellier
France

M. Gary Nicholls MBChB MD FRACP FRCP
(Glasgow, Edinburgh, London) FACC
Professor of Medicine
Christchurch School of Medicine
Christchurch Hospital
Christchurch
New Zealand

Eoin O'Brien FRCP FRCPI FRCP (Ed) MD
Professor of Cardiovascular Pharmacology
Blood Pressure Unit
Beaumont Hospital
Dublin
Ireland

Suzanne Oparil MD
Director, Vascular Biology and Hypertension
Program
Professor of Medicine, Professor of
Physiology and Biophysics
University of Alabama at Birmingham
Birmingham, AL
USA

Kathy Paizis MB BS PhD FRACP
Nephrologist
Department of Medicine
Flinders University
Flinders Medical Centre
Adelaide, SA
Australia

Gianfranco Parati MD
Professor of Medicine
University of Milan-Bicocca
S. Luca Hospital
Istituto Auxologico Italiano
Milan
Italy

Zdenka Pausova MD
Assistant Professor of Medicine
Research Centre
Centre hospitalier de l'Université de
Montréal
Montréal, QC
Canada

Achille C. Pessina MD PhD
Professor of Internal Medicine
Department of Clinical and Experimental
Medicine
University of Padua
Padua
Italy

Paddy A. Phillips MB BS DPhil FRACP MA FACP
Professor and Head of Medicine
Flinders University
Flinders Medical Centre
Adelaide, SA
Australia

Robert A. Phillips MD PhD
Director, Department of Medicine
Lenox Hill Hospital
New York, NY
USA

Thomas G. Pickering MD DPhil
Professor of Medicine
Cardiovascular Institute
Mount Sinai Medical Center
New York, NY
USA

Jürgen E. F. Pohl BSc MB BS FRCP (Retired)
Physician Emeritus
United Leicester University Hospitals
Medical Director, PPD Development
Leicester
UK

Richard A. Preston MD
Professor of Clinical Medicine
Director, Division of Clinical Pharmacology
University of Miami School of Medicine
Miami, FL
USA

B. N. C. Prichard MB BS MSc FRCP FACC FESC
FFPM
Professor of Clinical Pharmacology
University College London
London
UK

K. H. Rahn MD
Professor of Medicine
Chairman, Department of Medicine D
University of Münster
Münster
Germany

John L. Reid MA DM FRCP
Professor of Medicine and Therapeutics
University of Glasgow
Glasgow
UK

Jean Ribstein MD
Professor of Medicine
Médecine Interne et Hypertension Artérielle
Hôpital Lapeyronie
CHU
Montpellier
France

A. Mark Richards MB ChB MD PhD FRACP
Professor of Medicine
Christchurch School of Medicine
Christchurch Hospital
Christchurch
New Zealand

Takao Saruta MD PhD
Professor of Internal Medicine
Keio University School of Medicine
Tokyo
Japan

Yackoob K. Seedat MD (N. U. Irel.) PhD FRCP
(London) FRCP (Irel.) FACC FACP FCP (S. A.) FCCP
Professor of Research
Emeritus Professor of Medicine
Nelson R. Mandela School of Medicine
University of Natal
Durban
South Africa

Andrea Semplicini MD
Associate Professor of Therapeutics
Department of Clinical and Experimental
Medicine
Policlinico Universitario
Padua
Italy

Jan A. Staessen MD PhD
Academisch Consulent
Studiecoördinatiecentrum
Laboratorium Hypertensie
Departement Moleculair en Cardiovasculair
Onderzoek
Leuven
Belgium

Lutgarde Thijs MSc
Research Fellow
Hypertension Unit
UZ Gasthuisberg
University of Leuven
Leuven
Belgium

Johanne Tremblay PhD
Director, Laboratory of Cellular Biology of
Hypertension
Professor of Medicine
CHUM Research Centre
Montréal, QC
Canada

Tudor D. Vagaonescu MD PhD
Cardiology Fellow
UMDNJ Robert Wood Johnson Medical School
New Brunswick, NJ
USA

Bernard Waeber MD
Professor of Medicine
Division of Pathophysiology
University Hospital
Lausanne
Switzerland

Michael A. Weber MD
Professor of Medicine
State University of New York
Downstate College of Medicine
Brooklyn, NY
USA

Judith A. Whitworth AO DSc MD PhD BS (Melb.)
FRACP
Director and Howard Florey Professor of
Medical Research
John Curtin School of Medical Research
Australian National University
Acton, ACT
Australia

Ian B. Wilkinson MA BM BCh MRCP
Lecturer in Clinical Pharmacology and
Honorary Consultant Physician
Addenbrooke's Hospital
University of Cambridge
Cambridge
UK

Tim G. Yandle PhD
Scientific Officer
Endolab
Christchurch Hospital
Christchurch
New Zealand

Alberto Zanchetti MD
Professor of Medicine
Centro di Fisiologia Clinica e Ipertensione
University of Milan
Ospedale Maggiore
Istituto Auxologico Italiano
Milan
Italy

Peter A. van Zwieten MD PhD FESC MAE
Professor and Chairman
Department of Pharmacotherapy
Academic Medical Centre
Amsterdam
The Netherlands

Preface

Hypertension is a common condition that has adverse effects on a number of organ systems and contributes to many diseases. This makes hypertension of interest to physicians working in a variety of clinical fields, and is one of the many reasons that there has been such a large amount of research into the pathogenesis, diagnosis and treatment of hypertension. Therefore, it is not surprising that hypertension has been the subject of numerous research papers and books published over the last few decades.

The aim of the *Manual of Hypertension* is not to offer a comprehensive report on the multifold pathogenetic and pathophysiological data, hypotheses and theories on hypertension – although in many instances these have been fundamental in advancing knowledge of and forming current thinking on cardiac and vascular diseases. Readers requiring such information are referred to some excellent handbooks on hypertension published over the last few years. Rather, the editors of this Manual thought it useful to take a different approach to the subject. First, to provide the background essential to an understanding of how elevated blood pressure might originate, and why it represents a factor damaging to the cardiovascular system as a whole, and consequently to most organs of the body. Second, to focus on the practical diagnostic and therapeutic aspects of hypertension in a synthetic fashion with a uniform style. Although well known to the physician dealing with hypertensive patients on an everyday basis, he or she may find it useful to confront daily experience with accepted standards of practice in the management of a condition that: (i) presents with a wide range of clinical problems, and (ii) entails the often difficult choice between treatment options that vary in relation to factors as heterogeneous as therapeutic response and compliance, and the different types and magnitude of organ damage, cardiovascular risk factors, and associated non-cardiovascular or cardiovascular diseases. In this Manual, standard practice is outlined by well-known experts in clinical hypertension, who have endeavoured to make consultation as easy as possible. My fellow editors and I hope physicians will find it useful.

Giuseppe Mancia, 2001

Section 1

Epidemiology

1

Chapter

1.1

Update on hypertension as a cardiovascular risk factor

WB Kannel

1

Introduction

Epidemiologic investigations over the past five decades have identified a number of major, modifiable, independent factors that contribute to the development of atherosclerotic cardiovascular disease [1]. Elevated blood pressure ranks high among these in terms of prevalence, impact and attributable risk. Most of the hypertension in the general population has been characterized as 'benign essential hypertension' because of its uncertain etiology and lack of accompanying symptoms. However, prospective epidemiologic investigation has shown such characterization to be unjustified. These studies also indicate that hypertension is best conceptualized as an ingredient of a multivariable risk profile comprised of a number of metabolically linked risk factors with which elevated blood pressure tends to cluster and which profoundly influences the attendant risk [2].

Prevalence and trends

It is difficult to be precise about the trends in the prevalence of hypertension in the general population because the threshold for defining and treating elevated blood pressure has changed substantially over the years. The National Health and Examination Surveys (NHANES) suggest that the prevalence of hypertension has declined progressively since 1972 and that blood pressure distribution has shifted downward between 1960 and 1988 [3,4]. Consistent with this claim, awareness of hypertension, its treatment and control have also improved substantially [5]. Despite these favorable trends, hypertension remains a common disorder that is inadequately treated. Indeed, according to NHANES III, about 20% of the adult population (ages 18–74 years) has hypertension (140/90 mmHg) and in only 21% of those who have it is it under good control [6]. This amounts to some 30–40 million hypertensive Americans. Each year about two million new hypertensives are added to the pool of patients requiring treatment. The prevalence increases steeply with age so that at age 50–59 years 44% have the condition and at age 70 years or more two-thirds are afflicted [7,8]. The prevalence is higher in blacks and rises more steeply with age in women, so that it reaches or exceeds that of men beyond middle age [9]. In the Framingham Study cohort, the systolic blood pressure increased 20 mmHg and diastolic pressure 10 mmHg from age 30 years to age 65 years. The systolic pressures continued to rise into the eighties in women and the seventies in men [10]. Diastolic pressure peaks earlier and then declines beyond middle age, earlier in men than women – the result is a widened pulse pressure. These age trends in blood pressure, attributable to reduced arterial compliance, result in an increasing prevalence of isolated systolic hypertension with advancing age, whereas the prevalence of isolated diastolic pressure elevations decline. Indeed, about 65% of hypertension in the elderly is of the isolated systolic variety.

BOX 1.1.1 The Framingham Study

In the Framingham Study the average blood pressure of the cohort has declined steadily over the decades and elevated blood pressures are only one-third as prevalent as formerly [2]. However, if those with normalized pressures under treatment are included in the estimate, hypertension prevalence appears to have increased. This apparent lack of a decline in hypertension prevalence is very likely a product of earlier detection and treatment instituted at a lower level of pressure. No consistent trend in age-adjusted blood pressure, in either direction, has been noted in the Framingham Study cohorts not receiving treatment [7]. Two-thirds of the cohort who were originally normotensive developed some degree of hypertension over three decades of follow-up [8].

Examination of the incidence of hypertension in the Framingham cohort indicates that 25–50% of the cohort originally normotensive developed hypertension (> 140/90 mmHg) during 26 years of follow-up [11]. Those with absolutely normal pressures (<120/80 mmHg) developed hypertension at half the rate of those with high normal pressures (120–139/80–89 mmHg) [12]. The incidence of hypertension increased threefold with age in men from the third to fifth decade of age and eightfold in women [11]. After age 40 years, eight-year hypertension incidence rates were similar in men and women (about 14%).

Hypertension remains at epidemic proportions because the large numbers of susceptible persons continue to be exposed to causal environmental factors [6]. Treatment of existent hypertension is an important but inadequate response to the population burden of blood pressure-induced cardiovascular disease. Much of the excess morbidity and mortality attributable to hypertension arises from the segment of the population with modest blood pressure elevations that are too prevalent to justify indiscriminant expenditure for drug therapy considering the moderate average level of risk (Figure 1.1.1). Primary

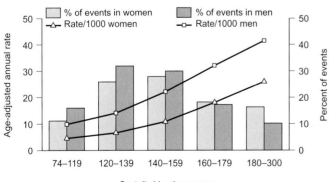

Fig. 1.1.1 Risk of cardiovascular events by level of systolic blood pressure. Subject aged 35–64 years. Framingham Study: 38-year follow-up. Reproduced with permission from Kannel WB. Cardiovascular risk assessment in hypertension. In: *Atlas of Heart Disease* (eds Braunwald E, Hollenberg N). Current Medicine: Philadelphia, 1994.

prevention is best achieved by a population approach designed to shift the entire distribution of blood pressure down to a more acceptable level [6]. Measures required include curbing of weight gain, reduction of salt intake, engineering of physical activity back into daily life, and curbing of excessive alcohol intake [6].

Classification and goals

All categorical classifications of 'hypertension' must be arbitrary because the blood pressure influences cardiovascular morbidity and mortality in a continuous graded fashion with no discernible critical values that separate normal from pathological pressures. It is, however, necessary to do so in order to designate indications and goals for therapy.

The goal of treatment is not simply to lower the blood pressure, but also to reduce hypertension-related morbidity and mortality by the least intrusive means. The JNC VI recommends a target blood pressure below 140/90 mmHg, and even lower if stroke is to be prevented, renal function preserved and progression of heart failure slowed. It is recommended that other modifiable risk factors for cardiovascular disease be sought out and controlled along with the blood pressure elevation [5]. This goal may be achieved by lifestyle modification or with medication depending on the severity of the blood pressure elevation, and the burden of associated risk factors or indications of target organ damage such as left ventricular hypertrophy, proteinuria, or overt cardiovascular disease.

Cardiovascular sequelae

Hypertension is a powerful risk factor for all of the major atherosclerotic cardiovascular disease outcomes including coronary disease, stroke, peripheral artery disease and heart failure [2]. Risk ratios are larger for all the other sequelae, but coronary disease is the most common and most lethal outcome (Figure 1.1.2). Indeed, the incidence of coronary disease in hypertensives is equal to that of all the other sequelae combined. The less than expected efficacy of antihypertensive therapy for coronary disease has led some to doubt the existence of a direct causal relationship of hypertension to the occurrence of coronary disease. However, the incidence of every clinical manifestation of coronary disease, including

---

BOX 1.1.2 Defining hypertension

The JNC VI classifies blood pressures as follows: <120/80 mmHg as optimal; <130/85 mmHg as normal; 130–139/85–89 mmHg as high–normal; 140–159 mmHg systolic or 90–99 mmHg diastolic as Stage 1; 160–179 mmHg or 100–109 mmHg as Stage 2; and >180 mmHg or >110 mmHg as Stage 3. Isolated systolic hypertension is also classified in three stages in persons with diastolic blood pressures of <90 mmHg who have systolic pressures of >140, >160 and >180 mmHg, respectively. These categories of blood pressure should be based on two or more readings at each of two or more examinations [5].

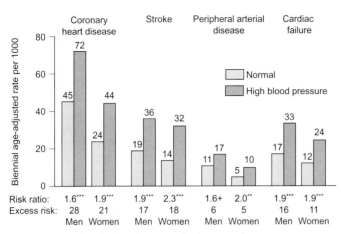

Fig. 1.1.2 Risk of cardiovascular events by hypertensive status. Framingham Study: 36-year follow-up. Subject aged 65–94 years. *P<0.05; **P<0.01; ***P<0.001; + NS.

angina pectoris, myocardial infarction, and sudden death is significantly increased in persons with hypertension and the risk is proportional to the severity of the hypertension (Table 1.1.1). Surprisingly, hypertension predisposes particularly to occult myocardial infarction [13]. This preference for unrecognized infarctions persists even after persons with possible confounding conditions such as diabetes, left ventricular hypertrophy and antihypertensive therapy are excluded. These data suggest that hypertensive individuals need to be routinely monitored by ECG examination for the unsuspected occurrence of a silent myocardial infarction.

Following a myocardial infarction, hypertension continues to have an adverse influence on mortality and reinfarction. Adjusting for other risk factors, each 25 mmHg increment in systolic blood pressure increases the risk of a mortality by 42% and of reinfarction by 53% [14]. The mean blood pressure at which reinfarctions occurred in the Framingham Study was only 146/87 mmHg, indicating the importance of controlling even mild hypertension. Because the blood pressure often drops after an acute myocardial infarction, it should be measured after it has stabilized. Patients whose blood pressures fall after an acute myocardial infarction and remain lower than before the infarction occurred, have a distinctly

Table 1.1.1 Risk of clinical manifestations of coronary heart disease (CHD) by blood pressure status. Age-adjusted risk ratio. Framingham Study: 40-year follow-up

Clinical manifestation	35–64 years		65–94 years	
	Men	Women	Men	Women
Myocardial infarction	1.95***	3.17***	1.79***	2.33***
Angina pectoris	2.03***	2.72***	1.40*	1.93***
Sudden death	2.60**	2.75**	1.86**	1.71*
Any coronary heart disease	2.13**	2.76***	1.63***	2.13**

* P<0.05 **P<0.01 ***P<0.001.

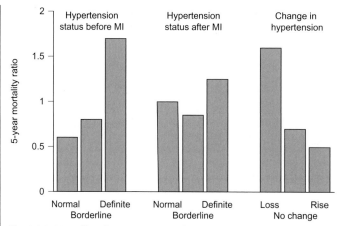

Fig. 1.1.3 Mortality after unrecognized myocardial infarction (MI). Reproduced with permission from Kannel WB *et al*. Blood pressure and survival after myocardial infarction. Framingham Heart Study. *Am Coll Cardiol* 1980;**45**:326–330.

poorer prognosis than those whose blood pressures remain stable (Figure 1.1.3), creating a J-curve of blood pressure mortality. Data from the Framingham Study indicate that it is important to ascertain the preinfarction blood pressure status of patients who sustain an infarction, because adverse outcomes are more closely related to the antecedent than the postinfarction blood pressure [14]. The preinfarction blood pressure should be used to determine the need to monitor the blood pressure after the infarction, and to decide whether antihypertensive therapy is likely to be needed.

BOX 1.1.3 Population impact

The impact of hypertension on the incidence of cardiovascular disease in the general population is best evaluated from the population attributable risk. This statistic takes into account both the prevalence of the risk factor (hypertension) and the strength of its impact (risk ratio) on cardiovascular disease. Because of its high prevalence in the general population and its sizeable risk ratio, approximately 35% of atherosclerotic events are attributable to hypertension. The odds ratio, or relative risk to the individual, increases with the severity of the hypertension, but the attributable risk is greatest for mild degrees of hypertension because of their greater prevalence than severe hypertension in the general population. Thus, the bulk of cardiovascular disease that arises from hypertension in the general population comes from those with relatively mild blood pressure elevations (Figure 1.1.1). About half the cardiovascular events in the general population are occurring at blood pressures below those recommended for treatment with antihypertensive medications. This indicates a need for vigorous non-pharmacologic treatment of persons with high–normal blood pressures and targeting of high-risk mild hypertensive persons for drug treatment based on their multivariate risk profile.

Investigation at the Framingham Study provides no support for the widely held contention that mild hypertension predisposes predominantly to atherothrombotic brain infarction whereas severe hypertension leads to intracerebral hemorrhage. The preponderance of strokes in the Framingham cohort with any severity of hypertension were brain infarctions and the proportion of such strokes in persons with mild hypertension (5%) was almost identical to that in those with severe hypertension [2]. With increasing severity of hypertension, the proportion of strokes attributable to brain infarction actually increased at the expense of subarachnoid hemorrhage and cerebral embolus, whereas the proportion due to intracerebral hemorrhage did not change.

Systolic hypertension

Until recently, it was widely and tenaciously held that blood pressure rises normally with age and that isolated systolic hypertension was largely an innocuous accompaniment to progressive arterial stiffening as age advanced. The term 'essential hypertension' was taken to mean that blood pressure was obliged to rise in order to maintain adequate perfusion of tissues supplied by a progressively more stenotic arterial circulation and that this effect may even be 'protective' in the very old. The prevalence of elevated blood pressure in general and isolated systolic hypertension in particular, does indeed rise with age in most populations, but this is neither inevitable nor beneficial. Moreover, it was feared that the elderly could not tolerate having blood pressure lowering because of orthostatic side effects, leading to reluctance to aggressively treat hypertension in the elderly. However, both the SHEP and SYST-EUR trials demonstrated that treatment of isolated systolic hypertension in the elderly was not only well tolerated but also highly efficacious in preventing cardiovascular events and prolonging life [15,16]

The elderly

Hypertension predisposes powerfully to the major cardiovascular problems that commonly afflict the elderly, doubling the risk [17]. Indeed, hypertension is a more important cause of excess risk than hypercholesterolemia, diabetes or smoking. The decreased risk ratio observed in the elderly is offset by their high cardiovascular disease incidence, resulting in a greater excess and attributable risk, making antihypertensive treatment actually more cost-effective in the elderly than in the middle-aged (Figure 1.1.4). Isolated systolic hypertension, the predominant type of hypertension in the elderly, has been shown to be dangerous, predisposing to strokes, coronary events and heart failure. As in the middle-aged, hypertension in the elderly clusters with hypercholesterolemia, diabetes, obesity, elevated triglyceride and left ventricular hypertrophy, all of which further enhance the risk. In addition 25% already have manifest cardiovascular disease which should impart a greater sense of urgency for treatment and influence the choice of therapy [17].

1

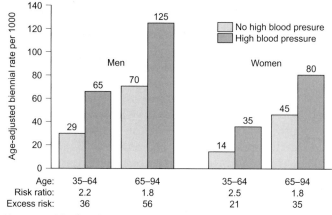

Fig. 1.1.4 Risk of cardiovascular disease in hypertension by age and sex. Framingham Study: 36-year follow-up. Reproduced with permission from Kannel WB. Hypertension. In: *Vascular Disease in the Elderly* (eds Aronow WS, Stemmer EA, Wilson SE), p. 181. Futura: Armonk, NY, 1997.

Antihypertensive trials indicate greater benefit of antihypertensive therapy in the elderly than in the middle-aged hypertensive patient and have conclusively demonstrated the benefit of treating isolated systolic hypertension [15,16]. Thus, hypertension is dangerous in the elderly, is readily controlled and when treated reduces the risk of cardiovascular sequelae.

Isolated systolic hypertension was in the past considered important only as an indicator of other conditions such as aortic regurgitation or hyperthyroidism. Increased peripheral resistance was considered the hallmark of essential hypertension and diastolic blood pressure was considered a better marker of peripheral resistance than systolic pressure and therefore it must be a superior indicator of the cardiovascular hazards of hypertension. As a result, recommendations for treatment and trials to examine the efficacy of antihypertensive treatment were based on diastolic blood pressure, further reinforcing the perception that the adverse effect of hypertension derives chiefly from the diastolic component of blood pressure. Framingham Study prospective investigations of the impact of the various components of blood pressure as risk factors for cardiovascular disease, beginning in 1971, provided no support for the contention that diastolic blood pressure was the chief determinant of the cardiovascular sequelae of hypertension [18]. All the cardiovascular consequences of hypertension, including coronary disease, stroke, peripheral artery disease and heart failure were shown to be more strongly related to systolic than diastolic pressure, at all ages in both sexes [2,19]. Cardiovascular disease risk gradients for comparable unit increases in blood pressure were greater for systolic than diastolic blood pressure (Table 1.1.2). Also comparing isolated elevations of systolic with isolated increases of diastolic pressure as risks for all cardiovascular disease sequelae, revealed larger risk ratios and incidence rates for systolic than diastolic hypertension as usually defined (Table 1.1.3). Furthermore, in

Table 1.1.2 Increase in risk of cardiovascular events per standard deviation increase in blood pressure parameter. Standardized increment in risk. Framingham Study: 30-year follow-up

Parameter	Men		Women	
	35–64 years	65–94 years	35–64 years	65–94 years
Systolic pressure	41%***	51%***	43%***	23%***
Mean arterial pressure	41%***	44%***	42%***	18%***
Pulse pressure	29%***	42%***	36%***	22%***
Diastolic pressure	35%***	30%***	33%***	9%†

† NS; ***$P<0.001$.

Table 1.1.3 Risk of cardiovascular events for isolated systolic vs. diastolic hypertension. Age-adjusted biennial rate per 1000. Framingham Study: 36-year follow-up

Outcome	35–64 Years				65–94 Years			
	ISH		IDH		ISH		IDH	
	Men	Women	Men	Women	Men	Women	Men	Women
Coronary disease	50	19	36	16	68	43	61	39
Stroke	10	5	7	4	52	30	14	21
Heart failure	12	3	5	4	37	23	19	19
Peripheral artery disease	12	15	8	4	22	12	4	5

ISH = isolated systolic hypertension; IDH = isolated diastolic hypertension.

persons whose diastolic blood pressure never exceeded 95 mmHg over 20 years of follow-up, risk of developing cardiovascular disease was strongly related to systolic blood pressure in a continuous graded fashion at all ages in both sexes [2].

Elevated systolic blood pressure, whether or not accompanied by an elevated diastolic pressure, is now an established risk factor for all the sequelae of hypertension. Even borderline isolated systolic hypertension merits consideration for treatment. Overreliance on diastolic blood pressure can be misleading, particularly in the elderly. The use of diastolic blood pressure to determine the need for treatment in persons with systolic hypertension is unwise. Clinical decisions and controlled trials have for too long emphasized the diastolic component of blood pressure. Surveys indicate that identification, treatment and control of systolic hypertension is suboptimal.

Left ventricular hypertrophy

Hypertension is a major determinant of left ventricular hypertrophy (LVH) in the general population, whether detected by ECG, chest X-ray or echocardiogram. The risk of developing significant hypertrophy increases with the level of blood pressure in a continuous graded fashion. Left ventricular mass increases with the level of blood pressure even within the high–normal range [20]. The systolic pressure exerts a greater influence than the diastolic pressure and even isolated systolic hypertension predisposes to hypertrophy.

Left ventricular
hypertrophy

Heart failure

Left ventricular hypertrophy cannot be taken as an incidental compensatory feature of hypertension since at any blood pressure those with hypertrophy are at a distinctly greater risk of all the cardiovascular sequelae of hypertension than those without [20,21]. Although a less sensitive indicator of anatomical hypertrophy, ECG-LVH is a powerful risk factor for adverse outcomes [22]. The risk increases with the degree of voltage elevation and the extent of repolarization abnormality. When repolarization abnormality accompanies the increased voltage, myocardial ischemia is also likely to be present [19]. Within five years 33% of men and 21% of the women with the condition were dead [23]. Those with a combination of ECG and chest film indications of hypertrophy have a greater risk than those with either alone [23]. There is no critical left ventricular mass that delineates compensatory from pathological hypertrophy; the risk of coronary disease, stroke and heart failure increases progressively with the left ventricular mass in a continuous graded fashion. ECG-LVH carries the same risk of adverse cardiovascular outcomes as ECG evidence of a myocardial infarction. Once a myocardial infarction has occurred, left ventricular hypertrophy independently contributes to recurrences and other adverse outcomes, and because of an association with ventricular ectopy, predisposes to sudden death. ECG-LVH is present in 22% of hypertensive persons who go on to develop heart failure, further increasing the hypertensive risk two- to threefold.

Left ventricular hypertrophy should be prevented or promptly corrected by vigorous treatment of the inciting blood pressure elevation. Observational data indicate that when ECG-LVH regresses there is a substantial 30–40% reduction in cardiovascular disease events (Table 1.1.4). However, controlled trials are needed to demonstrate the benefit of reversing left ventricular hypertrophy independent of the reduction in blood pressure that accompanies its reversal.

Heart failure

Hypertension is a major contributor to the incidence of heart failure in the general population, accounting for 39% of cases in men and 59% in women. Adjusting for age and other predisposing factors, compared to normotension, hypertension (>140/90 mmHg) imposes a twofold increased risk in men and threefold increase in women. Among

Table 1.1.4 Risk of cardiovascular events by change in ECG features of left ventricular hypertrophy. Framingham Study

Voltage change	Percent probability of events		Change in repolarization	Percent probability of events	
	Men	Women		Men	Women
None	10.7%	10.7%	None	9.8%	8.3%
Increase	13.8%	12.4%	Worse	12.1%	13.2%
Decrease	6.2%	7.2%	Improved	7.0%	11.2%
Percentage change in risk with improvement	–42%	–33%		–29%	+34%

BOX 1.1.4 Mechanisms of clustering

The mechanism whereby obesity and weight gain promotes atherogenic risk factors is reasonably well established [27]. Excess body fat has been shown to increase resistance to the action of insulin reducing uptake of glucose by the tissues [28]. Abdominal obesity, in particular, has been found to be associated with insulin resistance, hyperinsulinemia, lipoprotein lipase abnormality, elevated triglycerides, reduced HDL-cholesterol, and small-dense LDL. It may also promote increased resorption of sodium from the renal tubules, expanding the blood volume and inducing autonomic imbalance that results in hypertension. Furthermore, insulin resistance often eventuates in glucose intolerance and diabetes. All these features of insulin resistance induced by obesity jointly accelerate atherogenesis and may explain the tendency for all the major risk factors to cluster together (Figure 1.1.5). There is a great potential cardiovascular risk benefit to be achieved by weight control in hypertensive persons if we can learn how to achieve sustained weight control.

---

hypertensive persons myocardial infarction, valve disease, diabetes and left ventricular hypertrophy further increase the risk of failure two- to sixfold [24]. Epidemiologic evidence indicates that subclinical myocardial dysfunction is likely to be present in hypertensive persons when there is a low or falling vital capacity indicating diastolic dysfunction, a rapid resting heart rate compensating for a decreased stroke volume and left ventricular hypertrophy or cardiomegaly [25]. Survival following onset of heart failure in hypertensive persons remains unacceptably high with only 25–30% surviving five years. Preventive strategies against heart failure must continue to emphasize more aggressive control of hypertension using ACE inhibitors and other appropriate measures.

Clustering

There is a distinct tendency for other major risk factors to cluster with hypertension. These risk factors both promote its occurrence and influence its impact on the occurrence of cardiovascular disease [26]. Patients with hypertension tend to have a higher prevalence of dyslipidemia, glucose intolerance, left ventricular hypertrophy, obesity, more rapid heart rates and plasma fibrinogen [9]. They are also prone to have hyperinsulinemia, insulin resistance and hyperuricemia, leading some to consider hypertension as an ingredient of an insulin resistance syndrome [27]. Abdominal obesity appears to be a major promoter of this syndrome as well as the tendency of risk factors to cluster with hypertension (Figure 1.1.5). There is an increasing tendency for the specified risk factors to cluster with hypertension the greater the accompanying obesity, and weight changes are mirrored by accompanying changes in the cluster of risk factors (Table 1.1.5).

In any event, it is important to routinely test for these associated metabolically linked risk factors when evaluating a hypertensive patient, because hypertension occurs in isolation of these risk factors only about

Clustering

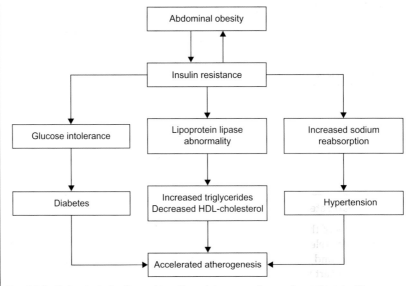

Fig. 1.1.5 Abdominal obesity and insulin resistance syndrome. Reproduced with permission from Kannel WB. Natural history of cardiovascular risk. In: *Atlas of Heart Disease*, Vol. 1 (eds Braunwald E, Hollenberg N), pp. 5–2–5–22. Current Medicine: Philadelphia, 1994.

Table 1.1.5 Risk factor clustering in Framingham Study offspring with elevated blood pressure according to BMI (subject ages, 18–74 years)

Men		Women	
BMI	Average number of risk factors	BMI	Average number of risk factors
<23.7	1.68 ± 0.91	<20.8	1.80 ± 0.87
23.7–25.5	1.85 ± 0.95	20.8–22.3	2.00 ± 1.02
25.6–27.2	2.06 ± 1.05	22.4–23.9	2.22 ± 1.06
27.3–29.5	2.28 ± 1.09	24.0–26.8	2.20 ± 0.99
>29.5	2.35 ± 1.08	>26.8	2.66 ± 1.09

Risk factors: Q_1 HDL-cholesterol; Q_5 total cholesterol; triglycerides; glucose.

20% of the time. Coexistence of hypertension with three or more of the atherogenic risk factors comprising the insulin resistance syndrome occurs at four to five times the rate expected by chance (Table 1.1.6). It is inefficient to single out hypertensive patients for treatment without consideration of the often associated cluster of risk factors. About 63–78% of coronary events in men and women, respectively, in the Framingham Study occurred in hypertensive persons with three or more accompanying risk factors. It is estimated from Framingham Study data that eliminating clusters of two or more risk factors in hypertensive men would reduce their risk of a coronary event 39%. In women, a 68% reduction should occur.

Table 1.1.6 Frequency of other risk factors in Framingham study offspring cohort with elevated blood pressure (Subject ages, 18–74 years)

Number of risk factors	Percent with specified number of risk factors		Observed/experimental ratio	
	Men	Women	Men	Women
None	24.4%	19.5%	0.74	0.59
One	29.1%	28.1%	0.71	0.69
Two or more	46.5%	52.4%	1.8	2.01
Three or more	22.5%	27.2%	4.5	5.4

Other risk factors: Q_5 total cholesterol, BMI, triglycerides, glucose, Q_1 HDL-cholesterol

---

BOX 1.1.5 Heart rate

Various features of the heart rate–cardiovascular disease relationship have been found to be relevant in evaluating risk. These include failure to reach target heart rate and peak heart rate achieved on the treadmill, chronotropic incompetence, heart rate variability and resting heart rate. Of these, only the resting heart rate has been examined specifically as a risk factor for cardiovascular outcomes in hypertension [29]. Increased heart rate is an underappreciated accompaniment to hypertension. Nor is it well recognized that high resting heart rates in normotensive persons are associated with increased risk of developing hypertension. In the Framingham Study, risk of developing cardiovascular disease in hypertensive persons was found to be related to their accompanying heart rate, the risk increasing in a continuous graded fashion with the heart rate [29]. Each 10 beat per minute increment in heart rate in hypertensive persons conferred a 14% increase in cardiovascular mortality and 20% increase in all cause mortality. Each 20 beat per minute increment in heart rate increased coronary mortality 16% in men and 12% in women. Cardiovascular events in persons with higher heart rates were more likely to be fatal than those in persons with lower heart rates. These findings may suggest that antihypertensive agents that reduce the heart rate may be particularly beneficial in reducing hypertensive cardiovascular mortality.

Multivariate risk

No one risk factor, including hypertension, appears to be essential for atherosclerotic cardiovascular disease to occur. The risk of the cardiovascular sequelae of raised blood pressure varies widely depending on the number and severity of often coexistent atherogenic risk factors. Judgement of the urgency for treatment to prevent cardiovascular sequelae must take into account not only the severity of the blood pressure elevation, but the coexistent burden of other atherogenic risk factors that usually accompany the hypertension. Epidemiologic data indicate that it is possible to target mildly hypertensive patients for drug therapy efficiently by means of multivariate risk assessment [9]. Such targeting of therapy can reduce the number of mildly hypertensive persons who have to be treated to prevent one event and also avoids needlessly alarming or falsely reassuring such patients.

Multivariate risk

For estimating hypertensive risk of a coronary event, the evaluation must include at a minimum, a blood lipid profile (total and HDL-cholesterol), blood glucose determination, an ECG to screen for left ventricular hypertrophy, and a smoking history. Convenient multivariate risk estimation has been aided by risk factor scoring charts distributed by the American Heart Association and other bodies [30].

To estimate the risk of a stroke, the most feared consequence of hypertension in an elderly patient, the risk factors to be assessed must include those for coronary disease plus the presence of atrial fibrillation and overt coronary disease or heart failure. The probability of a stroke in hypertensive patients can vary over an eightfold range depending on the number of these associated risk factors that are present (Figure 1.1.6).

Risk factor profiles for estimating the risk of peripheral artery disease in elderly hypertensive subjects have also been developed [31]. Estimating hypertensive risk of heart failure requires, in addition to ascertainment of the coronary risk factors, vital capacity determination, ascertainment of the resting heart rate, detection of heart murmurs denoting valvular disease, and *evaluation for the presence of a myocardial infarction*. The risk of heart failure in hypertensive persons varies over a wide range depending on the associated burden of these risk factors (Figure 1.1.7). Multivariate risk profiles are currently being produced to facilitate quantification of hypertensive propensity to develop heart failure.

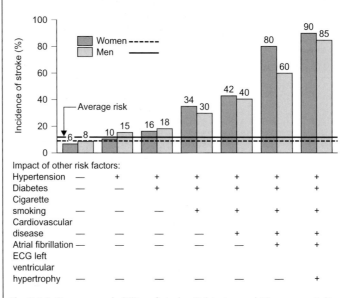

Fig. 1.1.6 Ten-year probability of stroke. Subjects aged 70 years, systolic blood pressure 160 mmHg. The Framingham Heart Study. Reproduced with permission from Wolf PA, D'Agostino RB, Belanger AJ, Kannel WB. Probability of stroke: A risk profile from the Framingham Heart Study. *Stroke* 1991;**22**:312–318.

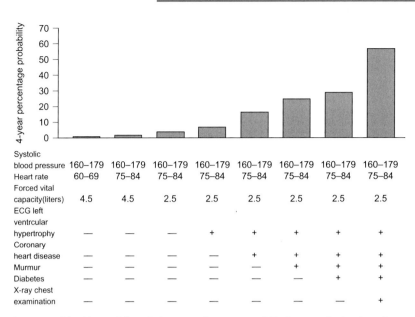

Fig. 1.1.7 Risk of heart failure in hypertensive men aged 60–64 years, by burden of associated risk factors. Framingham Study: 38-year follow up.

Summary

It is no longer appropriate to consider that the goal of antihypertensive therapy is simply to lower blood pressure. Approximately 60% of cardiovascular events occur in persons with high–normal or mild hypertension and among these, the bulk of events arise from those who have accompanying risk factors such as dyslipidemia and glucose intolerance. Since hypertension seldom occurs in isolation from other risk factors, to which it is metabolically linked, it is necessary routinely to assess all risk factors. More use should be made of multivariate risk formulations available for estimating the likelihood that hypertensive patients are high risk candidates for cardiovascular sequelae. Only in this way is it possible to efficiently estimate the hypertensive risk of cardiovascular events so that high-risk candidates can be appropriately targeted for treatment without needlessly alarming or falsely reassuring them.

More attention needs to be paid to systolic pressure because treatment based on this parameter is at least as effective as that based upon diastolic pressure alone [15,16]. When first encountered, hypertensive patients often already have overt cardiovascular disease which must be taken into account in choosing optimal therapy. Likewise, since most hypertension is accompanied by other risk factors, therapy should be individualized so that the antihypertensive therapy chosen does not aggravate these associated conditions. Therapy should be designed to improve the multivariate risk profile including correction of associated dyslipidemia, obesity, glucose intolerance, left ventricular hypertrophy and cigarette smoking.

References

References

1. Cupples LA, D'Agostino RB. Some risk factors related to the annual incidence of cardiovascular disease and death using pooled repeated measurements: the Framingham Study. 30 year follow-up. Section 34. DHHS publication No. NIH 83–2703. Springfield, VA: US Dept. Commerce, National Technical Information Service, 1987.
2. Kannel WB. Blood pressure as a cardiovascular risk factor. Prevention and treatment. *JAMA* 1996;**275**:1571–1576.
3. Drizd T, Dannenberg AL, Engle A. Blood pressure levels in persons 18–74 years of age in 1976–1980 and trends in blood pressure from 1960–1980 in the United States. Vital and Health Statistics 1986; 11(234). Dept. Health and Human Services Publication (PHS) 86–1684.
4. Burt VL, Whelton P, Roccella EJ *et al*. Prevalence of hypertension in the adult US population: results from the Third National Health and Nutrition Examination Survey 1988–1991. *Hypertension* 1995;**25**:305–313.
5. The Sixth Report of the Joint National Committee on Prevention, Detection, Evaluation and Treatment of High Blood Pressure. NIH Publication No. 98–4080, 1997.
6. Working Group Report on Primary Prevention of Hypertension: National High Blood Pressure Education Program. Bethesda, MD: National Institutes of Health, National Heart Lung and Blood Institute, 1993;93–2669.
7. Kannel WB, Garrison RJ, Dannenberg AL. Secular trends in blood pressure in normotensive persons: the Framingham Study. *Am Heart J* 1993;**125**:1154–1158.
8. Dannenberg AL, Garrison RJ, Kannel WB. Incidence of hypertension in the Framingham Study. *Am J Public Health* 1988;**7**:676–679.
9. Wilson PWF, Kannel WB. Hypertension, other risk factors and risk of cardiovascular disease. In: *Hypertension: Pathophysiology, Diagnosis and Management*, 2nd edn, eds Laragh JH, Brenner BM. pp. 99–114. Raven Press: New York, 1995.
10. Belanger AJ, Cupples LA, D'Agostino RB. Means at each examination and interexamination consistency of specified characteristics: Framingham Heart Study. 30 year follow-up. Washington, DC: US Dept. Health and Human Services. *Public Health Service, National Institutes of Health Document* 80–2970.
11. Garrison RJ, Kannel WB, Stokes J III, Castelli WP. Incidence and precursors of hypertension in young adults: the Framingham Offspring Study. *Prev Med* 1987;**16**:235–251.
12. Leitschuh M, Cupples LA, Kannel WB *et al*. High normal blood pressure progression to hypertension in the Framlington study. *Hypertension* 1991;**17**:22–27.
13. Kannel WB, Dannenberg AL, Abbott RD. Unrecognized myocardial infarction and hypertension: the Framingham Study. *Am Heart J* 1985;**109**:581–585.
14. Kannel WB, Sorlie P, Castelli WP, McGee D. Blood pressure and survival after myocardial infarction: the Framingham Study. *Am J Cardiol* 1980;**45**:326–330.
15. SHEP Cooperative Research Group. Prevention of stroke by antihypertensive drug treatment in older persons with isolated systolic hypertension: final results of the Systolic Hypertension in the Elderly Program (SHEP). *JAMA* 1991;**265**:3255–3264.
16. Staessen JA, Fagard R, Thijs L *et al*. A randomized double-blind comparison of placebo and active treatment for older patients with isolated systolic hypertension. The Systolic Hypertension in Europe (SYST-EUR) Trial Investigators. *Lancet* 1997;**350**:757–764.
17. Kannel WB. Hypertension in the elderly: epidemiologic appraisal from the Framingham Study. *Cardiol Elderly* 1993;**1**:359–363.
18. Kannel WB, Dawber TR, McGee DL. Perspectives on systolic hypertension. *Circulation* 1980;**61**:1179.
19. Kannel WB. Epidemiology of essential hypertension: the Framingham Experience. *Proc Royal Coll Phys Edinb* 1991;**21**:273–287.
20. Levy D, Garrison J, Savage DD *et al*. Prognostic implications of echocardiographically determined left ventricular mass in the Framingham Study. *N Engl J Med* 1990;**322**:1561–1566.
21. Kannel WB, Dannenberg AL, Levy D. Population implications of electrocardiographic left ventricular hypertrophy. *Am J Cardiol* 1987;**60**:851–931.

22. Levy D, Salomon M, D'Agostino RB *et al.* Prognostic implications of baseline electrocardiographic features and their serial changes in subjects with left ventricular hypertrophy. *Circulation* 1994;**90**:1786–1793.
23. Kannel WB, Cobb J. Left ventricular hypertrophy and mortality: results from the Framingham Study. *Cardiology* 1992;**81**:291–298.
24. Levy D, Larson MG, Vasan RS *et al.* The progression from hypertension to heart failure. *JAMA* 1996;**275**:1557–1562.
25. Kannel WB. Need and prospects for prevention of cardiac failure. *Eur J Clin Pharm* 1996; **49** Suppl:S3–S9.
26. Kannel WB. Cardioprotection and antihypertensive therapy: the key importance of addressing the associated coronary risk factors (the Framingham experience). *Am J Cardiol* 1996;**77**:6B–11B.
27. Reaven GM. Insulin resistance and compensatory hyperinsulinemia: role in hypertension, dyslipidemia and coronary heart disease. *Am Heart J* 1991;**121**:1283–1288.
28. Bergman RN. Lilly Lecture 1989. Toward physiological understanding of glucose intolerance. Minimal model approach. *Diabetes* 1989;**38**:1512–1527.
29. Gillman MW, Kannel WB, Belanger A, D'Agostino RB. Influence of heart rate on mortality among persons with hypertension: the Framingham Study. *Am Heart J* 1993;**125**:1148–1154.
30. Anderson KM, Wilson PWF, Odell PM, Kannel WB. Updated coronary risk profile. *Circulation* 1991;**83**:357–363.
31. Murabito JM, D'Agostino RB, Silbershatz H, Wilson PWF. Intermittent claudication. A risk profile from the Framingham Heart Study. *Circulation* 1997;**96**:44–49.

References

Results of intervention trials of antihypertensive treatment versus placebo, no or less intensive treatment

RH Fagard, JA Staessen and L Thijs

Introduction

Hypertension is an important cardiovascular risk factor. High blood pressure increases the incidence of fatal and non-fatal cardiovascular diseases such as stroke, coronary artery disease and heart failure. However, this association does not necessarily imply that high blood pressure should be reduced. Fortunately a number of controlled intervention trials, which compared antihypertensive treatment with placebo, no or less intensive treatment, have shown that drug therapy is beneficial. The purpose of the present chapter is to review such trials. Because of the large number of studies it would be desultory and confusing to describe fully and tabulate the design, methods and results of each trial separately. For the sake of clarity and simplicity, the present overview will be based on meta-analyses which have been performed on all trials available at the time of the overview [1,2] or which have addressed particular subgroups [3–7]. Table 1.2.1 lists these meta-analyses with mention of the included individual trials which involved at least 500 patients. Some have addressed patients with diastolic hypertension and reported the overall results in such trials [1], the results in younger and middle-aged patients [5] or in the elderly [7]. Others have reviewed trials on isolated systolic hypertension [6]. Analyses combining these two types of trials have assessed the results in men and women separately [3] or in the very elderly [4]. Table 1.2.2 summarizes some relevant characteristics of the larger individual studies.

Table 1.2.1 Survey of trials included in the various meta-analyses according to type of hypertension. Trials are given in chronological order of publication

Trial	Diastolic			Systolic	Diastolic + systolic	
	Collins* [1]	Mulrow** [5]	Thijs*** [7]	Staessen [6]	INDANA† [8]	INDANA†† [4]
Diastolic hypertension						
VA [16,17]	+	+				
VA – NHLBI [18]	+	+				
HDFP [19–21]	+	+			+	
ATTMH [22,23]	+	+	+			
OSLO [24]	+	+				
MRC1 [25]	+	+			+	
EWPHE [13]	+		+		+	+
COOPE [27]	+		+		+	+
STOP [28]			+		+	+
TOMHS [9]		+				
MRC2 [29]			+		+	
CASTEL [30]						+
Systolic hypertension						
SHEP [10]				+	+	+
SYST-EUR [11,26]				+		+
SYST-CHINA [12]				+		

* Includes six other small trials.
** Trials in primarily younger and middle-aged subjects; includes four other small trials.
*** Includes one more small trial.
† Results according to gender.
†† Results in the very elderly.

Meta-analyses of
intervention trials

Results of intervention
trials according to baseline
blood pressure

1

Table 1.2.2 Characteristics of individual trials

Trial	Patients n	Average age (years)	Random allocation	Type of trial	First-line drug	Control group
Diastolic hypertension						
VA [16,17]	523	51	+	DB	DIU	PLAC
VA – NHLBI [18]	1012	38	+	DB	DIU	PLAC
HDFP [19–21]	10940	51	+	Open	DIU	REF
ATTMH [22,23]	3427	50	+	SB	DIU	PLAC
OSLO [24]	785	45	+	Open	DIU	OBS
MRC1 [25]	17354	52	+	SB	DIU;BB	PLAC
EWPHE [13]	840	72	+	DB	DIU	PLAC
COOPE [27]	884	69	+	Open	BB	OBS
STOP [28]	1627	76	+	DB	DIU;BB	PLAC
TOMHS [9]	902	55	+	DB	DIU;BB;CCB; CEI;ABL	PLAC
MRC2 [29]	4396	70	+	SB	DIU;BB	PLAC
CASTEL [30]	655	74	+	Open	DIU + BB; CLON;NIF	FREE
Systolic hypertension						
SHEP [10]	4736	72	+	DB	DIU	PLAC
SYST-EUR [11,26]	4695	70	+	DB	CCB	PLAC
SYST-CHINA [12]	2394	67	–	SB	CCB	PLAC

DB: double-blind; SB: single-blind.
ABL: alpha-blocker; BB: beta-blocker; CCB: calcium-channel blocker; CEI: converting-enzyme inhibitor; CLON: clonidine; DIU: diuretic; NIF: nifedipine.
FREE: free therapy; OBS: observation; PLAC: placebo; REF: referred care

Meta-analyses of intervention trials

There can be no doubt that systematically reviewing previous work is an important step in scientific research. Methods have been developed to critically evaluate and statistically combine the results of intervention trials, as recently reviewed [8]. Such an analysis of analyses, termed 'meta-analysis', pools the findings of comparable trials to obtain an overall estimate of the effect. The procedure increases the number of observations and the power of the statistical analysis and provides a more precise estimate of the magnitude of the treatment effect. Although the method may be criticized, properly conducted meta-analyses are likely to be the best choice for reviewing previous work.

Results of intervention trials according to baseline blood pressure

The earliest intervention studies in the field of hypertension were conducted in patients with malignant hypertension. Though uncontrolled, these studies convincingly showed that such patients benefited from antihypertensive therapy and should, therefore, be treated, so that no randomized controlled trials have been undertaken in malignant hypertension. Such trials were first performed in patients with elevated diastolic pressure, and later on in elderly patients with isolated systolic hypertension. For the interpretation of trials according to baseline blood pressure we will make use of the results of meta-analyses in which these two types of hypertension have not been mixed.

Results of intervention
trials according to baseline
blood pressure

Diastolic hypertension

BOX 1.2.1 Meta-analysis

A meta-analysis should be conducted like a scientific experiment with a study protocol stating the hypothesis and the methods to be used, such as search procedures, inclusion and exclusion criteria for the selection of identified studies for the meta-analysis, data extraction and statistical analysis. The quality of any meta-analysis will depend heavily on the scientific validity of the individual studies. The meta-analysis of intervention trials relied mostly or even exclusively on randomized controlled trials of active treatment versus placebo, no or less intensive treatment. Randomization is considered essential because it guarantees the avoidance of bias. A further distinction between trials relates to the degree of blinding. In double-blind trials, the control group received placebo treatment which was indistinguishable from active therapy, so that both investigators and patients remained unaware of the actual treatment. It is conceivable, however, that some drug characteristics or side effects may have revealed the nature of the treatment in individual patients. Other trials were organized so that only the patients did not know to which group they belonged (single-blind design). Some trials were completely open, with just observation of the control group, or with referral of these patients to regular care or free therapy (Table 1.1.2). Publication bias is unlikely to pose problems, because large-scale intervention trials are usually published irrespective of outcome.

Most meta-analyses of intervention trials have been based on published summary data. However, when relevant information was missing investigators may have been contacted for missing data or for summary statistics which could not be calculated from published results. Another approach is the meta-analysis on individual patient data, as was done in the INDANA-project [2]. Its aim was to collect individual data from all randomized controlled trials assessing the efficacy of antihypertensive drug interventions versus placebo or no (or minimal) treatment on the basis of clinical outcomes for which the data were available.

Finally, the influence of antihypertensive treatment is usually expressed as an odds ratio, i.e. the ratio of an adverse event occurring among treated patients to the odds of its occurring among controls. The effect is significant if the 95% confidence limits of the odds ratio do not include 1.0. Definition and terminology of the considered outcome events may have differed slightly among meta-analyses. In the present review we will use the terminology as reported by the authors.

Diastolic hypertension

In 1990 Collins *et al.* published the results of a comprehensive meta-analysis of 14 unconfounded randomized controlled trials of at least one year duration of initially hypertensive patients (Table 1.1.1). The review included all randomized trials published before 1987, except those in which any effects of lowering blood pressure were deliberately confounded by differences between the treatment and control groups in some other risk factor interventions. The analysis presents the overall estimates for all randomized trials of the effects of antihypertensive treatment on stroke, on coronary heart disease, on vascular death and on non-vascular death. The overview involved nearly 37 000 individuals,

Results of intervention trials of antihypertensive treatment

Results of intervention
trials according to baseline
blood pressure

Diastolic hypertension

1

with a total of nearly 190 000 patient-years of follow-up. Baseline age averaged 52 years and 53% of the patients were male. Entry diastolic blood pressure was 90 mmHg or above in all but one trial, and averaged 99 mmHg. Among those attending follow-up for blood pressure measurement the diastolic blood pressure difference between those allocated treatment and those allocated control averaged about 5–6 mmHg. Information on systolic blood pressure available from some trials suggested that the net difference in systolic pressure was likely to have been about twice as great as the difference in diastolic pressure.

Figure 1.2.1 summarizes odds ratios and 95% confidence limits for the various endpoints. Total mortality was reduced significantly by active therapy (–14%; $P < 0.01$). Most deaths were vascular and most vascular deaths involved stroke or coronary heart disease. The proportional reduction of vascular mortality amounted to 21% ($P < 0.001$). Whereas fatal strokes were reduced significantly by 45% ($P < 0.001$), fatal coronary events were not (–11%; NS). Non-vascular mortality remained unchanged (–1%; NS). The reduction in the odds of any fatal or non-fatal stroke was 42% ($P < 0.001$) among subjects allocated antihypertensive treatment compared to those allocated control, whereas the proportional reduction in total coronary heart disease was 14% ($P < 0.01$). It should be noted, however, that coronary heart disease was more common than stroke in the studied populations, so that the absolute reduction in coronary heart disease was about half as big as the absolute reduction in stroke, despite the fact that the relative risk reduction of coronary heart disease was only one third of that of stroke.

Collins *et al.* [1] also analyzed trial results according to entry diastolic blood pressure. For example, when trials or strata in which all subjects had entry diastolic blood pressure below 110 mmHg were considered separately, the reduction in the odds of any fatal or non-fatal stroke was 41% ($P < 0.001$) and of vascular mortality 17% ($P < 0.05$). It was

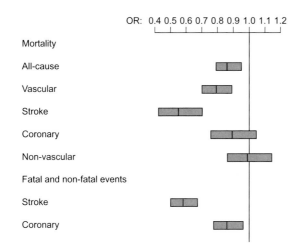

Fig. 1.2.1 Odds ratios (OR) and 95% confidence limits of fatal events and combined fatal and non-fatal events occurring among treated patients to the odds of its occurring among controls, in patients with diastolic hypertension. After Collins *et al.* [1] with permission.

1

Results of intervention
trials according to baseline
blood pressure

Diastolic hypertension

concluded that similar-sized proportional risk reductions were observed in mild, moderate and severe hypertension.

Finally, the authors noted that, in prospective observational studies, a long-term difference of 5–6 mmHg in usual diastolic blood pressure is associated with about 35–40% fewer strokes and 20–25% less coronary heart disease. The 42% reduction in stroke incidence in the trials suggests that virtually all the epidemiologically expected stroke reduction is observed within a few years of treatment. By contrast, only just over half the epidemiologically expected coronary heart disease reduction, i.e. 20–25%, appears in the trials.

BOX 1.2.2 Results in younger and middle-aged patients

Mulrow *et al.* [5] analyzed the results of trials on diastolic hypertension in primarily younger and middle-aged adults involving approximately 33 000 persons (Table 1.2.1). They also included the TOMHS-trial, which, in addition to randomization to active and placebo treatment, administered advice on lifestyle in all participants (The Treatment of Mild Hypertension Research Group [9]). As depicted in Figure 1.2.2, the meta-analysis revealed that treatment was better for all-cause (–17%) cardiovascular (–18%) and cerebrovascular mortality (–45%), but not for coronary heart disease mortality (–9%). As for combined morbidity and mortality, both cerebrovascular events (–33%) and coronary heart disease (–16%) were significantly reduced in these younger and middle-aged adults.

Therefore young and middle-aged patients benefited from antihypertensive treatment with regard to combined fatal and non-fatal cerebrovascular events and total coronary events; as for mortality, only cerebrovascular but not coronary events were significantly reduced.

BOX 1.2.3 Results in elderly

Thijs *et al.* [7] reported a meta-analysis of six randomized outcome trials of antihypertensive drug treatment in patients with diastolic hypertension, aged 60 years and over (Table 1.2.1). In case trials including younger as well as older patients, only the subgroups above the age of 60 years were considered. The analysis included a total of 8420 elderly patients, of whom 4253 were in the control groups and 4167 in the intervention groups. The analysis was restricted to mortality (Figure 1.2.3). Whereas all-cause mortality tended to decrease by 9%, cardiovascular, cerebrovascular and coronary mortality decreased significantly in the active treatment groups compared to the control groups, by respectively 22%, 33% and 26%. Furthermore, the significant overall decrease in cardiovascular, cerebrovascular and coronary mortality was not caused by any particular study. There was no significant influence on non-cardiovascular mortality (+11%).

The authors concluded that pharmacological treatment of elderly patients with combined systolic and diastolic hypertension decreased cardiovascular mortality whereas the incidence of fatal non-cardiovascular endpoints was not significantly affected.

1

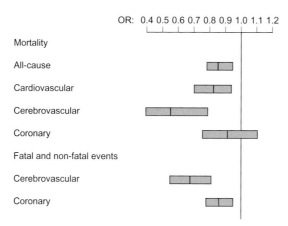

Fig. 1.2.2 Odds ratios (OR) and 95% confidence limits of fatal events and combined fatal and non-fatal events occurring among treated patients to the odds of its occurring among controls, in younger and middle-aged patients with diastolic hypertension. After Mulrow *et al.*[5] with permission.

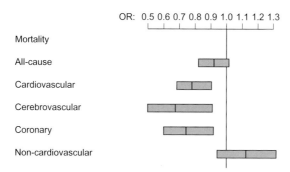

Fig. 1.2.3 Odds ratios (OR) and 95% confidence limits of fatal events occurring among treated patients to the odds of its occurring among controls, in elderly patients with diastolic hypertension. After Thijs *et al.*[7] with permission.

In conclusion, this overview of randomized drug trials indicates that antihypertensive therapy reduces all-cause and vascular mortality, as well as fatal and non-fatal stroke and coronary heart disease in patients with diastolic hypertension.

Systolic hypertension

Isolated systolic hypertension affects over 8–15% of all subjects older than 60 years and is rare at younger ages. Three placebo-controlled outcome trials on antihypertensive drug treatment of this disorder (Table 1.2.1), of whom two applied randomization [10,11] have been published and recently reviewed [6]. Entry systolic blood pressure was at least 160 mmHg in all trials, whereas the upper diastolic blood pressure was less than 90 mmHg in the SHEP trial [10] and less than 95 mmHg in SYST-EUR [11] and SYST-CHINA [12]. Average ages were 72, 70 and 67 years, respectively, and the percentage of males 43%, 33% and 64%. A

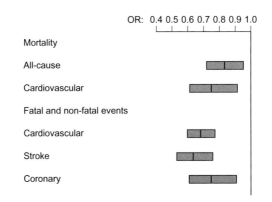

Fig. 1.2.4 Odds ratios (OR) and 95% confidence limits of fatal events and combined fatal and non-fatal events occurring among treated patients to the odds of its occurring among controls, in elderly patients with isolated systolic hypertension. After Staessen *et al.*[6] with permission.

total number of 11 825 patients were included. Figure 1.2.4 shows that all-cause mortality was reduced by 17% (*P* < 0.01) and cardiovascular mortality by 25% (*P* = 0.005). The reduction of all fatal and non-fatal cardiovascular events, strokes and coronary events amounted to, respectively, 32% (*P* < 0.001), 37% (*P* < 0.001) and 25% (*P* < 0.005).

The authors concluded that the pooled results of the three placebo-controlled trials in older patients with isolated systolic hypertension prove that antihypertensive treatment is beneficial if, on repeated measurements, systolic pressure is 160 mmHg or higher.

Results of intervention trials according to gender

Risk for cardiovascular events, particularly coronary heart disease, differed greatly between men and women. However, it is unclear from individual intervention trials whether the effect of antihypertensive treatment in reducing cardiovascular risk would depend on gender. This issue was explored by the INDANA working group, based on a meta-analysis of individual patient data from randomized controlled trials of systolic and of diastolic hypertension [3]. The overview was based on seven trials (Table 1.2.1), in which both men and women were enrolled. The total number of individuals was 40 777 of whom 49% were men. The odds ratios for all trials combined are shown in Figure 1.2.5, separately for men and for women. In women, odds ratios favoring treatment were statistically significant for fatal strokes (−29%; *P* < 0.05) and for combined fatal and non-fatal cardiovascular events (−26%; *P* = 0.001) and strokes (−38%; *P* < 0.001), but not for other outcomes. In men, odds ratios favoring treatment were statistically significant for all-cause (−12%; *P* = 0.01), cardiovascular (−20%; *P* < 0.001), stroke (−43%; *P* < 0.001) and coronary mortality (−17%; *P* < 0.001) and all fatal and non-fatal cardiovascular events (−22%; *P* <0.001), strokes (−34%; *P* <0.001) and coronary events (−18%; *P* < 0.001). The fact that statistical significance for coronary events or total mortality was not reached in women may be related to the lower rate of events in women and the

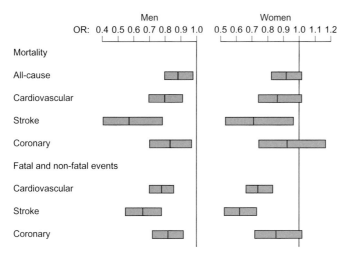

Fig. 1.2.5 Odds ratios (OR) and 95% confidence limits of fatal events and combined fatal and non-fatal events occurring among treated patients to the odds of its occurring among controls, in hypertensive men and women. After Gueyffier *et al.*[3] with permission.

subsequent lower statistical power. However, the risk ratios between the treated and control groups did not differ between men and women, regardless of outcome, and there were no significant interactions between treatment effect and gender. With regard to absolute risk, the authors could conclude that the size of the absolute risk reduction depended on the untreated risk but not on gender. In fact, the size of the absolute risk reduction appeared to be the same in women and in men with similar untreated risk. Finally, adjustment for risk factors such as age, blood pressure, smoking habits, serum cholesterol levels, presence of diabetes and history of stroke or myocardial infarction did not change these findings.

In conclusion, the proportional reduction of the cardiovascular risk appears to be similar in men and women. However, the quantification of benefit in term of absolute risk reduction showed that for women the benefit is seen primarily for strokes, whereas in men treatment prevented as many coronary events as strokes.

Results of intervention trials in the very elderly

Later on, the INDANA working group analyzed the summary statistics from participants in randomized controlled trials of antihypertensive drug treatment aged 80 years and over [4]. The meta-analysis included data from four trials on diastolic hypertension and two on systolic hypertension (Table 1.2.1). The very elderly subgroups represented about 15% of the participants in the various trials and involved 1670 subjects between 80 and 98 years of age, of whom 76% were women. As shown in Figure 1.2.6, all-cause and cardiovascular mortality were not significantly different between active treatment and control. However, the incidence of major cardiovascular events (-22%; $P = 0.01$), of fatal and nonfatal strokes (-34%; $P = 0.01$) and of heart failure (-39%; $P < 0.05$) were significantly

Results of intervention
trials in the very elderly

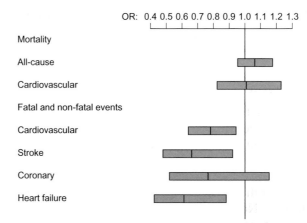

Fig. 1.2.6 Odds ratios (OR) and 95% confidence limits of fatal events and combined fatal and non-fatal events occurring among treated patients to the odds of its occurring among controls, in very old hypertensive patients. After Gueyffier *et al.*[4] with permission.

BOX 1.2.4 Absolute and relative benefit of treatment

The influence of antihypertensive treatment on outcome in intervention trials is usually expressed in terms of the relative risk of an event in the intervention group compared to the risk in the control group. However, the effect on absolute risk is of greater importance for public health, because it also takes into account the actual incidence rate of the event. For a similar or even lower relative risk reduction, more events may be prevented for common than for less common events; the same holds true for populations or subgroups at greater risk than for those with lower risk. For example, whereas the relative risk reduction for stroke appears to be about similar for mild, moderate and severe hypertension, for systolic and diastolic hypertension and for older and younger patients, the absolute risk reduction is larger in severe hypertension, in diastolic hypertension and in the elderly, because of the higher incidence in cerebrovascular events in these conditions. Similarly, whereas the relative risk reduction of coronary heart disease is only one-third of that of stroke, the absolute reduction in coronary heart disease reaches about 50% of the absolute reduction in stroke in Western populations, because of their higher incidence of coronary complications during follow-up.

The number of events avoided by antihypertensive therapy can be calculated from the difference between their occurrence rates in the active treatment group and in the control group. For example, in the SYST-EUR trial on isolated systolic hypertension in the elderly [11], active treatment prevented 29 strokes per 1000 patients treated for 5 years, whereas the prevention of cerebrovascular events amounted to 85 events per 1000 patient years in the EWPHE trial on systolic–diastolic hypertension in the elderly [13].

---

lower in the active treatment groups. There was only a non-significant tendency for a reduction in major coronary events (–23%).

Overall, the results suggest a significant benefit of treatment in very old patients for stroke, cardiovascular events and heart failure, but not for mortality. The authors noted, however, that the apparent beneficial results did not appear to be robust because of the relatively small number of subjects and that confirmation is needed through a properly designed trial in very old people of 80 years or more.

Drug treatment

Table 1.2.2 lists the first-line drug classes which have been used in the larger trials included in the various meta-analyses. In most trials the dose of the first drug could be increased and other drugs could be added in a stepped-care approach in order to achieve target blood pressure. Thiazide diuretics, possibly combined with a potassium-sparing agent, were used in the majority of the listed trials, followed by beta-blockers and calcium-channel blockers. No outcome trials are available in which other classes of drugs, such as converting-enzyme inhibitors, angiotensin II receptor antagonists or alpha-blockers have been compared with placebo or no treatment. However, comparative trials of two or more drug classes are currently being conducted or have recently been published; these trials are not discussed in this chapter. The results of the intervention trials inspired the Joint National Committee on the Prevention, Detection, Evaluation and Treatment of High Blood Pressure [14] to recommend diuretics and beta-blockers as first-line therapy in hypertension in general, unless there are compelling or specific indications for another drug, and calcium-channel blockers as alternative therapy to diuretics in isolated systolic hypertension in the elderly. The Guidelines Subcommittee of the World Health Organisation and the International Society of Hypertension [15] listed the strength of the evidence for reduction of cardiovascular events as one of the factors to be considered in the choice of the first-line drug for any particular patient.

Conclusions

The results of controlled intervention trials clearly show that pharmacological treatment is beneficial in patients with hypertension. Although the proportional reduction in events may be somewhat different in various categories of patients, benefit has been shown in mild, moderate and severe hypertension, in systolic and diastolic hypertension, in men and women, and in middle-aged, elderly and in very old patients. It is noteworthy that only a few years of intervention reduces the risk of stroke to the level expected on the basis of epidemiological observations. The reduction is somewhat less than expected for coronary heart disease, which could be related to interfering atherosclerotic processes or to adverse drug effects. Because the proportional risk reduction is rather similar in high- and low-risk individuals, the size of the absolute risk reduction in various categories of patients depends on the underlying rate of events. Therefore, the absolute risk reduction is in general greater in patients with more severe hypertension, in the elderly and in men. These results were achieved with predominantly diuretic-based regimens; some trials used beta-blockers or calcium antagonists as first-line therapy. It should be noted, however, that about one-fourth of all patients in the control group received antihypertensive drug treatment and that a variable number of patients in the active treatment groups did not comply with the therapy, so that the reduction in the odds of an event by antihypertensive therapy may even be greater than that reported in the controlled intervention trials.

Acknowledgements

The authors gratefully acknowledge the secretarial assistance of N. Ausseloos. R. Fagard is holder of the Prof. A. Amery Chair in Hypertension Research, founded by Merck Sharp and Dohme (Belgium).

References

1. Collins R, Peto R, MacMahon S *et al*. Blood pressure, stroke and coronary heart disease. Part 2. *Lancet* 1990;**335**:827–838.
2. Gueyffier F, Boutitie F, Boissel JP *et al*. INDANA: a meta-analysis on individual patient data in hypertension. Protocol and preliminary results. *Thérapie* 1995;**50**:353–362.
3. Gueyffier F, Boutitie F, Boissel JP *et al*. The effect of antihypertensive drug treatment on cardiovascular outcomes in women and men. Results from a meta-analysis of individual patient data in randomised controlled trials. *Ann Intern Med* 1997;**126**:761–767.
4. Gueyffier F, Bulpitt C, Boissel JP *et al*. Antihypertensive drugs in very old people: a subgroup analysis of randomised controlled trials. *Lancet* 1999;**353**:793–796.
5. Mulrow CD, Cornell JA, Herrera CR *et al*. Hypertension in the elderly. Implications and generalizability of randomized trials. *J Am Med Ass* 1994;**272**:1932–1938.
6. Staessen JA, Wang JG, Thijs L, Fagard R. Overview of the outcome trials in older patients with isolated systolic hypertension. *J Human Hypertension*. 1999;**13**:859–863
7. Thijs L, Fagard R, Lijnen P *et al*. A meta-analysis of outcome trials in elderly hypertensives. *J Hypertension* 1992;**10**:1103–1109.
8. Fagard RH, Staessen JA, Thijs L. Advantages and disadvantages of the meta-analysis approach. *J Hypertension* 1996;**14**(Suppl 2):S9–S13.
9. The Treatment of Mild Hypertension Research Group. TOMHS: a randomized, placebo-controlled trial of a nutritional–hygienic regimen along with various drug monotherapies. *Arch Intern Med* 1991;**151**:1413–1423.
10. SHEP Cooperative Research Group. Prevention of stroke by antihypertensive drug treatment in older persons with isolated systolic hypertension: final results of the Systolic Hypertension in the Elderly Program (SHEP). *J Am Med Ass* 1991;**265**:3255–3264.
11. Staessen JA, Fagard R, Thijs L *et al*. Randomised double-blind comparison of placebo and active treatment for older patients with isolated systolic hypertension. *Lancet* 1997;**350**:757–764.
12. Liu L, Wang JG, Gong L *et al*. Comparison of active treatment and placebo in older Chinese patients with isolated systolic hypertension. *J Hypertension* 1998;**16**:1823–1829.
13. Amery A, Birkenhäger W, Brixko P *et al*. Mortality and morbidity results from the European Working Party on High Blood Pressure in the Elderly Trial. *Lancet* 1985;**i**:1339–1354.
14. Joint National Committee on Prevention, Detection, Evaluation and Treatment of High Blood Pressure. The Sixth Report of the Joint National Committee on Prevention, Detection, Evaluation and Treatment of High Blood Pressure. *Arch Intern Med* 1997;**157**:2413–2446.
15. Guidelines Subcommittee 1999. World Health Organization – International Society of Hypertension Guidelines for the Management of Hypertension. *J Hypertension* 1999;**17**: 151–183.

16. Veterans Administration Cooperative Study Group on Antihypertensive Agents. Effects of treatment on morbidity in hypertension. Results in patients with diastolic blood pressure averaging 115 through 129 mmHg. *J Am Med Ass* 1967;**202**:1028–1034.

17. Veterans Administration Cooperative Study Group on Antihypertensive Agents. Effects of treatment on morbidity in hypertension. Results in patients with diastolic blood pressure averaging 90 through 114 mmHg. *J Am Med Ass* 1967;**213**:1143–1152.

18. Veterans Administration – National Heart, Lung and Blood Institute Study Group for Cooperative Studies on Antihypertensive Therapy: Mild Hypertension. Treatment of mild hypertension: preliminary results of a two-year feasibility trial. *Circulation Res* 1977;**40** (suppl I):180–187.

19. Hypertension Detection and Follow-up Program Cooperative Group. Five-year findings on the Hypertension Detection and Follow-up Program. I: Reduction in mortality of persons with high blood pressure, including mild hypertension. *J Am Med Ass* 1979;**242**:2562–2571.

20. Hypertension Detection and Follow-up Program Cooperative Group. Five-year findings on the Hypertension Detection and Follow-up Program. II: Mortality by race, sex and age. *J Am Med Ass* 1979;**242**:2572–2576.

21. Hypertension Detection and Follow-up Program Cooperative Group. Five-year findings on the Hypertension Detection and Follow-up Program. III: Reduction in stroke incidence among persons with high blood pressure. *J Am Med Ass* 1982;**247**:633–638.

22. Management Committee. The Australian therapeutic trial in mild hypertension. *Lancet* 1980;**i**:1261–1267.

23. Management Committee. Treatment of mild hypertension in the elderly. A study initiated and administed by the National Heart Foundation of Australia. *Med J Australia* 1981;**ii**:398–402.

24. Helgeland A. Treatment of mild hypertension: a five year controlled drug trial: the Oslo study. *Am J Med* 1980;**69**:725–732.

25. Medical Research Council Working Party. MRC Trial of treatment of mild hypertension: principal results. *Br Med J* 1985;**291**:97–104.

26. Staessen JA, Fagard R, Thijs L *et al*. Subgroup and per-protocol analysis of the randomized European trial on isolated systolic hypertension in the elderly. *Arch Intern Med* 1998;**158**:1681–1691.

27. Coope J, Warrender TS. Randomised trial of treatment of hypertension in elderly patients in primary care. *Br Med J* 1986;**293**:1145–1151.

28. Dalhöf B, Lindholm LH, Hansson L *et al*. Morbidity and mortality in the Swedish trial in old patients with hypertension (STOP-Hypertension). *Lancet* 1991;**338**:1281–1285.

29. MRC Working Party. Medical Research Council trial of treatment of hypertension in older adults: principal results. *Br Med J* 1992;**304**:405–412.

30. Casiglia E, Spolaore P, Mazza A *et al*. Effect of two different therapeutic approaches on total and cardiovascular mortality in a cardiovascular study in the elderly (CASTEL). *Japan Heart J* 1994;**35**:589–600.

References

Chapter

2.1

2

Experimental models of hypertension

AU Ferrari

2.1

Introduction

For most if not all diseases, the availability of experimental models is deemed essential to gain insight into etiology, pathophysiology and treatment. Hypertension is no exception and, indeed, many authorities believe the 'birth date' of a scientific approach to the disease to coincide with the Goldblatt experiment on canine renovascular hypertension in 1934 [1]. Since then, animal models have multiplied to an impressive (and perhaps exaggerated) number. Intensive experimental work allowed many aspects of the mechanisms, manifestations and complications of hypertension to be clarified, prevention strategies to be designed, and pharmacological and non-pharmacological therapeutic tools to be developed. Much of the knowledge obtained through models has been extremely useful to clinicians and thus benefited innumerable patients that could be effectively protected from the fatal and non-fatal complications of the disease.

In spite of these unquestionable scientific and practical successes, and the continuing clinical and experimental effort of thousands of investigators, the etiology of the disease has remained elusive. This is even more disappointing considering that hypertension is one of the most, if not the single most prevalent condition in Western societies, that its prevalence continues to rise, and that it is responsible for a large proportion of the increased cardiovascular risk of millions of individuals throughout the world. The basic reason why neither human nor experimental research have so far shed light on the cause of hypertension is its multifactorial nature. The pioneering mosaic theory elaborated by Page over 50 years ago [2] is still largely valid and rationally features the composite array of the factors that may determine a chronic elevation of blood pressure. Such factors may coexist, interact and contribute to the hypertensive state in a different way from patient to patient and from time to time within a single patient, which gives rise to a countless number of possible combinations. Thus, what is in scholarly circles referred to as 'essential hypertension' is by no means a single clinical entity but rather encompasses a variety of conditions whose etiology and pathophysiology may differ widely. This implies that 'the ideal model' of hypertension simply (and by definition) does not exist, whereas the effort, creativity and also good luck of basic hypertension investigators developed a number of different models, each of which is characterized by one or more etiologic component such as, for example, the renal, neural, hormonal, nutritional and psychosocial ones.

Somewhat paradoxically, the experimental models as a whole reproduced to some extent the fundamental characteristic found in the clinical arena: there are many animal lines, especially within the rat species, that develop high blood pressure either spontaneously or because of surgical, environmental or nutritional interventions, many of which have been very helpful to study hypertension mechanisms, complications or treatment, but whose correspondence with human forms of hypertension in terms of etiology and pathogenesis is, in most cases, largely uncertain.

Surgically and/or hormonally induced experimental hypertension

Goldblatt, Page and Grollmann hypertension

Development of chronic hypertension can be reproducibly induced by interfering in various ways with renal perfusion. Classically, stenosis of a main renal artery by a silver clip has been used (Goldblatt two-kidney, one-clip model). Variant procedures included the association of contralateral nephrectomy (one-kidney, one-clip model), positioning of bilateral renal artery clips (two-kidney, two-clip model), external compression of the renal parenchyma by inducing a perinephritic reaction via a cellophane wrap (Page hypertension, again with the unilateral, bilateral or unilateral + contralateral nephrectomy approaches) [3] or by application of special unilateral or bilateral figure-of-eight silk wires encompassing the renal poles (Grollman hypertension) [4]. The mechanisms responsible for the blood-pressure elevation in the Golblatt model and its variants and the complex pathophysiological changes observed during its course and reversal are discussed elsewhere in this book (see Chapter 4.1 on renovascular hypertension).

Aortic coarctation

Congenital aortic stenosis at the arch or less commonly at more distal sites along the artery's course is a clearcut example of 'experimentum naturae' and has been known to cause hypertension for many decades [5]. The rise in pressure was initially thought to depend on the mechanical obstruction by the narrowed lumen but was later recognized, as the 'Goldblatt' concept was established, to largely represent a further variant of renovascular hypertension [6]: the key experiment consisted in showing development of hypertension following placement of an aortic constriction between the renal arteries, reversal of the blood pressure elevation following removal of the kidney 'distal' to the constriction [7]. Replication of the naturally occurring aortic stenosis by various experimental tools (by means of periarterial collars, banding, single or multiple sutures, silver clips, etc.) has reproducibly generated hypertension in virtually all species tested, including dogs, rats, rabbits, baboons, etc.[8–10]. Pathophysiologically, aortic coarctation between the renal arteries mimics the two-kidney, one-clip model whereas coarctation above both renal arteries mimics the one-kidney, one-clip model.

Steroid-related models

Excess of both mineralocorticoid and glucocorticoid hormones promotes the development of hypertension. The first recognition of this phenomenon dates back to the late 1930s and early 1940s in patients with Addison's disease, treated by steriod-replacement therapy, and, soon after, in experimental dogs treated with 11-deoxycorticosterone

Surgically and/or
hormonally induced
experimental hypertension

Steroid-related models

Neurogenic and
psychogenic models

acetate (DOCA) [11]. The most widely used model of what is generally termed 'mineralocorticoid hypertension' makes use of dietary salt supplementation – usually 1% NaCl solution in place of tap water – plus unilateral nephrectomy, two additional measures that accelerate the development and increase the severity of hypertension and promote the development of renal and cardiac hypertrophy. The pathogenesis of mineralocorticoid hypertension is not entirely clear, but it is believed that a transient phase of sodium retention, followed by the so-called 'sodium escape', plays a major role, whereas the renin–angiotensin system is suppressed and provides little, if any, contribution. This is also indicated by the lack of an antihypertensive effect of ACE inhibitors in this model. A role of centrally-mediated sympathetic activation and of increased vasopressin secretion has been advocated by various studies but challenged by others. Interestingly, the Brattelboro rat model, that is congenitally devoid of vasopressin, fails to develop hypertension when treated with DOCA/salt.

Supplementation of many other steroid hormones, including cortisol, corticosterone, aldosterone, as well as androgens, also has hypertensinogenic effects. A peculiar variant of steroid-related hypertension is adrenal regeneration hypertension, that was discovered serendipitously by Skelton in the 1950s in the course of experiments related to androgen-dependent hypertension [12]. Removal of one adrenal gland plus enucleation of the contralateral adrenal gland (i.e. only leaving in place the adrenal capsule and the attached zona glomerulosa tissue) is followed by rapid development of hypertension. Although not well understood, this form of hypertension is probably caused by one or more corticosteroid substances produced *de novo* by the regenerating adrenal tissue under the stimulating influence of ACTH; indeed, hypophysectomy as well as administration of various inhibitors of the steroid synthetic pathways prevent the development of adrenal regeneration hypertension.

Neurogenic and psychogenic models

Hypertension by arterial baroreceptor denervation

Since the arterial baroreflex is the single most potent negative feedback system controlling blood pressure, the pressor effects of abolishing the afferent baroreceptor signal by carotid sinus and aortic nerve section has been extensively used to produce neurogenic hypertension. In-depth studies of this model have been performed in many species including dogs, rabbits, rats and cats. No matter which surgical technique is used, denervation is followed by an immediate and marked rise in blood pressure and heart rate. However, in the following hours/days there is a substantial attenuation of the degree of hypertension and an often complete regression of the tachycardia. Indeed, some authors have questioned whether this model is characterized by sustained hypertension, and believe it is associated with increased blood pressure variability around a largely average normal blood pressure level. This may be true in some species, such as the rabbit [13] and the cat, in which a normal average blood pressure level was found to persist even after the baroreceptor denervation was extended to cardiopulmonary afferent section by bilateral vagotomy [14]. However, in other species such as the rat and the dog, the prevailing consensus is that some degree of average blood pressure elevation does arise in most cases; in the dog it was reported that a slight increase in average blood pressure even develops after partial baroreceptor denervation (confined to aortic nerve section) [15].

Hypertension by lesions of the nucleus tractus solitarii

An alternative approach to study the effects of baroreceptor denervation has been to centrally ablate the first central relay station of baroreceptor afferents, i.e. the nucleus tractus solitarii. Using this approach, various groups largely reproduced the findings obtained with peripheral baroreceptor denervation, i.e. an immediate pronounced rise in mean blood pressure (indeed so pronounced as to frequently cause death by heart failure and pulmonary edema, especially in the rat) and its variability followed by a sustained although less marked degree of hypertension in the later stages, the blood pressure rise being mediated by a marked increase in efferent sympathetic nerve activity [16,17].

Hypertension by exposure to psychosocial distress

The popular concept that hypertension may be to a varying extent due to stressful life conditions has not been easy to substantiate experimentally. One of the few examples in this direction is the model developed by Henry in the mouse [18]: various rat colonies were exposed to prominent degrees of psychosocial stress due to unfavourable environmental conditions in which individuals had to compete for living space, access to food, and sexual activity. Such a stimulus proved to be effective in determining clearcut pressor responses. Even more importantly, if exposure to stress was maintained long enough, the blood-pressure rise became irreversible even after normal environmental conditions were restored, and the animals developed the well-known sequelae of hypertension such as myocardial fibrosis, coronary lesions, and interstitial nephritis.

Genetic models

Considering the evident tendency for essential hypertension to run in families, it is a logical experimental approach, in order to obtain an experimental model resembling as closely as possible the human essential hypertensive patient, to 'create' such a model using a selection procedure. This consists of identifying among randomly bred animals the ones displaying relatively higher arterial pressure values and breed them over subsequent generations until the blood pressure of the descendant population is consistently found to be elevated. Concomitantly, individuals from the same original parents showing lower blood pressure values are also bred to develop a proper 'control' normotensive progeny. Such a strategy was widely adopted in rodents (largely in the rat species) from the early 1950s and has given rise to the many 'traditional' models of genetically determined experimental hypertension. More recently, awareness of the limitations of the selection approach (due to potentially incomplete genetic homogeneity and to the confounding effect of genetic drift in establishing which genetic differences are truly important for hypertension (see below) along with the growing availability of techniques for genetic analysis and manipulation, opened the way to the production of a number of newer genetic models of hypertension in which the contribution of single 'candidate' genes or of given portions of the genome to the development of hypertension could be evaluated in a much more targeted fashion.

Major traditional models

The New Zealand genetically hypertensive (GH) rat

Thanks to the pioneering work of Prof. Smirk at the Otago Medical School, this was chronologically the first selected strain to consistently develop high blood pressure, which allowed extensive pathophysiological characterization [19]. The rise in blood pressure starts very early in life – probably at the fetal stage since by 2 days of age a 6-mmHg higher tail systolic pressure is observed in the animals from the GH strain compared to the normotensive (N) control rats. By the age of 6 weeks, the difference is up to 25 mmHg.

Over the first 15 generations of breeding, blood pressure was shown to progressively rise by about 2 mmHg per generation. This indicates that a large number of genes, most of which with weak hypertensinogenic potency, were aggregated during the breeding process thus giving rise to a distinctly polygenic model. Estimations by analysis of blood pressure distribution in backcross generations of crossbred animals suggest that at least five (presumably quite a few more) genes are involved in the etiology of genetic component of blood pressure in the GH rats.

As to the physiological derangements contributing to the genesis of hypertension in this model, evidence has been collected implicating a role for the sympathetic nervous system, for increased vascular reactivity, possibly via abnormalities in transmembrane calcium transport [20], and for renal (prostaglandin-mediated) dysfunction, but not for sodium retention or alterations in the renin–angiotensin system.

The spontaneously hypertensive (SHR) rat

Less than a decade after Smirk developed the GH rats, a second rat strain with genetically determined hypertension was established by the Japanese investigators Okamoto and Aoki by selectively breeding Wistar rats [21]. This strain had an enormous diffusion in the subsequent years and became the reference model for rat studies on hypertension, with hundreds of studies appearing each year in the literature making use of it to examine the widest range of topics in experimental hypertension, including (patho)physiology, genetics, pharmacology/therapy, and organ damage.

Although appropriately viewed by most authorities as the best animal model for 'essential' hypertension, its very genetic background initially posed some problems related to incomplete breeding of the hypertensive and even more so of the normotensive Wistar-Kyoto (WKY) control strain at the time the animals were distributed to experimental laboratories around the world. Despite the recurring reminders on the need of genetic standardization for at least the major hypertensive strains employed in research laboratories, there are still some genetically-based phenotypic differences among subcolonies of SHR even though each of them is nowadays fully inbred. Even more importantly (and intrinsic to the genetic selection strategy) there are many more differences between the genomes of SHR vs. WKY rats than is the number of genes actually involved in the etiology of hypertension; in other words, many genes that are most likely unrelated to hypertension have segregated together with the hypertension-related genes and are now consistently found to be different between the two strains – the so-called 'genetic drift' phenomenon – thus acting as potential confounders in the interpretation of many experimental results obtained with this model.

All the above considered, it is just impossible to attempt an even limited description of the pathophysiological characteristics of hypertension in the SHR. Studies on virtually all aspects addressed over the past 35 years were positive, in that the SHR was reported to carry the 'unfavorable' geno/phenotype concerning renal, hormonal, membrane, renin–angiotensin, neural, and behavioral features possibly involved in hypertension. How much and how many of these do indeed play an etiologic role remains to be established.

An interesting substrain of the SHR was selected by breeding the offspring of those SHR that died with a cerebrovascular infarction or hemorrage, giving rise to the 'stroke-prone' variant of the SHR, the SHR-SP strain [22].

The Dahl salt-sensitive hypertensive rat

A few years later, while pursuing an experimental tool helping to gain insight in the mechanisms underlying salt sensitivity, Lewis Dahl selectively bred rats for divergent responses to dietary sodium overload. The Brookhaven colony of salt-sensitive (S) rats developed high blood pressure if challenged with a high (8%) NaCl diet while remaining normotensive if this percentage was kept low (0.4%), whereas the control salt-resistant (R) strain remained normotensive on either salt intake [23]. In the pathophysiological characterization of these animals most attention was devoted to salt-regulating factors such as atrial natriuretic peptide and mineralocorticoid hormones and to the kidneys generally (including remarkable interstrain kidney transplant experiments) [24], but more recent evidence has pointed to the importance of neural factors [25, 26].

2

Other selectively bred genetic strains

Many more strains of rats were selectively bred to develop hypertension, either spontaneously, such as the Milan Hypertensive (MHS) and the Lyon hypertensive (LH) strains, or in response to dietary sodium such as the Sabra hypertensive (SBH) strain, each strain having been the focus of particularly intensive research in given areas such as transmembrane sodium transport (MHS) [27], obesity/insulin resistance (LH) [28] homeostatic adjustment to stressful stimuli (SBH) [29] and having accordingly contributed to expand understanding in these areas.

Newer genetic models

Congenic strains

Animals are defined as congenic when their genome is identical except for a segment of a chromosome: in other words, a chromosomal segment of interest, i.e. believed to carry one or more loci relevant to blood pressure, is transferred from one strain onto a recipient animal having a different genetic background. The principle upon which such 'transplant' can be accomplished is conceptually simple: an animal from the 'donor' strain is crossed with one from the 'recipient' strain and the offspring is subjected to genetic analysis to identify the individual that inherited the 'donor' chromosomal segment. Such an individual is again crossed with an inbred animal from the recipient strain and the segment of interest is again tracked in second backcross offspring. The procedure is repeated over ten backcross generations until the offspring is virtually genetically identical to the original recipient strain not subjected to any manipulation except for the chromosomal segment of interest [30]. At this time phenotypic studies (blood pressure measurement, pathophysiology, biochemistry, etc.) are performed and the possible differences observed can be reliably ascribed to the presence of the transferred chromosomal segment.

Recombinant inbred strains

A different strategy is used to obtain an array of inbred strains from the crossing of two different inbred progenitors, in principle, one hypertensive and one normotensive. The F2 animals are crossed with each other at random and each pair is subsequently bred to give rise to a further inbred strain, in which the genes relevant to blood pressure will segregate in many possible different combinations determining a range of genome-dependent blood pressure levels, the higher these are the higher the number of relevant genes inherited from the hypertensive progenitor. If some 20–30 lines of F2 inbred animals are developed, genetic analysis of the cosegregation of blood pressure with a marker for a candidate gene will provide information on the contribution of that gene to blood pressure, provided the gene markers are closely linked (in the order of few centimorgans) with the genes relevant to blood pressure [31]. This approach lends itself to particularly interesting strategies to define the relationships of blood pressure or other phenotypes of interest with fixed and at least partially known genomic patterns.

Genetically manipulated models

A different approach employed to assess the genetic influences is to develop animal strains in which a candidate gene has been manipulated. This may be of particular relevance to the genes coding for components of the renin–angiotensin system, adrenergic receptors, nitric oxide-forming enzymes, bradykinin, for example. The most commonly used approaches are the gene knockout technique, by which portions of the genome are deleted or functionally blocked, and the transgenic technique, by which supplemental genes are introduced in the fertilized oocyte to be incorporated in the embryonic cells and eventually be expressed postnatally and in the progeny. These techniques were originarily developed in the mouse species, which has been extensively characterized as far as genetics is concerned but is not ideal for physiological studies on the cardiovascular system. Significant effort was thus devoted to extend them to the rat species. The first example of successful implementation of transgenic technology in rats is a strain named TGR (mRen-2)27. In these animals, an extra renin gene derived from the mouse species has been introduced in the genome and gives rise to pathophysiologically interesting phenomena: animals that are homozygous for the transgene undergo a fulminant form of hypertension [32], whereas heterozygous animals develop a less dramatic although clearly sustained hypertensive condition. Of note, the presence of the transgene is associated with low circulating but exceedingly high tissue renin levels.

Conclusion

The range of the existing experimental models of hypertension is obviously far wider than can be encompassed in the present discussion. Although the rat species is by far the one most commonly employed, substantial work (including the seminal work of Harry Goldblatt) has been (and is currently being) done in dogs as well as in cats, rabbits and to a lesser extent in sheep and monkeys.

In addition, there is currently a trend, to create models reflecting as closely as possible emerging clinical entities such as cyclosporin-induced hypertension, or hypertension associated with other risk factors such as hyperlipidemia, diabetes mellitus (streptozotocin-treated spontaneously hypertensive rats), obesity (obese Zucker rats), and insulin resistance (fructose-fed rat).

Other areas in which a variety of experimental models proved to be extremely useful have been those relating both to complications and to treatment of hypertension. Collecting evidence from animal studies is a prerequisite for the development of any new antihypertensive drug. Damage to the heart, brain, kidneys and the arterial system at large, as well as its prevention by treatment, are extensively evaluated in models to advance pathophysiological knowledge and to evaluate the protective potential of drugs.

In conclusion, animal models of hypertension represent a multifaceted 'ensemble' of experimental tools. Although they have so far not allowed the continuing enigma of the cause(s) of hypertension to be solved, working with models has undoubtedly provided invaluable intellectual stimuli and in many cases a better understanding of hypertension mechanisms potentially operating in humans. New impetus in this direction has come from application of modern genetic and molecular biology techniques to experimental animal models. Animal experiments are also routinely and usefully employed in studies on the complications and the treatment of hypertension.

References

1. Goldblatt H, Lynch J, Hanzal RF, Summerville WW. Studies on experimental hypertension. 1. The production of persistent elevation od systolic blood pressure by means of renal ischemia. *J Exp Med* 1934;**59**:347–378.
2. Page IH. Pathogenesis of arterial hypertension. *J Am Med Ass* 1949;**140**:451–460.
3. Page IH. Production of persistent arterial hypertension by cellophane perinephritis. *J Am Med Ass* 1939;**113**:2046–2048.
4. Grollman A. A simplified procedure for inducing chronic renal hypertension in the mammal. *Proc Soc Exp Biol Med* 1944;**57**:102
5. Lewis T. Material relating to coarctation of the aorta of the adult type. *Heart* 1933;**16**:205–243.
6. Scott HW, Bahnson HT. Evidence for a renal factor in the hypertension of experimental coarctation of the aorta. *Surgery* 1951;**30**:206–217.
7. Rytand DA. The renal factor in arterial hypertension with coarctation of the aorta. *J Clin Invest* 1938;**17**:391–399.
8. Stanek KA, Coleman RG, Murphy WR. Overall hemodynamic pattern in coarctation of the abdominal aorta in conscious rats. *Hypertension* 1987;**9**:611–618.
9. Page IH. The effect of chronic construction of the aorta on arterial blood pressure in dogs: an attempt to produce coarctation hypertension. *Am Heart J* 1940;**19**:218–232.
10. Groenewald JH, Van Zyl JJW. Acute renal and systemic effects after experimental coarctation of the aorta in the baboon. *Invest Urol* 1970;**7**:299–312.
11. Kulman D, Ragan C, Ferrebee JW *et al*. Toxic effects of desoxycorticosterone esters in dogs. *Science* 1939;**90**:496–497.
12. Skelton FR. Development of hypertension and cardiovascular renal lesions during adrenal regeneration in the rat. *Proc Soc Exp Biol Med* 1955;**90**:342–346.
13. Saito M, Terui N, Numao Y, Kumada M. Absence of sustained hypertension in sino-aortic denervated rabbits. *Am J Physiol* 1986;H742–H747.
14. Ferrari A, Parati G, Ferrari MC *et al*. Controllo riflesso della pressione arteriosa nel gatto non anestetizzato. *Boll Soc It Cardiol* 1980;**25**:123–130.
15. Ito CS, Scher AM. Hypertension following denervation of aortic baroreceptors in unanesthetized dogs. *Circulation Res* 1979;**45**:26–34.
16. Nathan MA, Reis D. Chronic labile hypertension produced by lesions of the nucleus tractus solitarii in the cat. *Circulation Res* 1977;**40**:72–81.
17. Laubie M, Schmitt H. Destruction of the nucleus tractus solitarii in the dog: comparison with sino-aortic denervation. *Am J Physiol* 1979;**236**:H736–H743.
18. Henry JP, Meehan JP, Stephens PM. The use of psychosocial stimuli to induce prolonged systolic hypertension in mice. *Psychosom Med* 1967;**29**:408–432.
19. Smirk FH, Hall WH. Inherited hypertension in rats. *Nature* 1958;**182**:727–728.
20. Harris EL, Millar JA. Calcium efflux in cultured vascular smooth muscle cells from genetically hypertensive rats: effect of angiotensin II and vasopressin. *J Hypertension* 1988;**6**(Suppl 4):s234–s235.
21. Okamoto K, Aoki K. Development of a strain of spontaneously hypertensive rats. *Jpn Circ J* 1963;**27**:202–293.
22. Okamoto K, Yamori Y, Nagaoka A. Establishment of the stroke-prone spontaneously hypertensive rat (SHR). *Circulation Res* 1974;**34**:1143–1153.
23. Dahl LK, Heine M, Tassinari L. Role of genetic factors insusceptibility to experimental hypertension due to chronic excess salt ingestion. *Nature* 1962;**194**:480–482.

24. Dahl LK, Heine M. Primary role of renal homografts in setting chronic blood pressure levels in rats. *Circulation Res* 1975;**36**:692–696.
25. Takeshita A, Mark AL. Neurogenic contribution to hindquarter vasoconstriction during high sodium intake in Dahl strain of genetically hypertensive rats. *Circulation Res* 1978;**43**(suppl I):186–191.
26. Ferrari A, Gordon FJ, Mark AL. Impairment of cardiopulmonary baroreflexes in Dahl salt-sensitive rats fed low salt. *Am J Physiol* 1984;**247**:H119–H123.
27. Bianchi G, Ferrari P, Trizio D *et al*. Red blood cell abnormalities and spontaneous hypertension in the rat: a genetically determined link. *Hypertension* 1985;**7**:319–325.
28. Cohen R, Riou JP, Saquet J *et al*. Plasma lipids, ketone bodies and insulin in genetically hypertensive rats of the Lyon strain. *J Cardiovasc Pharmacol* 1983;**3**:1008–1014.
29. Ben Ishai D. The Sabra hypertension-prone and -resistant strains. In: *Handbook of Hypertension*, Vol. 4: *Experimental and Genetic Models of Hypertension* (ed. DeJong W), pp. 296–313. Elsevier Science. Amsterdam, 1984.
30. Hillel J, Schaap T, Haberfeld A *et al*. DNA fingerprints applied to gene introgression in breeding programs. *Genetics* 1990;**124**:783–789.
31. Pravenec M, Klir P, Kren V *et al*. An analysis of spontaneous hypertension in spontaneously hypertensive rats by means of new recombinant inbred strains. *J Hypertension* 1989;**7**:217–222.
32. Mullins JJ, Peters J, Ganten D. Fulminant hypertension in transgenic rats harbouring the mouse *Ren*-2 gene. *Nature* 1990;**344**:541–544.

Chapter

2.2

2

Hypertension as a genetic disease

P Hamet, Z Pausova, J Tremblay and AY Deng

2.2

Introduction

Hypertension is a disease that represents a major public health problem worldwide. It affects approximately 15–20% of the global population [1], exacting enormous social and economic costs. Many of the affected are even unaware of the onset of the disease. Considering the impact of hypertension on human health, the study of the disease is an active area of research. Following the recognition of the genetic component of hypertension, numerous key discoveries have been made in the study of both the primary and the secondary forms of hypertension. In this chapter, the approaches currently used to study the genetics of hypertension will be presented, followed by an overview of related research findings.

BOX 2.2.1 A primer on basic genetics

Commonly known as the 'blueprint of life', deoxyribonucleic acid or DNA is the genetic material present in all the cells of an organism. DNA contains heritable information that is essential for the development and propagation of a species. The basic chemical unit of DNA is the DNA base. There are four types of DNA bases: adenosine triphosphate (A), guanosine triphosphate (G), cytidine triphosphate (C), and thymidine triphosphate (T). DNA bases are joined together in strand-like fashion, and the ordered sequence is termed a 'DNA sequence'. DNA strands are further arranged into a DNA helix, and DNA helices are organized into higher structures known as chromosomes. A complete copy of the human genome is packaged into two pairs of 22 autosomal chromosomes and one sex chromosome.

DNA is composed of functional units known as genes. A gene is a DNA sequence that contains sufficient information for the synthesis of a protein. The DNA sequence of a gene is comprised of the coding sequence, which encodes the amino acid sequence of a protein, and regulatory sequences, which are required for the appropriate expression of the gene. There may be several DNA sequences for a single gene that can encode the same protein. Each variant DNA sequence is known as an 'allele'. Alleles that encode for 'normal forms' of the protein are known as 'wild-type alleles'. Alleles that encode for forms of the protein with altered structure or function are termed 'mutant alleles' and are said to carry a gene mutation. The region of a chromosome occupied by an allele of a particular gene is known as the gene 'locus'.

Many human traits (e.g. hypertension) are determined by the information encoded by genes. Individuals receive an allele for a trait-determining gene from each parent, and the allelic pair (genotype) determines the appearance of the trait (phenotype). 'Heterozygosity' refers to the presence of two different alleles at a gene locus, while 'homozygosity' describes the presence of two identical alleles at a gene locus. When only one allele of an allelic pair is necessary to cause a trait, the trait is said to be 'dominant'. When two copies of the same allele are required for the appearance of a trait, the trait is considered 'recessive'.

Early evidence for genetic components of hypertension: population studies

Family studies

The first report that hypertension may be genetically determined appeared in 1761. In that report, Morgagni noted that the father of one of his patients, who had died of a cerebral hemorrhage, had himself died of apoplexy [2]. Since then, the results of numerous population studies have revealed that hypertension occurs more frequently in individuals with a positive family history of the disease. This tendency is termed 'familial aggregation' or 'familial clustering'. The most recent studies suggest that the likelihood of individuals under the age of 55 to develop hypertension is almost fourfold greater when there is a positive family history than when there is no prior history of the disease [3,4].

Although family studies have shown that hypertension exhibits a high degree of familial aggregation, they do not conclusively demonstrate that this clustering has a genetic basis. Familial aggregation may also be due to shared environmental factors as well as inherited genetic determinants. In order to identify a genetic component for hypertension, twin studies have been used. In twin studies, monozygotic (MZ) and dizygotic (DZ) twins are tested for the tendency to share a particular trait, a condition termed 'genetic heritability'. MZ twins share 100% of their genes, while DZ twins share only 50% of their genes. When a trait is observed more frequently in MZ twins than DZ twins, a genetic determinant is strongly suggested. When a trait is observed with almost equal frequency between MZ and DZ twins, a genetic component cannot be concluded, and environment is suggested to be the determining factor. Twin studies on hypertension have consistently indicated that the incidence of high blood pressure is higher among MZ twins than DZ twins [5]. From these studies, the degree of genetic heritability of hypertension is estimated in the range of 44 to 49% [6].

Adoption studies

An alternative approach used to identify a genetic component of hypertension is the use of adoption studies. In studies relating to hypertension, adoption studies typically compare the frequency of the disease between natural and adopted children and their first-degree relatives. One of the largest adoption studies on hypertension was a survey of French-Canadian families, which compared the frequency of high blood pressure in natural and adopted individuals against that of their parents and siblings [7,8]. These studies indicated that the incidence of hypertension was approximately twofold greater in natural children compared to adopted children when either a parent or sibling was hypertensive.

2

BOX 2.2.2 The dual nature of hypertension

The results of family and adoption studies, amongst others, have established that hypertension is, in part, a genetically determined disease. However, understanding the genetic component of hypertension is a problem that has challenged researchers for decades. Of particular significance is a heated scientific debate between Sir Platt and Sir Pickering during the 1960s [5]. The issue was the mode of genetic transmission by which hypertension is propagated through family generations. Platt and colleagues argued that hypertension was inherited in a Mendelian fashion when measured by cardiovascular death. In their view, hypertension was a qualitative trait of discrete nature, being either present or absent in a given individual. Pickering and colleagues, on the other hand, held that hypertension was Gaussian in nature when assessed by measurements of blood pressure. They believed that the disorder was a quantitative trait, existing to varying degrees in individuals. In time, both men proved to be correct. Today, it is generally accepted that there are two forms of hypertension. 'Monogenetic hypertension' refers to hypertension syndromes that are caused by mutations within a single gene. 'Essential hypertension', the most common form of hypertension, is caused by the involvement of more than one gene.

Monogenetic forms of hypertension

Monogenetic forms of hypertension are rare forms of human hypertension that account for approximately 5% of all cases of the disease. At present, the genetic basis of hypertension is best understood in these hypertension syndromes [9,10]. Monogenetic forms of hypertension are considered simple traits because they display Mendelian modes of inheritance. They are caused by defects within a single gene that are sufficient to cause large changes in blood pressure.

Forms of monogenetic hypertension

Glucocorticoid-remediable hypertension

Glucocorticoid-remediable hypertension was the first monogenetic form of hypertension to be described. It is an autosomal dominant trait characterized by an overproduction of aldosterone and increased mineralocorticoid activity. Aldosterone interacts with the mineralocorticoid receptor in renal tubular cells and causes increased activity of epithelial sodium channels. The increased channel activity, in turn, increases salt and water retention and consequently elevates blood pressure. In individuals with glucocorticoid-remediable hypertension, aldosterone production is controlled by adrenocorticotropic hormone (ACTH) rather than angiotensin II. The causative genetic defect has been attributed to a chromosomal translocation (an exchange of DNA between chromosomes) between the genes encoding aldosterone synthase and steroid 11β-hydroxylase, two enzymes that are involved in adrenal steroid biosynthesis. The chromosomal translocation results in a hybrid gene that is comprised of the coding sequence of aldosterone synthase fused to the 5′ regulatory sequence of steroid 11β-hydroxylase, which permits regulation by ACTH [11,12]. As a result of regulation by ACTH, aldosterone is overproduced by the adrenal cortex with consequent increased salt and water reabsorption, and development of hypertension.

Syndrome of apparent mineralocorticoid excess

The syndrome of apparent mineralocorticoid excess is an autosomal recessive trait characterized by abnormally high circulating levels of cortisol. Cortisol is also capable of stimulating the renal mineralocorticoid receptor but is normally converted to a form known as cortisone that lacks this stimulatory capacity. The conversion of cortisol to cortisone is carried out by the enzyme 11β-hydroxysteroid dehydrogenase. In individuals with this syndrome, the observed increase in cortisol levels is caused by a decrease in 11β-hydroxysteroid dehydrogenase activity. Point mutations (single DNA base substitutions) in the gene that encodes 11β-hydroxysteroid dehydrogenase have been shown to be responsible for the decrease in enzyme activity and the increased stimulation of the mineralocorticoid receptor that leads to hypertension [13].

Liddle's syndrome

This autosomal dominant syndrome is caused by defects in sodium reabsorption. In individuals with Liddle's syndrome, the epithelial sodium channel is constitutively (continually) activated, resulting in increased sodium reabsorption and a consequent rise in blood pressure. Mutations in the genes encoding the β and γ subunits of the epithelial sodium channel have been shown to be responsible for this effect. Gene deletions (loss of DNA sequence from a gene) give rise to a truncated form of the channel that lacks the cytoplasmic carboxy-terminus, while gene insertions (addition of DNA sequence to a gene) lead to amino acid substitutions (changes in amino acid sequence of a protein) within the channel. Both of these gene defects increase the activity of the channel and consequently cause hypertension [14,15].

BOX 2.2.3 Other monogenetic forms of hypertension

Although the genetic mechanisms underlying monogenetic forms of hypertension are best understood for glucocorticoid-remediable hypertension, the syndrome of apparent mineralocorticoid excess, and Liddle's syndrome, additional monogenetic hypertension syndromes are known to exist. Information concerning the genes responsible for these forms is still preliminary and is summarized in Hamet *et al.*[10]

- *Female and male pseudohermaphroditism.* Female and male pseudohermaphroditism are disorders of sexual differentiation that share in common an autosomal recessive form of hypertension. Hypertension in the former has been attributed to mutations within the 11β-steroid hydroxylase gene, whereas mutations in the 17-hydroxylase gene have been implicated in the latter.

- *Gordon's syndrome.* This is characterized by a defect in renal ion transport. Similar to Liddle's syndrome, Gordon's syndrome is inherited in an autosomal dominant manner. Although the causal gene has yet to be identified, potential genes have been localized to regions on human chromosomes 1 and 17.
- *Hypertension and brachydactyly.* Hypertension accompanied by brachydactyly is an autosomal dominant form of severe hypertension. The gene responsible for this hypertension syndrome has been localized to a region of human chromosome 12.
- *Hypertension due to pheochromocytoma.* Several monogenetic forms of hypertension result from the overproduction of catecholamines caused by pheochromocytomas (tumors of the adrenal medulla). At least four distinct hypertension syndromes are characterized by pheochromocytomas. These include familial pheochromocytoma, multiple endocrine neoplasia types IIA and IIB, von Hipple–Lindau syndrome and neurofibromatosis type 1. They all share in common an autosomal dominant mode of inheritance.

Phenotypic variability of monogenetic hypertension syndromes

Although the cause of monogenetic forms of hypertension has generally been attributed to a single gene defect, it is commonly observed that individuals with the same genetic defect vary in the severity of the disease [9,10]. This phenomenon is known as 'varying penetrance'. Varying penetrance has been observed, for example, in individuals who carry the same predisposing allele for glucocorticoid-remediable hypertension [16]. A number of factors have been proposed to account for this apparent inconsistency between genotype and phenotype. Environmental factors (non-genetic factors), such as salt and diet, have been suggested to influence the expression or activity of genes that are capable of causing a particular hypertension syndrome. Locus heterogeneity (the ability of several genes to cause the same trait independently) is another possible factor and has been implicated in a monogenetic hypertension syndrome known as Gordon's syndrome [17]. In addition, an important determinant of varying penetrance appears to be allelic variation (the ability of several alleles of a single gene to cause the same trait). For instance, different mutations in the gene encoding 11β-hydroxysteroid dehydrogenase can cause the syndrome of apparent mineralocorticoid excess [13,18]. Some of these gene mutations are associated with variable enzyme activity and thus variable penetrance. In addition to alleles that can produce less severe forms of hypertension, other alleles that can cause hypotension have been identified. Mutations have been found within the genes coding for the subunits of the epithelium sodium channel, the same channel that is mutated in Liddle's syndrome, that can cause an autosomal recessive form of hypotension known as pseudohypoaldosteronism type 1 (PHA-1) [19]. Variable penetrance may occur when individuals carry a copy of a hypertension-causing and a hypotension-causing allele [9].

Essential hypertension: animal models of hypertension

Essential hypertension accounts for the vast majority of cases of hypertension. However, in contrast to monogenetic forms of hypertension, the genetic mechanisms underlying essential hypertension are less well understood. Essential hypertension is considered a complex trait because it displays familial aggregation without a clear pattern of Mendelian inheritance. Several factors may contribute to the complex pattern of inheritance for essential hypertension. First, it is generally accepted that essential hypertension is caused by the interactions of several genes and is therefore polygenic. Second, essential hypertension may be determined by the interaction of a few major genes or many minor genes. Third, essential hypertension may be caused by different combinations of genes, a condition known as genetic heterogeneity. Lastly, essential hypertension is a trait that is influenced significantly by environmental factors as well as genetic determinants.

BOX 2.2.4 Rationale for the use of animal models

The use of inbred animal strains figures prominently in studying the genetic determinants of hypertension. Model animal strains that exhibit hypertension are considered a less complex model for studying the disease for two main reasons. In contrast to human subjects, animal strains can be bred so that only differences in genes related to hypertension can be studied. In addition, animal models can be analyzed in controlled settings where numerous variables, such as population size and environmental conditions, can be predetermined [20].

Although a number of different animals have been used to study essential hypertension, the rat is the most common animal model for several practical advantages. Rats provide sizeable litters in relatively short gestation periods, can be subjected to a variety of experimental conditions, and are fairly inexpensive to breed. Since rats have a relatively short life span, they also provide the opportunity to study the natural history of hypertension. Hypertension in rats and humans share a similar pathophysiology of the disease, series of complications, and response to antihypertensive treatments [20,21].

The inbred strain

The majority of rat models of hypertension that are currently in use are inbred strains. Inbred strains are generated in order to fix a trait (e.g. hypertension) and to obtain a genetically homogeneous test population. The generation of a hypertensive inbred rat strain begins with the selection of hypertensive animals from outbred strains (randomly bred strains). These hypertensive progenitors are crossed (mated) to produce the first filial generation (F_1). F_1 offspring that are hypertensive are selected for brother–sister matings to give rise to the F_2 generation. This process of selective breeding is continued until all the offspring display the trait of interest. At this point, the trait is considered fixed. Selective

2

brother–sister matings are then continued in order to obtain genetic homogeneity, which is the presence of identical alleles at each gene locus. The degree of genetic homogeneity achieved with each subsequent round of inbreeding is approximately 12.5%, and 20 rounds of inbreeding (F_{20}) are considered sufficient to obtain a fully inbred strain [22]. Control strains for hypertensive animal strains are derived in a similar manner by selectively breeding normotensive animals.

Inbred rat strains have facilitated the analysis of essential hypertension by allowing only differences in genes that cause hypertension to be studied. At the same time, though, the use of inbred rat strains poses several limitations on such studies. When an inbred rat strain is selectively bred to obtain genetic homogeneity, alleles for every locus are fixed simultaneously. As a result, a single allele for a hypertension-causing gene is selected. In addition, a single allele at all other loci is selected, and the combination of these alleles determines the genetic background in which hypertension-causing genes are expressed. However, the nature of essential hypertension dictates that genetic heterogeneity (the presence of other interactive genes) is an important component of the disease. Thus, genetic homogeneity may exclude the effects of other alleles for genes directly or indirectly related to hypertension. This effect is the major drawback of using inbred strains to study essential hypertension.

BOX 2.2.5 Inbred rat models of essential hypertension

During the 1960s and 1970s, a number of investigators developed inbred rat models of essential hypertension by selective breeding. Currently, there are six major inbred hypertensive rat strains that are in common use [21,47]

Spontaneously hypertensive rat (SHR). The spontaneously hypertensive rat (SHR) was generated from the mating of hypertensive progenitors selected from a colony of Wistar rats in Kyoto University. A fully inbred strain was obtained by selective breeding for high blood pressure and is currently beyond its 80th generation. The SHR is a widely used animal model for hypertension. A related inbred rat model, the spontaneously hypertensive stroke-prone (SHR-SP) rat, is employed as a model of hypertension, stroke, and cardiovascular disease. The Wistar-Kyoto (WKY) rat, which was generated by selective breeding of normotensive progenitors, was created several generations after the SHR and is a commonly used control strain [20].

New Zealand strain of genetically hypertensive rat (GH). The New Zealand strain of genetically hypertensive (GH) rat originates from a colony of albino rats at the University of Otago Medical School. The GH rat was obtained by selective inbreeding for elevated blood pressure and is past its 60th generation of inbreeding. The GH rat serves as a model of hypertension and cardiac hypertrophy. A normotensive control strain (N rat) has been bred alongside GH rats.

Inbred Dahl salt-sensitive (SS/Jr) and salt-resistant (SR/Jr) rats. The inbred Dahl salt-sensitive (SS/Jr) and salt-resistant (SR/Jr) rats are derived from an animal colony in Brookhaven National Laboratory in the United States. They were generated by selective breeding for a tendency to develop hypertension or to remain unaffected in response to dietary salt loading. They are distinct from the Dahl salt-sensitive (DSS) and Dahl salt-resistant (DSR) strains, which were inbred for only a limited number of generations. After the seventh generation of inbreeding, the DSS and DSR rats were outbred in order to maintain viability, and this process of bidirectional selection has continued to the present day. The SS/Jr rat serves as a model for salt sensitivity of blood pressure. When SS/Jr rats are maintained on a high-salt diet, they die within eight weeks of hypertension. When they are maintained on a low-salt diet, they die within six months of a spontaneous form of hypertension. The SS/Jr and SR/Jr rats are beyond the 35th and 46th generation of inbreeding respectively.

Sabra hypertensive-prone (SBH) and hypertensive-resistant (SBN) rats. The Sabra hypertensive-prone (SBH) and hypertensive-resistant (SBN) rats represent inbred strains derived from albino rats maintained at the Hebrew University of Jerusalem. They were generated by crossing progenitors that either developed hypertension or remained unaffected after being maintained on a high-salt diet for a month. Offspring were selectively bred for salt sensitivity or salt resistance of blood pressure for 20 generations. The SBH rat is used to study the role of sodium and catecholamines in hypertension.

Lyon model of genetic hypertension. The Lyon model of hypertension is comprised of three inbred rat strains that are descended from a colony of Sprague-Dawley rats. These are the Lyon hypertensive (LH), the Lyon low blood pressure (LL), and the Lyon normotensive (LN) rat strains. All three strains are derived from progenitors that were classified according to blood pressure. The strains are beyond the 28th generation of selective inbreeding. In contrast to other rat models of hypertension, the Lyon model permits the distinction between genetic variations that are responsible for hypertension (variation between LH and LL as well as LH and LN) as opposed to those that are not (variation between LH and LL and LN).

Milan hypertensive (MHS) and normotensive (MHN) rats. The Milan hypertensive strain (MHS) and Milan normotensive strain (MNS) are descended from a colony of Wistar rats that were maintained in Milan, Italy. These strains have been generated simultaneously by selective breeding for high and low blood pressures. The MHS rat was considered a fully inbred strain at the 21st generation of inbreeding, whereas the fully inbred MNS rat was obtained at the 26th generation. The MHS rat is used as a model of mild hypertension.

Additional normotensive rats. In addition to the normotensive rats already mentioned, the following inbred rat strains are often employed as control strains: AxC Irish (ACI), Brown Norway (BN), Donryu (DRY), Fischer (F344), and Lewis (LEW) rats.

F_2-segregating population

The F_2-segregating population is an animal experiment often used in the study of essential hypertension. F_2 hybrids are derived from crossing inbred hypertensive and normotensive progenitors to produce an F_1 generation. All members of the F_1 generation are heterozygous at every locus. Members of the F_1 offspring are then intercrossed to produce a segregating F_2 population. In contrast to animals of the F_1 generation, F_2

2

hybrids display a random distribution of alleles across their loci due to the independent assortment of alleles.

The F_2-segregating population offers an important advantage over inbred animal strains in studies of essential hypertension. Unlike an inbred animal strain, an F_2-segregating population is comprised of animals that express hypertensive-causing genes in a variety of genetic backgrounds. The effects of such genetic heterogeneity on hypertension is reflected in the range of blood pressure values observed among the animals of a single F_2-segregating population. F_2-segregating populations have been widely used in studies that have implicated numerous genes in essential hypertension.

Recombinant inbred strain

The recombinant inbred strain (RIS) is generated by an initial random crossing of F_2-segregating hybrids, followed by subsequent brother–sister matings for at least 20 generations in order to fix the random distribution of alleles achieved during the initial cross. The RISs derived from all combinations of F_2 matings collectively represent a panel of most independent assortment events [22]. When a RIS panel is generated from hypertensive and normotensive progenitors, the animals display a wide spectrum of intermediate blood pressure values.

A RIS panel offers practical advantages over both the inbred animal strain and the F_2-segregating population in studies of essential hypertension. In contrast to the inbred animal strain, the use of a RIS panel allows the effects of genetic heterogeneity on hypertensive-causing genes to be assessed. In addition, a RIS panel can be propagated indefinitely in comparison to an F_2-segregating population. A RIS panel also permits longitudinal studies of a trait. For instance, an analysis of a RIS panel has indicated a positive correlation between kidney weight at birth and the risk of hypertension later in life [23]. At present, only a single RIS panel, developed in Prague from SHR and BN progenitors, is available for use in studies relating to essential hypertension [24].

Congenic and related strains

The congenic animal strain is an inbred animal model that is gaining prominence in studies of essential hypertension. Congenic animal strains are generated to narrow the chromosomal region that contains a trait-causing gene by transferring a chromosomal region from a donor animal to a recipient animal. Congenic animals are generated by crossing inbred progenitors that differ in the trait of interest to produce an F_1 generation. An F_1 animal (the donor) is then mated to either progenitor (recipient) in a process called 'backcrossing'. For instance, if the transfer of a chromosomal region containing a hypertension-causing gene to a normotensive animal is desired, the F_1 animal is backcrossed to the normotensive progenitor. The opposite can also be performed. Backcrossing is continued for at least eight generations. At this stage, the

Hypertension as a genetic disease

Essential hypertension:
animal models of
hypertension

Congenic and related
strains

2

genetic background of the congenic animal is more than 99% of the recipient, but the chromosomal region that contains the trait-determining gene is still present. An ideal congenic animal is one that differs from the recipient animal in only the chromosomal region containing the trait-determining gene [22]. In studies relating to hypertension, congenic animal strains have generally been used to confirm the role of genes in essential hypertension that had been initially identified with the use of F_2 hybrids or a RIS panel [25].

There are two additional animal strains that are closely related to the congenic animal strain. A consomic animal strain is an animal that is derived from the transfer of an entire chromosome from a donor animal to a recipient animal [22]. A consomic animal strain, generated from the transfer of the Y chromosome from a SHR progenitor to a WKY background, has indicated the presence of one or more genes on the Y chromosome that can increase blood pressure [26]. A double congenic animal strain is an animal strain that has been obtained from the simultaneous transfer of two chromosomal regions containing trait-determining genes [27]. In one study, a double congenic animal strain derived from SS/Jr rats was used to demonstrate that angiotensin-converting enzyme (ACE) can modify the expression of the atrial natriuretic peptide receptor A and thus influence the onset of salt-sensitive hypertension [28].

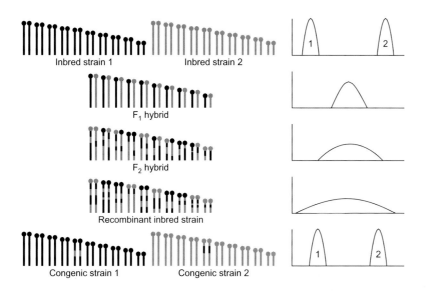

Fig. 2.2.1 Schematic representation of effects of genetic heterogeneity on blood pressure values in animals derived from normotensive (1) and hypertensive (2) inbred strains. The x-axis indicates number of animals, and the y-axis represents blood pressure values. Only 10 of the 20 chromosomes comprising the rat genome are illustrated.

Essential hypertension: tools of genetic analysis

The goal of using any animal model to study essential hypertension is to identify the genetic differences between hypertensive and normotensive animals that can account for the disease. In the past, these animals were generally compared for differences in visible traits. This trait would then be further analyzed to determine its Mendelian pattern of inheritance in order to infer information relating to hypertension-causing genes. However, such studies met with little success since differences in such traits were often subtle and difficult to distinguish. Nowadays, with the application of molecular biology to genetic analysis, genetic differences between hypertensive and normotensive animals can be determined by genetic mapping. Genetic mapping involves examining DNA directly in order to map a trait (phenotype) to a chromosomal region (genotype). Mapping the genes that cause essential hypertension can be carried out in a number of ways.

Linkage analysis

Linkage analysis is a commonly used method of genetic mapping. It is based on the premise that a marker locus in proximity to a disease-causing locus will co-segregate (travel) with the disease-causing locus in affected individuals. The closer these loci are to each other, the more frequently they will co-segregate since the likelihood of recombination (exchange of DNA between pairs of chromosomes) is decreased. When a marker locus and a disease locus co-segregate above what is considered a random frequency, they are considered linked. Linkage is measured in terms of a lod score, which is the logarithm of the distance between the marker and disease loci (θ). Generally, a lod score of 3 (1000:1) indicates 95% probability of linkage between loci [29,30].

A marker locus can be evaluated with the use of DNA polymorphisms (differences in the DNA sequences between individuals). The two main types of DNA polymorphisms routinely used in linkage analysis are the restriction fragment-length polymorphism (RFLP) and the variable-number tandem repeat (VNTR). RFLP results from differences in the number of sites for a restriction enzyme within the marker locus among individuals, and VNTR occurs when certain DNA sequences are repeated in numbers that are variable among individuals. VNTRs may be short (microsatellites and simple sequence length polymorphisms, SSLPs) or longer (minisatellites). Differences in the lengths of VNTRs within the marker locus can be determined by performing the polymerase chain reaction (PCR) and gel electrophoresis (techniques that amplify DNA, separate it according to length, and visualize it) on DNA isolated from test subjects.

Linkage analysis on hypertensive rat models has only become possible in recent years. This is due to the increased availability of known DNA polymorphisms as a result of efforts to determine the DNA sequence of the rat genome. Linkage analysis can be carried out on any animal model used in the study of essential hypertension.

2

BOX 2.2.6 Establishing linkage in human populations

The use of linkage analysis is generally most useful in studies of single-gene disorders, such as monogenetic forms of hypertension. In such studies, a model of Mendelian inheritance (*parametric model*) can be tested by charting the path of a single causative gene within affected families. Since the effects of the gene are either present or absent in family members, co-segregation of disease-causing alleles can be readily detected. However, linkage analysis is less useful in studies of essential hypertension, which results from the effects of several genes. Since the contributions of the genes are smaller, disease-causing alleles may not be easily detected by linkage analysis. To detect linkage between essential hypertension and its causative genes, alternative methods of linkage analysis are employed. These methods are termed *non-parametric models* since they are not based on prior assumptions of inheritance.

Allele-sharing methods represent alternative methods of linkage analysis that search for differences in the frequency of alleles in families with affected members. The three main types of allele sharing methods are affected sib-pair analysis, discordant sib-pair analysis, and extended family analysis.

- *Affected sib-pair analysis* measures the degree of allele sharing in pairs of siblings who both exhibit the disease. Normally, the likelihood of siblings to share an allele for any gene is 50%. When affected siblings share an allele more often than is expected by chance, it is said that there is excessive allele sharing. The excessively shared allele may serve as a marker for the disease or be the disease-causing gene itself. Affected sib pairs are considered identical by descent (IBD) when the shared allele has been inherited from the same parent or identical by state (IBS) when the origin of the shared allele is unknown [29,30].
- *Discordant sib-pair analysis* examines allelic frequency in pairs of siblings comprised of an unaffected and an affected member. In this type of analysis, when an allele is present in only one of the siblings, it is considered related to the disease-causing gene.
- *Extended family analysis* is similar to affected sib-pair analysis except that excessive allele sharing is measured between an affected individual and his/her affected second degree relatives (such as uncles, aunts, and cousins).

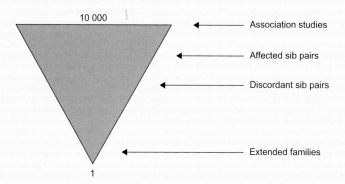

Fig. 2.2.2 The relative number of subjects generally required for these study designs is represented above. Association studies require the largest number of subjects, while extended family analyses require the fewest.

BOX 2.2.6 *Continued*

Association analysis is an alternative method of linkage analysis that
compares the frequency of alleles between affected and non-affected
individuals. If an allele is found more often in individuals with the disease
than in individuals without the disease, then the allele is said to be in
'linkage disequilibrium' with a disease-causing allele [29,30].

Candidate gene approach

The candidate gene approach is a genetic mapping technique that is
based on prior knowledge of the function of a protein encoded by a
gene. Candidate genes generally encode components of biochemical or
physiological systems that are defective in the disease. The gene that is
considered most likely to be involved in the disease process is analyzed
for differences in DNA sequence between affected and control subjects.
There are two different ways in which the candidate gene approach can
be performed. In the positional candidate approach, the candidate gene
is selected based on prior information on both the function and the
chromosomal localization of the gene. The latter information is generally
drawn from previous genetic mapping studies; a DNA marker within
the candidate gene locus is evaluated to determine if an allele of the
marker has co-segregated with the disease. In the independent
candidate gene approach, a candidate gene is selected for function but
without any prior knowledge of chromosomal position. Whatever
approach is used, affected and control subjects are then examined to
determine if the candidate gene exhibits allelic variation that can
account for the disease.

The use of the candidate gene approach in identifying hypertension-
causing genes has met with some success in animal models. Candidate
gene studies on hypertension have generally focused on components
of the renin–angiotensin system. For example, analysis of an F_2-
segregating population derived from SS/Jr and SR/Jr rats has
indicated the presence of an RFLP within the renin gene that co-
segregates with the salt-sensitivity of blood pressure [31,66]. Several
alleles have been identified in a locus containing the steroid 11β-
hydroxylase gene that also co-segregate with the salt-sensitivity of
blood pressure [32]. Variant alleles for a locus containing the atrial
natriuretic peptide receptor A gene (*Gca*) have also been found to co-
segregate with blood pressure in an F_2-segregating population derived
from SS/Jr rats and WKY rats [33]. In addition, the candidate gene
approach has been used to demonstrate a role for the α-adducin gene
in essential hypertension [34].

Despite these successes, the usefulness of the candidate gene
approach in finding hypertension-causing genes is limited. First, the
technique can test only known genes, which account for approximately
5–10% of all possible genes. In addition, the candidate gene approach is
limited by the fact that there are many potential candidate genes for

essential hypertension. When a candidate gene is shown to co-segregate with high blood pressure, several other candidate genes may be present within its flanking DNA sequences. For example, although several alleles for the *Gca* gene locus were found to co-segregate with blood in SS/Jr rats [33], further analysis of the locus indicated the presence of five other candidate genes in the region [35].

Total genome scanning

Total genome scanning, also known as 'random genome scanning' or 'interval mapping', represents an alternative gene mapping technique to the candidate gene approach. It tests the possibility that a locus affecting either a quantitative trait (quantitative trait locus or QTL) or qualitative trait is close to a marker locus. In total genome scanning, polymorphic markers are evaluated in affected populations in order to identify polymorphisms that co-segregate with the trait of interest. Once such markers have been identified, the DNA sequences flanking the markers can be examined for the presence of any candidate genes.

The success of total genome scanning depends upon the availability of genetic markers that can be tested (Table 2.2.1). For this reason, total genome scanning has only recently been used in the study of essential hypertension as an increasing number of marker loci for the rat have been identified. At present, several QTLs for essential hypertension have been reported and summarized [10]. Rat chromosome 1 contains a QTL that has been reported in four different rat models. This QTL contains the *Sa* gene, which is considered a candidate gene, since it has been shown to be more highly expressed in SHR versus WKY normotensive controls. The QTL on chromosome 1 also contains genes encoding the γ and β subunits of the epithelial sodium channel, which have been implicated in Liddle's syndrome. A QTL on rat chromosome 2 is in proximity to the candidate genes, *Gca* and carboxypeptidase B. A specific region of rat chromosome 4 contains QTLs for SHR hypertension, insulin resistance, and hypertriglyceridemia [84,85]. Using cDNA microarrays, congenic mapping and radiation hybrid mapping, a defective SHR gene, Cd36 (encoding fatty acid translocase), was identified at the peak of linkage to these QTLs [86]. Although evidence has been provided that CD36 plays a role in defective carbohydrate and lipid metabolism in SHR [86], analysis of Cd36 genotypes in SHR and SHR-SP strains indicates that the defective variant of Cd36 was not critical to the initial selection for hypertension in the SHR model [87]. Rat chromosome 10 contains a QTL that lies in the vicinity of the genes encoding ACE, Na$^+$, K$^+$-ATPase β_2 subunit, and inducible nitric oxide synthase. Rat chromosome 8 has also been reported to contain a QTL that may mediate neonatal and adult heart weight. A human chromosomal region that is syntenic (containing the same group of genes) to the QTL on rat chromosome 8 contains the DNA-mismatch repair gene. This gene is considered a candidate gene since the results from several studies indicate that SHR neonates exhibit a greater degree of DNA synthesis and polyploidy.

2

Table 2.2.1 Summary of hypertension-causing genes implicated in essential hypertension by the candidate gene approach or total genome scanning

Gene	Chromosome	Animal population(s) used in genetic analysis	Reference
Sa	1	F_2 hybrids from SHR and LEW rats	[54]
		F_2 hybrids from SHR and WKY rats	[55]
		F_2 hybrids from SS/Jr and LEW rats	[56]
Kallikrein	1	RIS panel from SHR and BN rats	[57]
Atrial natriuretic peptide receptor (*Gca*)	2	F_2 hybrids from SS/Jr and WKY rats	[33]
		F_2 hybrids from GH and BN rats	[58]
		Congenic strains from SS/Jr and WKY or MNS rats	[59]
Angiotensin II Receptor AT1B	2	F_2 hybrids from LH and LN rats	[35]
		F_2 hybrids from SS/Jr and WKY rats	[60]
Carboxypeptidase B	2	F_2 hybrids from SHR-SP and WKY rats	[61]
		F_2 hybrids from LH and LN rats	[62]
α-Adducin	4	F_2 hybrids from MHS and MNS rats	[34]
Neuropeptide Y	4	F_2 hybrids from SHR and WKY rats	[63]
Steroid 11β-hydroxylase	7	F_2 hybrids from SS/Jr and SR/Jr rats	[32]
Angiotensin-converting enzyme (*Ace*)	10	F_2 hybrids from SHR-SP and WKY rats	[48,49]
		Congenic strain from SHR-SP and WKY rats	[64]
		F_2 hybrids from GH and BN rats	[58]
		Double congenic strain from SS/Jr and SS/Jr rats	[28]
Heat-shock protein 27 (*hsp27*)	12	F_2 hybrids from SHR and WKY rats	[65]
		RIS panel from SHR and BN rats	[65]
Renin	13	F_2 hybrids from SS/Jr and SR/Jr rats	[31,66]
		F_2 hybrids from SHR and LEW rats	[67]
		Congenic strain from SS/Jr and SR/Jr rats	[68]
		F_2 hybrids from LH and LN rats	[62]
		F_2 hybrids from GH and BN rats	[58]
Heat-shock protein 70 (*hsp70*)	20	RIS panel and congenic strains from SHR and BN rats	[69]
Unknown	X	F_2 hybrids from SHR-SP and WKY rats	[49]
Unknown	Y	F_2 hybrids from SHR and WKY rats	[70]
		Consomic strains from SHR and WKY rats	[26,71]
		F_2 hybrids from SHR-SP and WKY rats	[72]

Total genome scanning, like the candidate gene approach, is also limited in usefulness. In order to produce results, a large number of genetic markers must be used, otherwise many false negatives may be obtained [29]. For example, when total genome scanning is conducted on F_2-segregating populations, 100–200 F_2 hybrids are typically examined for polymorphisms in approximately 500 genetic markers. However, by using many genetic markers to decrease the number of false negatives, total genome scanning may be hampered by the large number of possible candidate genes involved in essential hypertension [25].

BOX 2.2.7 The story of ACE: a positional candidate gene paradigm

In 1991, two independent groups led by Jacob and Hilbert simultaneously reported the discovery of a gene involved in hypertension by genetic mapping [48,49]. The studies carried out were based on the observation that SHR-SP rats were susceptible to developing hypertension in response to salt-loading and set out to identify the gene responsible for this effect. The causative gene that was identified by both groups was the gene encoding angiotensin-converting enzyme (ACE). ACE is an enzyme that is positively regulated by the renin–angiotensin system. It is responsible for the conversion of angiotensin I into angiotensin II, which acts as a stressor and stimulates vasoconstriction and an increase in blood pressure.

The two groups used a similar approach to find *Ace*, namely, total genome scanning. Both initiated their studies by using the same F_2-segregating population from a cross of SHR-SP and WKY progenitors. Linkage analysis was then conducted on the F_2 hybrids to find marker loci that co-segregated with the salt-sensitivity of blood pressure. However, owing to a scarcity of rat genetic markers, the groups first had to generate a large set of polymorphic markers. Jacob *et al.*[48] generated 290 markers based on VNTRs shared by mice and humans and, they reasoned, rats. Hilbert *et al.* [49] developed a 181 genetic marker system based on VNTRs and an RFLP in the renin gene. In both cases, when linkage analysis was carried out, a potential QTL was localized to rat chromosome 10 (Bp1). By comparative mapping, the Jacob group found that this region was syntenic with mouse chromosome 11 and human chromosome 17. The Hilbert group arrived at the same result with the use of somatic cell hybrids. Of particular interest to both groups of investigators was the presence of the *Ace* gene within Bp1. The groups proceeded to sequence the *Ace* genes in both the SHR-SP and WKY rats. The result was the identification of a variant allele in SHR-SP rats that was shown to co-segregate with the salt-sensitivity of blood pressure.

Despite the linkage of ACE to essential hypertension in a rat model, the role of ACE in human essential hypertension remains ambiguous, as summarized by Cusi and Bianchi [50]. A variant allele of the *Ace* gene has been shown to produce a form of ACE that persists at high levels in serum. However, this allele has not been conclusively proven to be important in essential hypertension, being only variably associated with the incidence of cardiovascular disease. However, one large affected sib-pairs study has indicated linkage of a marker that lies in close proximity to the ACE locus on human chromosome 17 to hypertension. It seems that for the time being, the story of *Ace* is awaiting an ending.

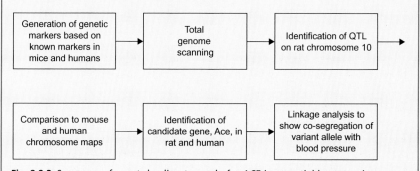

Fig. 2.2.3 Sequence of events leading to a role for ACE in essential hypertension.

Etiology and pathophysiology

2.2

Essential hypertension:
animal models of
hypertension

Transgenics

Transgenics

Once a candidate gene or a QTL for essential hypertension has been identified, its function can be tested in a transgenic animal model. Transgenics involves the introduction of new genetic material, a transgene, into the germline (sex cells) of an animal so that every cell of the transgenic animal will carry the new genetic material. With the use of transgenic technology, the function of a gene can be evaluated in two main ways. By causing the overexpression of the gene, the effects of gene addition can be observed in the transgenic animal. Similarly, by disrupting the normal expression of the gene (a 'knockout'), the impact of gene subtraction can be assessed in the transgenic animal (Table 2.2.2).

In classical transgenics, the transgene is inserted into the genome indiscriminately by random insertion. However, it is now possible to introduce a transgene at a particular site within the genome and to even express it within specific tissues by gene-targeted homologous recombination. Although transgenics is most often performed in mice, the generation of any transgenic animal is in principle the same. First, fertilized oocytes are obtained from a donor female animal, and the transgene is introduced into the oocytes. The manipulated oocytes are then transferred into a pseudopregnant female, which has been obtained by mating to a sterilized male. Fifty percent of the F_1 offspring are heterozygous for the transgene. A series of crosses with the F_1 hybrids carrying the transgene are conducted to generate animals that are

Table 2.2.2 Summary of gene engineering studies on essential hypertension

Animal used	Gene manipulation	Effect on blood pressure in transgenic animal	Reference
Rat	Overexpression of renin-2	Fulminant hypertension	[37]
Mouse	Overexpression of one to four copies of angiotension	Correlative increase in hypertension with gene copy	[73]
Mouse	Overexpression of angiotensinogen	Hypertension	[74]
Mouse	Overexpression of renin and angiotensinogen	Hypertension	[75]
Mouse	Overexpression of Na^+–H^+ exchanger	Hypertension in response to salt loading	[76]
Mouse	Overexpression of kallikrein	Hypotension	[77]
Mouse	Knockout of angiotensinogen	Hypotension	[73]
Mouse	Knockout of angiotensin-converting enzyme (ACE)	Hypertension after salt loading	[78]
Mouse	Knockout of atrial natriuretic peptide (ANP)	Hypertension after salt loading	[79]
Mouse	Knockout of atrial natriuretic peptide receptor A (ANP receptor), *Gca*	Hypertension resistant to salt	[80]
Mouse	Knockout of angiotensin type II receptor AT1B	Hypotension	[81]
Mouse	Knockout of endothelin-1	Embryonic lethality in homozygotes. Hypertension in heterozygotes	[82]
Mouse	Knockout of endothelial nitric oxide synthase	Hypertension	[83]

homozygous for the transgene. The transgenic animals are then
maintained by continual inbreeding (brother–sister matings) [22].

Until recently, the generation of transgenic rats was uncommon since
certain inherent features of the rat were not amenable to the transgenic
techniques that were designed primarily for the mouse [36]. Transgenic
techniques have now been adapted for the rat, although it is still not
possible to generate gene 'knockouts' in rats. The first transgenic rat to
be created in hypertension research was the transgenic rat carrying the
renin gene [37].

Gene hunt and beyond

Although essential hypertension is a genetically determined disease, it is
also influenced significantly by the environment. The environmental
component of essential hypertension varies between 30 and 60% [3]. In
complex traits such as essential hypertension, the environment generally
does not produce independent effects that are simply additive to the
effects of genetic factors. Instead, the environment interacts with genetic
factors to determine the outcome of the disease. For example,
individuals who have a genetic predisposition to salt sensitivity of blood
pressure will display different degrees of hypertension depending on
whether they are on a high-salt or a low-salt diet. Several candidate
genes have been proposed to mediate the effects of environmental
factors on essential hypertension. They are known as genes of
environmental susceptibility.

BOX 2.2.8 Evolution: the missing link in essential hypertension?

The importance of environment in the development of essential hypertension
is widely recognized, but why is this so? The evolution of modern society
may be the answer to this question. It has been argued that the human
genome has incurred very little change since the emergence of *Homo sapiens*
almost 35 000 years ago [51]. During this time, however, civilization has
transformed radically from a preagricultural hunter–gatherer society to a
technologically advanced modern one. The lifestyle of the typical
hunter–gatherer centered around the search for food. This physically active
lifestyle necessitated a diet that was rich in protein and potassium yet low in
fat and salt. With the irregular availability of food, short periods of feasting
were often the norm. The metabolic mechanisms determined by the human
genome evolved to accommodate these needs. Today, however, the lifestyle
of modern humans is far more convenient than it was tens of thousands of
years ago. As a result, physical activity is on the decrease, whereas
consumption of food (often laden with fat and sodium) is on the rise. It is
possible then that metabolic mechanisms necessary for the survival of
hunter–gatherers may, in fact, be etiological to many modern chronic
diseases, such as hypertension. Likewise, other physiological mechanisms,
such as the 'fight or flight' response and increased glomerular filtration rate
and kidney size, may have contributed to the survival of the hunter–gatherer
but actually predispose the modern human to disease.

Stress

One of the most important environmental factors that contribute to essential hypertension is stress. It has been frequently shown that individuals who have a positive family history of hypertension exhibit higher blood pressure responses than individuals of normotensive descent when subjected to mental and physical stresses [38]. The heritability of the stress component in hypertensive individuals has also been suggested by twin studies that evaluated blood pressure responses after mathematical testing (i.e. mental stress)[6].

Several candidate genes have been suggested to mediate the effects of stress in hypertension [10,39–41]. Body temperature and blood pressure increase in response to stress. Total genome scanning of the RIS panel derived from SHR and BN progenitors revealed two QTLs for body temperature-response to stress on rat chromosomes 10 and 12. The QTL on chromosome 12 contains the heat-shock protein 27 (*hsp27*) gene. A variant allele of the gene was identified in SHR that co-segregated with left ventricular hypertrophy upon comparison to WKY and BN normotensive controls. Several stress-related candidate genes are also located on rat chromosome 20. They are the heat-shock protein 70 (*hsp70*) and tumor necrosis factor (*TNF*) genes. Hsp 70 has been shown to be expressed more in hypertensive versus normotensive human and animal subjects, whereas the *TNF*-containing QTL co-segregates with elevated blood pressure in response to the TNF receptor agonist endotoxin.

Diet

Salt has long been recognized as an important environmental factor in essential hypertension. Studies have shown that animals maintained on a low-salt diet develop hypertension when switched to a high-salt diet. In addition, both hypertensive and normotensive human subjects are sensitive or resistant to the blood pressure-raising effects of salt [42]. Salt sensitivity to blood pressure may also be dependent on other environmental factors such as stress and the consumption of alcohol and other dietary ions[43].

The most common animal model used to study the role of salt in essential hypertension is the SS/Jr rat. When SS/Jr rats are maintained on a high-salt diet for more than four weeks, they die due to complications induced by high blood pressure. In contrast, SR/Jr rats can survive the same high-salt diet for more than a year. Genetic studies conducted on the Dahl rats have identified QTLs for salt sensitivity of blood pressure on several chromosomes, and the results of these studies have been summarized [10,27,41]. A QTL on rat chromosome 13 has been shown to contain an allele of the renin gene that co-segregated with salt-sensitive blood pressure in an F_2-segregating population. However, the significance of this finding remains controversial as a result of additional studies. In one report, a congenic rat strain carrying this chromosomal region from the SS/Jr rat actually exhibited a decrease in blood pressure in comparison to the

SR/Jr progenitor. Another report showed that the transfer of the salt-resistant allele from the SR/Jr rat to the SS/Jr rat actually increased blood pressure in the congenic animal. Additional QTLs for salt sensitivity to blood pressure have been localized to rat chromosomes 2 and 10. The QTL on chromosome 2 lies near the *Gca* gene that encodes for atrial natriuretic peptide receptor A. *Gca* is considered a candidate gene since SS/Jr rats exhibit defective natriuretic and diuretic responses mediated by atrial natriuretic peptide. The QTL on rat chromosome 10 contains the candidate gene encoding for ACE, and the effect of the QTL has been confirmed by examining congenic strains derived from SHR-SP and WKY rats.

2

Obesity

Body weight is considered another environmental factor that influences the susceptibility to essential hypertension [10,41]. Population studies have indicated that there is a significant correlation between body weight and blood pressure. These studies have also shown that body weight reduction results in a significant decrease in blood pressure.

It has been demonstrated that body weight is regulated by the products of the *ob* and *db* genes, which encode for leptin and the leptin receptor respectively [44,45]. The current understanding is that circulating leptin, which is produced by adipose tissue, transmits information to the hypothalamus via the interaction with the leptin receptor and there regulates energy intake and expenditure. Leptin resistance is observed in most obese individuals. Leptin has been suggested to be a possible link between obesity and hypertension since chronic infusions of leptin in rats cause an increase in blood pressure.

Another feature of excessive body weight has been linked to essential hypertension. Obese individuals who are hypertensive often display glucose intolerance and dyslipidemia. These traits can both be caused by insulin resistance and/or excessive insulin secretion (e.g. hyperinsulinemia). The possible role for insulin in essential hypertension is supported by the results of population studies indicating that insulin resistance, hyperinsulinemia, and resulting dyslipidemia occur frequently in families with hypertensive individuals. Further, medications that alleviate insulin resistance appear to decrease blood pressure independently of body weight, suggesting a role for insulin resistance in essential hypertension independent of obesity.

The candidate gene that has been proposed to be responsible for influencing insulin sensitivity of hypertension is the *TNF* gene. TNF has been shown to inhibit intracellular signaling events from the insulin receptor. TNF also plays a role in apoptosis, which has also been implicated in essential hypertension. Studies have shown that apoptosis is higher in hypertensive rats relative to normotensive rats. Cardiomyocytes also undergo apoptosis in response to pressure overload. In addition, apoptosis of smooth muscle cells contributes to the regression of vascular hypertrophy in response to administration of certain antihypertensive drugs.

BOX 2.2.9 Detecting and preventing risk factors by molecular diagnosis

As an understanding of the genetic mechanisms that underlie hypertension slowly emerges, an increasing number of candidate genes have been associated with the regulation of blood pressure. However, the nature of essential hypertension necessitates the identification of other genes that act in concert with blood pressure-regulating genes to cause the disease. Possible interacting genes have generally been thought to be genes for risk factors associated with hypertension. One goal of treating and preventing hypertension, which is not yet achievable, is determining whether individuals express the genes that could predispose them to the development of essential hypertension. However, integrate genetic studies on hypertension and risk-related disorders are still few in number. In at least one case, the role of a widely accepted risk factor for essential hypertension has already been challenged.

- *Obesity*. Obesity has long been considered a risk factor for the development of hypertension. However, transgenic animals with a disrupted leptin gene do not display alterations in blood pressure [52].
- *Type II diabetes*. Type II diabetes is another well-known risk factor for hypertension. However, a study of whether genetic mutations that contribute to type II diabetes may also increase the risk of hypertension is not yet available.
- *Atherosclerosis*. Atherosclerosis is a condition that is commonly associated with hypertension. Numerous genetic mutations have been identified that contribute to atherosclerosis, including mutations in the genes encoding ApoE, the HDL and LDL receptors, and MTHFR that lead to homocysteinemia. There is evidence that cholesterol level may be an indicator for blood pressure since hypertriglyceridemic rats are hypertensive [53]. The close relationship between atherosclerosis and hypertension warrants studies on whether genetic mutations that predispose to elevated cholesterol levels increase the risk of hypertension in individuals.

Pharmacogenetics

Perhaps one of the greatest benefits to come from studies on the genetics of hypertension will be the identification of genes that dictate an individual's response to medication. This area of study, known generally as pharmacogenetics, is aimed at identifying genes that are responsible for the blood pressure response to antihypertensive medication and has been summarized [46]. The rational design of most antihypertensive drugs is based on targeting specific components of physiological systems involved in blood pressure regulation. However, these drugs have met with variable success when administered to patients with hypertension. The range in efficacy appears to be influenced by genetic differences that lie at both the population and the individual level. For instance, white hypertensive subjects consistently show a better response than black hypertensive subjects to ACE inhibitors and beta-blockers, suggesting that racial genetic composition may be important in the efficiency of these drugs. At the individual level, it has been observed that there is a preferential response of individuals with low-renin hypertension to calcium-channel blockers. Similarly, 'non-modulators' respond particularly well to treatment with ACE inhibitors. Therefore, the goal of pharmacogenetics is to identify genes that control the response to a particular medication and to determine which alleles of these genes can predispose to drug sensitivity or drug resistance.

Pharmacogenetics has already been successfully applied in certain forms of monogenetic hypertension. For instance, the drug amiloride is effective in reducing blood pressure in individuals with Liddle's syndrome. Amiloride inhibits the activity of the renal tubular epithelial sodium channel, which is overactive in individuals with this form of hypertension. In addition, individuals with glucocorticoid-remediable hypertension can be treated with glucocorticoids, such as dexamethasone. Dexamethasone alleviates the symptoms of this syndrome by decreasing the expression of the hybrid aldosterone gene that is responsible for the increase in blood pressure.

The application of pharmacogenetics to essential hypertension has been more challenging. The first total genome search for genetic determinants of the response to calcium-channel blockers was performed on a cross of LH and LN rats. A QTL was identified on chromosome 2, which contains the gene for calmodulin-dependent protein kinase II delta, a regulator of calcium homeostasis. However, this QTL failed to co-segregate with blood pressure in the Lyon rat. Variants of the ACE and angiotensin genes have also been tested for the blood pressure response to the antihypertensive drugs nifedipine, lisinopril, and atenolol. However, no relationship was found between any of the variants and the efficacy of these drugs. Another study has indicated a lack of predictive response between a variant angiotensin allele and ACE inhibitors, beta-blockers, and calcium blockers. Perhaps the best potential for pharmacogenetics is the α-adducin gene in which mutations have been identified that may influence the response to diuretics.

Despite these challenges, pharmacogenetics continues to represent the most rational approach for treating hypertension. If successful, pharmacogenetics will be able to offer treatment to responsive hypertensive individuals with some expectation of benefit, without subjecting non-responsive individuals to potential side effects of treatment.

References

1. James GD, Baker PT. Human population biology and hypertension. In: *Hypertension: Pathophysiology, Diagnosis, and Management* (eds Laragh JH, Brenner BM), pp. 137–145. New York: Raven Press, 1990.
2. Morgagni JB. *De sedibus et causus Morboreum per Anatomen Indegatis*, Vol. I. Venice: Remondiana, 1761.
3. Williams RR, Hunt SC, Hasstedt SJ *et al.* Are there interactions and relations between genetic and environmental factors in predisposing to high blood pressure? *Hypertension* 1991;**18** (Suppl I):I29–I37.
4. Hunt SC, Williams RR, Barlow GK. A comparison of positive family history definitions for defining risk of future diseases. *J Chron Dis* 1986;**39**:809–821.

References

5. Ward R. Familial aggregation and genetic epidemiology of blood pressure. In: *Hypertension: Pathophysiology, Diagnosis, and Management*, 2nd edn. (eds Laragh JH, Brenner BM), pp. 67–88. New York: Raven Press, 1995.

6. Feinleib M, Garrison RJ, Faraiz R *et al*. The NHLBI twin study of cardiovascular disease risk factors: methodology and summary of results. *Am J Epidemiol* 1977;**106**:284–295.

7. Biron P, Mongeau JG. Familial aggregation of blood pressure and its components. *Pediatr Clin* 1978;**25**:29–33.

8. Biron P, Mongeau JG, Bertrand D. Familial aggregation of blood pressure in 558 adopted children. *Can Med Ass J* 1976;**115**:773–774.

9. Lifton RP. Molecular genetics of human blood pressure variation. *Science* 1996;**272**:676–680.

10. Hamet P, Pausova Z, Adarichev V *et al*. Hypertension: genes and environment. *J Hypertension* 1998;**16**:397–418.

11. Lifton RP, Dluhy RG, Powers M *et al*. Hereditary hypertension caused by chimeric gene duplications and ectopic expression of aldosterone synthase. *Nature Genet* 1992;**2**:66–74.

12. Pascoe L, Curnow KM, Slutsker L *et al*. Glucocorticoid-suppressible hyperaldosteronism results from hybrid genes created by unequal crossovers between CYP11B1 and CYP11B2. *Proc Natl Acad Sci USA* 1992;**89**:8327–8331.

13. Mune T, Rogerson FM, Nikkila H *et al*. Human hypertension caused by mutations in the kidney isozyme of 11β-hydroxysteroid dehydrogenase. *Nature Genet* 1995;**10**:394–396.

14. Shimkets RA, Warnock DG, Bositis CM *et al*. Liddle's syndrome: heritable human hypertension caused by mutations in the beta subunit of the epithelial sodium channel. *Cell* 1994;**79**:407–414.

15. Hansson JH, Nelson-Williams C, Suzuki H *et al*. Hypertension caused by a truncated epithelial sodium channel gamma subunit: genetic heterogeneity of Liddle syndrome. *Nature Genet* 1995;**11**:76–82.

16. Dluhy RG, Lifton RP. Glucocorticoid-remediable aldosteronism (GRA): diagnosis, variability of phenotype and regulation of potassium homeostasis. *Steroids* 1995;**60**: 48–51.

17. Mansfield TA, Simon DB, Farfel Z *et al*. Multilocus linkage of familial hyperkalaemia and hypertension, pseudohypoaldosteronism type II, to chromosomes 1q21-42 and 17q11-q21. *Nature Genet* 1997;**16**:202–205.

18. Wilson RC, Krozowski ZS, Li K *et al*. A mutation in the *HSD11B2* gene in a family with apparent mineralocorticoid excess. *J Clin Endocrinol Metab* 1995;**80**:2263–2266.

19. Chang SS, Grunder S, Hanukoglu A *et al*. Mutations in subunits of the epithelial sodium channel cause salt wasting with hyperkalemic acidosis, pseudohypoaldosteronism type 1. *Nature Genet* 1996;**12**:248–253.

20. Rubattu S, Struk B, Kreutz R *et al*. Animal models of genetic hypertension: what can we learn for human hypertension? *Clin Exp Pharmacol Physiol* 1995;Suppl 2:S386–S393.

21. Lovenberg W, Horan M (eds) Genetic rat models for hypertension: guidelines for breeding, care, and use. *Hypertension* 1987;**9**(Suppl I):I40–I42.

22. Silver LM. *Mouse Genetics: Concepts and Applications*. Oxford University Press: Oxford, 1995.

23. Hamet P, Pauvosa Z, Dumas P *et al*. Newborn and adult recombinant inbred strains: a tool for the search of genetic determinants of target organ damage in hypertension. *Kidney Int* 1998;**53**:1488–1492.

24. Pravenec M, Kren V, Zicha J, Kunes J. An analysis of spontaneous hypertension in spontaneously hypertensive rats by means of new recombinant inbred strains. *J Hypertension* 1989;**7**:217–222.

25. Rapp JP, Deng AY. Detection and positional cloning of blood pressure quantitative trait loci: is it possible? *Hypertension* 1995;**25**:1121–1128.

26. Ely DL, Daneshvar H, Turner ME *et al*. The hypertensive Y chromosome elevates blood pressure in F_{11} normotensive rats. *Hypertension* 1993; **21**:1071–1075.

27. Deng AY. In search of hypertension genes in Dahl salt-sensitive rats. *J Hypertension* 1998; **16**:1707–1717.

28. Rapp JP, Garret MR, Deng AY. Construction of a double congenic strain to prove an epistatic interaction on blood pressure between rat chromosomes 2 and 10. *J Clin Invest* 1998;**101**:1591–1595.

29. Lander ES, Schork NJ. Genetic dissection of complex traits. *Science* 1994;**265**:2037–2048.
30. Ghosh S, Collins FS. The geneticist's approach to complex disease. *Ann Rev Med* 1996;**47**:333–353.
31. Rapp JP, Wang S-M, Dene H. Effect of genetic background on cosegregation of renin alleles and blood pressure in Dahl rats. *Am J Hypertension* 1990;**3**:391–396.
32. Cicila GT, Rapp JP, Wang JM *et al*. Linkage of 11 beta-hydroxylase mutations with altered steroid biosynthesis and blood pressure in the Dahl rat. *Nature Genet* 1993;**3**:343–356.
33. Deng AY, Rapp JP. Cosegregation of blood pressure with angiotensin converting enzyme and atrial natriuretic peptide receptor genes using Dahl salt-sensitive rats. *Nature Genet* 1992;**1**:267–272.
34. Bianchi G, Tripodi G, Casari G *et al*. Two point mutations within adducin genes are involved in blood pressure variation. *Proc Natl Acad Sci USA* 1994;**91**:3999–4003.
35. Deng AY, Dene H, Rapp JP. Mapping of a quantitative trait locus for blood pressure on rat chromosome 2. *J Clin Invest* 1994;**94**:431–436.
36. Hoffmann S, Paul M, Urata H *et al*. Transgenic rats and experimental hypertension. In: *Hypertension: Pathophysiology, Diagnosis, and Management*, 2nd edn. (eds Laragh JH, Brenner BM), pp. 1301–1308. Raven Press: New York, 1995.
37. Mullins JJ, Peters J, Ganten D. Fulminant hypertension in transgenic rats harbouring the mouse *Ren-2* gene. *Nature* 1990;**344**:541–544.
38. Widgren BR, Wikstrand J, Berglund G, Andersson OK. Increased response to physical and mental stress in men with hypertensive parents. *Hypertension* 1992;**20**:606–611.
39. Hamet P. Environmental stress and genes of hypertension. *Clin Exp Pharmacol Physiol* 1995;Suppl. 2:S394–S398.
40. Hamet P. Environmentally-regulated genes of hypertension. *Clin Exp Hypertension* 1996;**18**:267–278.
41. Pausova Z, Tremblay J, Hamet P. Gene-environment interactions in hypertension. *Curr Hypertens Rep* 1999;1:42–50.
42. Weinberger MH. Salt sensitivity: does it play an important role in the pathogenesis and treatment of hypertension. *Curr Opin Nephrol Hypertension* 1996;**5**:205–208.
43. Hamet P, Mongeau E, Lambert J *et al*. Interactions among calcium, sodium and alcohol intake as determinants of blood pressure. *Hypertension* 1991;**17** (Suppl):I150–I154.
44. Zhang Y, Proenca R, Maffel M *et al*. Positional cloning of the mouse obese gene and its human homologue. *Nature* 1994;**372**:425–431.
45. Tartaglia LA, Dembrski M, Weng X *et al*. Identification and expression cloning of a leptin receptor, OBR. *Cell* 1995;**83**:1263–1271.
46. Hamet P. Genes and hypertension: where we are and where we should go. *Clin Exp Hypertens* 1999;**21**:947–960.
47. Koike G, Jacob HJ. Hypertension. In: *Principles of Molecular Medicine* (ed. Jameson JL), pp. 145–155. Humana Press, Totowa, NJ 1998.
48. Jacob HJ, Lindpainter K, Lincoln SE *et al*. Genetic mapping of a gene causing hypertension in the stroke-prone spontaneously hypertensive rat. *Cell* 1991;**67**:213–224.
49. Hilbert P, Lindpainter K, Beckmann JS *et al*. Chromosomal mapping of two genetic loci associated with blood-pressure regulation in hereditary hypertensive rats. *Nature* 1991;**353**:521–529.
50. Cusi D, Bianchi G. A primer on the genetics of hypertension. *Kidney Int* 1998; **54**:328–342.
51. Eaton SB, Konner M, Shostak M. Stoneager in the fast lane: chronic degenerative diseases in evolutionary perspective. *Am J Med* 1988;**84**:739–749.
52. Lusis AJ, Weinreb A, Drake TA. Genetics of atherosclerosis. In: *Comprehensive Cardiovascular Medicine* (ed. Topol EJ), pp. 2763–2787. Lipincott-Raven: Philadelphia, 1998.
53. Kunes J, Mazeaud MM, Devynck MA, Zicha J. Platelet hypoaggregability in hereditary hypertriglyceridemic rats: relation to plasma triglycerides. *Thromb Res* 1997;**88**:347–353.
54. Iwai N, Kurtz TW, Inagami T. Further evidence of the *SA* gene as a candidate gene contributing to the hypertension in spontaneously hypertensive rat. *Biochem Biophys Res Commun* 1992;**188**:64–69.
55. Samani NJ, Lodwick D, Vincent M *et al*. A gene differentially expressed in the kidney of the spontaneously hypertensive rat cosegregates with increased blood pressure. *J Clin Invest* 1993;**92**:1099–1103.

2

References

56. Harris EI, Dene H, Rapp JP. SA gene and blood pressure cosegregation using Dahl salt-sensitive rats. *Am J Hypertension* 1993;**6**:330–334.
57. Pravenec M, Kren V, Kunes J *et al*. Cosegregation of blood pressure with a kallikrein gene family polymorphism. *Hypertension* 1991;**17**:242–246.
58. Harris EL, Phelan EL, Thompson CM *et al*. Heart mass and blood pressure have separate genetic determinants in the New Zealand genetically hypertensive (GH) rat. *J Hypertension* 1995;**13**:397–404.
59. Deng AY, Dene H, Rapp JP. Congenic strains for the blood pressure quantitative trait locus on rat chromosome 2. *Hypertension* 1997;**30**:199–202.
60. Deng AY, Rapp JP. Evaluation of the angiotensin II receptor *AT1B* gene as a candidate gene for blood pressure. *J Hypertension* 1994;**12**:1001–1006.
61. Clark JS, Jeffs B, Davidson AO *et al*. Quantitative trait loci in genetically hypertensive rats: possible sex specificity. *Hypertension* 1996;**28**:898–906.
62. Dubay C, Vincent M, Samani NJ *et al*. Genetic determinants of diastolic and pulse pressure map to different loci in Lyon hypertensive rats. *Nature Genet* 1993;**3**:354–357.
63. Katsuya T, Higaki J, Zhao Y *et al*. Neuropeptide Y locus on chromosome 4 cosegregates with blood pressure in the spontaneously hypertensive rat. *Biochem Biophys Res Commun* 1993;**192**:261–267.
64. Kreutz R, Hubner N, James MR *et al*. Dissection of a quantitative trait locus for genetic hypertension on rat chromosome 10. *Proc Natl Acad Sci USA* 1995;**92**:8778–8782.
65. Hamet P, Kaiser MA, Sun Y *et al*. HSP27 locus cosegregates with left ventricular mass independently of blood pressure. *Hypertension* 1996;**28**: 1112–1117.
66. Rapp JP, Wang SM, Dene H. A genetic polymorphism in the renin gene of Dahl rats cosegregates with blood pressure. *Science* 1989;**243**:542–544.
67. Kurtz TW, Simonet L, Kabra PM *et al*. Cosegregation of the renin allele of the spontaneously hypertensive rat with an increase in blood pressure. *J Clin Invest* 1990;**85**:1328–1332.
68. St Lezin E, Wong A, Wang JM *et al*. *Hypertension* 1993;**22**:421 (Abstract).
69. Hamet P, Kong D, Pravenec M, *et al*. Restriction fragment length polymorphism of *hsp70* gene, localized in the RT1 complex, is associated with hypertension in spontaneously hypertensive rats. *Hypertension* 1992;**19**:611–614.
70. Ely DL, Turner ME. Hypertension in the spontaneously hypertensive rat is linked to the Y chromosome. *Hypertension* 1990;**16**:277–281.
71. Turner ME, Johnson ML, Ely DL. Separate sex-influenced and genetic components in spontaneously hypertensive rat hypertension. *Hypertension* 1991;**17**:1097–1103.
72. Davidson AO, Schork N, Jaques BC *et al*. Blood pressure in genetically hypertensive rats: influence of the Y chromosome. *Hypertension* 1995;**26**:452–459.
73. Kim HS, Krege JH, Kluckman KD *et al*. Genetic control of blood pressure and the angiotensinogen locus. *Proc Natl Acad Sci USA* 1995;**92**:2735–2739.
74. Kimura S, Mullins JJ, Bunnemann B *et al*. High blood pressure in transgenic mice carrying the angiotensinogen gene. *EMBJO J* 1992;**11**:821–827.
75. Fukamizu A, Sugimura K, Takimoto E *et al*. Chimeric renin–angiotensin system demonstrates sustained increase in blood pressure of transgenic mice carrying both human renin and human angiotensinogen genes. *J Biol Chem* 1993;**268**:11617–11621.
76. Kuro-o M, Hanaoka K, Hiroi Y *et al*. Salt-sensitive hypertension in transgenic mice overexpressing Na⁺–proton exchanger. *Circulation Res* 1995;**76**:148–153.
77. Wang M, Xiong W, Yang Z *et al*. Human tissue kallikrein induces hypotension in transgenic mice. *Hypertension* 1994;**23**:236–243.
78. Krege JH, John SW, Lagenbach LL. Male–female differences in fertility and blood pressure in ACE-deficient mice. *Nature* 1995;**375**:146–148.
79. Veress AT, Chong CK, Field LJ, Sonnenberg H. Blood pressure and fluid–electrolyte balance in ANF-transgenic mice on high- and low-salt diets. *Am J Physiol* 1995; **269**:R186–R192.
80. Lopez MJ, Wong SK, Kishimoto I *et al*. Salt-resistant hypertension in mice lacking the guanylyl cyclase-A receptor for atrial natriuretic peptide. *Nature* 1995;**378**:65–68.
81. Ito M, Oliverio MI, Mannon PJ *et al*. Regulation of blood pressure by the type 1A angiotensin II receptor gene. *Proc Natl Acad Sci USA* 1995;**92**:3521–3525.
82. Kurihara Y, Kurihara H, Suzuki H *et al*. Elevated blood pressure and craniofacial abnormalities in mice deficient in endothelin-1. *Nature* 1994;**368**:703–710.

83. Huang PL, Huang Z, Mashimo H *et al.* Hypertension in mice lacking the gene for endothelial nitric oxide synthase. *Nature* 1995;**377**:239–242.

84. Aitman TJ, Gotoda T, Evans AL *et al.* Quantitative trait loci for cellular defects in glucose and fatty acid metabolism in hypertensive rats. *Nature Genet* 1997;**16**:197–201.

85. Pravenec M, Gauguier D, Schott JJ *et al.* Mapping of quantitative trait loci for blood pressure and cardiac mass in the rat by genome scanning of recombinant inbred strains. *J Clin Invest* 1995;**96**:1973–1978.

86. Aitman TJ, Glazier AM, Wallace CA *et al.* Identification of Cd36 (Fat) as an insulin-resistance gene causing defective fatty acid and glucose metabolism in hypertensive rats. *Nature Genet* 1999;**21**:76–83.

87. Pravenec M, Zidek V, Simakova M *et al.* Genetics of Cd36 and the clustering of multiple cardiovascular risk factors in spontaneous hypertension *J Clin Invest* 1999;**103**:1651–1657.

References

The renin–angiotensin system

MG Nicholls, AM Richards and TG Yandle

Introduction

In 1898, Tigerstedt and Bergman isolated a pressor substance from rabbit kidney which they termed 'renin'[1]. This turned out to be an enzyme which is released from the juxtaglomerular apparatus under the control of a constellation of input signals, into the circulation, where it acts on angiotensinogen (renin substrate) from the liver forming the biologically inactive decapeptide angiotensin I, which in turn is converted, by angiotensin-converting enzyme (ACE), to the active octapeptide, angiotensin II (Figure 2.3.1).

The above description is of the circulating renin–angiotensin system. In addition, there are renin–angiotensin systems functional within many tissues and organs although some, at least, are dependent on delivery of kidney-based renin. In the heart, for example, renin uptake from the circulation leads ultimately to the formation of local tissue angiotensin II. Alternative pathways of angiotensin II production, independent of ACE (via chymase for example), are found in some organs.

Angiotensin II, whether the product of ACE or other enzymes, has numerous biologic actions mostly via the AT_1 receptor but AT_2

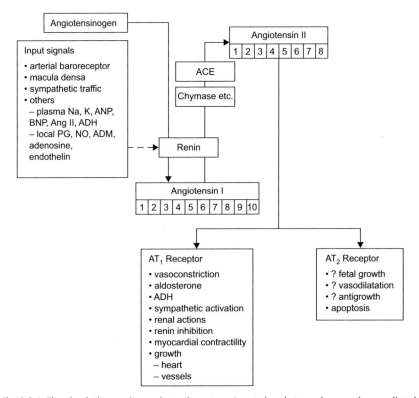

Fig. 2.3.1 The circulating renin–angiotensin system. Input signals to renin secretion are listed, as are the actions of angiotensin II via its two receptor types. Angiotensin I is composed of ten amino acids and eight for angiotensin II. Na = sodium; K = potassium; ANP = atrial natriuretic peptide; BNP = brain natriuretic peptide; Ang II = angiotensin II; ADH = antidiuretic hormone; PG = prostaglandins; NO = nitric oxide; ADM = adrenomedullin.

receptors may play a role in fetal tissue development and act as a counterbalance to some of the effects of AT_1 stimulation (Figure 2.3.1). Although hotly disputed in earlier times, it is now clear that the renin–angiotensin system, through its diverse actions, is vital to the maintenance of arterial pressure, blood volume and electrolyte balance in normal subjects especially when challenged by loss of body fluid or in states of low blood pressure. Far from acting in isolation, the system works in concert with other pressor, fluid-maintaining systems most obviously the sympathetic nervous system, and is a counterbalance to vasodilating, natriuretic systems particularly the cardiac natriuretic peptides.

Biologic responses to angiotensin II vary according to circumstances. Its pressor effect is heightened by sodium loading (for example, with a high sodium diet) but is attenuated in volume-deplete states. The opposite is true for aldosterone secretion where the response to angiotensin II is magnified in sodium deplete states and diminished with sodium loading. Temporal profiles are also important in that the pressor effect of angiotensin II is gradually incremental: a barely-pressor response to low dose angiotensin II may evolve into severe hypertension if the infusion is continued over days or weeks. This is the 'slow-pressor' effect of angiotensin II [2]. Such basic physiological observations are vital in interpreting the importance of a given level of circulating renin or angiotensin II.

In recent years awareness of the trophic, and possibly toxic, actions of the renin–angiotensin system has increased [3]. Angiotensin II, at least under some circumstances, contributes to cardiac and vascular hypertrophy, thereby enhancing the tendency for blood pressure to rise in hypertensive states. There is a school of thought that hypertensive patients with activation of the renin–angiotensin system suffer greater cardiovascular consequences than similarly hypertensive subjects in whom renin is 'normal' or suppressed. This could be explained by the experimentally well described toxic actions of angiotensin II.

In this chapter we describe measurement of activity of the renin–angiotensin system and summarise the role of this system in various forms of hypertension.

Assessing activity of the renin–angiotensin system
Plasma angiotensin II

Accurate measurement of plasma angiotensin II requires expertise and attention to detail, as outlined by Nussberger and Brunner [4]. These measurements are particularly difficult in patients taking an ACE inhibitor when angiotensin II levels initially at least, are low and angiotensin I levels (which cross-react with most angiotensin II antibodies) are high. Numerous factors can modify levels of angiotensin II (Table 2.3.1). Because of the technical difficulties, angiotensin II is generally only measured in research laboratories with a special interest in the renin–angiotensin system.

Table 2.3.1 Factors affecting plasma levels of renin and angiotensin II

Factor	Effect
Patient age	Renin levels fall with aging
Body posture	Levels rise on standing
Diet sodium intake	Levels elevated with sodium restriction
Time of day	Levels fall through daytime
Medications	*Renin levels rise* with diuretic, ACE inhibitors, angiotensin II receptor blockers *Renin suppressed* by beta-blockers, α-methyldopa-like drugs
Other	Meal-time, phase of menstrual cycle

Plasma renin

A technically simpler approach is to measure plasma levels of renin, either renin concentration (when an excess of renin substrate is added to the plasma sample) or plasma renin activity (PRA, when endogenous substrate is utilized). Either way, the level of angiotensin I (generated during an *in vitro* incubation step) is an index of the level of renin in the plasma sample. Care is required for accurate measurements of renin, as outlined by Poulsen and Nielsen [5]. Furthermore, interpretation of renin levels, as with angiotensin II, should take into account a number of factors (Table 2.3.1). Blood sampling for renin measurements must be carried out under conditions determined by the local laboratory which should earlier have defined its normal range under the same circumstances.

Documentation of high levels of plasma renin is vital for the diagnosis of renin-secreting tumour, and low plasma renin is central to the differentiation of primary aldosteronism from essential hypertension (see below). Whereas some clinical centres use renin measurements also under other circumstances (predicting blood pressure response to surgical intervention in unilateral renal artery stenosis for example), many more laboratories only make use of renin measurements in hypertensive patients for research purposes.

Plasma sodium concentration

Experience from the early days of renin measurements has shown there is an inverse, if not always close, relationship between activity of fhe renin-angiotensin system and plasma sodium concentration (Figure 2.3.2). In hypertensive patients with gross activation of the renin–angiotensin system (as is often seen in malignant hypertension and the hyponatremic–hypertensive syndrome), plasma sodium concentration is usually towards the lower limit of the normal range or frankly low (Figure 2.3.2). This reflects the ability of high levels of angiotensin II to stimulate water intake (by augmenting thirst) and inhibit water loss via a direct action on the kidney and indirectly by enhancing pituitary antidiuretic hormone release.

Whilst plasma sodium does not provide an entirely accurate index of renin levels, it does give a useful clinical caution, particularly in patients

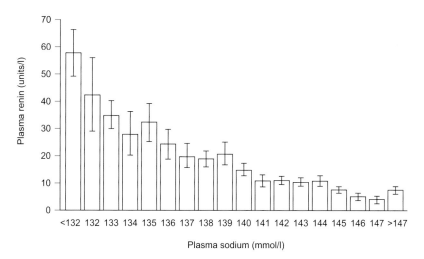

Fig. 2.3.2 Relationship between plasma renin concentration and plasma sodium in 253 patients with essential hypertension or various forms of secondary hypertension. Some patients were receiving antihypertensive medication. After Brown *et al*. [8], with permission.

with severe hypertension. When antihypertensive drug treatment is considered urgent in a patient whose plasma sodium concentration is low–normal or frankly reduced, the renin–angiotensin system is probably activated and care must be exercised with the first dose of an ACE inhibitor or angiotensin II receptor blocker. Volume depletion, sometimes obvious in such patients, may warrant volume repletion (cautious intravenous saline) prior to administration of an ACE inhibitor or angiotensin II receptor blocker to avoid a first-dose hypotensive response.

On the other hand, the hypertensive patient with a high–normal or elevated plasma sodium concentration, is likely to have a low renin level in which case minerlaocorticoid-type hypertension (especially primary aldosteronism, but also secretion of a mineralocorticoid other than aldosterone or licorice intake) should be suspected. Under such circumstances, monotherapy with blockers of the renin–angiotensin system is unlikely to have a major initial effect on blood pressure.

Blood pressure response to blockade of the renin–angiotensin system

The advent of specific blocking drugs has greatly assisted in understanding the role of the renin–angiotensin system in hypertensive patients. Experience has shown that where plasma renin levels are high, a vigorous initial fall in arterial pressure is seen with administration of one or other of the blocking drugs – ACE inhibitors or angiotensin II receptor blockers. The first-dose response, then, provides an index of activity of the renin–angiotensin system although few now use these drugs for this purpose.

2

The renin–angiotensin system in hypertension
Secondary forms of hypertension
Renin-secreting tumor [6]

Primary reninism is caused most often by a juxtaglomerular cell tumor, occasionally by renal cell carcinomas and rarely by non-renal malignant tumors (ovarian neoplasms, adenocarcinoma of the pancreas, soft-tissue sarcoma, oat cell carcinoma of the lung, etc (Figure 2.3.3).

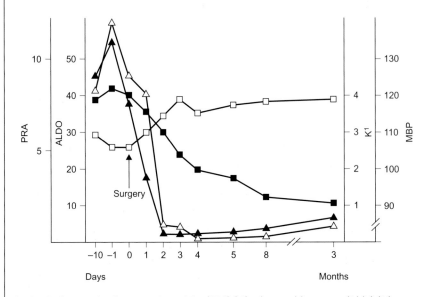

Fig. 2.3.3 Changes in plasma renin activity (PRA) (▲), plasma aldosterone (Aldo) (△), plasma potassium (K+) (□), and mean blood pressure (MPB) (■) with removal of a renin–secreting tumor of the kidney in a 23-year-old male. From Pedrinelli *et al.* [31], with permission.

BOX 2.3.1 Juxtaglomerular cell tumors

Primary reninism due to renal juxtaglomerular cell tumors is not common (approximately 40 cases reported up to 1993), but is important from a number of viewpoints. It is normally a curable form of hypertension. In regards to pathophysiology, the disorder demonstrates that autonomous overproduction of renin results in hypertension usually of considerable severity, and hypokalemia secondary to elevated aldosterone production. Documentation of a raised plasma renin level (and where possible a raised pro-renin) is vital to the diagnosis. Elevated renin levels in one renal vein (or one branch of a renal vein) combined with radiologic identification of a solid tumor (either by computerized tomography or ultrasound) should lead to removal of the tumor with normalization of blood pressure and plasma renin levels, and correction of hypokalemia.

Unilateral renal artery stenosis/occlusion/renal segmental infarction [7]

Reduction or cessation of blood flow to a segment, or to the whole, of a kidney with retention of normal flow to the other kidney, is one of the commoner forms of secondary hypertension. In most cases it is due to atheromatous renal vascular disease, but fibromuscular hyperplasia and rarer pathologies can also be involved. It is generally considered that the renin–angiotensin system is central to the pathophysiology of this form of hypertension. If man is like the experimental rat, there are typically three phases to the development of hypertension in unilateral renal ischemia (Figure 2.3.4). In phase one when the stenosis or occlusion develops, arterial pressure rises in parallel with an increase in circulating renin produced by the ischemic kidney. In phase two, arterial pressure remains elevated but circulating levels of renin fall towards, and sometimes into, the 'normal' range. There is a new heightened relationship between blood levels of renin (and angiotensin II) and arterial pressure, presumably as a result of the 'slow pressor' effect of angiotensin II [2] due to its trophic effects on blood vessels and heart over time, and a positive cumulative balance of body sodium which enhances its pressor activity. In this phase, as in phase one, removal of the stenotic lesion or administration of angiotensin II blocking drugs reverses the hypertension.

In phase three, blood pressure remains high but there is no longer clear elevation of plasma renin. Furthermore, relief of the ischemic lesion or administration of angiotensin II blocking agents may not reduce arterial pressure. The pathophysiology of phase three is disputed but probably involves the development of vascular lesions in the contralateral kidney or the evolution of trophic and toxic lesions within

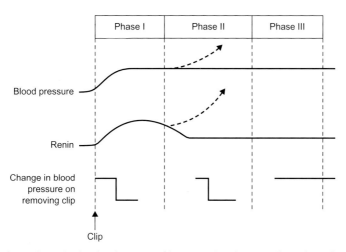

Fig. 2.3.4 Three phases in the development of hypertension due to unilateral renal ischemia (Goldblatt, two-kidney, one-clip hypertension). Arrows in phase two indicate the course in the hyponatremic–hypertensive syndrome. Reproduced from Brown *et al*. [32], with permission.

the cardiovascular system which respond minimally if at all to removal of the initiating lesion.

As might be anticipated from the discussion so far, peripheral plasma renin levels do not provide a good screening test for unilateral renal ischemia as a cause for hypertension. Some have found, however, that raised peripheral plasma renin predicts a good response of blood pressure to surgery, as does a high ratio (≥ 1.5 or ≥ 2.0) of renin in renal vein plasma from the ischemic, versus non-ischemic kidney – especially if there is also complete suppression of renin production from the non-ischemic kidney.

Apart from the three classical stages of hypertension due to unilateral renal ischemia, an additional phase, as indicated by the broken arrows in Figure 2.3.4, can develop in phase two or presumably phase one: the hyponatremic–hypertensive syndrome (Figure 2.3.5 and 2.3.6) [8,9]. This underrecognized disorder, most commonly seen in heavy smoking asthenic women, is characterized by severe supine hypertension but postural hypotension (reflecting body volume depletion), hyponatremia and commonly hypokalemia with extreme activation of the renin–angiotensin system. The hypertension secondary to segmental renal ischemia or infarction (due to trauma, thrombosis, embolus or aneurysm) can evolve into the hyponatremic–hypertensive syndrome. In some cases, the hypertension resolves, presumably with death of previously ischemic renin–secreting cells [10].

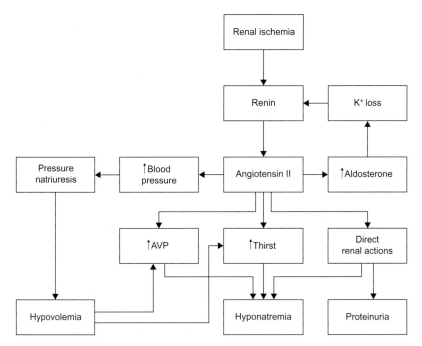

Fig. 2.3.5 Pathophysiology of the hyponatremic–hypertensive syndrome due to unilateral renal ischemia. AVP = arginine vasopressin.

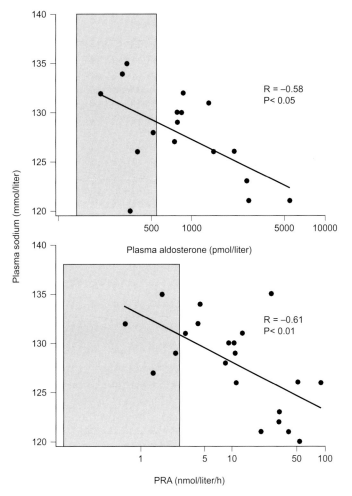

Fig. 2.3.6 Relationship between plasma sodium levels and plasma renin activity (PRA, lower panel) and plasma aldosterone (upper panel) in patients with the hyponatremic–hypertensive syndrome due to renal ischemia. The cross-hatched areas indicate normal ranges. From Agarwal *et al.* [9], with permission.

Bilateral renal artery stenosis, or stenosis to a single kidney [7]

Evidence from animal studies would suggest that the early rise in arterial pressure is accounted for by release of renin from both kidneys when bilateral renal artery stenosis is present. However, this early phase is supplanted by expansion of body sodium content and normal or even low levels of plasma renin and angiotensin II. In some cases, sodium retention can progress to pulmonary edema [11]. Treatment with blockers of the renin–angiotensin system (ACE inhibitors or angiotensin II receptor blockers) can, especially when combined with diuretics, induce azotemia which, fortunately, is reversible. Correction of ischemia on one side (by angioplasty, stent or surgery) can result in a natriuresis through the now non-ischemic kidney, and hypertension which is more easily controlled with or without agents which block the renin–angiotensin system.

2

BOX 2.3.2 Hyponatremic–hypertensive syndrome

It is presumed that, with the development of critical renal ischemia, a particularly vigorous release of renin results in a rapid elevation of arterial pressure which induces a natriuresis from the non-ischemic kidney. This induces further release of renin from the ischemic kidney which enhances aldosterone secretion thereby leading to hypokalemia (Figure 2.3.5). The hyponatremia, which relates to the degree of activation of the renin–angiotensin system (Figure 2.3.6), is believed to result from stimulation of thirst and antidiuretic hormone secretion together with a direct effect of angiotensin II on the kidney to retain water in excess of sodium (Figure 2.3.5). Initial management of such patients can be complicated by a potentially dangerous hypotensive response to drugs which block the renin–angiotensin system (ACE inhibitors or angiotensin II receptor blockers). Rational therapy includes cautious intravenous volume replacement prior to administration of such drugs. Definitive treatment might be correction of ischemia by angioplasty or stent placement, removal of a shrunken ischemic kidney or segment of kidney, or long-term antihypertensive drug treatment.

Scleroderma renal crisis

This important if uncommon disorder is almost always accompanied by marked hyperreninemia reflecting multiple ischemic lesions in both kidneys. The advent of ACE inhibitors revolutionized management in that the blood pressure is, in most cases, readily controlled and the otherwise relentless decline in renal function is halted [12] (Figure 2.3.7). The microvascular disease within the kidney stimulates vigorous and presumably rapid activation of the renin–angiotensin system which not only elevates arterial pressure but presumably accelerates the

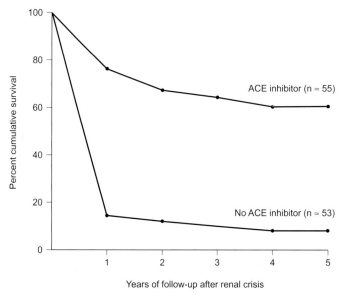

Fig. 2.3.7 Survival in patients with scleroderma renal crisis who were (n = 55) or were not (n = 53) treated with an ACE inhibitor. After Steen *et al.* [12], with permission.

microvascular process within the kidney. This 'vicious cycle' can, usually, be readily broken by blockade of the renin–angiotensin system. Whereas activation of the renin–angiotensin system is not the primary event, it is clearly an essential element in the pathophysiology.

Malignant hypertension

Most, but by no means all patients with malignant hypertension, exhibit considerable, and often gross, activation of the renin–angiotensin system [13]. It is likely that high levels of angiotensin II contribute to the vasculotoxicity associated with progressive renal failure and retinopathy, although the level of blood pressure and the rapidity with which it rises are probably dominant in this regard. Many patients develop hyponatremia and hypokalemia, and some are volume depleted. As with the hyponatremic–hypertensive syndrome caused by unilateral renal ischemia, there may be a place for cautious volume repletion prior to or during administration of ACE inhibitors or angiotensin II receptor blockers to avoid a first-dose hypotensive response. Anecdotal reports suggest that such volume repletion, presumably in part through suppression of activity of the renin–angiotensin system, can itself reduce arterial pressure (Figure 2.3.8).

Diabetes mellitus [14]

The renin–angiotensin system undergoes complex changes in diabetes mellitus, and variations are seen before and during the onset of complications, and with the development of hypertension. In the early uncomplicated stages of diabetes, the components of the renin–angiotensin system are relatively normal. Later, activity of the renin–angiotensin system remains normal or is slightly suppressed, although pro-renin and plasma ACE activity tend to be elevated. The development of nephropathy, retinopathy or neuropathy is usually accompanied by elevated levels of plasma pro-renin. In patients with nephropathy, plasma levels of active renin and angiotensin II are in the normal or low range.

In diabetics with hypertension, there is a trend for excessive sodium retention (exchangeable body sodium is increased by approximately 10% on average), and whereas active renin and angiotensin II levels are suppressed, pressor responsiveness to administered angiotensin II is enhanced.

The possibility that the renin–angiotensin system, whether the 'classic' circulating system or tissue-based, is involved in the development of diabetic complications receives some support from studies using ACE inhibitors. Blood pressure control has tended to be superior in ACE inhibitor-treated diabetics than in those receiving alternative antihypertensives, which makes interpretation of outcomes difficult. Nevertheless, current evidence points to superior protection against diabetic nephropathy [15] in patients given ACE inhibitors versus alternative antihypertensive drugs, and these drugs probably protect against retinopathy [16]. Intriguingly, ACE inhibition has also been reported to slow the development of diabetic neuropathy [17]. More work is required in this area, but it does seem possible that the

2

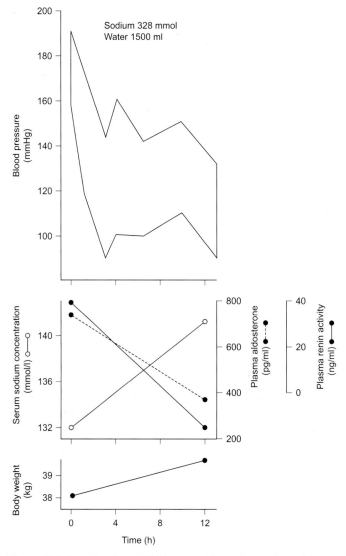

Fig. 2.3.8 Effect of infusion of sodium chloride over 12 hours in a patient with essential hypertension who entered the malignant phase. Note the fall in renin, aldosterone and arterial pressure. From Kaneda *et al.* [33], with permission.

renin–angiotensin system is involved in the evolution of diabetic complications especially in hypertensive patients. In theory, blockade of AT_1 receptors in hypertensive diabetics might prove especially protective in that such agents will not only block AT_1 receptors with all expected benefits, but in addition will stimulate AT_2 receptors with potentially beneficial results.

Primary aldosteronism

In classical primary aldosteronism and in other mineralocorticoid forms of hypertension (including that due to licorice ingestion) renin and

The renin-angiotensin system

The renin–angiotensin
system in hypertension

Secondary forms of
hypertension

Essential hypertension

2

angiotensin II levels in plasma are extremely low, suppressed by expansion of extracellular and circulating volume in part via release of cardiac natriuretic peptides. Documentation of a low plasma renin level, and in many laboratories a high plasma aldosterone:renin ratio, is vital in differentiating primary aldosteronism from essential hypertension [18]. Acute administration of blockers of the renin–angiotensin system has no effect on arterial pressure confirming that the hypertension is independent of the renin–angiotensin system. Accordingly, monotherapy in the longer term with blockers of the renin–angiotensin system has no place in routine management.

Other secondary forms of hypertension

The renin–angiotensin system is one factor contributing to hypertension in chronic renal failure, polycystic kidney disease, pheochromocytoma, aortic coarctation and possibly in pre-eclampsia and during administration of oral contraceptives.

Essential hypertension [19]

The role of the renin–angiotensin system in the development and maintenance of high blood pressure in patients with essential hypertension is controversial. Amongst essential hypertensives, plasma renin is distributed in a unimodal fashion, hence division into high, normal and low renin subgroups is essentially arbitrary. The fall in plasma renin with aging is exaggerated in essential hypertensives, and responsiveness of plasma renin to a variety of stimuli including diuretics, is reduced compared to normotensive subjects. Furthermore, there is an inverse association between the level of arterial pressure (particularly systolic readings) and the level of plasma renin. African-American hypertensives have lower plasma renin levels than Caucasians, and in women the renin levels tend to be lower than in men.

A small proportion of essential hypertensives, especially younger patients, have circulating renin levels above those of age-matched normotensive volunteers. It appears that such patients have increased sympathetic outflow in general and to the kidney in particular, resulting in enhanced renin secretion [20].

Whilst there is little doubt that the renin–angiotensin system contributes to the maintenance of arterial pressure in essential hypertensives, it is but one amongst many contributors. Indeed, there is a complex interplay between the renin–angiotensin system and, for example, body sodium and fluid status, the level of sympathetic activity (globally and to key organs such as heart and kidney as well as to blood vessels), and an array of endothelial-produced factors including nitric oxide, prostaglandins, endothelin, adrenomedullin, and potassium. Certainly, renin stimulation limits the decline in arterial pressure with dietary sodium restriction in hypertensive and normotensive subjects (Figure 2.3.9) [21]. The fact that arterial pressure falls in a majority of essential hypertensives during treatment with ACE inhibitors or angiotensin II receptor blockers points to a contributory role of the

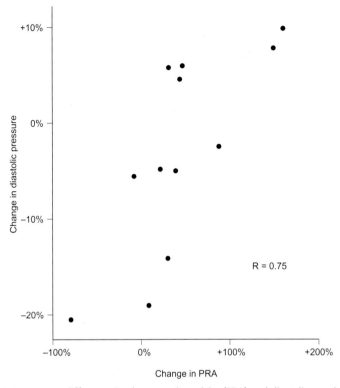

Fig. 2.3.9 Percentage difference in plasma renin activity (PRA) and diastolic arterial pressure recordings between a 'normal' sodium diet (180 mmol/day) and a sodium-restricted diet (80 mmol/day) in 12 patients with mild essential hypertension. For PRA, the mean level from hourly venous samples over 24 hours on each of the two diets was used to calculate percentage differences, and for blood pressure the mean intra-arterial diastolic recording over 24 hours was used. From Richards *et al.* [34], with permission.

renin–angiotensin system. Equally however, arterial pressure usually falls with extreme diet sodium restriction or diuretic administration, beta- or postsynaptic α_1-blockade, centrally-acting α_2-agonist drugs, calcium-channel blockers, endothelin antagonists, etc. some of which activate, rather than suppress activity of the renin–angiotensin system. It is now quite clear, therefore, that whereas the renin–angiotensin system is one contributor to the level of blood pressure (more so in Caucasians than Blacks), it is not the primary cause of the hypertension nor is it the sole determinant of the level of arterial pressure in established essential hypertension.

If, indeed, angiotensin II in plasma is toxic within the physiologic or pathophysiologic range, one should see increased cardiovascular complications in essential hypertensives who have high, rather than low levels of plasma renin, and antihypertensive drugs which reduce angiotensin II formation or actions should be more protective than drugs which enhance angiotensin II production. Data from New York over three decades suggest that plasma levels of renin do indeed predict, independent of other known risk factors, some complications of hypertension, most obviously myocardial infarction [23,24] (Figure 2.3.10).

BOX 2.3.3 **Cardiovascular trophic/toxic effects of angiotensin II**

Another disputed area is the cardiovascular trophic and toxic effects of the renin–angiotensin system in essential hypertension. High infusion rates of angiotensin II in animals have trophic and toxic effects on blood vessels and heart. In man, a number of workers have documented a positive association between activity of the renin–angiotensin system and left ventricular mass under a variety of circumstances. Reversal of left ventricular hypertrophy in essential hypertension is arguably faster and more complete with ACE inhibitors than alternative drug groups [22] lending further credence to the premise that angiotensin II has a trophic action on the myocardium.

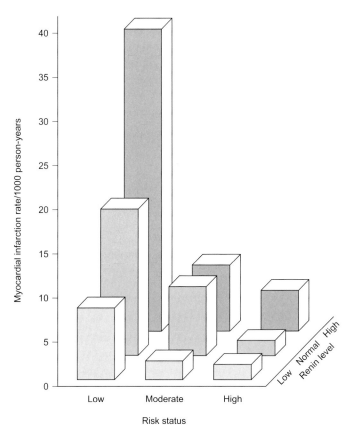

Fig. 2.3.10 Incidence of myocardial infarction per 1000 person-years by cardiovascular risk status and renin level from a study of 2902 hypertensive patients followed on average for 3.6 years. 'High'-risk status indicates two or more risk factors (smoking, cholesterol ≥6.3 mmol/liter, left ventricular hypertrophy); 'moderate', one risk factor; 'low', no risk factors. From Alderman *et al.* [24], with permission.

The same group also report that a low dietary intake of sodium (as assessed by diet recall or measurement of urinary sodium excretion), which stimulates renin release, is associated with an increased risk of myocardial infarction in hypertensive men [25], and higher total and cardiovascular mortality in a representative sample of 11 346 American

2

adults approximately 16% of whom had hypertension [26]. These results, which are consistent with angiotensin II having toxic effects on the cardiovascular system, have, however, been criticized on methodological grounds. Further, there is contrary information which suggests no relationship between the activity of the renin–angiotensin system and the cardiovascular complication rate in patients with hypertension.

An overview of antihypertensive drug trials comparing beta-blockers (which suppress activity of the renin–angiotensin system) and diuretics (which stimulate the renin system) show similar or greater cardiovascular protection with the latter, at least in the elderly [27]. Perhaps the ideal study in this regard would be one comparing an antihypertensive drug which specifically inhibits angiotensin II formation or action and one of similar antihypertensive efficacy but which augments its formation. In this regard, the CAPPP study suggests there are no major differences in the cardiovascular complication rate in essential hypertensives receiving an ACE inhibitor versus those receiving diuretic-based treatment: the exception being a lesser incidence of diabetes in those randomized to the ACE inhibitor [28]. Of course, longer term studies in younger patients might be required to show any important difference between such disparate therapeutic approaches.

BOX 2.3.4 Genotype and essential hypertension

In regards to the pathophysiology of essential hypertension and to its cardiovascular complications, there have been suggestions that various genotypes, particularly for ACE and angiotensin I receptors, might be relevant. In theory some genotype characteristics could favor a greater tissue formation or accumulation of angiotensin II than alternative genotypes. The various genotypes would not necessarily be detected by routine measurements of plasma levels of renin. Most emphasis has been focussed on the ACE gene polymorphism, accounted for by the presence (insertion, I) or absence (deletion, D) of a 287 basepair sequence in a non-coding section of the ACE gene. Since plasma and tissue levels of ACE track with the genotype (DD > ID > II) the formation of angiotensin II (and perhaps bradykinin) may be greater in tissues for DD than ID and especially the II genotype. Any relation between ACE genotype and cardiovascular disease remains under discussion and dispute [30]. Some reports are that one genotype is overrepresented in essential hypertensives compared with normotensives, but there are more contrary reports. There is also a disputed association between the ACE genotype and the prevalence of left ventricular hypertrophy in essential hypertension. Additional reports, again requiring further investigation, are of a linkage between the angiotensinogen gene and essential hypertension, and between the same gene and the blood pressure response to ACE inhibition. Finally, a plethora of studies have recently reported on statistical associations between genotypes for ACE, AT_1 receptor and angiotensinogen and the various complications of diabetes mellitus. Unfortunately, there is no clear pattern to these reports and therapeutic implications are unclear.

2

Renin profiling

Renin profiling could, in theory, find a place in determining which types of antihypertensive agent would prove most efficacious in an individual with essential hypertension. For example, diuretics might be preferred in patients exhibiting low renin whereas blockers of the renin–angiotensin system or beta-blockade may be especially effective in those with higher renin levels. Current evidence, however, is disappointing in this regard. Age and race were apparently better predictors of the blood pressure response to antihypertensive drugs in an American population than was renin profiling [29].

Therapeutics in hypertension and the renin–angiotensin system

As has been mentioned already, there is evidence that in patients with hypertension, those with activation of the renin–angiotensin system might have a greater risk of cardiovascular complications than others with normal or suppressed activity. If indeed this is so, non-pharmacologic maneuvers which activate renin release or drug treatment which stimulates renin might be associated with a worse cardiovascular outcome than therapeutic endeavors which suppress the system or block its actions.

This is an area of ongoing debate and uncertainty. On the one hand studies can be quoted to suggest that a high salt intake (which will suppress renin) exacerbates the hypertension in many patients and may have effects beyond those on blood pressure, e.g. to increase left ventricular mass and to increase the risk of hypertensive complications, particularly stroke. On the contrary, as noted above, other studies suggest that patients on a low dietary sodium intake (which will augment renin release) are at greater risk of cardiovascular events than those on a higher salt intake.

In regard to antihypertensive drug treatment, there is evidence, mentioned earlier in this chapter, that ACE inhibitors reverse left ventricular hypertrophy more rapidly and perhaps more completely than alternative antihypertensives, most of which have neutral or stimulating effects on the renin-angiotensin system. However, there is no evidence currently to suggest that ACE inhibitors are more effective in reducing mortality. Head-to-head comparisons of drugs which stimulate versus those which inhibit the renin–angiotensin system are needed. In fact, such studies are underway many using angiotensin II AT_1-receptor-blocking drugs for comparison with a diuretic, beta-blocker or calcium-channel antagonist. Interpretation of the outcomes in regard to the 'toxicity' of the renin–angiotensin system may prove difficult. For example, if drugs which block the angiotensin AT_1 receptor more effectively protect against stroke or cardiac failure than beta-blockers (which suppress renin secretion), is stimulation of the AT_2 receptor germane to such cardiovascular protection? If so, the ideal approach might be to block the AT_1 receptor, thereby inhibiting the actions of

Therapeutics in
hypertension and the
renin–angiotensin system

References

2

angiotensin II which promote vasoconstriction, myocardial contractility, sodium retention and cardiovascular growth, whilst augmenting the contrary effects of angiotensin via its AT_2 receptor (Figure 2.3.1).

References

1. Robertson JIS. Renin and angiotensin: a history review. In: *The Renin–Angiotensin System* (eds Robertson JIS, Nicholls MG), pp. 1.1–1.18. Gower Medical Publishing: London, 1993.
2. Lever AF. The fast and the slowly developing pressor effect of angiotensin II. In: *The Renin–Angiotensin System* (eds Robertson JIS, Nicholls MG), pp. 28.1–28.9. Gower Medical Publishing: London, 1993.
3. Gavras I, Gavras H. Angiotensin II – possible adverse effects on arteries, heart, brain, and kidney: experimental, clinical, and epidemiological evidence. In: *The Renin–Angiotensin System* (eds Robertson JIS, Nicholls MG), pp. 40.1–40.11. Gower Medical Publishing: London, 1993.
4. Nussberger J, Brunner HR. Measurement of angiotensins in plasma. In: *The Renin–Angiotensin System* (Robertson JIS, Nicholls MG), pp. 15.1–15.13. Gower Medical Publishing: London, 1993.
5. Poulsen K, Nielsen AH. The measurement of renin. In: *The Renin–Angiotensin System* (eds Robertson JIS, Nicholls MG) pp. 13.1–13.12. Gower Medical Publishing: London, 1993.
6. Lindop GBM, Leckie BJ, Mimran A. Renin–secretin tumors. In: *The Renin–Angiotensin System* (eds Robertson JIS, Nicholls MG), pp. 54.1–54.12. Gower Medical Publishing: London, 1993.
7. Robertson JIS. Renin and the pathophysiology of renovascular hypertension. In: *The Renin–Angiotensin System* (eds Robertson JIS, Nicholls MG), pp. 55.1–55.34. Gower Medical Publishing: London, 1993.
8. Brown JJ, Davies DL, Lever AF, Robertson JIS. Plasma renin concentration in human hypertension. 1: Relationship between renin, sodium and potassium. *Br Med J* 1965; **ii**:144–148.
9. Agarwal M, Lynn KL, Richards AM, Nicholls MG. Hyponatremic–hypertensive syndrome with renal ischemia. An under-recognized disorder. *Hypertension* 1999;**33**:1020–1024.
10. Elkik F, Corvol P, Idatte J-M, Ménard J. Renal segmental infarction: a cause of reversible malignant hypertension. *J Hypertension* 1984;**2**:149–156.
11. Pickering TG, Herman L, Devereux RB *et al*. Recurrent pulmonary oedema in hypertension due to bilateral renal artery stenosis: treatment by angioplasty or surgical revascularisation. *Lancet* 1988;**ii**:551–552.
12. Steen VD, Costantino JP, Shapiro AP, Medsger TA Jr. Outcome of renal crisis in systemic sclerosis: relation to availability of angiotensin converting enzyme (ACE) inhibitors. *Ann Intern Med* 1990;**113**:352–357.
13. Robertson JIS Renin and malignant hypertension. In: *The Renin–Angiotensin System* (eds Robertson JIS, Nicholls MG), pp. 60.1–60.10. Gower Medical Publishing: London, 1993.
14. Weidmann P, Ferrari P, Shaw SG. Renin in diabetes mellitus. In: *The Renin–Angiotensin System* (eds Robertson JIS, Nicholls MG), pp. 75.1–75.26. Gower Medical Publishing: London, 1993.
15. Kasiske BL, Kalil RSN, Ma JZ *et al*. Effect of antihypertensive therapy on the kidney in patients with diabetes: a meta-regression analysis. *Ann Intern Med* 1993; **118**:129–138.
16. Chaturvedi N, Sjolie A-K, Stephenson JM *et al*. Effect of lisinopril on progression of retinopathy in normotensive people with type 1 diabetes. *Lancet* 1998;**351**:28–31.
17. Malik RA, Williamson S, Abbott C *et al*. Effect of angiotensin-converting enzyme (ACE) inhibitor trandolapril on human diabetic neuropathy: randomised double-blind controlled trial. *Lancet* 1998;**352**:1978–1981.
18. Ganguly A. Primary aldosteronism. *N Engl J Med* 1998;**339**:1828–1834.

References

19. Swales JD. The renin–angiotensin system in essential hypertension. In: *The Renin–Angiotensin System* (eds Robertson JIS, Nicholls MG), pp. 62.1–62.12. Gower Medical Publishing: London, 1993.

20. Esler M, Julius S, Zweifler A *et al*. Mild high renin essential hypertension. *N Engl J Med* 1977;**296**:105–111.

21. Volpe M, Lembo G, Morganti A *et al*. Contribution of the renin–angiotensin system and of the sympathetic nervous system to blood pressure homeostasis during chronic restriction of sodium intake. *Am J Hypertension* 1988;**1**:353–358.

22. Schmieder RE, Martus P, Kingbeil A. Reversal of left ventricular hypertrophy in essential hypertension. A meta-analysis of randomized double-blind studies. *J Am Med Ass* 1996;**275**:1507–1513.

23. Alderman MH, Madhavan S, Ooi WL *et al*. Association of the renin–sodium profile with the risk of myocardial infarction in patients with hypertension. *N Engl J Med* 1991;**324**:1098–1104.

24. Alderman MH, Ooi WL, Cohen H *et al*. Plasma renin activity: a risk factor for myocardial infarction in hypertensive patients. *Am J Hypertension* 1997;**10**:1–8.

25. Alderman MH, Madhavan S, Cohen H *et al*. Low urinary sodium is associated with greater risk of myocardial infarction among treated hypertensive men. *Hypertension* 1995;**25**:1144–1152.

26. Alderman MH, Cohen H, Madhavan S. Dietary sodium intake and mortality: the National Health and Nutrition Examination Survey (NHANES I). *Lancet* 1998;**351**:781–785.

27. Lever AF, Ramsay LE. Treatment of hypertension in the elderly. *J Hypertension* 1995;**13**:571–579.

28. Captopril Prevention Project (CAPP) in Hypertension. *Lancet* 1999;**353**:611–616.

29. Preston RA, Materson BJ, Reda DJ *et al*. Age–race subgroup compared with renin profile as predictors of blood pressure response to antihypertensive therapy. *J Am Med Ass* 1998;**280**:1168–1172.

30. Harrap SB. Genetics of coronary disease: beginning the long journey. *Lancet* 1994;**344**:901–902.

31. Pedrinelli R, Graziadei L, Taddei S *et al*. A renin-secreting tumor. *Nephron* 1987;**46**:380–385.

32. Brown JJ, Cuesta V, Davies DL *et al*. Mechanism of renal hypertension. *Lancet* 1976;**i**:1219–1221.

33. Kaneda H, Yamauchi T, Murata T *et al*. Treatment of malignant hypertension with infusion of sodium chloride; a case report and a review. *Tohoku J Exp Med* 1980;**132**:179–186.

34. Richards AM, Nicholls MG, Espiner EA *et al*. Blood-pressure response to moderate sodium restriction and to potassium supplementation in mild essential hypertension. *Lancet* 1984;**i**:757–761.

Chapter

2.4

2

Etiology and pathophysiology of hypertension: neural factors

M Esler

Introduction

Approximately a hundred years ago Geisbock proposed that the nervous system might be involved in the development of essential hypertension [1]. The historical antecedent to the emergence of this clinical hypothesis was the description of the pressor nerves [2], and the subsequent isolation of an adrenal medullary pressor principle, epinephrine (adrenaline) [3], which for a time was thought to be their neurotransmitter. Eventually, von Euler demonstrated that the sympathetic nervous transmitter was in fact norepinephrine (noradrenaline) and not epinephrine [4].

The neural hypothesis of hypertension received support from investigation of the effects of intravenous infusion of norepinephrine, which raised blood pressure and increased total peripheral vascular resistance, replicating the hemodynamic features of essential hypertension, as it was understood at the time. von Euler was the first to apply clinically neurochemical measurements of transmitter release, based on urinary norepinephrine excretion rates, in an attempt to quantify the level of sympathetic nervous activity present in patients with essential hypertension [5].

In the last decade it has become possible to test rigorously, and in fact confirm, the 'neural hypothesis' of essential hypertension etiology, using methods for quantifying sympathetic nervous tone in individual organs. What follows is an outline of these methods, a description of the syndrome of neural essential hypertension, discussion of its possible causes, and analysis of the impact of high sympathetic nervous tone on development of the complications of hypertension, and of the proposition that these adverse effects might be specifically reversed by antihypertensive drugs and non-pharmacological measures which reduce sympathetic activity in hypertensive patients.

BOX 2.4.1 Measurement of sympathetic nervous activity in hypertensive patients

Responses in the sympathetic nervous system typically show regional differentiation which can be detected in clinical research only by techniques which assess organ-specific sympathetic function [6]. For this reason, measurement of the excretion of the sympathetic nervous neurotransmitter, norepinephrine, in urine is now largely obsolete as a test of human sympathetic nervous activity, while assay of the plasma concentration of norepinephrine has also fallen into disfavor.

Clinical methods for assessing regional sympathetic nervous system function Measurement of rates of sympathetic nerve firing and of norepinephrine release to plasma provide the most secure basis for studying regional sympathetic nervous function in patients with hypertension (see Figure 2.4.1):

Clinical microneurography
This technique provides a method for studying nerve firing rates in subcutaneous sympathetic nerves (Figure 2.4.1). The technique involves the insertion of fine tungsten electrodes through the skin, with positioning of the

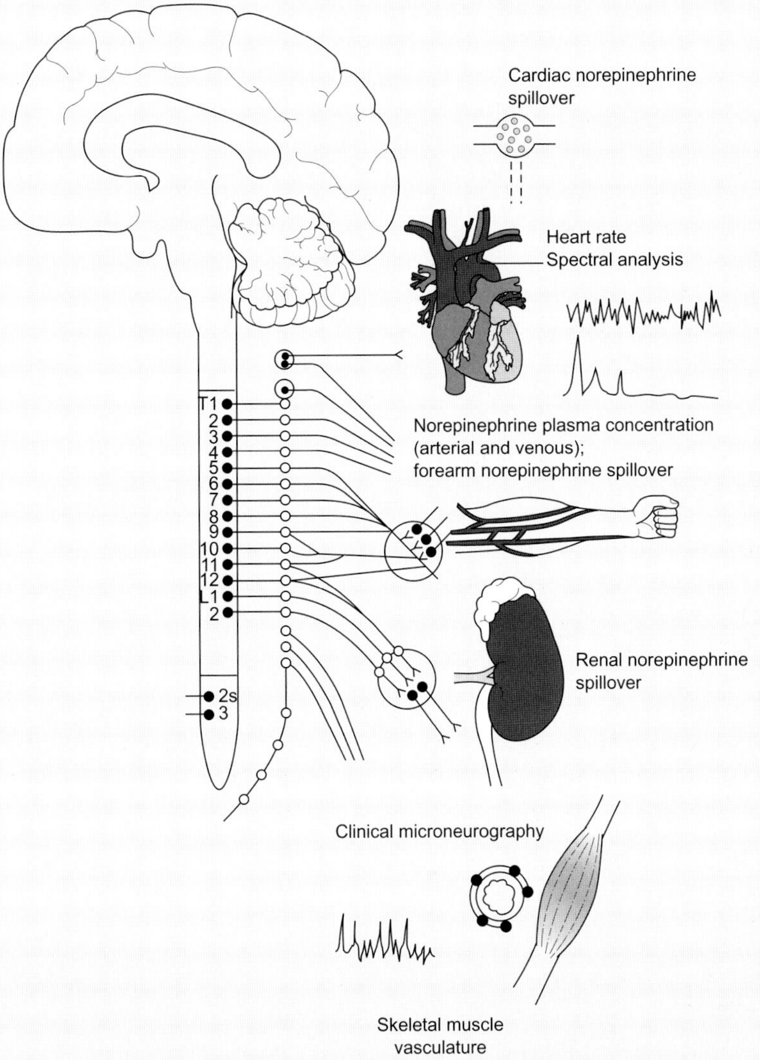

Fig. 2.4.1 The available methods for studying regional sympathetic nervous system activity in man. Clinical microneurography provides a method for studying nerve firing rates in subcutaneous sympathetic nerves. Norepinephrine spillover rate measurements provide quantification of the rate of flux of the sympathetic neurotransmitter, norepinephrine, to plasma from individual organs. Heart rate power spectral analysis techniques are commonly applied as an alternative, non-invasive method for studying sympathetic function in the heart, but are unreliable as a measure of cardiac sympathetic firing.

electrode tip in sympathetic fibres of, most commonly, the common peroneal nerve near the fibular head. Multifiber recordings of 'bursts' of nerve activity, are generated [7].

Norepinephrine spillover rate measurements
Sympathetic neurotransmitter release can be studied clinically using radiotracer-derived measurements of the appearance rate of norepinephrine in plasma from individual organs [6] (Figure 2.4.1). Microneurographic

2

methods do not give access to sympathetic nerves of internal organs. With infusion of tritiated norepinephrine and regional blood sampling from the coronary sinus and renal veins, neurotransmitter release from the heart and kidneys can be measured [6].

Heart rate power spectral analysis

Spectral analysis techniques are commonly applied as an alternative, non-invasive method for studying sympathetic function in the heart. With this technique, mathematical partitioning allows identification of individual, superimposed rhythms producing cyclical variation in heart rate and arterial pressure. The autonomic nervous system provides the principal effector mechanism for heart rate variability. Although the low-frequency heart rate variability (approximately 0.1 Hz) derives in part from the influence of the cardiac sympathetic nerves, it is very misleading when used as a measure of cardiac sympathetic firing [8,9].

The syndrome of neural essential hypertension

Evidence drawn from a number of sources, utilizing the electrophysiological and neurochemical techniques described above, provides compelling evidence that overactivity of the sympathetic nervous system is present in a substantial proportion of patients with essential hypertension. Nerve firing rates in postganglionic sympathetic fibers passing to skeletal muscle blood vessels are commonly increased [10,11]. There is also increased spillover of the sympathetic neurotransmitter, norepinephrine, from the heart and kidneys, providing evidence of stimulated sympathetic outflow to these organs [6,12] (Figure 2.4.2). This increased cardiac and renal sympathetic nerve firing provides a plausible mechanism for the development of hypertension, through the regulatory influence of the sympathetic nervous system on renin release, glomerular filtration rate and renal tubular sodium reabsorption, and on cardiac pumping performance and myocyte growth.

Could sympathetic activation in hypertensive patients just be an artefact of the measurement process?

There have been some misgivings that sympathetic nervous activation in hypertension might, perhaps, simply represent an alerting response in the laboratory, perhaps contributed to by anxiety resulting from recent diagnostic labelling of patients as 'hypertensive' [13]. Unlike in mental stress reactions, however, the sympathetic nervous activation present in essential hypertension spares the sympathetic innervation of the skin [11] and hepatomesenteric circulation [12], and is not accompanied by increased adrenal medullary secretion of epinephrine. In a mental stress response, epinephrine secretion is increased, the sympathetic outflow to skeletal muscle vasculature typically is unchanged or reduced while that to skin is increased, and hepatomesenteric sympathetic tone is increased [14–16].

2

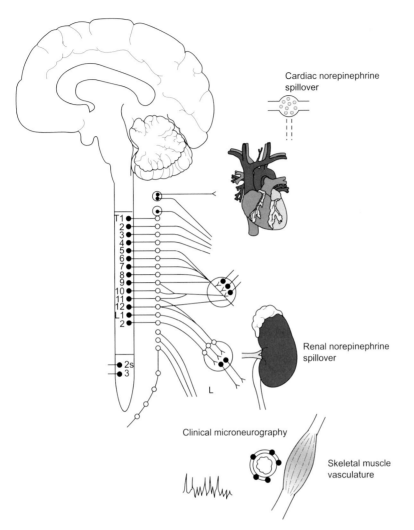

Cardiac norepinephrine spillover

Renal norepinephrine spillover

Clinical microneurography

Skeletal muscle vasculature

Fig. 2.4.2 The defining characteristic of neural essential hypertension is a preferential activation of the sympathetic nervous outflows to the heart, kidneys and skeletal muscle vasculature.

Characteristics of patients with neural essential hypertension

The patients with neural essential hypertension typically are young (the majority are less than 40 years) men and women with milder grades of hypertension. Typical features of the syndrome (Table 2.4.1) are the sympathetic nervous activation, manifest as an increase in muscle sympathetic nerve firing and high rates of spillover of norepinephrine from the kidneys and heart, coupled with the peripheral expression of this sympathoexcitation evident in a high plasma renin activity (due to an elevated rate of renal renin release), commonly a high heart rate and elevated cardiac output, and in some patients isolated systolic

2

Table 2.4.1 Typical features of the syndrome of neural essential hypertension

Aged less than 40 years
Mild hypertension
High rates of muscle sympathetic nerve firing
Increased spillover of norepinephrine from the heart, kidneys
Adrenal medullary secretion of epinephrine normal
High heart rate, with or without increased cardiac output
Isolated systolic hypertension
Elevated renal renin release and plasma renin activity

hypertension [10–12,17,18]. The neural basis of the isolated systolic hypertension is adrenergic augmentation of left ventricular contractility, perhaps accompanied by a neurogenic reduction in the compliance of the arterial tree. The higher heart rates and widened pulse pressure (accompanying isolated systolic hypertension) are now thought to be of particular clinical significance, as there is evidence that both are independent risk factors for cardiovascular disease [19,20], conferring risk additional to that deriving from hypertension alone.

Rigorous testing of this neural model of essential hypertension pathogenesis is under way with ongoing research involving such matters as the possible genetic determinants, and the CNS mechanism underlying chronic activation of the sympathetic outflows [21]. Follow-up studies are needed to ascertain whether progression occurs, from mild neurogenic hypertension in young adults to the more severe established hypertension of later years, in which neural activity is not increased [12]. An additional important priority will be to ascertain what adverse effects additional to the blood pressure elevation, such as myocardial hypertrophy, hyperlipidemia and atherosclerosis, might derive directly from the sympathetic nervous activation (see below).

Causes of neural essential hypertension

The specific causes of the increased sympathetic activity in essential hypertension remain unclear, although genetic and lifestyle influences appear to be involved.

Genetics

The heritability of sympathetic overactivity in primary human hypertension has been little studied. The limited research undertaken so far for single-gene abnormalities involving the sympathetic nervous system has been unsuccessful in patients with high blood pressure. Normotensive young men with a family history of hypertension do have higher rates of norepinephrine spillover to plasma than young men with a negative family history of hypertension [22]. Sympathetic nervous activity does appear to be heritable in healthy subjects with normal blood pressure. In monozygotic twins [23], skeletal muscle sympathetic nerve firing rates were found to be almost identical in individual pairs, unlike in randomly paired groupings of unrelated subjects in whom a wide range of nerve firing rates was evident.

Lifestyle influences on blood pressure

Stress and behavior

While studies substantiating a role for experimental stress in causing hypertension in laboratory animals are interesting and important, it is another matter to demonstrate that essential hypertension is due to psychosocial conflict. Clinical, epidemiological and laboratory research does, however, provide increasingly strong support for the notion that behavioral and psychological factors are of importance in the pathogenesis of human hypertension [17,24–26]. Of particular importance in this regard are epidemiologically based observations made on human populations who demonstrate blood pressure elevation soon after migration [24], and long-term follow-up studies of human populations, such as cloistered nuns, living in secluded and unchanging environments, in whom blood pressure does not show the expected rise with age [25]. Long-term neural effects of stress on renal function could possibly be the principal blood pressure-elevating mechanism [27].

Research on the possible psychosomatic origins of essential hypertension, in addition to focussing on the external stress as the stimulus, has assessed personality characteristics of hypertensive patients which determine responsiveness to these external influences. As a group hypertensive patients commonly exhibit a behavioral pattern, suppression of hostility, that is particularly associated with activation of the sympathetic nervous system [17,26]. Young hypertensive patients with suppression of hostility tend to have the neural syndrome of essential (see above) [17,26].

Obesity and increased dietary energy intake

Patients with primary hypertension are commonly overweight. An excessive dietary energy load is known to stimulate the sympathetic nervous system and elevate arterial pressure. There is selective activation of the sympathetic nerves to the kidneys and skeletal muscle vasculature in human obesity [28] (see below).

Physical inactivity

An additional factor possibly contributing to sympathetic nervous overactivity in hypertensive patients is sedentary lifestyle. Regularly performed physical exercise produces long-term lowering of blood pressure [29]. The blood pressure-lowering effects of exercise are only seen in previously sedentary people. This antihypertensive effect of exercise is most probably caused by inhibition of the sympathetic nervous system [29], especially the sympathetic nerves of the kidneys [30].

Is this neural hypertension? – the diagnostic dilemmas

When associated with elevated blood pressure, the clinical features in some other disorders may suggest a possible diagnosis of neural

2

2

Table 2.4.2 Diagnostic alternatives to neural essential hypertension

Panic disorder
'White coat hypertension'
Pheochromocytoma
'Labile hypertension'

essential hypertension (Table 2.4.2). If blood pressure appears to be highly variable, or if heart rate is high, neural mechanisms are often thought to be operating. Heightened blood pressure variability, in fact, is not a typical feature of the syndrome of neural essential hypertension, which has other phenotypic markers (Table 2.4.1).

Panic disorder

The symptomatology and blood pressure peaks of panic attacks can cause confusion. Sympathetic nervous activity, epinepherine secretion, heart rate and blood pressure do increase during panic attacks [15], but patients with panic disorder typically have both normal blood pressure and normal sympathetic nervous activity between attacks [15].

White coat hypertension

Another form of anxiety, the situational anxiety of 'white coat hypertension' [31], may also masquerade as neural essential hypertension, especially if heart rates are high in the clinic. Such people showing an alerting response to medical examination, with blood pressure elevation, need to be differentiated from neural essential hypertension, in which the hypertension on 24-hour ambulatory blood-pressure monitoring is sustained.

Pheochromocytoma

Persistent tachycardia in patients with catecholamine-secreting tumors can also cause diagnostic uncertainty in the present context. The need to identify patients with possible pheochromocytoma, and confirm the diagnosis by measurement of urinary excretion of catecholamines and their metabolities is self-evident. It is unusual for the level of sympathetic activation in neural essential hypertension to be such that urinary norepinephrine values are so elevated as to create diagnostic difficulty.

'Labile hypertension'

Sometimes the term 'labile hypertension' is equated with neurogenic hypertension. Labile hypertension, however, does not exist. It is a misnomer typically applied to patients with borderline blood pressure elevations [32]. In those with borderline hypertension, blood pressure recorded in the clinic, while showing the usual degree of variability, creates an illusion of greater fluctuation or variability than normal by oscillating around the cutoff point for the diagnosis of established

---

BOX 2.4.2 A special case: obesity-related hypertension

Patients with primary hypertension are commonly overweight. Since positive energy balance initiates thermogenesis by stimulation of the sympathetic nervous system, the sympathetic activation seen in essential hypertension could perhaps represent an adaptive response to overeating [34].

Renal sympathetic tone is high in obesity, independent of blood pressure There is selective activation of the sympathetic nerves to the kidneys and skeletal muscle vasculature in normotensive human obesity, but suppression of the cardiac sympathetic outflow [28] (see Figure 2.4.3). The possible importance of activation of the renal sympathetic outflow in the pathogenesis of obesity-related hypertension is illustrated in a recent study on dogs made obese by overfeeding, where renal denervation prevented the development of hypertension [35]. Increased renal sympathetic activity in human obesity may be a *necessary* cause for the development of hypertension (and predisposes to hypertension development), but apparently is not a *sufficient* cause.

Cardiac sympathetic tone is suppressed in the normotensive but not the hypertensive obese In patients with obesity-related hypertension, there is a comparable elevation of renal norepinepherine spillover to that present in the normotensive obese, but without suppression of cardiac sympathetics, as here cardiac norepinephrine spillover is more than double that of normotensive obese and 25% higher than in healthy volunteers [36] (see Figure 2.4.3). The discriminating feature of the obese who develop hypertension is this absence of the adaptive suppression of cardiac sympathetic outflow seen in the normotensive obese.

---

hypertension. While the earlier suggestion was that spontaneous variability of arterial pressure was greater in borderline hypertension, 24-hour ambulant blood-pressure monitoring in borderline hypertension has disclosed unremarkable pressure traces, with blood pressure fluctuation no greater than in healthy subjects [33].

The contribution of high sympathetic activity to cardiovascular risk

While the sympathetic activation present in human hypertension no doubt contributes to the blood pressure elevation, it seems to have additional adverse consequences in hypertensive patients which go beyond this. Neural vasoconstriction can have undesirable metabolic effects, in skeletal muscle impairing glucose delivery to muscle, causing insulin resistance and hyperinsulinemia [37], and in liver retarding postprandial clearing of lipids, contributing to hyperlipidemia.

Effects of high sympathetic tone in the heart

Similarly, high sympathetic nervous activity in the heart of hypertensive patients may be deleterious. A growth-promoting effect of norepinephrine on cardiac myocytes has been demonstrated *in vitro* [38].

The contribution of high
sympathetic activity to
cardiovascular risk

Effects of high sympathetic
tone in the heart

2

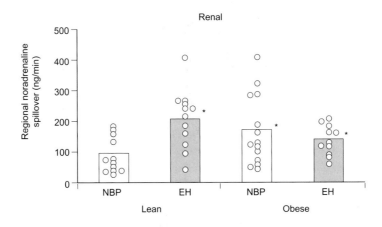

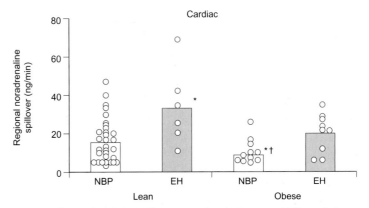

Fig. 2.4.3 Regional norepinephrine spillover rates for the heart and kidneys in lean and obese subjects with either normal blood pressure (NBP) or high blood pressure (EH). Norepinephrine spillover from the heart and kidneys was increased in hypertensive lean patients, compared with normotensive lean subjects, providing evidence of increased cardiac and renal sympathetic nervous activity. Renal norepinephrine spillover was increased in the obese, independent of blood pressure. In contrast, cardiac sympathetic tone was significantly reduced only in the obese with normal blood pressure. *$P < 0.05$ difference from lean normotensives; †$P < 0.05$ comparison between obese normotensives and hypertensives.

A trophic effect of sympathetic activation in the human heart is probable in hypertensive patients, perhaps contributing to the development of left ventricular hypertrophy. The importance of neural mechanisms in arrhythmogenesis is well established, with stimulation of the cardiac sympathetic outflow predisposing to ventricular tachycardia and ventricular fibrillation in a variety of experimental models of arrhythmia development. Increased cardiac sympathetic nerve firing, as measured by cardiac norepinephrine spillover, has also been demonstrated to commonly underlie clinical ventricular tachyarrhythmias [39]. A comparable proarrhythmic effect is probable in hypertension also, although in hypertensive patients the relative contributions of left ventricular hypertrophy, which promotes reentrant arrhythmias, increased cardiac sympathetic activity and coronary atherosclerosis to the arrhythmia development to which they are prone is uncertain at this stage.

Effects of antihypertensive drugs on sympathetic nervous activity

Effects of antihypertensive drugs on sympathetic nervous activity

A special place for antiadrenergic therapies in neural hypertension?

Antiadrenergic drugs for essential and secondary hypertension with high sympathetic tone?

Changes commonly occur in sympathetic nervous system function during drug treatment of hypertension, representing in some cases therapeutic sympathetic inhibition by the drug, and in others reflex adaptations opposing a drug's efficacy. Examples of the former are the reduction in sympathetic nerve firing with clonidine [6], and of the latter, the reflex sympathetic activation produced by some slow channel calcium-influx blockers [40]. As sympathetic nervous system activation in patients with essential hypertension might have adverse effects, it is pertinent to ask whether additional stimulation of the sympathetic nervous system by antihypertensive drugs is undesirable, and conversely, whether specific inhibition of the sympathetic nervous activation commonly present in hypertensive patients is beneficial. This issue has been brought into recent focus by claims that vasoactive calcium-channel blockers may be harmful, in rapidly releasable pharmaceutical formulations, and perhaps increase cardiac risk by stimulating sympathetic activity in the heart [40].

A special place for antiadrenergic therapies in neural hypertension?

Antiadrenergic drugs for essential and secondary hypertension with high sympathetic tone?

Given that sympathetic activation in hypertensive patients seems to contribute to clinical adverse events in hypertension, might it be appropriate to specifically recommend drugs reducing sympathetic tone in hypertensive patients in whom sympathetic nervous activation is present? Using this reasoning, with essential hypertension in young adults, obesity-related hypertension, pregnancy hypertension [41], hypertension accompanying renal failure [42], and perhaps renovascular hypertension [43,44] antiadrenergic agents might have a special place in therapy because the hypertension in each instance is in part neurogenic. Conversely, in variants of hypertension in which sympathetic nervous activity is normal, essential hypertension in the elderly [12] and post-transplantation hypertension [45,46], or reduced, primary aldosteronism [43] and Cushing's syndrome [47], antiadrenergic agents would have little to recommend them. Such a logical 'tailoring' of antihypertensive drug therapy for the existing pathophysiology would be expected to lead to greater efficacy in reducing the cardiovascular complications of hypertension, with lesser incidence of adverse drug effects. The current high level of interest shown by many pharmaceutical companies in 'pharmacogenetics' illustrates the pervasive influence of ideas such as this.

2

Non-pharmacologic therapies lowering sympathetic activity

This line of reasoning can also be extended to non-pharmacological therapies. The two non-pharmacological measures most commonly applied in the treatment of obesity-related hypertension, dietary calorie restriction and an exercise program are well known to suppress sympathetic nervous system activity. With negative energy balance from calorie restriction, sympathetic tone and blood pressure is lowered [48]. Aerobic exercise training preferentially reduces renal sympathetic activity [30], and could be especially efficacious in obesity-related hypertension because of this specific neurophysiological effect.

Matching of antihypertensive therapy to neural pathophysiology: theoretically appealing but premature

Given our present state of knowledge, however, matching of antihypertensive therapy to the pathophysiology of the hypertension in an individual patient (or for that matter pharmacogenetic information) cannot be the primary therapeutic principle, in part because knowledge of both hypertension pathophysiology and the precise mechanisms of drug action remains imperfect. Further, overriding clinical considerations commonly apply in the choice of initial therapy, including the presence of coexisting illnesses carrying particular pharmaceutical recommendations [49], the potential surgical cure of a secondary hypertension, or the intolerance of elderly patients for postural hypotension in the face of inhibition of neurocirculatory reflexes. This point being made, the important and actively researched but to this stage incompletely answered question remains: of all antihypertensive therapies, would those inhibiting the sympathetic nervous system best reduce cardiovascular risk?

References

1. Geisbock F. Cited in The nervous system. In: *Arterial Hypertension* (eds Julius S, Esler M), p. xii. Charles C Thomas, Springfield, IL, 1976.
2. Bernard C. Influence du grand sympathique sur la sensibilité et sur la calorification. *Compte Rendu Soc Biol (Paris)* 1851;**3**:163–183.
3. Elliot TR. The action of adrenaline. *J Physiol (Lond)* 1905;**32**:401–467.
4. von Euler US. A specific sympathetic ergone in adrenergic nerve fibres (sympathin) and its relation to adrenaline and noradrenaline. *Acta Physiol Scand* 1946;**12**:73–97.
5. von Euler US, Hellner S, Purkhold A. Excretion of noradrenaline in the urine in hypertension. *Scand J Clin Lab Invest* 1954;**6**:54–59.
6. Esler M, Jennings G, Lambert G *et al*. Overflow of catecholamine neurotransmitters to the circulation: source, fate and functions. *Physiol Rev* 1990;**70**:963–985.
7. Vallbo AB, Hagbarth K-E, Torebjork HE, Wallin BG. Somatosensory, proprioceptive and sympathetic activity in human peripheral nerves. *Physiol Rev* 1979;**59**:919–957.
8. Kingwell BA, Thompsom JM, Kaye DM *et al*. Heart rate spectral analysis, cardiac norepinephrine spillover and muscle sympathetic nerve activity during human sympathetic nervous activation and failure. *Circulation* 1994;**90**:234–240.
9. Eckberg DL. Spectral balance: a critical appraisal. *Circulation* 1997;**96**:3224–3232.

References

10. Grassi G, Colombo M, Seravalle G *et al*. Dissociation between muscle and skin sympathetic nerve activity in essential hypertension, obesity, and congestive heart failure. *Hypertension* 1998;**31**:64–67.
11. Anderson EA, Sinkey CA, Lawton WJ, Mark AL. Elevated sympathetic nerve activity in borderline hypertensive humans: evidence from direct intraneural recordings. *Hypertension* 1989;**14**:177–183.
12. Esler M, Jennings G, Korner P *et al*. The assessment of human sympathetic nervous system activity from measurements of norepinephrine turnover. *Hypertension* 1988;**11**:3–20.
13. Rostrup M, Mundal HH, Westheim A, Eide I. Awareness of high blood pressure increases arterial plasma catecholamines, platelet norepinephrine and adrenergic responses to mental stress. *J Hypertension* 1991;**9**:159–166.
14. Callister R, Suwarno NO, Seals DR. Sympathetic activity is influenced by task difficulty and stress perception during mental challenge in humans. *J Physiol* 1992;**454**:373–387.
15. Wilkinson DJC, Thompson JM, Lambert GW *et al*. Sympathetic activity in patients with panic disorder at rest, under laboratory mental stress and during panic attacks. *Arch Gen Psychiatry* 1998;**55**:511–520.
16. Kaye DM, Cox H, Lambert G *et al*. Regional epinephrine kinetics in severe heart failure: evidence for extra-adrenal, non-neural release. *Am J Physiol* 1995;**269**:H182–H188.
17. Esler M, Julius S, Zweifler A *et al*. Mild high-renin essential hypertension: a neurogenic human hypertension? *N Engl J Med* 1977;**296**:405–411.
18. Julius S, Pascual A, London R. Role of parasympathetic inhibition in the hyperkinetic type of borderline hypertension. *Circulation* 1971;**44**:413–418.
19. Benetos A, Rudnichi A, Thomas F *et al*. Influence of heart rate on mortality in a French population. Role of age, gender and blood pressure. *Hypertension* 1999;**33**:44–52.
20. Darne B, Girerd X, Safar M *et al*. Pulsatile versus steady component of blood pressure: a cross-sectional analysis and a prospective analysis on cardiovascular mortality. *Hypertension* 1989;**13**:392–400.
21. Ferrier C, Jennings GL, Eisenhofer G *et al*. Evidence for increased noradrenaline release from subcortical brain regions in essential hypertension. *J Hypertension* 1993;**11**:1217–1227.
22. Ferrier C, Cox H, Esler M. Elevated total body noradrenaline spillover in normotensive members of hypertensive families. *Clin Sci* 1993;**84**:225–230.
23. Wallin BG, Kunimoto MM, Sellgren J. Possible genetic influence on the strength of human muscle nerve sympathetic activity at rest. *Hypertension* 1993;**22**:282–284.
24. Poulter NR, Khaw KT, Hopwood BEC *et al*. The Kenyan Luo migration study: observations on the initiation of the rise in blood pressure. *Br Med J* 1990;**300**:967–972.
25. Timio M, Verdechioa P, Rononi M *et al*. Age and blood pressure changes: a 20 year follow-up study of nuns of a secluded order. *Hypertension* 1988;**12**:457–461.
26. Perini C, Muller FB, Rauchfleisch U *et al*. Hyperadrenergic borderline hypertension is characterized by suppressed aggression. *J Cardiovasc Pharmacol* 1986;**8** (Suppl 5):53–56.
27. Koepke JP, Jones S, DiBona GF. Stress increases renal nerve activity and decreases sodium excretion in Dahl rats. *Hypertension* 1988;**11**:334–338.
28. Vaz M, Jennings G, Turner A *et al*. Regional sympathetic nervous activity and oxygen consumption in obese normotensive human subjects. *Circulation* 1997;**96**:3423–3429.
29. Jennings G, Nelson L, Nestel P *et al*. The effects of changes in physical activity on major cardiovascular risk factors, hemodynamics, sympathetic function, and glucose utilization in man: a controlled study of four levels of activity. *Circulation* 1986;**73**:30–40.
30. Meredith IT, Frieberg P, Jennings GL *et al*. Regular exercise lowers resting renal but not cardiac sympathetic activity in man. *Hypertension* 1991;**18**:575–582.
31. Pickering TG, James GD, Boddie C *et al*. How common is white coat hypertension? *J Am Med Ass* 1988;**259**:225–228.
32. Esler M. Hyperadrenergic and 'labile' hypertension. In: *Textbook of Hypertension* (ed. Swales J), pp. 741–749. Blackwell: London 1994.
33. Mancia G, Ferrari G, Gregorini L *et al*. Blood pressure and heart rate variabilities in normotensive and hypertensive human beings. *Circulation Res* 1983;**53**:96–104.

References

34. Landsberg L. Diet, obesity and hypertension: an hypothesis involving insulin, the sympathetic nervous system, and adaptive thermogenesis. *Q J Med* 1986;**236**:1081–1090.
35. Kassab S, Kato T, Wilkins FC *et al*. Renal denervation attenuates the sodium retention and hypertension associated with obesity. *Hypertension* 1995;**25**:893–897.
36. Rumantir MS, Vaz M, Jennings GL, Collier G *et al*. Neural mechanisms in human obesity-related hypertension. *J Hypertension* 1999;**17**:1125–1133.
37. Julius S, Gundrandsson T, Jamerson K, Andersson O. The interconnection between sympathetics, microcirculation and insulin resistance in hypertension. *Blood Pressure* 1992;**1**:9–19.
38. Mann DL, Kent RL, Parsons B, Cooper G. Adrenergic effects on the biology of the adult mammalian cardiocyte. *Circulation* 1992;**85**:790–804.
39. Meredith IT, Esler MD, Jennings GL, Esler MD. Evidence of a selective increase in cardiac sympathetic activity in patients with sustained ventricular arrhythmias. *N Eng J Med* 1991;**325**:618–624.
40. Ruzicka M, Leenen FHH. Relevance of intermittent increases in sympathetic activity for adverse outcome on short acting calcium antagonists. In: *Hypertension. Pathophysiology, Diagnosis and Management* (eds Laragh JH, Brenner BM), pp. 2815–2825. Raven Press: New York, 1995.
41. Schobel HP, Fischer T, Heuszer K *et al*. Pregnancy induced hypertension: a state of sympathetic overactivity. *N Engl J Med* 1996;**335**:1480–1485.
42. Converse RL Jr, Jacobsen TN, Toto RD *et al*. Sympathetic overactivity in patients with chronic renal failure. *N Engl J Med* 1992; **327**:1912–1918.
43. Miyajima E, Yamada Y, Yoshida Y *et al*. Muscle sympathetic nerve activity in renovascular hypertension and primary aldosteronism. *Hypertension* 1991;**17**:1057–1062.
44. Grassi G, Cattaneo BM, Seravalle G *et al*. Baroreflex control of sympathetic nerve activity in essential and secondary hypertension. *Hypertension* 1998;**31**:68–72.
45. Kaye D, Thompson J, Jennings G, Esler M. Cyclosporine therapy after cardiac transplantation causes hypertension and renal vasoconstriction without sympathetic activation. *Circulation* 1993;**88**:1110–1118.
46. Rundqvist B, Elam M, Eisenhofer G, Friberg P. Normalization of total body and regional sympathetic hyperactivity in heart failure after heart transplantation. *J Heart Lung Transplant* 1996;**15**:516–526.
47. Mannelli M, Lanzillotti R, Pupilli C *et al*. Adrenal medullary secretion in Cushing's syndrome. *J Clin Endocrinol Metab* 1994;**78**:1331–1335.
48. Jung RT, Shetty PS, Barrand M *et al*. Role of catecholamines in hypotensive response to dieting. *Br Med J* 1979;**i**:12–13.
49. Zweifler A, Esler M. Factors influencing the choice of antihypertensive agents. *Postgrad Med* 1976;**60**:18–85.

2.5

2

Cell membrane and ion-transport abnormalities in hypertension

A Semplicini and A Monari

Introduction

The basic abnormality of essential hypertension is an imbalance between total peripheral resistance and plasma volume. The former stems from an abnormal regulation of contractility of vascular smooth muscle cells in resistance arteries, and the latter from an abnormal regulation of extracellular fluid volume. Both may depend on abnormalities of the plasma membrane which separates the intracellular from the extracellular space. Therefore, the structure and function of the cell membrane may play a key role in the pathogenesis of essential hypertension.

Interest in this hypothesis has stimulated clinical and experimental research, which has already identified the role of specific abnormalities of membrane transport in the pathogenesis of rare forms of hypertension (Liddle's syndrome, licorice abuse, syndrome of apparent mineralocorticoid excess). Studies have also been conducted in humans and experimental animals to gain further insight into the pathogenesis of essential hypertension. However, they have been conducted in cells, such as the circulating blood cells, that express different transport proteins and which may not be involved in the regulation of arterial pressure. Such studies have nevertheless considerably improved our understanding of cell pathophysiology, while sometimes leading to conflicting results. In this chapter we have tried to summarize these.

BOX 2.5.1 The plasma membrane

The cell membrane consists of a lipid bilayer effecting compartmentalization of the internal cellular milieu (cytoplasm, organelles, nucleus, etc.) from the external milieu, i.e. the interstitium in pluricellular organisms. It creates a dynamic structure whereby the cell, besides maintaining its individuality and homeostasis, can interact with the adjacent cells, and, through particular signals and specific membrane structures, with the organism as a whole.

To permit this complex function, the structure of the cell membrane is altered by the presence of a number of molecules other than lipids (proteins, as a major component, with their versatility of structure–function, but also glycolipids and glycoproteins) that are inserted in the lipid bilayer (see Figure 2.5.1). The traffic of hydrophilic molecules, by themselves impermeable through the hydrophobic lipid bilayer, is made possible by the presence of specific protein structures called 'transporters'.

The mode of transport of molecules across the plasma membrane is defined according to the energy source:

- *Active transport*, is where the energy required to overcome the concentration gradient is derived from the hydrolysis of high-energy phosphate compounds (ATP).
- *Selective channels*, which may open to permit unidirectional flow of specific ions in response to specific stimuli (see Figure 2.5.2)
- *Facilitated diffusion* whereby energy stored in an electrochemical or concentration gradient is used to transport the molecule of interest and is associated with the movement of other molecules or ions that flow along their electrochemical or concentration gradient in the same direction (*cotransport* or *symport*) or in the opposite direction (*countertransport* or *antiporter* or *exchange*) (see Figure 2.5.3 and 2.5.4).

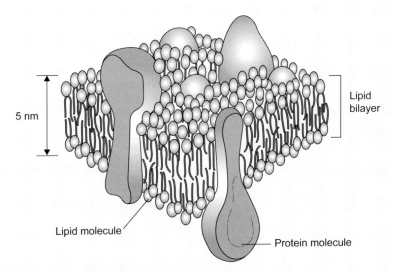

Fig. 2.5.1 The plasma membrane.

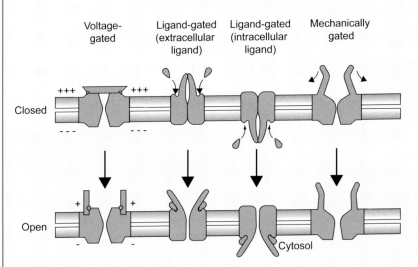

Fig. 2.5.2 Different ways of channel gating.

The velocity of ion transport across the cell membrane is dependent upon the number of transporter units, affinity for the transported species and velocity of translocation, all of which can be specifically modulated by intra- and extracellular signals. The signal transduction cascade of ion transport is activated by extracellular signals (*systemic*, such as hormones and neurosignalling molecules, and *local*, autocrine–paracrine molecules such as prostaglandins, nitric oxide, physical factors such as stretch and flux conditions). They interact with specific cellular receptors to transduce the external and specific signal to the intracellular complex of pathways that mediate a finite number of responses. They consist of membrane-bound steps (phospholipases, G-proteins, protein kinases), cytoplasmatic steps (second messengers such as inositoltriphosphate, Ca^{2+}, cAMP, cGMP, nitric oxide, and their targets, such as protein kinases), and nuclear steps (where a

113

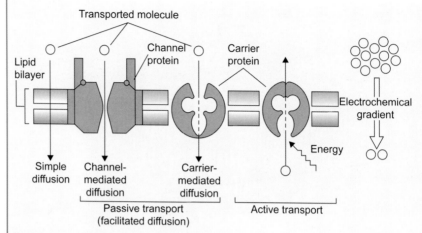

Fig. 2.5.3 Transmembrane transport systems.

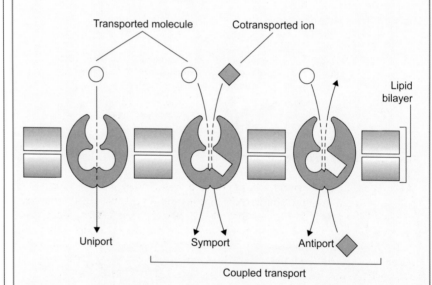

Fig. 2.5.4 Different ways of co- and countertransport through the membrane.

transcription response is evoked). Some of the steps in the signal-transduction system, which regulate transmembrane ion transport, have been investigated in depth in the search for the possible cause of abnormal ion transport in hypertension.

The protein kinase C (PKC) pathway is one of the signal transduction systems involved in the regulation of ion transport across the cell membrane. Protein kinase C is an intracellular, cytoplasmatic ATPase that effects the phosphorylation of a number of intracellular target proteins when recruited to the membrane and activated by the interaction with diacylglycerol (DAG), which is itself formed by the phospholipase C (PLC)-mediated hydrolysis of PIP2. PLC activation is initiated by the interaction of specific signals with their membrane receptors, which then activate PLC through a G-protein (see Figure 2.5.5). Overstimulation of PKC has been associated with stimulation of Na^+–H^+ exchange in hypertension [1].

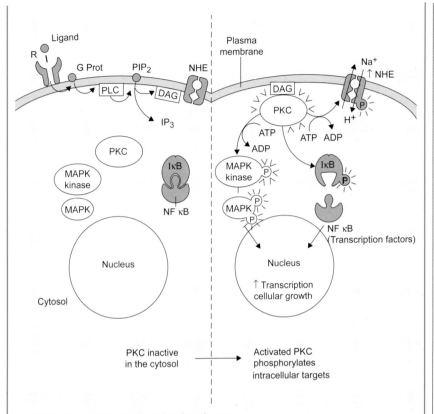

Fig. 2.5.5 The protein kinase C (PKC) pathway.

G-proteins are a numerous collection of proteins divided into two main groups: the trimeric G-proteins and the monomeric G-proteins. The former are interposed between the seven transmembrane domain receptors to connect them in a positive–stimulatory or negative–inhibitory way to downstream intracellular effectors, such as adenylate or guanylate cyclases, phospholipases, and protein kinases. The monomeric G-proteins are linked to the tyrosine kinase activity of the single spanning receptors of growth factors and to a number of other receptors. Polymorphism of G-proteins has been associated with abnormal regulation of Na^+–H^+ exchange in hypertension (see below) [2].

Finally, the MAPK (mitogen-activated protein kinase) family of proteins, the final common way of transmission of the growth/hypertrophic signals to cells and then to their nuclei, have been shown to be involved in the abnormal regulation of ion transport (see Figure 2.5.6). At least three families are involved in the modulation of cell growth/death: the ERK1–2 (extracellular response kinases) family, the JNK (*Jun N-terminus kinase*) family and the p38 family. Their abnormal activation may be involved in the development of cardiac and vascular hypertrophy in hypertension, in part at least through the activation of ion transport.

A physical way of initiating a cellular response is also emerging: the stretch imposed on the cell membrane and its intrinsic proteins (that behave as mechanoceptors) by sheer stress or lateral tension. The stretch-activated stimuli converge on intracellular targets common to other signals (channel opening, growth, protein synthesis, inflammatory signals) by steps involving

Introduction
Calcium and magnesium homeostasis
Intracellular calcium

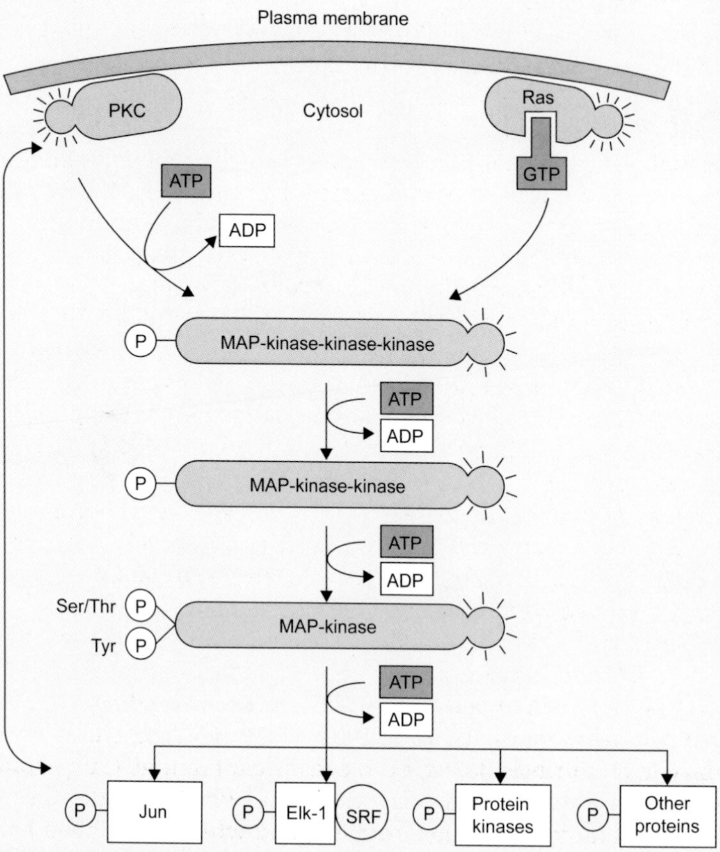

Fig. 2.5.6 The MAPK cascade.

the cytoskeleton and its regulatory proteins. Adducin is one of the cytoskeleton and its regulatory proteins. Adducin is one of the cytoskeleton regulatory proteins that is related to the development of hypertension in the Milan hypertensive rat model and in some humans with essential hypertension. The hypertensive strain differs from the normotensive rat for a mutation in the adducin sequence that affects the actin assembly and the activity of sodium channels and electrolyte traffic through the tubular epithelial cells in the proximal nephron [3]. The hyperactivity of sodium transport in the mutated strain results in sodium-sensitive hypertension. This polymorphism is also under investigation in human hypertension, with interesting results.

Calcium and magnesium homeostasis

Intracellular calcium

Intracellular Ca^{2+} is a major determinant of vascular smooth muscle cell contraction and a key element of cellular response to agonists, acting as a second messenger. In resting cells it is kept constant by a balance between a variety of Ca^{2+} – mobilizing and Ca^{2+} homeostatic mechanisms, mediated by Ca^{2+} channels and Ca^{2+} pumps located in the plasma membrane and intracellular organelles. Activation of vascular smooth muscle cells by different external stimuli disturbs the balance between Ca^{2+} mobilization and Ca^{2+} homeostasis, increasing intracellular calcium (Ca^{2+}_i) and inducing vascular smooth muscle cell contraction.

Essential components of the Ca^{2+} homeostatic mechanisms are (1) plasmalemma Ca^{2+} ATPase, which pumps Ca^{2+} out of the cell, (2) the Na^+–Ca^{2+} exchanger, which extrudes Ca^{2+} against the concentration gradient in exchange for Na^+ which enters the cell along the concentration gradient, and (3) the sarcoplasmic reticulum Ca^{2+} ATPase, which sequestrates Ca^{2+} in intracellular organelles (Figure 2.5.7).

As noted, the balance between these two opposite mechanisms maintains a Ca^{2+} concentration which is constantly lower by an order of four, in respect to the extracellular concentration in the resting cell. However, data in experimental animals and humans with hypertension suggest disruption in Ca^{2+} homeostasis. Much of the evidence comes from circulating blood cells (platelets, erythrocytes, lymphocytes and thymocytes), which have elevated intracellular Ca^{2+} levels and/or larger Ca^{2+} transients to agonists, but evidence for an abnormal Ca^{2+} balance has also been gathered in vascular smooth muscle cells.

The abnormalities associated with primary hypertension include increased cell Ca^{2+}_i, increased Ca^{2+} uptake and decreased Ca^{2+} removal. Ca^{2+}_i may be higher in hypertension due to reduced binding of Ca^{2+} to the inner cell membranes, to low activity of Ca^{2+} ATPase, either secondary to an intrinsic defect, or to extrinsic inhibition. Ca^{2+}_i could also be high for a reduced Na^+–Ca^{2+} exchange, which extrudes Ca^{2+} from the cell against its concentration gradient, and which is inhibited by an increased cell Na^+ concentration. Despite extensive investigations in the last two decades, a unifying explanation for abnormal Ca^{2+} metabolism in hypertension still does not exist.

Magnesium

Magnesium plays a pivotal role in controlling neuronal activity, cardiac excitability, neuromuscular transmission, muscular contraction, vasomotor tone, blood pressure, and peripheral blood flow, through its biochemical cellular activities. By competing with Ca^{2+} for membrane-binding sites and by modulating calcium binding and release from the sarcoplasmic reticulum membranes, Mg^{2+} can act to maintain low resting Ca^{2+} levels and trigger muscle contraction and relaxation. Moreover, it controls membrane permeability and the electrical properties of cellular membranes.

Many studies with different techniques have shown inadequate dietary intake, inadequate cellular metabolism, through extracellular as well as intracellular Mg^{2+} deficiency in experimental animals and humans with arterial hypertension. Mg^{2+} deficiency may increase Ca^{2+} activity and may induce endothelial cell dysfunction as well as free-radical formation and contribute to hypertension and accelerated atherosclerosis.

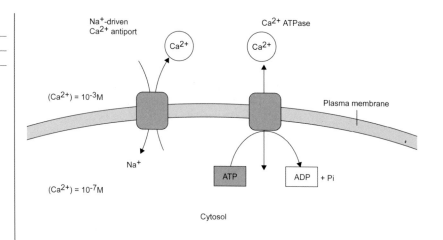

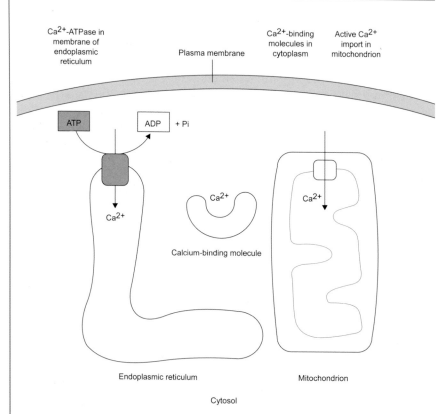

Fig. 2.5.7 Diagram of the systems involved in calcium homeostasis (across the membrane, upper panel, intracellular organelles, lower panel).

Sodium homeostasis

The relationships between Na^+ intake and the development of hypertension in animal models and in humans with salt-sensitive hypertension have prompted investigations between total body Na^+ and

2

blood pressure. Exchangeable Na$^+$ in essential hypertensives is normal. Therefore a great deal of research has been devoted to the study of cell Na$^+$ and cell membrane Na$^+$ transport.

Cellular Na$^+$ content is increased in many cell types (erythrocytes, lymphocytes) in primary hypertension both in humans and animals. This may be due to increased Na$^+$ influx or decreased Na$^+$ extrusion.

The principal determinant of the unequal distribution of Na$^+$ between the intra- and extracellular compartment is Na$^+$, K$^+$–ATPase, wich operates an electrogenic exchange between Na$^+$ and K$^+$, extruding three Na$^+$ ions from the intracellular compartment for every two K$^+$ imported, with the hydrolysis of one molecule of ATP for each exchange (Figure 2.5.8). This maintains a low intracellular concentration of Na$^+$ and a high concentration of K$^+$. This unequal distribution is the principal driving force for almost all the other ion and molecule fluxes (co- and countertransport) between the two compartments. It is therefore not surprising that alterations in the structure or mode of function of the Na$^+$ pump were at first investigated as a possible site for the pathogenesis of hypertension. No conclusive results have been found however, possibly because major changes in this key molecule would be incompatible with life itself. However, some authors have recognized a role for regulatory molecules, secretion of which would be increased in sodium-overload states. This could mediate the hypertensive effect in this condition through the inhibition of the pump which would then determine the changes in the intracellular cation concentration of calcium, eventually responsible for hypertension. It is therefore possible that the Na$^+$ pump is inhibited in some clinical conditions characterized by Na$^+$ and water overload and secretion of inhibiting substances (endogenous ouabain).

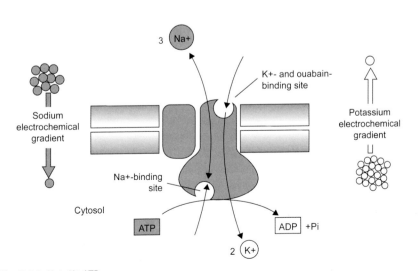

Fig. 2.5.8 Na$^+$, K$^+$-ATPase.

Ouabain-like factors (OLF)

In the late 1970s it was proposed that, in conditions of defective Na^+ and water excretion, high Na^+ intake expands extracellular fluid volume and stimulates secretion of endogenous inhibitors of the cell membrane Na^+–K^+ pump, known as 'digitalis-like' or 'ouabain-like' factors (OLF), which correct Na^+ retention, by blocking renal Na^+ reabsorption. However, the widespread inhibition of the ubiquitous Na^+–K^+ pump induces peripheral vasoconstriction, sympathetic stimulation and arterial hypertension by increasing intracellular Na^+ and Ca^{2+} (Figure 2.5.9).

The most widely known inhibitors of the Na^+–K^+ pump, the cardiotonic digitalis glycosides, are synthesized by plants, while bufodieneolides can be found in plants and in toad skin, venom and plasma. However, ion-transport experiments also support the existence of inhibitors of Na^+ transport in the biological fluids of mammals. Plasma from hypertensive patients inhibits ouabain-sensitive ion transport in white cells and vascular tissue. Circulating Na^+ pump inhibitors were found in the plasma of rats and pigs with volume-expanded, low-renin hypertension (one-kidney one-wrap, one kidney one-clip, reduced renal mass, deoxycorticosterone acetate (DOCA)-salt). Other techniques have shown elevated levels of humoral inhibitors of

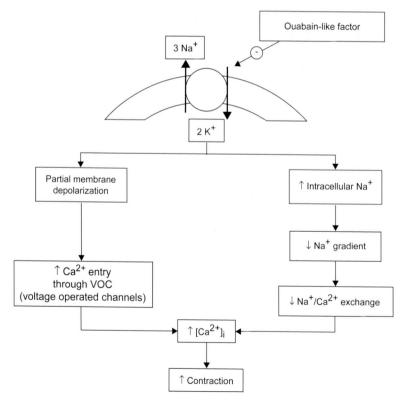

Fig. 2.5.9 Hypothetical pathogenesis of hypertension in sodium-overload states following hyperproduction of ouabain-like factors (OLF).

the Na^+, K^+–ATPase in genetically hypertensive Milan rats and also in hypertensive or salt-loaded patients. Ouabain has been identified in human plasma and mass spectrometry has convincingly shown that it is indeed identical to plant ouabain. Ouabain immunoreactivity is also high in primary hyperaldosteronism and it decreases after surgical removal of the adenoma. Finally, ouabain is increased in patients with congestive heart failure and its plasma levels are inversely related to cardiac index and mean pressure. That is, the more severe the cardiac decompensation, the higher is the plasma ouabain, which suggests a role for endogenous ouabain in the control of extracellular fluids.

Endogenous ouabain exerts cardiodynamic and vasculotonic actions similar to plant ouabain. In isolated guinea pig heart, it induces a reversible and dose-dependent increase of maximal tension and of the rate of its development. In guinea-pig aortic strips, a subthreshold dose of endogenous ouabain increases histamine-induced contraction and this effect lasts even after ouabain washout. The acute administration of cardiac glycosides may be thought to be associated with a short-term vasopressive action or hypertension. On the contrary, in patients with heart failure, chronic digoxin treatment is not associated with any increase in pressure. Only in rats with subtotal nephrectomy does ouabain raise blood pressure in proportion to the reduction in renal mass.

The role of endogenous ouabain in essential hypertension is unknown. It has already been mentioned that ouabain pretreatment increases the pressor effect of norepinephrine in normotensive controls. However, in hypertensives the pressor effect is diminished, particularly in low renin hypertensives. This can be taken as indirect evidence for high ouabain levels in low-renin hypertensives with volume-expanded hypertension.

Na–K–2Cl cotransport

Na–K–2Cl cotransport is a widely distributed transport protein that catalyzes electroneutral-coupled transport of Na^+, K^+ and Cl^- in both inward and outward directions across the cell membrane. It does not require energy and it is inhibited by loop diuretics (furosemide and bumetanide). Important roles of Na–K–2Cl cotransport are to maintain the Cl^- ion concentration far from equilibrium (in vascular smooth muscle cells) and to mediate the polarized movements of ions leading to net ion extrusion (glands) or reabsorption (kidney) (Figure 2.5.10).

In the medullary thick ascending limb, the cotransport system accounts for almost all luminal sodium reabsorption. The cotransport is also well characterized in non-epithelial cells, such as red blood cells, in which it is near equilibrium and inward and outward fluxes have similar magnitude. In vascular smooth muscle cells, it catalyzes a very small Na^+ flux and it is more likely involved in the regulation of cell Cl^- concentration.

Increased cotransport activity has been found in erythrocytes of human and rat models of primary hypertension and it has been

Sodium homeostasis

Ouabain-like factors (OLF)

Na–K–2Cl cotransport

121

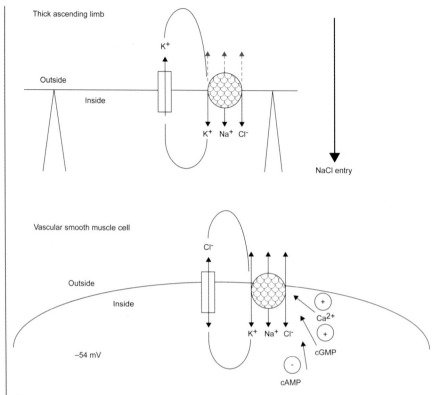

Fig. 2.5.10 Na–K–2Cl cotransport functioning.

proposed as a genetic maker of increased sodium reabsorption in the thick ascending limb of Henle. This was confirmed in the Milan hypertensive rat strain (MHS). However, cotransport activity is reduced in vascular smooth muscle cells, probably due to circulating inhibiting substances, where it may be associated with slight depolarization of the cell membrane and increased membrane excitability.

Cell pH

A tight regulation of cell pH is essential for the normal cell function. This is made possible by intracellular buffers and cell membrane proteins which transport H^+ or HCO_3^- to compensate for any change in cell pH.

Anion exchange

Two types of anion exchange are involved in the regulation of cell pH. One is a Na^+-driven Cl^-–HCO_3^- exchange, which consists of two exchangers: one extruding one H^+ for each Cl^- imported on one side, the other being a Na^+–HCO_3^- exchange. Both of these exchanges are pH_i sensitive, increasing in their activation as the intracellular pH falls. A second system provides a Na^+-independent HCO_3^-–Cl^- exchanger similar to the band 3 protein of red blood cells and operating in nucleated cells to pump out bicarbonate when intracellular pH becomes too alkaline.

None of these systems has been convincingly demonstrated as a possible determinant of hypertension.

Sodium–proton exchange

The sodium–hydrogen exchanger is a plasma membrane glycoprotein that mediates the exchange of intracellular H^+ for extracellular Na^+ with a 1:1 stoichiometry (Figure 2.5.11). In mammalian cells several isoforms of the protein have been identified and are designed NHE-1 to 5.

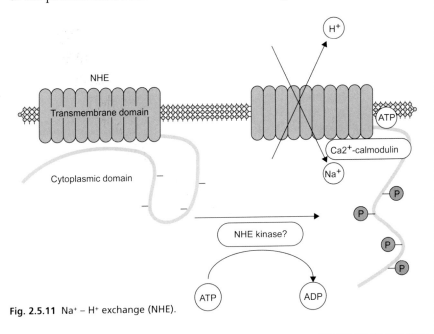

Fig. 2.5.11 $Na^+ - H^+$ exchange (NHE).

BOX 2.5.2 Sodium–proton exchange

The Na^+–H^+ exchanger isoform 1 (NHE-1) is a ubiquitous membrane transporter that has a 'housekeeping' role in the regulation of cell pH (pH_i), cell volume and cell proliferation. NHE-1 is present in all mammalian cells and it is activated by a wide variety of stimuli including growth factors, phorbol esters, insulin and hormones and it is regulated by several intracellular kinases such as Ca^{2+}-calmodulin, cAMP-dependent kinase, protein kinase C and the mitogen-activated protein kinase (MAPK).

NHE-2 is present in the brush border membrane of some epithelia, but its function is not clear. NHE-3 is present in the brush border membrane of jejunum, ileum, colon and kidney; its expression is stimulated by glucocorticoids. NHE-3 is involved in transepithelial Na^+ absorption, and is inhibited by all stimuli which activate protein kinase A (PKA). In kidney tubule epithelia, NHE-3 is responsible for Na^+ reabsorption and plays an important role in the regulation of salt balance. NHE-4 and NHE-5 have been recently characterized, but their tissue distribution and their physiological functions are unknown.

Cell pH

Sodium–proton exchange

Sodium–lithium exchange

Recent studies demonstrate that the mitogen-activated protein kinases (MAPK) is involved in the NHE regulation. MAPK are a family of ubiquitous serine/threonine kinases which play an important role in various signal-transduction pathways, including insulin, growth factors, tumor promoters, cytokines, osmotic shock and stress. Another common signal-transduction pathway for many agonists is the activation of phospholipase C, with release of diacylglycerol (DAG) leading to activation of protein kinase C (PKC), which activates NHE.

Several hormones (i.e. insulin, angiotensin II, endothelin-1) and growth factors (i.e. epidermal growth factor, platelet-derived growth factor, thrombin) induce an enhancement of the exchanger activity through G-proteins, modification of cell Ca^{2+}, and protein kinases which affect the signal-transduction system and protein phosphorylation.

The activity of NHE is increased in different cell types in hypertensive patients, suggesting that its abnormal function may be involved in the pathophysiology of hypertension. The abnormal activation of the transporter in hypertension does not seem to be due to gene overexpression, but it seems to be caused by a post-translational modification of NHE protein, such as phosphorylation. These abnormalities are conserved in Epstein–Barr virus immortalized lymphoblasts from patients with essential hypertension, and are found in vascular smooth muscle cells from spontaneously hypertensive (SHR) rats suggesting that they are not due to the hypertensive milieu, but are secondary to a defective regulation, possibly caused by intra- or extracellular factors. Among them, the stimulating action of insulin has to be acknowledged. In fact, insulin increases NHE activity *in vitro* and the kinetic abnormalities, found in hypertensives, are more pronounced in insulin-resistant hypertensives.

The abnormal activity of isoform 3 of the NHE (NHE-3) may lead to significant changes of kidney proximal tubule reabsorption of Na^+, contributing to developing hypertension. Moreover, enhanced NHE-1 activity has been associated to left ventricular hypertrophy, vascular remodelling, and diabetic nephropathy. This 'proliferative phenotype' may be due to excessive cell alkalization, which stimulates protein synthesis, or to upregulation of upstream kinase signalling.

Epidemiological and experimental studies have shown that an increase of NHE is associated with an higher cardiovascular risk, through increased sodium reabsorption and blood pressure and/or increased cardiac and vascular remodelling.

Sodium–lithium exchange

In 1975, a ouabain-insensitive Na^+–Li^+ exchange (or countertransport or antiport, NLE) in human red cells was first documented. Later, interest in the clinical measurement of NLE in hypertension was raised by the finding by Canessa *et al.* [4] who showed increased red cell NLE in patients with essential hypertension and not in patients with secondary hypertension and normotensive controls. They suggested that the activity of NLE was heritable and that an increased NLE could be a genetic marker of susceptibility to hypertension.

It was first proposed that NLE reflects Na^+–Na^+ exchange. Subsequently, it has been hypothesized that NLE represents a mode of functioning of cell membrane Na^+–H^+ exchange. Increased NLE could therefore reflect the abnormal kinetic properties of the Na^+–H^+ exchanger, accounting for the relationship between NLE and hypertension. In favor of this hypothesis is experimental evidence gathered in some laboratories, but the issue of the relationship between NLE and NHE has not been resolved.

The red cell membrane NLE operates in either direction across the cell membrane. It binds either Li^+ or Na^+ on one side of the membrane and exchanges the transported species for either Li^+ or Na^+ on the opposite side in a stoichiometric ratio of 1:1. It is ATP independent and the energy for uphill translocation is derived from the disequilibrium of Na^+ across the cell membrane, maintained by the Na^+ pump.

In the general population, NLE is unimodally distributed. It is higher in males than in females and correlated to body weight, body mass index and blood pressure. NLE is higher in Whites compared to Blacks and in Chinese compared to either Europeans or non-Chinese Asians. It is ten times slower in cord blood than in adulthood but later there is no change with aging.

After the first report by Canessa *et al.*, many other laboratories have confirmed the increased activity of red cell NLE in patients with essential hypertension, due either to increased maximal velocity of translocation or abnormal affinity for the transported ions.

NLE is increased in a subset of 40–50% of hypertensives, more so in severe and drug-resistant patients than in others. NLE is increased in normotensive offsprings of hypertensive parents, who are prone to develop hypertension later in life, and longitudinal studies have shown that the higher the NLE, the larger the increase of arterial pressure with age.

Overweight, hyperlipidemia, reduced glucose tolerance, reduced physical activity, type A behavior, smoking and caffeine consumption are more common among hypertensives than normotensives and are additive in increasing the risk attributable to hypertension and independently correlated to the activity of NLE. Actually, some of the covariables (body weight, plasma lipids, serum uric acid, alcohol consumption, reduced physical activity) are more strongly related to NLE than to blood pressure itself.

There are suggestions that increased NLE reflects proximal tubule Na^+ retention and salt sensitivity in patients with non-modulating hypertension (strong family history for hypertension, blunted vascular, renin and adrenal response to sodium load and angiotensin II infusion, reduced ability to handle a sodium load, which favors salt sensitivity).

Hypertension is often associated with insulin resistance, hyperinsulinemia and overt diabetes. NLE is inversely correlated with insulin sensitivity, both in patients with essential hypertension and insulin-dependent (IDDM) and non-insulin-dependent diabetes mellitus (NIDDM).

Cell pH

Sodium–lithium exchange

Cellular potassium

In patients with IDDM and high NLE, the reduced insulin sensitivity could result in poor metabolic control and favor the development of microalbuminuria and diabetic nephropathy. Increased NLE also predicts the development of target organ damage in hypertensive patients. Hypertensives with high NLE display greater interventricular septum, posterior and relative wall thickness than patients with low NLE on echocardiography. Moreover, the former have greater kidney volume, glomerular filtration rate, and proximal sodium reabsorption. Finally, an increased NLE is associated with vascular remodelling and it prevents its correction by antihypertensive treatment.

In conclusion, among the various alterations of cation transport reported in hypertension, an increase in red cell NLE is the one that has been most widely investigated and confirmed. The pathophysiological significance of this finding is still not clear. We do not even know if it is primary or secondary to other alterations in cell metabolism. It seems unlikely that alterations of NLE are secondary to genetically determined alterations of NHE-1.

Altered phosphorylation of the transporter, secondary to protein kinase activation or phosphatase inactivation, is another possibility. In fact, angiotensin II, insulin and growth factors activate NHE through direct or indirect activation of membrane protein kinases.

Cytoplasmic calcium is increased in various cells of hypertensive patients (see above) and the links between cytoplasmic calcium and NHE are strong. Intracellular Ca^{2+} activates NHE and NLE while NHE on its own modulates free cytoplasmic Ca^{2+}. It is therefore likely that the high NLE and NHE of many hypertensive patients reflects a genetically determined alteration of the phosphorylation state of the cell membrane and/or increased cytoplasmic calcium.

Whatever the pathophysiological relevance of NLE may be for the development of hypertension, its measurement could be of some clinical use. Its association with severe and drug-resistant hypertension, insulin resistance, vascular and cardiac hypertrophy, hyperlipidemia and obesity, positive family history for hypertension and for major cardiovascular accidents, suggests that high NLE could be considered a biochemical marker for increased cardiovascular risk.

Cellular potassium

Several studies have suggested that (1) the lower the potassium intake, the higher the blood pressure in the population, and, (2) that potassium supplementation may reduce blood pressure in animals and humans ingesting large amounts of sodium. These observations have prompted investigations on K^+ homeostasis in hypertension.

Only 2% of total body K^+ is in the extracellular space. However, even if a much larger amount is absorbed daily, the extracellular cation concentration must vary within a narrow range to allow normal neuromuscular function. This is made possible by an efficient regulation of extracellular K^+ concentration, which involves renal and extrarenal mechanisms (insulin, glucagon, epinephrine, mineralocorticoids and changes in acid–base balance), which promote K^+ excretion or K^+ shift from the extracellular to the intracellular compartment.

Increased plasma membrane permeability for K^+ as well as for other cations has been reported in patients with hypertension and in hypertensive experimental animal models. However, total body K^+ is not different in Dahl salt-sensitive rats and in stroke-prone SHR rats, despite the protective effect of a high K^+ diet against hypertension and stroke in these animals. The high K^+ diet has no effect on K^+ content in the skeletal muscle, aortic wall, bone and plasma. It is therefore conceivable that dietary K^+ content exerts its protective effect either by increasing urinary Na^+ excretion, or promoting vasodilation, or preventing endothelial damage and reducing oxidative stress.

Gene polymorphism of cell membrane ion transport associated with abnormal blood pressure regulation

Liddle's syndrome

Patients with Liddle's syndrome present with early and typically moderate-to-severe hypertension. The pathogenesis of hypertension in Liddle's syndrome entails increased renal reabsorption of salt and water as in hyperaldosteronism-mediated syndromes. However, mineralocorticoid levels are extremely suppressed in these patients and antagonism of mineralocorticoid receptors has no effect on blood pressure. On the contrary, renal transplantation has corrected the defect in a Liddle's syndrome patient, which suggests that the defect in these patients is intrinsic to the kidney.

Linkage analysis has localized the genes causing Liddle's syndrome to a small segment of chromosome 16 [5]. This segment contains two genes of particular interest: the genes encoding the β and γ subunits of the amiloride-sensitive epithelial Na^+ channel (ENaC). This channel is composed of at least three subunits and normal channel activity requires all of them (the α subunit gene is located on chromosome 12). Reabsorption of sodium through the ENaC is regulated by aldosterone, and normally this regulated step appears to be the major determinant of net renal sodium reabsorption. Examination of these genes in patients with Liddle's syndrome has revealed mutations in genes encoding either the β and γ subunits of the channel. These mutations result in deletion of the cytoplasmic –COOH terminus of the subunits or in introduction of amino acid substitutions into a short proline-rich segment of the –COOH terminus. Expression in *Xenopus* oocytes of ENaC containing these mutant subunits produces a markedly increased whole-cell Na^+ current. This increased activity *in vivo* leads to increased sodium reabsorption and explains the hypertension seen in patients.

Investigation of the mechanism of these 'gain of function' mutations has indicated that the short proline-rich segments of the ENaC subunits are the critical targets for the activating mutations. It appears that these mutations result in an inability to remove active channels from the

2

2

apical surface, a function that is likely to be mediated by the binding of another protein to the proline-rich segment.

Bartter's and Gitelman's syndromes

Two forms of autosomic recessive syndromes characterized by systemic hypokalemic alkalosis and low blood pressure have been described and associated with derangements in the function of the renal handling of salt – Bartter's and Gitelman's syndromes.

Patients with Bartter's syndrome present at an early age with severe volume depletion, hypokalemia, metabolic alkalosis, hyperreninemia, hyperaldosteronism, and normal–low blood pressure, resistance to the pressure effects of norepinephrine and angiotensin II, and hyperplasia of the juxtaglomerular apparatus. The clinical symptoms are weakness, muscle cramps, polyuria and abdominal pain, excessive urinary loss of potassium, sodium, chloride, magnesium and calcium, with increased renal production of PGE_2. Recently, molecular genetic approaches and linkage analysis have demonstrated that frameshift or non-conservative missense mutations in the gene encoding for the bumetanide-sensitive Na–K–2Cl (NKCC2) cotransporter co-segregate with the disease.

Gitelman's syndrome is characterized by hypokalemic alkalosis, hypocalciuria, renal salt wasting, low serum magnesium levels and an activated renin–angiotensin system, and commonly presents with neuromuscular abnormalities. The gene causing Gitelman's syndrome has been mapped to a region of chromosome 16 containing the gene encoding the renal thiazide-sensitive $Na^+ – Cl^+$ cotransporter. This ion transporter is present on the apical membrane of renal tubular epithelium in the distal convoluted tubule and mediates electroneutral reabsorption of sodium and chloride.

Patients with Gitelman's syndrome present with a diverse array of non-conservative missense mutations, premature termination codons and splice site mutations in the $Na^+–Cl^+$ cotransporter or the NKCC2 gene that co-segregates with the disease and results in loss of cotransporter function. This finding demonstrates that the primary defect in these patients is renal salt wasting, but manifestations of the disease may derive from other abnormalities.

Dahl rats

Dahl rats represent an animal model of sodium-sensitive hypertension extensively studied, although no conclusive evidence supports a single determinant of this trait. One of the pathogenetic factors relevant in this model is an abnormality of function in the Na–K–2Cl cotransporter, that has been confirmed, however, only in circulating erythrocytes. More recent evidence points to an abnormal regulation of the renal handling of loop chloride reabsorption possibly secondary to a disruption in levels of renal cytochrome P450-arachidonic acid metabolites (with loss of a tonic inhibitory effect of 20-HETE, in the salt-sensitive strain). An analogous dysfunction could explain the sodium-sensitive trait in some essential hypertensives.

References

1. Aviv A. The links between cellular Ca^{2+} and Na^+–H^+ exchange in the pathophysiology of essential hypertension. *Am J Hypertension* 1996; **9**(7):703–707.
2. Siffert W, Rosskopf D, Siffert G *et al*. Association of a human G-protein beta-3 subunit variant with hypertension. *Nature Genet* 1998;**18**(1):45–48.
3. Manunta P, Barlassina C, Bianchi G. Adducin in essential hypertension. *FEBS Lett* 1998; **430**(1–2):41–44
4. Canessa M, Adragna N, Solomon HS *et al*. Increased sodium–lithium countertransport in red cells of patients with essential hypertension. *N Engl J Med* 1980;**302**(14):772–776.
5. Lifton RP. Molecular genetics of human blood pressure variation. *Science* 1996;**272**(5262):676–680.

Blood pressure measurement

Chapter

3.1

Initial diagnostic testing and risk stratification of the patient with hypertension

TD Vagaonescu and RA Phillips

Introduction

Arterial hypertension is the most frequent reason for attendance at a clinic in Europe and the USA. Since the assessment of the patient with hypertension may vary from a simple clinical examination that focuses on the cardiovascular status of the patient to an extensive multisystem evaluation that involves expensive invasive procedures, it is important to understand the rationale behind the various laboratory procedures before ordering them. Along with the initial assessment that includes physical examination and simple laboratory tests (Table 3.1.1), the following questions should be answered (see also Figure 3.1.1):

- Is the patient really hypertensive?
- Is the hypertension essential or secondary?
- What is the degree of target organ damage?
- What is the total cardiovascular risk profile?
- Are there any associated cardiovascular or metabolic diseases?
- Is the patient adhering to lifestyle modification?

The answers to these questions help determine whether further assessment is necessary and help guide the therapeutic plan. The decision to order a specific test should be individualized to the specific patient and should always follow a thorough clinical assessment of the patient; ordering 'everything' to be 'thorough', from urinary metanephrines to a magnetic resonance angiogram is a shotgun approach and is bad medicine.

Essential versus secondary hypertension

Essential hypertension is the most frequently encountered form of hypertension, accounting for 95% of all cases of hypertension; the remaining 5% is secondary hypertension, which can be identified and often successfully treated. The patient with essential hypertension commonly presents with an unremarkable clinical examination and often with a family history significant for arterial hypertension. In the patient with newly diagnosed grade 1, or stage 1 hypertension, it is frequently helpful to obtain repeated home blood pressures and/or ambulatory blood pressure monitoring (ABPM) to be certain that the patient does not have 'white coat' hypertension and that treatment is necessary. If there is no reason to suspect secondary hypertension and blood pressure can be easily controlled, no further laboratory tests other than those listed in Table 3.1.1 are required for the etiologic diagnosis of

Table 3.1.1 Routine tests for essential hypertension

Definitely indicated	Selectively indicated
Serum electrolytes with uric acid	Home blood pressure monitoring
Creatinine	Ambulatory blood pressure monitoring
Urinalysis	Echocardiogram
Electrocardiogram	
Lipid profile	

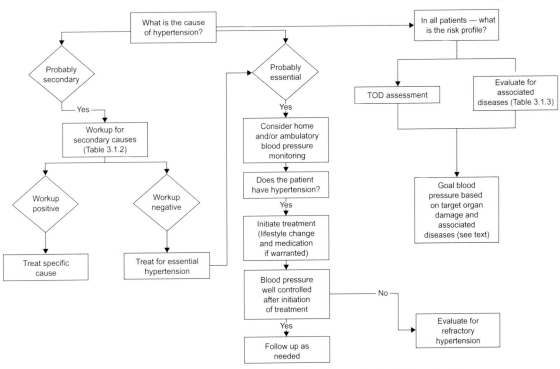

Fig. 3.1.1 Schema for initial diagnostic testing and risk stratification of the patient with hypertension.

arterial hypertension. If history, initial physical examination or simple laboratory tests suggest otherwise, further investigations should be ordered based on a specific suspected diagnosis (see Table 3.1.2).

Target organ damage assessment

The degree of injury to various organs and systems, i.e. 'target organ damage' as a result of elevated blood pressure, should be quantified in every patient; this helps to risk stratify the hypertensive patient and to guide treatment. Every patient with arterial hypertension should have a funduscopic examination as part of initial evaluation. It is useful to tell the patient during the examination that this is the only 'window' that allows direct visualization of hypertension-induced vessel damage. 'Copper wiring' and arteriovenous nicking are specific retinal changes of arterial hypertension, while others may also be found in various other diseases ('cotton wool spots' in diabetes, systemic lupus erythematosus, AIDS; flame-shaped intraretinal hemorrhages in diabetes, retinal vein occlusion, blood dyscrasias; 'silver wiring' in diabetes, collagenoses, arterial occlusive diseases). In selected cases such as retinal vein or artery occlusion, or optic disk swelling, the patient should also be referred to an ophthalmologist.

When the history or examination is consistent with stroke, transient ischemic attacks or carotid bruits, further non-invasive evaluation of the cerebral circulation is warranted. The cerebral vasculature can be

Target organ damage assessment

135

Table 3.1.2 Testing for secondary hypertension

Possible secondary cause of hypertension	Clinical hints suggesting condition	Initial testing for condition	Additional testing
Renovascular disease	Age of onset less than 20 or more than 60 years Smoking history Atherosclerotic vascular disease Abdominal bruit Severe, accelerated or malignant hypertension ACE-inhibitor induced reversible creatinine elevation	Captopril-enhanced isotopic nephrogram Duplex sonography (renal arteries) MRA (renal arteries)	Renal arterogram if initial tests are suggestive or conflicting
Renoparenchymal disease	Known pre-existent renal disease (uni/bilateral) Chronic renal failure Known use of analgesics Family history of polycystic kidney disease Palpable abdominal mass	Serum creatinine Urinalysis Urinary microalbumin and total protein Renal ultrasonography	Renal biopsy
Cushing's syndrome	Long-term corticosteroid therapy Truncal obesity with moon facies, buffalo hump Fatigability and proximal muscle weakness Hirsutism Skin striae and ecchymoses	24 hour-urinary free-cortisol level Dexamethasone suppression test	Adrenal CT/MRI scan ACTH sampling (plasma, inferior petrosal sinus, after corticotropin-releasing factor stimulation)
Primary hyperaldosteronism	Muscle weakness and fatigue Polyuria and polydipsia	Serum electrolytes Supine and erect aldosterone PRA and cortisol. 24-hour urine for aldosterone Plasma aldosterone (before and after saline loading)	Adrenal CT/MRI scan Adrenal veins sampling for aldosterone
Pheochromocytoma	Spontaneous sudden onset of hypertension, headache, profuse sweating, palpitations Severe hypertension associated with anesthesia or surgery Marked orthostatic blood pressure associated with severe supine hypertension Familial history of phakomatoses Known thyroid or parathyroid tumor Family history of type II multiple endocrine neoplasia (MEN II)	Urine sample for catecholamines or their metabolites (metanephrines, vanillylmandelic acid homovanillic acid Supine plasma catecholamines (basal and 2 hours after 0.3 mg clonidine)	Adrenal CT or MRI scan ^{131}I-MIBG imaging ^{111}Indium–octreotide scan
Coarctation of the aorta	Young age Headache, epistaxis, cold extremities and claudication with exercise Femoral pulses are diminished and delayed when compared with the radial, brachial or carotid pulses Arterial pulsations in the posterior intercostal spaces Ejection murmur at the left sternal border and in the interscapular area Difference in blood pressure between upper and lower extremities	Chest X-ray ECG Sonogram and Doppler of aortic arch	MRI of thorax Aortic (and coronary) angiography

investigated with Doppler flow studies of the extra-and intracranial arteries, ultrasound of the carotid arteries and magnetic resonance angiography (MRA) of the cerebral arteries. Computed tomography (CT) or magnetic resonance imaging (MRI) scans document previous cerebrovascular accidents.

Hypertensive heart disease can be confirmed by a clinical examination that elicits history of dyspnea, heart failure, angina, myocardial infarction or coronary revascularization, and by a prominent point of maximal impulse (PMI) or S_4 or S_3. In all patients with hypertension, an electrocardiogram should be obtained to ascertain the presence of atrial fibrillation, left atrial and left ventricular hypertrophy, intraventricular conduction delay or prior myocardial infarction. Indeed, because regression of left ventricular hypertrophy (LVH) is associated with improved prognosis, it could be argued that a 'limited echocardiogram' to measure left ventricular mass should be a routine part of the clinical evaluation of all patients with hypertension.

Hypertension-induced renal dysfunction (nephrosclerosis) can be quantified by measurement of creatinine or the presence of microalbuminuria, or proteinuria. Hypertensive renal disease places the patient in a high-risk category for cardiovascular disease and, therefore warrants aggressive treatment of blood pressure (see targets below) to slow the progression of renal disease, and to prevent further cardiovascular complications.

Evaluation of other cardiovascular risk factors

Arterial hypertension is the leading cause of LVH and congestive heart failure, and is a major risk factor for atherosclerosis. During the initial 'workup' of the hypertensive patient the cardiovascular risk profile should also be assessed. The information necessary to do this can be obtained from history and physical examination and laboratories:

- The presence of clinical cardiovascular disease which includes myocardial infarction, angina, stroke, transient ischemic attack or peripheral arterial disease.
- Family history significant for coronary artery diseases in a first-degree female relative under the age of 65 or a first-degree male relative under the age of 55.
- History of smoking within the past year.
- History of dyslipidemia or diabetes mellitus.
- Sedentary lifestyle, dietary habits, depression and ability to cope with stress.
- Body mass index.
- Fasting blood sugar.
- Lipid profile: cholesterol, triglycerides, LDL-cholesterol and HDL-cholesterol.
- C-reactive protein levels, fibrinogen and the lipoprotein Lp(a) may emerge in the next few years as risk factors that are routinely measured.

Associated diseases in
patients with hypertension
Optimal blood pressure
goals and resistant arterial
hypertension

3

It is controversial whether the determination of plasma renin activity (PRA) (normalized for the urinary sodium) should be part of the routine risk assessment. There is good evidence that elevated PRA is a predictor of future ischemic heart disease that is independent of smoking history, glucose level or cholesterol. However, perhaps because the PRA level has not yet been incorporated into standard risk formula, such as the Framingham Risk Score, it is not standard practice to obtain it. In addition, some advocate that a PRA level may streamline antihypertensive selection. However, choosing initial drug therapy based on age and race is at least as effective as that based on a renin profile.

Associated diseases in patients with hypertension

Hypertension can present as an isolated disease or in association with other disorders such as diabetes mellitus, renal dysfunction, atherosclerosis, gout and obesity. If the clinical examination and initial routine laboratory tests present enough clues to suggest the presence of the above-mentioned diseases, further testing is warranted (see Table 3.1.3).

Optimal blood pressure goals and resistant arterial hypertension

Optimal control of blood pressure is as follows:

- Below 140/90 mmHg in patients with uncomplicated hypertension.
- Below 130/85 mmHg in patients with clinical cardiovascular disease, diabetes mellitus or renal insufficiency.
- Below 125/75 mmHg in hypertensive patients with renal insufficiency and proteinuria in excess of 1 g/24 hours.

In patients who remain above these goals despite adherence to a triple drug regimen that includes a diuretic and near maximal doses of medications, the patient should be reassessed. Indeed, many patients with resistant hypertension have normal blood pressure on ambulatory or home blood pressure monitoring, and require no additional medications.

Table 3.1.3 Testing for diseases associated with arterial hypertension

Associated disease	Clinical clues	Initial test
Diabetes mellitus	Polyuria, polydipsia, weight loss despite polyphagia	Fasting blood sugar, glycosylated hemoglobin Urine analysis, urinary microalbumin and total protein
Hyperuricemia	Arthritis, kidney stones	Serum uric acid Urine analysis
Obstructive sleep apnea	Disruptive snoring, excessive daytime hypersomnolence and fatigue, upper body obesity	Sleep studies
Atherosclerosis	History of cardiovascular disease	Fasting lipid profile Fibrinogen?, Lp(a)?, homocysteine? C-reactive protein?

Conclusion

The evaluation of the patient with elevated blood pressure relies mainly on the history and clinical examination. Routine tests (see Table 3.1.1) are recommended to assess target organ damage and the risk profile of the patient. Home blood pressure and/or ambulatory monitoring are often very helpful and can change the course of treatment, especially in grade 1 or stage 1 hypertension. Optional tests should be requested in selected patients if the initial history, physical or simple laboratory tests suggest a possible curable cause of the arterial hypertension or for better cardiovascular risk stratification. Some of the tests may be repeated in the follow up of the hypertensive patient if, after clinical reassessment, they are considered to be helpful in providing better blood pressure control.

Further reading

1. Phillips RA, Diamond JA. Non-invasive modalities for evaluating the hypertensive patient: focus on left ventricular mass and ambulatory blood pressure monitoring. *Prog Cardiovasc Dis* 1999; **41**:397–440.
2. Izzo JL, Jr, Black HR, eds. *Hypertension Primer*, 2nd edn. The Council on High Blood Pressure Research, American Heart Association: Dallas, TX, 1999.
3. The Sixth Report of the Joint National Committee on Prevention, Detection, Evaluation, and Treatment of High Blood Pressure. *Arch Intern Med* 1997;**157**:2413–2446.
4. Williams GH. Hypertensive vascular disease. In: *Harrison's Principles of Internal Medicine*, 14th edn. (eds Fauci AS, Braunwald E, Isselbacher KJ *et al.*), pp. 1380–1394. New York, McGraw-Hill: 1998.
5. Black HR. Approach to the patient with hypertension. In: *Primary Cardiology.* (eds Goldman L, Braunwald E), pp. 129–143. WB Saunders: Philadelphia 1998.
6. Frohlich ED. Hypertension and hypertensive heart disease. In: *Classic Teachings in Clinical Cardiology. A Tribute to W. Proctor Harvey.* (ed. Chizner MA), pp. 1249–1274. Laennec Publishing, Cedar Grove, NJ, 1998.
7. Kaplan NM. *Clinical Hypertension*, 7th edn. Williams and Wilkins: Baltimore, MD, 1998.
8. Krakoff LR. *Management of the Hypertensive Patient*. Churchill Livingstone. New York, 1995.

3

Chapter

3.2

3

Home blood pressure

J-M Mallion

Introduction

The principles of blood pressure measurement have not changed for over a century. In 1896 Riva-Rocci described the first mercury manometer. In 1905 the Russian surgeon Nikolai Korotkoff proposed the use of the auscultation method and the concept of systolic blood pressure (SBP) and diastolic (DBP) pressure was established.

Over time, and with the establishment of various recommendations, the basic method evolved but remained almost the exclusive domain of the doctor in his surgery, but in recent years the development of self-measurement has become widespread. The first description of home measurement was by Brown around 1930 when he described the use of the technique in a young man over a period of three years. Other key dates were the integration of the sphygmomanometer and cuff in 1967 and, in 1975, the first electronic sphygmomanometers for self-measurement. In 1985 the first oscillometric measure was described and finally in 1992 the first possibilities of measurement at the wrist and in the finger.

It is of interest to examine the elements which led to the use of home measures instead of surgery-based measures or other measures such as ambulatory measurement of blood pressure (AMBP). These elements include:

- The discovery in 1940 by Ayman and Goldshine that the blood pressure levels at home were lower than those found in the surgery.
- The cumulation of studies over the years, which have revealed that such data can yield interesting information of a diagnostic, prognostic and therapeutic nature.
- The advancement of technology with the appearance of reliable automatic devices that are easy to use by the patient and relatively low priced.

In this chapter we will discuss the conditions and methods of measurement without discussing the choice of machines. We will also discuss normal or reference values, and the usefulness for diagnostic, prognostic and therapeutic applications.

Definition

Self blood pressure measurement can be defined as the measurement by the subject himself or herself of his or her blood pressure BP in a conscious and voluntary manner. This measure is usually carried out in the home and is thus called 'home blood pressure' (HBP). Of course the blood pressure can, and should be measured by the patient in other circumstances.

Technique – measurement conditions

HBP should be considered as a medical act, which means that the doctor and the patient must respect certain recommendations. Some of these recommendations are the same as for taking blood pressure readings in the surgery. Others are related to informed consent by the subject and will render the technique inapplicable if the subject is incapable of understanding it. [1–7]

Measurement technique

The subject is informed of the necessity of placing the cuff on the skin and not on the clothes which could act as a tourniquet. The subject must also correctly position the cuff so that the center of the inflatable section of the cuff can be placed in the middle third of the arm opposite the humeral artery. The subject also needs to know how to identify manually the lower border of the cuff placed 3 cm above the bend of the elbow. It is necessary to obtain good support during the inflation of the cuff and ensure proper use of the bulb system. The reduction of the cuff inflation should be at a constant speed and ought to be by means of a deflation button or indeed be automatic.

BOX 3.2.1 Measurement conditions

These are dependent on factors which influence blood pressure levels such as the diurnal cycle with blood pressure higher by day than by night and the variations related to activity such as static or dynamic exercise or psychosensorial influences related to mental activity, emotion, alcohol consumption, or medications (sympathicomimetics or antidepressants).

Whatever the objectives of the measurement it is necessary to carry out the readings under strict conditions as follows.

- Reading should be before meals, after five minutes rest in a calm and relaxed environment.
- The subject should not take alcohol or tobacco.
- After the placement of the cuff, the arm should be situated at the level of the heart (below this level the blood pressure is overestimated and vice versa).
- The ideal position, which should always be recommended to the subject, is sitting with the arm extended and resting on a table. If the cuff cannot be inflated automatically, then it should be placed on the opposite arm to that which inflates the cuff.

Instruction of the patient is a medical act and thus implies a level of competence and the investment of time. It should be carried out by a doctor or a nurse and should include some simple explanations about blood pressure and its variations and consequences as well as the ideal conditions of measurement and an explanation of the equipment to use.

In a more formal setting we could envisage an interview with more detailed instructions and the use of written support material. Also possible would be the formation of groups for instruction and training, perhaps with video support. Not all patients are capable of benefiting from such intervention for various reasons which have to be evaluated, such as their level of education and social class, the level of medical support, age, motivation and the amount of time available for the measures, as well as the training time.

Results

Results are valid when a sufficient number of recordings have been acquired. It is recommended that three successive measures be obtained at each time. At least two measurements during the day before meals and between 6 a.m. and 8 a.m. in the morning and between 6 p.m. and 8 p.m. in the evening are recommended.

During the week, two estimations per day for at least three or four days should be completed, taking into account days of activity and of rest.

Over longer periods (months or years) this frequency should be adapted in relation to the clinical state of the subject. When a diagnosis of hypertension has been made or when antihypertensive treatment has been commenced, the frequency could be once or twice a month. It could be once or twice every three to six months in subjects without any particular diagnostic problems or in whom the treatment is well tolerated.

It is very important that the results of SBP and DBP and of heart rate be recorded and shown at each consultation. This record is kept by the patient.

Reference values

Established 'normal values' do not exist and only one paper [8] has addressed the topic in this context, using epidemiological data. Furthermore, these data cannot be widely applied as the data concerns cerebrovascular events in a Japanese population.

The data from studies to date have been subject to a meta-analysis performed by Thijs *et al.* [9] and refer to 17 studies of which nine referred to normotensive populations. The results of this meta-analysis need to be interpreted with particular caution for a variety of reasons (Table 3.2.1). The studies were carried out on a variety of subjects including volunteers, students and occupational groups. Likewise, the equipment used varied with automatic machines in some cases and using auscultatory or oscillometric methods in others. The values accepted for upper values differ little whether calculated by parametric or non-parametric methods and Thijs *et al.* [9] accepts 135–137 mmHg for the SBP and 86–89 mmHg for DBP. The reference value proposed in the recommendations of the JNCVI 1997 are 135/85 mmHg. The last recommendations of WHO [7] are still lower (around 125/80 mmHg).

In any case the following points are crucial [10–12]: that blood pressure at any age is higher in men and increases with age and is also lower in the morning than the evening and higher in the winter compared to the summer [13]. These values are lower than those obtained in the surgery and this difference is greater for the SBP. In relation to the other methods of measurement, the values obtained in the surgery are higher than those found at home depending on whether the subject is well versed in the procedure and used to frequent recordings in which case these differences may be small or not evident. This is particularly the case in hypertensive subjects on long-term treatment [14].

3

Table 3.2.1 Description of studies included in the meta-analysis*

Source	Subjects	n†	Age (years) (range)	Men (%)	Home BP monitoring device‡	Frequency of measurements		
						days§	Time	Sequence‖
Bättig et al. (1989)	NT	41	? (19–68)	?	Sysditon	14	M+E	1 (?)
Beckman et al. (1981)	NT, military enlistment center	22	22 (21–24)	100	SK-Test 2001	14	M+A	1 (L)
Brody and Rau (1994)	Healthy volunteers	80 (80)	31 (22–53)	57	Sanoquell 320661	7	E	1 (S)
De Gaudemaris et al. (1994)	Students, workers, non-workers	390 (318)	38 (20–59)	54	Tensiopuls UA516	3	M+E	3 (S)
Imai et al. (1993)	Population	871 (707)	46 (7–98)	43	HEM 401C	3–28	M	1 (S)
James et al. (1988)	NT volunteers	14	24 (?–?)	40	?	6	M+E	3 (S)
Johnson (1989)	NT	24	20 (19–25)	100	Marshall	28	M+E	1 (S)
Joossens et al. (1971)	White-collar workers	39 (?)	? (17–65)	49	?	63	M+E	2 (L+E)
Julius et al. (1974)	NT	49	25 (?–?)	100	?	7	M+E	1 (S)
Julius et al. (1992)	Population	937 (840)	30 (18–38)	?	Marshall (104)	7	M+E	1 (S)
Kawabe et al. (1994)	NT students	72	16 (15–17)	100	EW 255	1	M+E	3 (S)
Kesteloot et al. (1980)	Volunteers	758 (?)	39 (20–59)	44	Auto-test SK, Presso-stabil	3	M+E	2 (L+E)
Kjeldsen et al. (1993)	Healthy	40 (40)	32 (20–40)	100	HC 1401	7	?	2 (S)
Mancia et al. (1995)	Population	1438 (1225)	46 (25–64)	49	HP 5331	1	M+E	1 (S)
Mengden et al. (1990)	Employees	122 (61)	43 (?–?)	62	Sysditon	7	M+E	1 (?)
Saito et al. (1990)	NT	25	21 (18–24)	100	EW 255	7	M+E	3 (S)
Weisser et al. (1994)	Population	503 (?)	47 (20–90)	53	OM 1	14	M+E	1 (S)

* BP, blood pressure; NT, normotensive; M, morning; E, evening; A, afternoon; and ?, data not available.
† Total number of participants (number of normotensives).
‡ The manufacturers (and their locations) are Sysditon (Friederich Bosh, GmbH, Juningen, Germany); SK-Test 2001 (Speidel & Keller, Germany); Sanoquell 320661 (Bosh + Sohn, Germany); Tensiopuls UA 516 (OCEM Co, Rambouillet, France); HEM 401C (Omron Life Science Co Ltd, Kyoto, Japan); Marshall (Marshall Products Inc, Lincolnshire, Il); EW255 (National, Osaka, Japan); Auto-test SK (Presso-Stabil); Norelco HC 1401 (North American Philips Co, Stanford, CA; HP 5331 (Philips, Tokyo, Japan); and OMI (Boehringer Mannheim, Switzerland).
§ Number of days during which self-recorded BPs were obtained.
‖ Number of measurements obtained consecutively in the sitting (S), lying (L), or erect (E) position.

Reference values

The values found are fairly similar to those obtained by ambulatory recordings over the daytime [12] (Figure 3.2.1). This difference between the measures at home and in the surgery is found in normotensives and hypertensives and is also the case for both men and women. It does not seem that patients classed as 'anxious' (outside formal scales) are more susceptible to having higher values in the surgery. For elderly subjects, the increase with age is less important with self-measurement than in the surgery but lower than ambulatory recordings. It seems also that the difference is greatest in hypertensive subjects perhaps because hypertensive subjects are more apprehensive about the clinic visit than normotensives. Heart rate measures are also higher in the surgery. In any case a significant correlation is found between the values measured in the surgery and self-measurement and also between self-measurement and ambulatory values.

The reproducibility of self-measurement is satisfactory over a short period both for measures carried out at home and at work [3]. Over longer periods of about a year, the reproducibility of measures outside the surgery is greater than clinic measures [15].

3

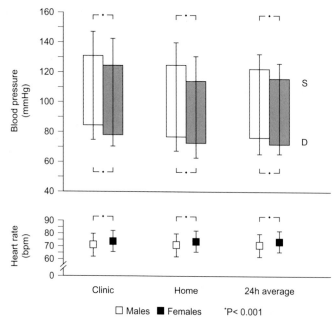

Fig. 3.2.1 Clinic, home and 24-hour average blood pressure and heart rate in men (*n* = 708) and women (*n* = 730). Data are shown as means ±SD.

Diagnostic data

Mild or moderate hypertension

It is important to identify clearly patients with mild to moderate hypertension. The most recent recommendations indicate that the diagnosis of hypertension cannot be confirmed except by a consultation. Two or more readings 2 minutes apart should be averaged. If the first two readings differ by more than 5 mmHg additional readings should be obtained and averaged. These measures should be repeated at least three times over a period of one month.

In practice, these recommendations are not always easy to follow because of the shortage of doctors' time and because of patient indisposition. Thus self-measurement seems an interesting alternative in a number of cases to confirm genuine hypertension [16]. Nagai *et al* appreciate the prevalence of hypertension by this way [17].

White coat or clinical hypertension

White coat hypertension is an entity which is defined as the presence of elevated blood pressure in the doctor's office but which is normal outside this setting. There is a current consensus which defines white coat hypertensives as those subjects who in the surgery have blood pressure values >140/90 mmHg and outside the surgery at <135/85 mmHg.

Most authors prefer ambulatory measures over the daytime to define reference values outside the surgery because of the possibility of numerous measures over prolonged periods under resting conditions and during periods of activity.

The use of self-measurement in the home is also useful for identifying the subject with white coat hypertension. It should be noted that it was by this means that the white coat effect was first identified and in this context that the 'blood pressure lowering effect of home recording' was noted [16–19].

Generally, there is a good concordance between blood pressure data from AMBP and self-measurement results in 80% of subjects [3]. Identical results cannot be expected from the two methods, however, as they are performed under different conditions. In particular, self-measurement is carried out after five minutes rest in a seated position while automatic blood pressure recording can be in the upright or seated position as well as during rest or activity. As in the case of AMBP, the frequency of the white coat effect is variable and depends on the reference values used. For example, in the Tecumseh study [18], the reference values were elevated and white coat hypertension occured in 7% of that population compared to the much larger incidence (30%) noted by Nagai *et al.* [17] where the reference values for home blood pressure is low at 131/79 mmHg. It is clear that one of the major indications for home measurement is the identification of white coat hypertension while the use of AMBP has other advantages and applications, such as a disturbance of the diurnal rhythm of blood pressure.

Hypertension and pregnancy

The occurrence of hypertensive disorders in pregnancy is common. Hypertension is one of the major causes of morbidity and mortality for the mother and the baby accounting for 15.5% of maternal deaths directly [20]. Several attempts at classification have been made in order to differentiate these disorders and to more easily identify patients at risk. Currently, there is no means of detecting this problem at an early stage and once the diagnosis of hypertension has been established there is no means of quickly identifying which mother is going to develop pre-eclampsia or eclampsia. The only possibility is regular and close supervision in order to reduce the risks of early intervention. In this situation, the use of self-measurement could reduce the frequency of visits and hospitalizations and, while motivating the expectant mother, allow her greater liberty. By this means the blood pressure can be controlled daily but these measures should be linked with parallel measures of weight as well as daily estimation of proteinuria by use of dipsticks [20].

Prognostic data

The usefulness of data from measurement of blood pressure in the surgery has been widely useful for the evaluation of morbidity and mortality. The use of ambulatory measurements or self-measurement is no longer controversial. Investigation of the effects of blood pressure measured in the surgery does not show any correlation between the

3

level measured and the end-organ effects on the kidneys or heart as, for example, left ventricular hypertrophy (LVH) or microalbuminuria. In contrast, such correlations have been found in numerous studies investigating blood pressure by ambulatory measures but few studies using self-measures have been performed. Mancia *et al.* [21] have shown a significant correlation between the level of LVH as measured by echocardiography and self-measures, although the level of correlation is less than that found by ambulatory measures. In both cases the level of correlation was less than 0.50.

As regards mortality the only data are those of Imai *et al.* [22] for overall cardiac mortality and those of Sakuma *et al.* [8] for mortality by cerebrovascular accident (Figure 3.2.2). A population of 1789 subjects had both surgery levels of blood pressure and self-measures plus ambulatory levels and were followed for 5.1 ± 2.2 years. As regards general cardiovascular mortality, Kaplan–Meier survival curves showed significant differences in the survival distribution between home systolic blood pressure and home diastolic blood pressure levels. Individuals in the highest quintile showed the poorest survival. Such a trend was not observed for the screening of blood pressure. There was a J-shaped relationship between the baseline home diastolic pressure level and the relative hazard ratio for cardiovascular mortality. Such a trend was also observed in home systolic blood pressure. However, no such trend was observed for screening of blood pressure.

BOX 3.2.2 Compliance

All the studies examining the level of compliance of hypertensive subjects are in agreement that after a year of follow up, on average, only 50% of subjects take their treatment in a regular manner. This poor compliance seems peculiar to hypertensive populations perhaps because it seems innocuous and that patients can pass many years without any obvious effects. Thus they are not motivated to take tablets regularly, which could cause some side effects. The analysis of predictive factors for non-compliance such as age, sex, social class, level of education, intelligence, etc. is not doubt of interest but does not provide a solution to the problem. The use of self-measurement may encourage compliance, but the few studies carried out are fairly old and based on measurement systems which were not automated [23]. These studies have shown an improvement in compliance related to a better awareness of their disorder and the antihypertensive effects of the doses prescribed. To date it has not been shown formally that this improvement in compliance leads to a better control of blood pressure. A study by Myers [24] draws attention to the possibility of reporting bias with certain subjects recording only the blood pressure values 'of interest' and thus it is recommended using technology with a memory. Teletransmission may also be used for self-measures of blood pressure. This can be done directly by modem or by a system of exchange of information with recording of other elements such as compliance and the consumption of medications and the presence of possible secondary effects. This mode of approach seems to lead to better compliance and to an important reduction in blood pressure in non-compliant subjects [25].

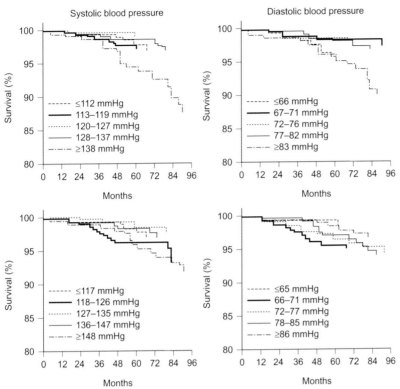

Fig. 3.2.2 Kaplan–Meier estimate of event probability (cardiovascular and cerebrovascular mortality) based on home (*n* = 1789) blood pressure levels. Blood pressure levels were classified into quintiles and survival rate is illustrated for each quintile.

Therapeutic applications and therapeutic trials

Therapeutic applications

It is necessary to differentiate the uses and the practical applications of this method of blood pressure measurement. In ordinary practice in the doctor's surgery and during randomized trials performed to examine the benefits of treatment. In daily practice the interest of this tool derives from data acquired previously.

- The elimination of poor precision and operator errors plus the possibility of multiple measures during the day or over time in reproducible conditions of rest or activity.
- The demonstration of a white coat effect which could lead to a diagnosis of hypertension and lead to the introduction of treatment.
- The uncovering of a falsely resistant hypertension when treatment is incorrectly given to patients with white coat hypertension.
- The possibility of improving compliance in patients who accept the principle of self-measurement. They are more involved in the follow up of their treatment as they can appreciate immediately the effect on their blood pressure benefits to be achieved. Ultimately, one could envisage that the patient could learn to modulate his or her own

treatment according to self-measurement results but care has to be taken that the situation is correctly managed.

Therapeutic trials

The reflections noted above are also valid in the context of clinical trials but with the proviso that the doctor should not be led to overestimate the benefits since the results are not subject to blinded trials. However, the use of self-measurement could improve precision and the sensitivity of therapeutic studies by reducing the standard deviation and the mean difference and improve the correlation coefficients between blood pressure measures. By decreasing the variability of the blood pressure values obtained, the sample size of hypertension trials designed to detect even minor blood pressure changes, can be reduced [26,27].

Thus we could reduce the number of patients required to detect a difference of 5 mmHg in DBP from 88 to 23 mmHg in the context of a trial in parallel groups in comparison to measures in the doctor's surgery[28]. Even if the number of trials using self-measurement is limited, the results are concordant on a number of points. Studies are practically possible even involving such large numbers as 1000 or 2000 patients. The use of home blood pressure measurement increases the power of cooperative trials allowing either study of fewer subjects or detecting a smaller difference in blood pressure. The use of measures taken in the morning and the evening allows some assessment of the peak trough effects if the time of the recording is well noted as well as the time of taking the medication. Thus the duration of action of a treatment can be better appreciated. So we should consider that this type of measure could be a good choice in chronopharmacology studies in hypertension [27,28].

At the dawn of the 21st century, one cannot discuss medical innovation without attention to cost [29]. Theoretically, self-measurement should reduce costs because of more precise and reproducible blood pressure values by allowing repeated measures. This should reduce the number of consultations and allow better use of therapeutic interventions with more precise assessment of effects. Several studies have confirmed this impression.

Summary

Self-measurement of blood pressure at home has developed enormously in recent years and this has been in large part driven by technological development with non-cumbersome lightweight automatic electronic devices. Nonetheless, it is crucial that the technique be recognized as a medical intervention and that the doctor needs to be involved at several levels:

● advice on choice of material;
● decisions about type and conditions of recordings;
● interpretation of results.

For each of these steps there now exists precise recommendations and rules. Reference values have recently been revised at 125/85 mmHg for the WHO [7] and are lower than normal surgery values. The advantages of the technique in diagnosis are well defined: more data than from measurement in the surgery, identification of the white coat effect, and follow up of high-risk pregnancy. As regards prognosis, currently active studies may yield results but it already appears that the method is superior to surgery estimates.

The therapeutic applications of self-measurement are many:

- it verifies the reality of hypertension before treatment;
- repeated untroublesome measurement for the patient and the doctor; and
- more objective, repeated and reproducible results in research trials, allowing a smaller population to be studied.

More generally, it seems that self-measurement may lead to better compliance in patients who can adapt to it because of their greater participation in their treatment. This may lead to better blood pressure control. Thus, this technique is about to undergo widespread development particularly as the technology of the equipment develops.

References

1. O'Brien E, O'Malley K, Fitzgerald D. The role of home and ambulatory blood pressure recording in the management of hypertension. *J Hypertension* 1985;**3** (Supp 1):35–39.
2. Mallion JM, Asmar R, Poggi L, Safar M. Pression artérielle, automesure, recommandations, Société Française d'Hypertension Artérielle, Groupe de la Mesure. *Arch Mal Cœur* 1989;**S2**:1001–1005.
3. Padfield PL, Stewart MJ, Gough K. The role of self-measurement of blood pressure in the management of hypertension. *Blood Pressure Monitoring* 1996;**1**(Supp 2):S15–S18.
4. Pickering TG. Recommendations for the use of home (self) and ambulatory blood pressure monitoring. *Am J Hypertension* 1995;**9**:1–11.
5. Celis H, De Cort P, Fagard R *et al.* For how many days should blood pressure be measured at home in older patients before steady levels are obtained *J Human Hypertension* 1997;**11**:673–677.
6. The Sixth Report of the Joint National Committee on Prevention, Detection, and Treatment of High Blood Pressure. NIH Publication No 98–4080;1997.
7. 1999 World Health Organization – International Society of Hypertension Guidelines for the Management of Hypertension. Guidelines Subcommittee. *J Hypertension* 1999;**17**:151–183.
8. Sakuma M, Imai Y, Tsuji I *et al.* Predictive value of home blood pressure measurement in relation to stroke morbidity: a population-based pilot study in Ohasama, Japan. *Hypertension Res* 1997;**20**:167–174.
9. Thijs L, Staessen JA, Celis H *et al.* Reference values for self-recorded blood pressure. *Arch Intern Med* 1998;**158**:481–488.
10. Mengden T, Bättig B, Edmonds D *et al.* Self-measured blood pressure at home and during consulting hours: are there any differences? *J Hypertension.* 1990;**8**(Supp 3):S15–S19.
11. De Gaudemaris R, Phong Chau N, Mallion JM. Home blood pressure: variability, comparison with office readings and proposal for reference values. *J Hypertension,* 1994;**12**:831–838.
12. Mancia G, Sega R, Bravi C *et al.* Ambulatory blood pressure normality: results from the PAMELA study. *J Hypertension* 1995;**13**:1377–1390.
13. Minami J, Ishimitsu T, Kawano Y, Matsuoka H. Seasonal variations in office and home blood pressures in hypertensive patients treated with antihypertensive drugs. *Blood Pressure Monitoring* 1998;**3**:101–106.

References

14. Kjeldsen SE, Hedner T, Jamerson K *et al*. Hypertension optimal treatment (HOT) study. Home blood pressure in treated hypertensive subjects. *Hypertension* 1998;**31**:1014–1020.

15. Sakuma M, Imai U, Nagai K *et al*. Reproducibility of home blood pressure measurements over a 1-year period. *Am J Hypertension* 1997;**10**:798–803.

16. Kleinert HD, Harshfield GA, Pickering TG *et al*. What is the value of home blood pressure measurement in patients with mild hypertension? *Hypertension* 1984;**6**:574–578.

17. Nagai K, Imai Y, Tsuji I *et al*. Prevalence of hypertension and rate of blood pressure control as assessed by home blood pressure measurements in a rural Japanese community, Ohasama. *Clin Exp Hypertension* 1996;**18**(5):713–728.

18. Julius S, Mejia A, Jones K *et al*. White coat versus sustained borderline hypertension in Tecumseh, Michigan. *Hypertension* 1990;**16**:617–623.

19. Hall CL, Higgs CMB, Notarianni L. Value of patient-recorded home blood pressure series in distinguishing sustained from office hypertension: effects on diagnosis and treatment of mild hypertension. *J Human Hypertension* 1990;**4**(Supp 2):9–13.

20. Rushbrook J, Shennan A. Self monitoring of blood pressure in pregnancy. *Prof care mother Child* 1997;**7**(4):88–90.

21. Mancia G, Zanchetti A, Agebiti Rosei E *et al*. Ambulatory blood pressure is superior to clinic blood pressure in predicting treatment induced regression of left ventricular hypertrophy. *Circulation* 1997;**95**:1464–1470.

22. Imai Y, Ohkubo T, Tsuji I *et al*. Prognostic value of ambulatory and home blood pressure measurements in comparison to screening blood pressure measurements: a pilot study in Ohasama. *Blood Pressure Monitoring* 1996;**1**(Supp 2):S51–S58.

23. Edmonds D, Foerster E, Groth H *et al*. Does self-measurement of blood pressure improve patient compliance in hypertension? *J Hypertension* 1985;**3**(Supp 1):31–34.

24. Myers MG. Self measurement of blood pressure at home. The potential for reporting bias. *Blood Pressure Monitoring* 1998;**3**(Supp 1):S19–S22.

25. Triedman RH, Kasis LE, Jette A *et al*. A telecommunication system for monitoring and counseling patients with hypertension impact on medication adherence and blood pressure control. *Am J Hypertension* 1996;**9**:285–292.

26. Bobrie G, Dutrey-Dupagne C, Vaur L *et al*. Mise en évidence de différences dans l'effet de deux antihypertenseurs par automesure tensionnelle: comparaison du trandolapril et du périndopril. *Thérapie* 1997;**52**:187–193.

27. Vaur L, Dubroca I, Dutrey-Dupagne C *et al*. Superiority of home blood pressure measurements over office measurements for testing antihypertensive drugs. *Blood Pressure Monitoring* 1998;**3**:107–114.

28. Mengden T, Bättig B, Vetter W. Self-measurement of blood pressure improves the accuracy and reduces the number of subjects in clinical trials. *J Hypertension* 1991;**9**(Supp 6):S336–S337.

29. Wilson M, Cziraky MJ, Kalmanowicz J. The usefulness of home blood pressure monitoring in the managed care setting. *Blood Pressure Monitoring* 1998;**3**(Supp 1):S23–S27.

3.3

Ambulatory blood pressure monitoring

G Parati and G Mancia

Limitations of conventional clinic blood pressure measurements

In spite of its time-honored, and yet undisputable usefulness in clinical practice, blood pressure (BP) measurement in the physician's office by the traditional Riva Rocci–Korotkoff technique is affected by several problems [1,2]. These include a limited accuracy in a number of conditions, such as in obese subjects, pregnant women, children and elderly individuals (particularly for diastolic blood pressure), and the estimation of only a fraction of values of the pressure waves that occur over a 24-hour period. Indeed, a heart rate of 72 beats/min results in 103 680 pulse waves during 24 hour. This clearly underlines the limited ability of isolated cuff readings obtained in a clinic environment to fully quantify the actual blood pressure load exerted on the heart and blood vessels over the day and night. Such a limitation is further emphasized by the pronounced variability that characterizes BP in daily life, as clearly shown by studies carried out by means of 24-hour intra-arterial ambulatory BP monitoring techniques [3].

As illustrated in Figure 3.3.1, both fast and slow fluctuations occur continuously over the day and night, in response to different behavioral challenges, the magnitude of which is greater amongst hypertensive subjects (Figure 3.3.2) [4]. A further problem affecting

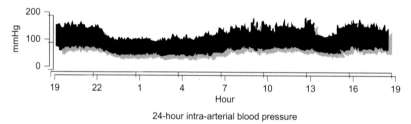

24-hour intra-arterial blood pressure

Fig. 3.3.1 Original intra-arterial ambulatory blood pressure tracing illustrating a normal 24-hour blood pressure profile.

Box 3.3.1 The 'white coat' effect

In a group of hospitalized patients we have provided the first direct quantification of the effects on BP of cuff measurements by a doctor. This was done by recording BP intra-arterially for 24 hours. As shown in Figure 3.3.3, the doctor's appearance was accompanied by an immediate rise in patient's BP and heart rate, presumably elicited by an alerting reaction. The BP rise reached its maximum at 2–4 minutes after the start of the visit, with a subsequent decline, although intra-arterial BP throughout the visit remained higher than pre-visit BP values [5,6]. In the group of subjects included in our study, the peak systolic and diastolic intra-arterial BP increases recorded during the physician's visit were on average 27 and 14 mmHg, respectively, with an extremely large interindividual difference (Figure 3.3.4) [7]. This clearly emphasizes that taking BP readings in a hurry only during the first few minutes of a consultation by a physician should be carefully avoided to prevent an important overestimation of patient's actual BP levels.

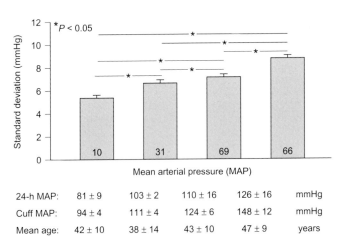

24-h MAP:	81 ± 9	103 ± 2	110 ± 16	126 ± 16	mmHg
Cuff MAP:	94 ± 4	111 ± 4	124 ± 6	148 ± 12	mmHg
Mean age:	42 ± 10	38 ± 14	43 ± 10	47 ± 9	years

Fig. 3.3.2 Blood pressure variability is shown as the standard deviation of 24-hour average blood pressure values obtained by ambulatory intra-arterial blood pressure monitoring in 10 normotensive subjects, 31 borderline hypertensive patients, 69 mild and 66 more severe hypertensive patients. 24-hour mean arterial pressure (MAP) ± SEM and mean office cuff values (±SEM) are shown at bottom. (From [4] modified, by permission.)

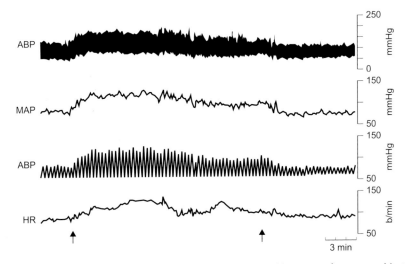

Fig. 3.3.3 Original tracing of intra-arterial blood pressure and heart rate from one subject over a 15-minute period when a doctor was at the bedside and measured blood pressure by the cuff method four times. Arrows indicate the beginning and the end of the visit. ABP, pulsatile arterial blood pressure; MAP, mean arterial pressure; ABP, arterial blood pressure integrated over 10-second periods. (From [5], by permission.)

sphygmomanometric BP readings is represented by the alerting reaction and pressure rise induced in the patient by the physician's visit, commonly known as the white coat effect. This phenomenon was described by Riva Rocci in his pioneering paper and its possible clinical relevance was suggested in 1940 by Ayman and Goldshine, who observed in 34 hypertensives that BP values recorded by the patient at home were invariably lower than the BP values recorded by the physicians at their offices, and that these differences were not transient but could persist over observation periods of several months.

3

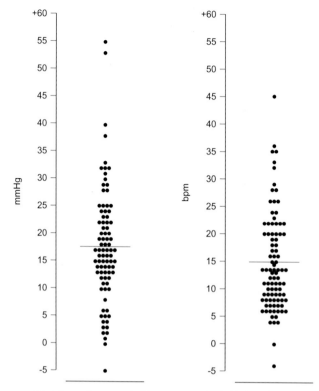

Maximal change in mean arterial pressure and HR with doctor's visit (*n*=88)

Fig. 3.3.4 Peak increase in intra-arterial mean arterial pressure (MAP, left) and heart rate (HR, right) in 88 patients during a visit by a physician measuring blood pressure with a sphygmomanometer. The intra-arterial blood pressure and HR values observed during the physician's visit were compared with those observed 4 minutes before the visit. Data are shown for individual patients (points) and as average changes for the group as a whole (horizontal lines). (From [9], by permission.)

The possibility of introducing correction factors for this phenomenon in individual subjects is made difficult by the above-mentioned high between-subject variability in such a pressor reaction and by the finding that the individual BP increases do not show any relationship with the patients' usual BP levels (either normal or elevated), with their age, their spontaneous BP variability over 24 hours, or their BP and heart rate response to laboratory tests aimed at assessing the subject's reactivity to stress [5–8]. Thus the error in BP estimation due to such a 'white coat effect' is both widely different among subjects and almost completely unpredictable in any given individual. Indeed, when we evaluated the effects of four repeated visits by the same physician on intra-arterial BP and heart rate over a 48-hour period in 35 subjects there were no significant differences in the average BP peaks observed during the four visits, indicating that no easy attenuation of this response and therefore no reduction in the error of overestimation can be expected with the simple repetition of the physician's visit, at least within relatively short time-windows [6]. However, in the same paper, we were able to observe that the peak BP and heart rate increases observed during the visit were

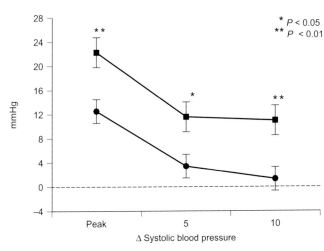

Fig. 3.3.5 Line graphs show rises in intra-arterial systolic blood pressure (SBP), during the visit of a physician (■) and nurse (●) in charge of measuring blood pressure with a sphygmomanometer. Data are shown as mean ± SEM changes from control values taken 4 minutes before the visit and refer to 30 subjects under 24-hour intra-arterial blood pressure monitoring. The nurse's visit preceded the physician's visit in 15 subjects and followed it in the remaining 15. (Modified from [6], by permission.)

significantly less if a nurse, rather than a physician, was in charge of BP measurement (Figure 3.3.5).

Other methods for blood pressure measurement

In the attempt to overcome the above limitations of the traditional Riva Rocci–Korotkoff method, a number of different approaches have been proposed over the years aimed at obtaining a more precise definition of subjects' 'true' BP level. Amongst them is the use of the so-called 'basal' BP, obtained after prolonged rest in absence of external stimuli, proposed by Smirk and coworkers in 1944 to replace the 'casual' BP measured by the doctor in his or her office. However, such an approach has not been generally employed for obvious technical difficulties and also because it does not lead to any important progress in the clinical evaluation of hypertensive patients. Other investigators have, on the other hand, proposed the use of BP values recorded under physical exercise or in response to laboratory stressors, values which were claimed to have a higher predictive value on either the development of stable hypertension or of cardiovascular complications than isolated office readings. In this instance, however, conflicting data are available on the actual clinical relevance of 'stress' BP obtained by such a procedure.

Much better results have been obtained with two other approaches, which are now widely used in clinical practice, namely home BP measurements and 24-hour ambulatory BP monitoring. In both instances BP is assessed out of the physician's office thus, in principle, offering a chance to avoid the problems of the 'white coat effect'.

This chapter will focus on the latter approach, i.e. on ambulatory blood pressure monitoring.

Techniques for ambulatory blood pressure monitoring

Intra-arterial technique

BP is recorded via a catheter inserted into a peripheral artery (usually the radial or the brachial), which is connected to a pressure transducer positioned at the heart level. Intra-arterial recordings are commonly performed under controlled laboratory conditions. A method for ambulatory intra-arterial BP recording in humans under daily-life conditions was made available in the late sixties by Bevan *et al.* in Oxford [3]. Use of such a technique has offered us valuable information on the variability that characterizes BP over 24 hours [4–8] and on the various mechanisms underlying the modulation of such changes. Its major advantages consist in the precision of the BP values so obtained and in the availability of a beat-to-beat assessment of BP variability. Its limitations are represented by the invasiveness and costs of the procedure, which do not allow its routine use in a clinical setting but restrict its application to a research environment.

Automatic or semi-automatic non-invasive techniques

Non-invasive techniques are certainly more suited to everyday use, and a number of different methods have been proposed to obtain BP quantification through the classic 'occlusion technique', but in absence of the direct intervention of a physician or a nurse and also during daily life activities.

Microphonic techniques

These techniques couple automatic or semi-automatic (i.e. triggered by the patient) cuff inflations with microphonic recording of Korotkoff sounds. Both the sounds and the cuff pressure are stored on a tape or on RAM cards and systolic and diastolic BP values are derived from the combined analysis of these signals. The first device based on this technique that was developed for ambulatory BP monitoring is the semi-automatic (i.e. cuff inflation had to be operated by the patient himself) Remler device, through which pioneering information on the clinical and prognostic value of ambulatory BP monitoring could be obtained. A number of fully automatic devices have since been developed both for home and ambulatory measurements, their major advantage being the theoretical possibility of providing BP values close to those measured by the physician with the Riva Rocci–Korotkoff method. A possible disadvantage is that the accuracy of the values so obtained can be limited by external noise and vibrations, which may disturb microphonic recordings, and by the possible displacement of the microphone, particularly in ambulatory conditions. The accuracy of microphonic BP reading can be improved by combining the recording of Korotkoff sounds with that of other signals, such as an ECG lead, that might guarantee the synchronization of the sounds recorded with the cardiac cycle, thus improving the signal-to-noise ratio.

Oscillometric method

The development of the oscillometric technique dates back to the times of Marey (1885) and Erlanger (1903). Its theoretical background is still based on some empirical considerations, in particular on the assumption that the maximal oscillation in the cuff air pressure observed during deflation corresponds to the mean intra-arterial pressure. Systolic and diastolic BP values are then computed through a specific algorithm. This technique is now largely used for both home and ambulatory BP recorders because of its simplicity, free from the methodological problems related to use of a cuff-associated microphone. As for microphonic devices, however, in this case careful validation through international protocols and 'local' validation by comparison with traditional measurements on the patient's arm is necessary to guarantee the accuracy of the BP values obtained [9].

Other methods

All the above methods only provide BP measurements on a discontinuous basis, usually at 15–20-min intervals. This offers reliable information on average BP levels over a given relatively wide time window. However, it cannot allow accurate assessment of the rapid and short-lasting changes in BP which occur spontaneously or in response to a number of laboratory tests that are commonly employed to assess the cardiovascular effects of neural influences. Until a few years ago this could be achieved only with the use of intra-arterial catheters, a procedure not free from risks and inconveniences to the patients. In the early seventies, a Czech physiologist, Ian Penaz, described a new approach which represents a major step forward in the field of non-invasive BP monitoring, based on the principle of vascular unloading. This approach makes use of a small cuff wrapped around a finger of the hand, which contains an infra-red photoplethysmograph and is connected with a computer-operated proportional pneumatic valve, a source of compressed air and an electropneumatic transducer. This device was later improved by Wesseling and coworkers in Amsterdam, resulting in a BP monitor called Finapres (from Finger Arterial PRESsure, Ohmeda, CO). In a number of validation studies this device was shown to provide BP values close to those simultaneously obtained through intra-arterial recordings, during anesthesia as well as at rest or under laboratory tests known to induce rapid and often marked BP changes [10] (Figure 3.3.6).

A portable version of this device is now also available, named Portapres (TNO, Amsterdam), which allows continuous non-invasive BP monitoring in ambulant subjects, all over 24 hours, with acceptable accuracy [11] (Figure 3.3.7).

Given the peripheral site of pulse detection with both Finapres and Portapres, a difference in pulse waveform is to be expected as compared to more proximal intra-arterial recordings. This is responsible for some

Techniques for ambulatory
blood pressure monitoring

Automatic or semi-
automatic non-invasive
techniques

3

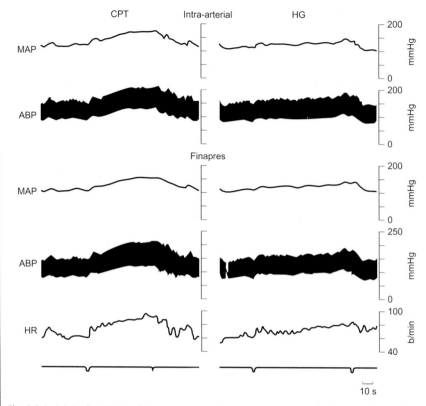

Fig. 3.3.6 Original tracings of intra-arterial and finger blood pressure (Finapres) from one subject during a cold pressor test and a hand-grip exercise. MAP, mean arterial pressure; ABP, pulsatile arterial pressure. (From [10], by permission.)

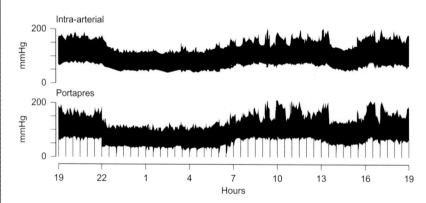

Fig. 3.3.7 Original ambulatory blood pressure recordings simultaneously obtained in the same subjects with the intra-arterial method (upper tracing) and with the Portapres device (lower tracing). Vertical bars at the bottom of Portapres tracing refer to between-finger shifts at 30-min intervals.

overestimation of intra-arterial systolic BP and of its variability, either as assessed as the standard deviation of the average value of the recorded signal, or as assessed in the frequency domain by power spectral analysis. Because of the systematic nature of this overestimation, however, correction factors can be applied, and a digital filter is now available to reconstruct the brachial pulse waveform out of finger pulse waveforms [12].

Methodological advantages of ambulatory blood pressure monitoring over isolated office readings

Evidence is available that analysis of 24-hour ambulatory BP recordings can yield a rich body of information on different aspects that characterize subjects' BP in daily life. This includes quantification of 24-hour, daytime or night-time average BP values, the BP fluctuations between day and night, the difference between clinic and 24-hour or daytime average BP and the different components of overall 24-hour BP variability. A number of studies have shown that the quantification of several of these parameters may allow a more precise diagnostic and prognostic evaluation of hypertensive patients than that allowed by office BP readings (see below) [7,9,13,14].

3

BOX 3.3.2 Technical advantages of ABPM vs clinic BP

Ambulatory BP recordings are characterized by a number of important technical advantages [9]. First 24-hour average BP values are more reproducible than isolated office readings, a reproducibility which, at least in part is a function of the higher number of BP values so obtained [15]. This represents an important advantage in clinical pharmacology, because an increased reproducibility of BP values may offer the chance to reduce the number of patients to be recruited in a study.

Secondly, non-invasive automatic ambulatory BP monitoring, although requiring repeated cuff inflations throughout the day and night and thus unavoidably worsening sleep quality, does not usually prevent the occurrence of a physiological nocturnal BP reduction. This was clearly shown by performing ambulatory intra-arterial blood pressure monitoring for 48 hours in a group of 17 hypertensive patients [16]. For 24 hours, the intra-arterial recording was coupled with non-invasive automatic blood pressure monitoring, while for the other 24-hour subperiod intra-arterial monitoring was carried out alone. The separate analysis of the two intra-arterial recordings did not show any significant difference in the degree of the nocturnal BP reduction based on whether simultaneous automatic BP monitoring was operative or not.

Thirdly, automatic and semi-automatic cuff inflations do not trigger any alerting reaction and pressure rise in the patients, and thus represent useful methods to avoid the inconveniences of the 'white coat effect' (see above). This, again, was shown by performing intra-arterial BP recordings in a number of patients during which non-invasive blood pressure measurements were delivered automatically or semiautomatically, i.e. triggered by the subject (Figure 3.3.8) [17].

Lastly, ambulatory BP monitoring is also largely unaffected by any placebo effect, no differences being found between 24-hour average BP values obtained at baseline and under placebo. A small placebo effect can be observed, however, during the first 4–8 hours of the recording, possibly due to an emotional reaction to the whole procedure the first time a patient is exposed to ambulatory BP monitoring [18].

Methodological
advantages of ambulatory
blood pressure monitoring
over isolated office
readings

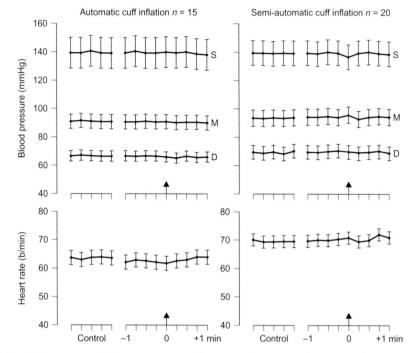

Fig. 3.3.8 Intra-arterial blood pressure and heart rate during the minute immediately preceding the beginning of cuff inflation (–1 to 0), the minute immediately after cuff inflation (0 to 1) and the 1-min control period 5 min before cuff inflation. Values measured every 15 s are shown. Data refer to hypertensive subjects in whom intra-arterial blood pressure was monitored for several hours in combination with automatic ($n = 15$) or semi-automatic ($n = 20$) non-invasive blood pressure monitoring in the contralateral arm. Automatic and semiautomatic blood pressure readings were obtained every 10 min. Data were averaged in each subject and mean $\pm$ SEM calculated for the group as a whole. M, mean arterial pressure; S, systolic; D, diastolic. Arrows refer to the time of cuff inflation. (From [17], by permission.)

The methodological advantages of ambulatory blood pressure monitoring need, however, to be considered vis-à-vis some methodological problem still waiting for an optimal solution. First, although the discontinuous nature of automatic blood pressure readings provided by these techniques does not prevent the reliable calculation of the 24-hour average BP values, intermittence of BP measurements does represent a major problem in the assessment of BP variability, because all fast BP changes are missed, and the resulting calculation of the standard deviation of the 24-hour BP values, i.e. a measure of overall BP variability, is prone to errors anytime automatic BP readings are taken at intervals longer than 10 minutes throughout the 24 hours [7,9]. Second, the accuracy of automatic BP measurements obtained in ambulant subjects may not be invariably guaranteed, even when using devices validated at rest according to International Guidelines. Again, this can be shown by the simultaneous performance of intra-arterial and automatic BP recordings over the 24 hours in ambulatory conditions. Widely employed devices, such as the Spacelabs 90202 and 90207 or the AM5600, have been tested in such a way, and the results show that

3

while 24-hour average values of systolic and mean arterial pressure are similar, non-invasive devices overestimated 24-hour intra-arterial diastolic BP significantly. When hourly, rather than 24-hour average values are considered, the discrepancy between systolic or diastolic BP obtained invasively and non-invasively is much wider than that usually reported when comparing intra-arterial with non-invasive measurements in resting conditions [19], a problem that emphasizes both the need for care in performing ambulatory BP recordings and the need for adequate signal editing to remove possible artifacts before proceeding to data analysis.

Clinical value of ambulatory blood pressure monitoring

The above-mentioned methodological advantages offered by ambulatory BP monitoring, have contributed to the large diffusion of this technique in a clinical setting, a diffusion that has been further stimulated by the growing amount of evidence collected on the diagnostic and (possibly) prognostic superiority of ambulatory BP values as compared to office BP readings. In particular, several parameters derived from the analysis of ambulatory BP recordings have been reported to have a clinical value.

24-hour average blood pressure

A large number of studies have shown that the organ damage associated with hypertension is more closely related to 24-hour average systolic or diastolic BP than to corresponding isolated clinic values [7,13,14,20] (Figure 3.3.9). This is, in particular, the case for left ventricular hypertrophy, although clear-cut evidence is also available for other types of cardiac damage (alterations in left ventricular function) and for extracardiac damage, for example, involving the brain (number of lacunae as quantified by nuclear magnetic resonance), the kidney (microalbuminuria and/or changes in renal function) and the small and large arteries (wall thickening and plaques). A recent example comes for the baseline data of the ELSA Study (European Lacidipine Study on Atherosclerosis) in which carotid artery wall abnormalities, as measured by ultrasonography, were related first to age and then to 24-hour average BP values (systolic and pulse pressure), the latter relationships being closer than those with the corresponding clinic BP values [21].

However, most of these data come from cross-sectional studies, and a major limitation in this field that persists is the limited number of prospective controlled studies proving the superior ability of 24-hour average BP to predict cardiovascular morbidity and mortality, as compared to clinic blood pressure, although most evidence has surfaced from uncontrolled observational studies only [22]. A controlled study (the SAMPLE Study, for Study on Ambulatory Pressure and Lisinopril Evaluation, see above) has recently been completed on the ability of ambulatory versus clinic BP control by treatment to predict regression of

3

163

Clinical value of
ambulatory blood pressure
monitoring

24-hour average blood
pressure

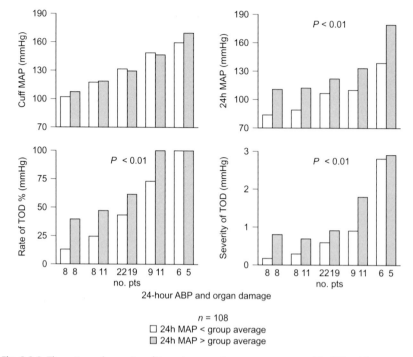

Fig. 3.3.9 The rate and severity of target organ damage was assessed in 108 subjects divided into five groups according to the increasing value of their clinic mean arterial pressure (MAP). The subjects in each group were further subdivided into two classes according to whether their 24-hour average blood pressure (intra-arterial recording) was below or above the average 24-hour mean value of the group. Note that within each group the two classes had a similar clinic MAP, but that the rate and the severity of target organ damage was less in the class in which 24-hour average MAP was lower. (From [13], by permission.)

echocardiographic left ventricular hypertrophy, i.e. an organ damage that frequently accompanies hypertension and increases its cardiovascular risk [14]. The results clearly show that regression of left ventricular hypertrophy was more closely predicted by treatment-induced changes in 24-hour hour average than in clinic BP, supporting the prognostic superiority of the former vs the latter approach (Figure 3.3.10) [14].

A few important questions need to be addressed in this field, however. Indeed, it should be clarified whether the greater ability of 24-hour average BP to correlate with organ damage or to predict its regression is due to either the greater clinical value of daily life BP versus a pressure taken in an artificial environment such as the doctor's office or just to the advantages of average values versus single values, as far as elimination of meaningless 'noise' and increase in reproducibility are concerned. We have shown, for example, that averages of multiple clinic pressure values have the same reproducibility as 24-hour average BP [23]. Furthermore, Fagard *et al.* have shown that when the number of clinic BP measurements is increased, its average correlation with left ventricular mass arises to the same degree as ambulatory BP average [24]. Thus the possibility that the advantage of ambulatory BP is

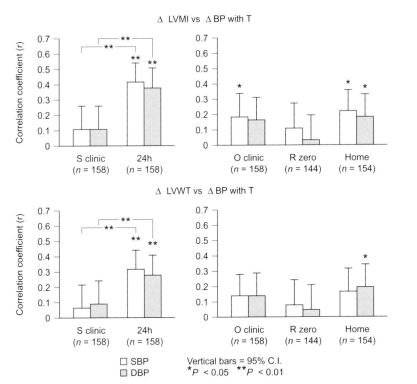

Clinical value of
ambulatory blood pressure
monitoring

24-hour average blood
pressure

3

Fig. 3.3.10 Average correlation coefficients between different blood pressures measured in the SAMPLE Study and left ventricular mass index (LVMI). Correlations are calculated for entry values and for changes induced by 12 months of treatment. Numbers in parentheses refer to the number of subjects used for correlations. Vertical bars indicate 95% confidence limits. Open histograms refer to systolic blood pressure (SBP), hatched histograms diastolic (D)BP. 24 h, 24-hour average BP; O, orthostatic BP; S, supine BP, R zero, random zero BP; T, treatment with lisinopril + hydrochlorothiazide when needed. (From [14], by permission.)

obtained in a simpler and cheaper fashion, just by increasing the number of clinic BP measurements, cannot be ruled out.

Moreover, in the general population clinic and 24-hour average BP correlate with each other but the correlation coefficient is about 0.6–0.7 [25]. Furthermore, in hypertensive patients the effects of treatment on clinic BP and 24-hour average BP correlate with each other with a correlation coefficient that is only about 0.5. This means that large differences may exist between clinic and average ambulatory pressures in any given individual. However, on average these two pressures tend to change in parallel [14], which suggests that in the hypertensive population at large there may be little advantage in assessing treatment based on ambulatory versus clinic blood pressure, because an average reduction of one means reduction of the other as well. This is indeed supported by Staessen *et al.* [26] who have recently shown regression of left ventricular hypertrophy to be similar in a group treated with the guidance of clinic versus another treated with the guidance of ambulatory blood pressure.

From a practical point of view, it is of relevance to assess whether the clinical information provided by 24-hour average BP can be obtained by shorter ambulatory recordings, with an advantage for cost and time. However, in a large number of hypertensive patients under 24-hour ambulatory intra-arterial BP monitoring, we have previously shown that no time-window within the 24 hours can consistently estimate 24-hour average blood pressure. Yet, in the SAMPLE Study regression of left ventricular hypertrophy was similarly predicted by 24-hour average BP and by daytime average BP, night-time average BP, 2-hour average and peak and trough BP values [14]. Thus it is indeed plausible that as far as clinical evaluations are concerned, shorter BP-monitoring times may be enough.

Additional information that can be obtained from ambulatory BP monitoring

Day versus night blood pressure

In recent years, this issue has received a large deal of attention from investigators who have frequently defined hypertensive patients as dippers or non-dippers based on a reduction in night-time BP respectively greater or smaller than 10% as compared to day-time values. The clinical importance of this phenomenon, however, is far from being established because, although several studies have reported non-dippers to have a greater organ damage and possibly a greater incidence of cardiovascular morbid events than dippers [27], other studies have been negative [14,28]. Moreover, the classification of hypertensive individuals into dippers and non-dippers has been shown to be poorly reproducible [14]. Finally, we have observed [14,28] that day-time and night-time blood pressures are closely related to each other and that this is the case also for day and night BP changes induced by treatment. Thus BP values during the day and night are not truly independent variables. We have also observed in the SAMPLE Study that (1) left ventricular mass index before treatment correlated to a similar degree with day and night blood pressure, (2) regression of left ventricular hypertrophy during treatment correlated to a similar degree with treatment-induced changes in day and night blood pressures and (3) in either condition cardiac structural alterations did not bear any relationship with day and night BP differences. These findings suggest that how BP is distributed between the day and night is not important, vis-à-vis the overall BP 'load' throughout the 24 hours. This may not apply however to the specific types of hypertensive subjects in whom the day–night BP difference is peculiarly disrupted, i.e. those who reproducibly have no nocturnal hypotension at all and those who are 'extreme' dippers. The former situation may reflect a clinically severe condition and/or a marked abnormality of autonomic cardiovascular regulation. The latter may directly lead to a organ damage by underperfusion.

BP variability

BP is highly variable over 24 hours and more so in hypertensive than normotensive subjects [4,29]. At any given 24-hour average blood

3

Clinical value of
ambulatory blood pressure
monitoring

Additional information
that can be obtained from
ambulatory BP monitoring

pressure, organ damage has been shown to be greater or to progress faster when 24-hour BP standard deviation is greater [13,30,31] (Figure 3.3.11). This has led to the hypothesis that the consequences of hypertension on the cardiovascular system may also depend to some degree on the extent of BP variations. Experimental support for such a hypothesis has been provided by a study in rats, showing in a prospective fashion, that the development of aortic atherosclerosis is more pronounced in animals with an experimentally induced increase in BP variability [32]. This has led to the concept that the effect of drug treatment should be so homogeneous over the 24 hours as to avoid a pharmacologically-dependent increase in BP variability. To quantify how homogeneous and balanced the BP effect of antihypertensive drugs can be over 24 hours, a number of mathematical indices have been proposed. The most popular one is the trough-to-peak ratio, i.e. the ratio

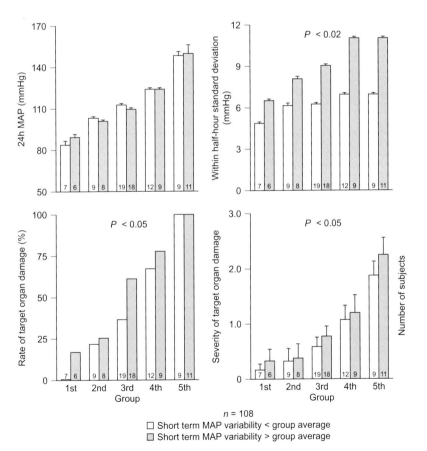

n = 108
☐ Short term MAP variability < group average
☐ Short term MAP variability > group average

Fig. 3.3.11 The rate and severity of target organ damage was assessed in 108 subjects divided into five groups according to the increasing value of their 24-hour average mean arterial pressure (MAP). The subjects in each group were further subdivided into two classes according to whether their within-half-hour standard deviation of MAP (short-term variability) was below or above the average short-term variability of the group. Note that within each group the two classes had a similar 24-hour MAP, but that the rate and the severity of target organ damage was less in the class in which short-term variability was lower. (From [13], by permission.)

Clinical value of
ambulatory blood pressure
monitoring

Additional information
that can be obtained from
ambulatory BP monitoring

3

between the drug-induced BP changes at trough (just before next dosing) and those at the time of the peak effect. When applied to the analysis of 24-hour ambulatory BP recordings in individual subjects, however, due to interference by spontaneous BP variability, the trough : peak ratio is affected by problems such as a poor reproducibility, and a non-normal dispersion of what sometimes are meaningless values [33]. Given the large diffusion of ambulatory BP monitoring in the evaluation of antihypertensive drugs, a new index has been more recently proposed to assess the 24-hour distribution of the antihypertensive effect over 24 hours, which takes into account the dispersion of such an effect over the whole 24-hour period. This index, termed 'smoothness index', is simply obtained by computing the ratio between the average of the 24-hourly changes in BP induced by treatment and the standard deviation of such an average change [34] (Figure 3.3.12). Data obtained from the SAMPLE study [34] have shown that, at variance from the trough : peak ratio, the smoothness index is related to the degree of BP variability under treatment and, most importantly, it correlates with the clinical benefit provided by antihypertensive treatment, namely, in this study, with the degree of regression of left ventricular hypertrophy (Figure 3.3.13).

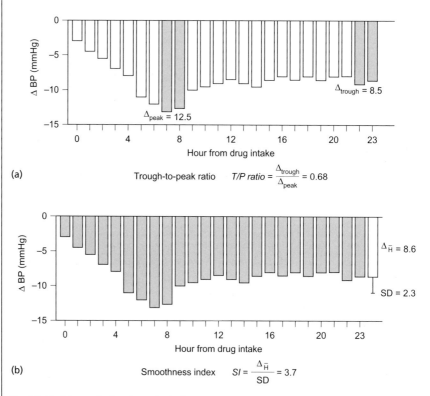

Fig. 3.3.12 Schematic drawing which illustrates the calculation of trough:peak ratio (**a**) and smoothness index (SI) (**b**) from hourly blood pressure (BP) values obtained before and during treatment by 24-hour ambulatory blood pressure recordings. BP, blood pressure; $\triangle H$, average of 24-hourly BP reductions induced by treatment; $SD_{\triangle H}$, standard deviation of the average hourly BP reduction. (From [34], by permission.)

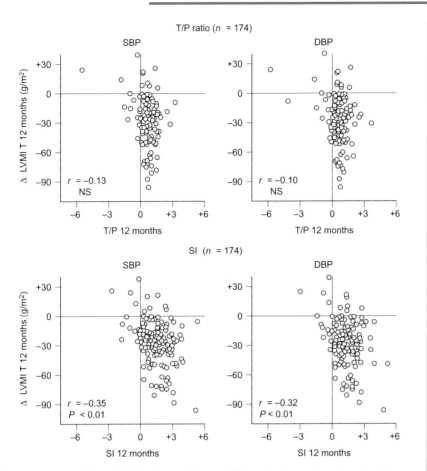

Fig. 3.3.13 Dots refer to individual correlation coefficients between trough:peak ratio (upper panels) or smoothness index (SI, lower panels) and the treatment-induced reduction in left ventricular mass index (LVMI). Data obtained after 12 months of treatment are shown separately for systolic and diastolic blood pressure. The *r* values between SI and LVMI are negative because an increase in SI was associated with a greater reduction in LVMI. (From [34], by permission.)

However, further evidence is needed to test the hypothesis that BP variability does indeed represent an independent additional risk factor on a firmer basis. This will not be easy to collect because, as mentioned above, when obtained through the intermittent BP sampling employed by automatic non-invasive BP monitoring devices, the true standard deviation of all BP values occurring over 24 hours is not accurately reflected. Beat-to-beat ambulatory monitoring is thus needed for this purpose, with obvious difficulties for most laboratories. New devices which allow ambulatory beat-to-beat BP monitoring to be obtained non-invasively may help however, in reaching this goal [11] (see above).

Conclusions

Based on these observations, ambulatory BP monitoring appears to represent a potentially useful means to improve diagnosis of hypertension, evaluate the risk inherent to a BP elevation and assess the efficacy of treatment. This is supported by the growing evidence that 24-hour average BP relates to the adverse consequence of hypertension on its target organs more closely than clinic BP and that improvement of organ damage is more effective when 24-hour ambulatory BP is controlled by treatment. However, ambulatory BP monitoring should not yet be a routine procedure, but rather be used as a source of supplementary information in selected cases. Specific conditions where ambulatory BP monitoring may be of use are when diagnosis of hypertension is uncertain, in particular because of the possible interference by a pronounced 'white coat effect', when treatment is seemingly ineffective despite multiple drug administration, when there is a chance of hypotensive episodes without or during treatment and when sustained disruption of the normal circadian BP profile is suspected. It cannot be doubted, however, that ambulatory BP monitoring is a tool of major importance for hypertension research. This is the case in the field of clinical pharmacology and in the investigation of normal and deranged mechanism for cardiovascular control, where computer analysis of BP variability may offer deeper insights.

References

1. Mancia G. Methods for assessing blood pressure values in humans. *Hypertension* 1983;**5**(Suppl. III), III5–III13.
2. Grim CM, Grim CE. Blood pressure measurement. In: *Hypertension Primer*, 2nd edn. (eds Izzo Jr JL, Black HR) pp. 295–298. Lippincott Williams & Wilkins, American Heart Association: Dallas, TX, 1999.
3. Bevan AT, Honour AJ, Stott FD. Direct arterial pressure recordings in unrestricted man. *Clin Sci* 1969;**36**:329–344.
4. Mancia G, Ferrari A, Gregorini L *et al.* Blood pressure and heart rate variabilities in normotensive and hypertensive human beings. *Circulation Res* 1983;**53**:96–104.
5. Mancia G, Bertinieri G, Grassi G *et al.* Effects of blood pressure measurements by the doctor on patients' blood pressure and heart rate. *Lancet* 1983;**ii**:695–698.
6. Mancia G, Parati G, Pomidossi G *et al.* Alerting reaction and rise in blood pressure during measurements by physician and nurse. *Hypertension* 1987;**9**:209–215.
7. Mancia G, Di Rienzo M, Parati G. Ambulatory blood pressure monitoring. Research and clinical applications. *Hypertension* 1993;**21**:510–524.
8. Parati G, Pomidossi G, Casadei R *et al.* Comparison of the cardiovascular effects of different laboratory stressors and their relationship with blood pressure variability. *J Hypertension* 1988;**6**:481–488.
9. Parati G, Mutti E, Ravogli A *et al.* Advantages and disadvantages of non-invasive ambulatory blood pressure monitoring. *J Hypertension* 1990;**8** (Suppl. 6):S33–S38.
10. Parati G, Casadei R, Groppelli A *et al.* Comparison of finger and intra-arterial blood pressure monitoring at rest and during laboratory testing. *Hypertension* 1989;**13**:647–655.
11. Imholz BPM, Langewouters GJ, van Montfrans GA *et al.* Feasibility of ambulatory, continuous 24-hour finger arterial pressure recordings. *Hypertension* 1993;**21**:65–73.
12. Gizdulich P, Imholz BPM, van den Meiracker DH *et al.* Finapres tracking of systolic blood pressure and baroreflex sensitivity improved by waveform filtering. *J Hypertension* 1996;**14**:243–250.
13. Parati G, Pomidossi G, Albini F *et al.* Relationship of 24-hour blood pressure mean and variability to severity of target-organ damage in hypertension. *J Hypertension* 1987;**5**:93–98.

References

14. Mancia G, Zanchetti A, Agabiti-Rosei E *et al.* for the SAMPLE Study Group: Ambulatory blood pressure is superior to clinic blood pressure in predicting treatment-induced regression of left ventricular hypertrophy. *Circulation* 1997;**95**:1464–1470.

15. Trazzi S, Mutti E, Frattola A *et al.* Reproducibility of non-invasive and intra-arterial blood pressure monitoring. Implications for studies on antihypertensive treatment. *J Hypertension* 1991;**9**:115–119.

16. Villani A, Parati G, Groppelli A *et al.* Noninvasive automatic blood pressure monitoring does not attenuate nighttime hypotension. *Am J Hypertension* 1992;**5**:744–747.

17. Parati G, Pomidossi G, Casadei R, Mancia G. Lack of alerting reactions to intermittent cuff inflations during non-invasive blood pressure monitoring. *Hypertension* 1985;**7**: 597–601.

18. Mutti E, Trazzi S, Omboni S *et al.* Effect of placebo on 24 hour non-invasive ambulatory blood pressure. *J Hypertension* 1991;**9**:361–364.

19. Groppelli A, Omboni S, Parati G, Mancia G. Evaluation of noninvasive blood pressure monitoring devices Spacelabs 90202 and 90207 versus resting and ambulatory 24-hour intra-arterial blood pressure. *Hypertension* 1992;**20**:227–232.

20. Mancia G, Omboni S, Parati G. Lessons to be learned from 24 hour ambulatory blood pressure monitoring. *Kidney Int* 1996;**49** (Suppl. 55):S63–S68.

21. Zanchetti A, Bond MG, Hennig M *et al.* on behalf of the ELSA Study Group. Risk factors associated with alterations in carotid intima-media thickness in hypertension: baseline data from the European Lacidipine Study on Atherosclerosis. *J Hypertension* 1998;**16**:949–961.

22. Verdecchia P, Porcellati C, Schillaci G *et al.* Ambulatory blood pressure: an independent predictor of prognosis in essential hypertension. *Hypertension* 1994;**24**:793–801.

23. Mancia G, Ulian L, Parati G, Trazzi S. Increase in blood pressure reproducibility by repeated semi-automatic blood pressure measurements in the clinic environment. *J Hypertension* 1994;**12**:469–473.

24. Fagard RH, Staessen JA, Thijs L. Relationships between changes in left ventricular mass and in clinic and ambulatory BP in response to anti-hypertensive therapy. *J Hypertension* 1997;**15**(12 Pt 1):1493–1502.

25. Mancia G, Sega R, Bravi C *et al.* Ambulatory blood pressure normality: results from the PAMELA Study. *J Hypertension* 1995;**13**:1377–1390.

26. Staessen JA, Byttebier G, Buntinx F *et al.* Anti-hypertensive treatment based on conventional or ambulatory blood pressure measurement. A randomized controlled trial. Ambulatory Blood Pressure Monitoring and Treatment of Hypertension Investigators. *J Am Med Soc* 1997;**278**(13):1065–1072.

27. O'Brien E, Sheridan J, O'Malley K. Dippers and non-dippers (letter). *Lancet* 1988; **ii**:397.

28. Omboni S, Parati G, Palatini P *et al.* Reproducibility and clinical value of nocturnal hypotension: prospective evidence from the SAMPLE study. Study on Ambulatory Monitoring of Pressure and Lisinopril Evaluation. *J Hypertension* 1998;**16**(6):733–738.

29. Mancia G, Parati G, Di Rienzo M, Zanchetti A. BP variability. In: *Handbook of Hypertension*, Vol. 17: *Pathophysiology of Hypertension*. (eds Zanchetti A, Mancia G), pp. 117–169. Elsevier Science: Amsterdam, 1997.

30. Frattola A, Parati G, Cuspidi C *et al.* Prognostic value of 24-hour BP variability. *J Hypertension* 1993;**11**:1133–1137.

31. Palatini P, Penzo M, Racioppa A *et al.* Clinical relevance of night-time BP and of day-time BP variability. *Arch Intern Med* 1992;**152**:1855–1860.

32. Sasaki S, Yoneda Y, Fujita H *et al.* Association of blood pressure variability with induction of atherosclerosis in cholesterol-fed rats. *Am J Hypertension* 1994;**7**:453–459.

33. Omboni S, Fogari R, Palatini P *et al.* Reproducibility and clinical value of the trough-to-peak ratio of the anti-hypertensive effect: evidence from the SAMPLE study. *Hypertension* 1998;**32**(3):424–429.

34. Parati G, Omboni S, Rizzoni D *et al.* The smoothness index: a new, reproducible and clinically relevant measure of the homogeneity of the blood pressure reduction with treatment for hypertension. *J Hypertension* 1998;**16**:1685–1691.

3.4

3

Special blood pressure measuring devices

E O'Brien

3

Introduction

Sphygmomanometry has evolved over nearly three centuries, but conventional sphygmomanometry, the technique with which we are all so familiar in clinical practice, was introduced just over a century ago by Riva-Rocci [1]. However, as we enter the new millennium a number of developments, not least being the availability of accurate automated devices, herald the demise of so-called classic sphygmomanometry and the dawning of a new era in blood pressure measurement. This new age will see the introduction of innovative technologies that will allow not only accurate non-invasive measurement of blood pressure but also an assessment of blood pressure as a dynamic phenomenon, the effects of which are as dependent on the waveform and velocity characteristics as on the level of the generated pressure within the cardiovascular system.

Blood pressure measurement provides a figure, or set of figures, to the measurer, which then form the basis for a decision, the exact nature of which is influenced by the reason for measurement, which may be clinical, therapeutic, research, or epidemiological, just to mention a few of the more common requirements for blood pressure measurement. So the measurement technique is always 'special' at least to the measurer, who rightly demands accurate and reproducible results. In considering how best to define a 'special blood pressure-measuring device,' I have taken the view that what may be regarded as 'special,' or avant-garde today will be passé tomorrow, and that it is necessary therefore to view blood pressure measurement as an evolving discipline, albeit one subject to change. To appreciate the developments that are influencing measurement, it is necessary to identify the point of departure from an established technique to a new methodology. In short, we must be prepared to glance back before looking forward.

Traditional sphygmomanometry

When sphygmomanometry was first introduced, it was regarded as so innovative – so 'special' – as to have little future; one commentator, writing in 1895, while acknowledging that 'the middle-aged and successful physician may slowly and imperceptibly lose the exquisite sensitiveness of his finger tips through repeated attacks of gouty neuritis,' doubted if the sphygmomanometer would be welcomed by 'the overworked and underpaid general practitioner, already loaded with thermometer, stethoscope, etc., etc., …'[2]. And yet the technique, modified by Korotkoff's addition of the stethoscope in 1908, has lived on for over a century, earning the reputation of having contributed more to cardiovascular science than any other measurement technique in clinical medicine[3].

The technique, however, is now under threat mainly because of the proposed banning of mercury from clinical use, but also because automated devices can now provide measurements that are not subject to the observer error of the traditional technique. The environmental call to ban mercury is because mercury is not merely a toxic substance but one that is bioaccumulable, and therefore persistently toxic. Much of the many tons of mercury supplied for the manufacture of sphygmomanometers and then distributed throughout the world to hospitals and countless individual doctors is never returned for disposal, but finds its way into the environment through evaporation, or dispersion in sewage and solid waste, most seriously damaging the marine environment. Ecologists and environmentalists resolved to reduce mercury in the environment to 'levels that are not harmful to man or nature before the year 2000'[1]. The mercury thermometer has been replaced in many countries, and in most Scandinavian countries and the Netherlands, where the use of mercury is no longer permitted in hospitals, the mercury sphygmomanometer is being relegated to the museum shelves. However, in other countries, the move to ban mercury from hospital use has been resisted – for the moment – on the grounds that the once common alternative, the aneroid sphygmomanometer, becomes inaccurate with use and should not, therefore, be substituted for the mercury instrument[1,4]. Of course, banning mercury from the wards raises another issue of considerable importance for clinical medicine: if we no longer have mercury, the argument that we measure what we see – the millimeter of mercury – is scarcely credible and the medical stance against its replacement with the *Système International* (SI) unit, the kilopascal, is no longer tenable[5,6].

The passing of the mercury sphygmomanometer should not in itself be a cause for concern. In fact, it might be argued that the sooner we rid ourselves of this most inaccurate technique, on which we base so many important decisions of management, the better. This is not to blame the mercury sphygmomanometer, but rather to impugn the most fallible part of the whole procedure – the human observer[7]. But if the mercury column is no longer available, what are the alternatives? In the past, the aneroid sphygmomanometers have been regarded as a reasonable substitute for the mercury sphygmomanometer, but because they become inaccurate with use without the operator being aware of such inaccuracy, and because they have not been subjected to independent validation, they are not generally recommended[8]. Automated devices, in their many guises, have performed badly in validation studies in the past[9], but recently, their record in this regard has been improving[10]. Before considering, therefore, how best to measure blood pressure without the mercury manometer, it is timely to review the state of the market in relation to automated devices in general.

The Working Group on Blood Pressure Monitoring of the European Society of Hypertension (ESH) published its recommendations on blood pressure measuring devices in the *British Medical Journal* (*BMJ*) in 2001 to guide the would-be purchaser through a complex market[10]. In the *BMJ* report, devices were assessed on the basis of published evidence of independent validation according to the British Hypertension Society (BHS) and Association for the Advancement of Medical Instrumentation (AAMI) protocols. The ESH is planning to update the *BMJ* report at regular intervals on its website.

Validation standards

In 1987, the AAMI published a standard for sphygmomanometers, which included a protocol for the evaluation of the accuracy of devices, and this was followed in 1990 by the protocol of the BHS[10]. Both protocols have since been revised[11,12], and as the two can be reconciled, the joint criteria are applied in most published validation studies. The criteria for fulfillment of the BHS protocol are that the test devices must achieve at least grade B for systolic and for diastolic pressures; the criteria for fulfillment of the AAMI protocol are that the test device must not differ from the mercury standard by a mean difference greater than 5 mmHg or a standard deviation greater than 8 mmHg.

Criteria for recommendation

The following criteria were used to designate devices according to accuracy in the *BMJ* report[10]:

'*Recommended*' – a device that fulfills the AAMI criteria for both systolic and diastolic pressures and achieves a BHS grade B or A for both systolic and diastolic blood pressures.

'*Not recommended*' – a device that fails the AAMI criteria for either systolic or diastolic pressure, and achieves a BHS grade C or D for either systolic or diastolic pressure.

'*Questionable recommendation*' – a device for which there is doubt about the strength of evidence, as may occur in the following circumstances: (i) when a device fulfills the criteria of one protocol but not the other, it may be best not to recommend the device for clinical use until a confirmatory study is performed; (ii) when the validation results are presented in abstract form only without sufficient detail being available to appraise the methodology, it may be best to withhold an opinion until the full results have been published, or at least provided to a would-be purchaser by the manufacturer; (iii) when the conditions of the protocols have not been fully adhered to (listed as 'protocol violation'); (iv) when a device fulfills the AAMI criteria for intra-arterial validation, it may be best to await a validation against indirect blood pressure measurement before recommending the device general clinical use; the BHS protocol does not advocate validation using direct intra-arterial measurement.

Identification of devices

The *BMJ* review was based on a follow-up of two previous surveys, and computerized search programs were used to identify validation studies in the literature up to December 1999. Blood pressure measuring devices were divided into two broad categories: *manual sphygmomanometers*, to include mercury and aneroid devices, and *automated sphygmomanometers*, to include devices for clinical use in hospitals, for self blood pressure measurement, and for ambulatory blood pressure measurement. With increasing pressure for a ban on mercury, a large market for alternative devices to the mercury sphygmomanometer has been created. Some devices for self-measurement

Table 3.4.1 Alternative devices to the mercury sphygmomanometer

Validated
1. Modified Omron HEM-705CP
2. Modified A & D UA-767
3. Omron HEM-907
4. WELCH ALLYN VITAL SIGNS monitor
5. BPM-100

Non-validated
6. GREENLIGHT 300
7. ACCUSPHYG
8. FINOMETER

of blood pressure have been successively modified for clinical use by increasing the length of tubing, and others are being developed but have not yet been validated; these devices are listed in Table 3.4.1[10].

Manual (mercury and aneroid) sphygmomanometers

These devices are listed in Table 3.4.2[10]. One model of the many mercury sphygmomanometers available, the PyMah, has been validated according to both protocols and was given the designation 'recommended.' As mercury sphygmomanometers generally adhere to a simple basic design with standard components, it is probably reasonable to assume that most, if not all, mercury sphygmomanometers would be of similar accuracy. The standard aneroid sphygmomanometer has only been formally validated recently according to the calibration procedure of the BHS protocol, and the results support reservations about aneroid devices because of their susceptibility to becoming inaccurate with use without this being apparent to the user.

Automated sphygmomanometers

Devices for clinical use in hospitals

These devices are listed in Table 3.4.3 [10].

Devices for self-measurement of blood pressure

There are a large number of automated devices for self-measurement of blood pressure, virtually all of which use the oscillometric technique. Formerly these devices used automated inflation and deflation of a cuff

Table 3.4.2 Manual devices which have been subjected to validation by the BHS and AAMI protocols. Grades A–D according to BHS protocol: A, best agreement with mercury standard; D, worst agreement with mercury standard. After O'Brien *et al.*[10]

Device	AAMI	BHS	Circumstance	Recommendation
PyMah Mercury	Passed	A/A	At rest	Recommended
Hawksley RZS: US model	Failed	B/D	At rest	Not recommended
Hawksley RZS: UK model	Failed	C/D	At rest	Not recommended
Aneroid device	n/a	Failed	In use; abstract only	Questionable recommendation

RZS = random zero sphygmomanometer; n/a = not applicable.

Table 3.4.3 Automated blood pressure measuring devices for clinical use in hospitals which have been subjected to validation by the BHS (devices must achieve at least grade B/B) and AAMI (mean difference ≤ 5 mmHg, SD ≤ 8mmHg) protocols. Grades A–D according to BHS protocol: A, best agreement with mercury standard; D, worst agreement with mercury standard. After O'Brien *et al.*[10]

Device	Mode	AAMI	BHS	Circumstance	Recommendation
Datascope Accutorr Plus	Osc	Passed	A/A	At rest	Recommended
CAS Model 9010	Osc	Passed	n/a	At rest in adults	Recommended
				Neonates	Recommended
Tensionic Mod EPS 112	Osc	Passed	B/A	At rest; abstract only	Questionable recommendation
Colin Pilot 9200	Tonometry	Passed	n/a	At rest; intra-arterial	Questionable recommendation
Dinamap 8100	Osc	Failed	B/D	At rest	Not recommended

Osc = oscillometric, Aus = auscultatory, n/a = not applicable.

Automated
sphygmomanometers

Devices for
self-measurement of
blood pressure

Automated devices for
upper arm measurement

applied to the upper arm over the brachial artery, but recently the technique has been used to measure blood pressure over the radial artery at the wrist; however, as they become inaccurate if the arm is not kept at heart level during measurement, there is reluctance to recommend them, regardless of accuracy.[10] Devices for measurement of blood pressure by occluding a digital artery in the finger are also available, but because the problem of limb position is even more critical and there is the additional problem of peripheral vasoconstriction affecting accuracy, this technique is no longer recommended, and these devices have not been considered in this review.

Automated devices for upper arm measurement

These devices are listed in Table 3.4.4[10].

Table 3.4.4 Automated blood pressure measuring devices for self-measurement of upper arm blood pressure which have been subjected to validation by the BHS (devices must achieve at least grade B/B) and AAMI (mean difference ≤ 5 mmHg, SD ≤ 8mmHg) protocols. Grades A–D according to BHS protocol: A, best agreement with mercury standard; D, worst agreement with mercury standard. After O'Brien *et al.*[10]

Device	Mode	AAMI	BHS	Circumstance	Recommendation
Omron HEM-400C	Osc	Failed	Failed	At rest	Not recommended
Philips HP5308	Aus	Failed	Failed	At rest	Not recommended
Philips HP5306/B	Osc	Failed	Failed	At rest	Not recommended
Healthcheck CX-5 060020	Osc	Failed	Failed	At rest	Not recommended
Nissei Analogue Monitor	Aus	Failed	Failed	At rest	Not recommended
Systema Dr MI-150	Osc	Failed	Failed	At rest	Not recommended
Fortec Dr MI-100	Osc	Failed	Failed	At rest	Not recommended
Philips HP5332	Osc	Failed	C/A	At rest	Not recommended
Nissei DS-175	Osc	Failed	D/A	At rest	Not recommended
Omron HEM-705CP	Osc	Passed	B/A	At rest	Recommended
Omron HEM-706	Osc	Passed	B/C	At rest	Not recommended
Omron HEM-403C	Osc	Failed	C/C	Protocol violation	Not recommended
Omron HEM-703CP	Osc	Passed	n/a	Intra-arterial	Questionable recommendation
Omron M4	Osc	Passed	A/A	Abstract only; detail missing	Questionable recommendation
Omron MX2	Osc	Passed	A/A	Abstract only; detail missing	Questionable recommendation
Omron HEM-722C	Osc	n/a	A/A	Protocol violation	Questionable recommendation
		Passed	A/A	Rest/elderly	Recommended
Omron HEM-735C	Osc	Passed	B/A	Rest/elderly	Recommended
Omron HEM-713C	Osc	Passed	B/B	At rest	Recommended
Omron HEM-737 Intellisense	Osc	Passed	B/B	At rest	Recommended
Visomat OZ2	Osc	Passed	C/B	At rest	Not recommended

Osc = oscillometric, Aus = auscultatory, n/a = not applicable.

Note in the first seven devices, grading criteria that had not been established though BHS protocol was in operation.

Table 3.4.5 Automated blood pressure measuring devices for self-measurement of blood pressure at the wrist which have been subjected to validation by the BHS (devices must achieve at least grade B/B) and AAMI (mean difference ≤ 5 mmHg, SD ≤ 8mmHg) protocols. Grades A–D according to BHS protocol: A, best agreement with mercury standard; D, worst agreement with mercury standard. After O'Brien *et al*.[10]

Device	AAMI	BHS	Circumstance	Recommendation
Omron R3	n/a	C/C	At rest; protocol violation	Not recommended
	Fail	D/D	At rest	Not recommended
Boso-Mediwatch	n/a	C/C	At rest; protocol violation	Not recommended
Omron Rx	Failed	B/B	At rest; abstract publication	Questionable recommendation

n/a = not applicable.

Automated devices for wrist measurement

These devices are listed in Table 3.4.5[10]. These devices have been validated against brachial arterial measurements.

Devices for ambulatory blood pressure measurement

There are two techniques for measuring ambulatory blood pressure: the commonly used method of intermittent measurement of blood pressure over the 24-hour period, and the developing method of continuous waveform analysis.

Devices dependent on intermittent blood pressure measurement

These devices are listed in Table 3.4.6[10]. Many of these devices have been validated in special groups, such as the elderly and pregnant women, and in differing circumstances, such as during exercise and in various postures.

Devices for continuous non-invasive finger blood pressure monitoring

The Portapres (TNO, Amsterdam), a portable recorder for 24-hour ambulatory monitoring, can provide beat-to-beat blood pressure monitoring that gives waveform measurements similar to intra-arterial recordings [10].

An automated alternative to mercury

From a review of the literature, it is evident that there are very many 'special' devices on the market, and that the accuracy of most of these has not been determined. Furthermore, of those that have been evaluated, rather few have fulfilled the requirements of the BHS and AAMI validation protocols.

Manufacturers of blood pressure measuring devices have failed to identify the need for reasonably priced accurate automated devices in clinical practice – a need which becomes all the more acute with the impending ban on mercury. Soundings from the manufacturing industry suggest that notice is now being taken of the need for an accurate

Table 3.4.6 Ambulatory blood pressure measuring devices which have been subjected to validation by the BHS (devices must achieve at least grade B/B) and AAMI (mean difference ≤ 5 mmHg, SD ≤ 8mmHg) protocols. Grades A–D according to BHS protocol: A, best agreement with mercury standard; D, worst agreement with mercury standard. After O'Brien et al.[10]

Device	Mode	AAMI	BHS	Circumstance	Recommendation
Accutracker II (30/23)	Aus	Passed	A/C	At rest	Not recommended
CH-DRUCK	Aus	Passed	A/A	At rest	Recommended
Daypress 500	Osc	Passed	A/B	At rest	Recommended
DIASYS 200	Aus	Passed	C/C	At rest	Not recommended
DIASYS Integra	Aus	Passed	B/A	At rest	Recommended
	Osc	Passed	B/B	At rest	Recommended
ES-H531	Aus	Passed	A/A	At rest	Recommended
	Osc	Passed	B/B	At rest	Recommended
Medilog ABP	Aus	Passed	n/a	At rest	Questionable recommendation
Meditech ABPM-04	Osc	Passed	B/B	At rest	Recommended
Nissei DS-240	Osc	Passed	B/A	Abstract only; detail missing	Questionable recommendation
OSCILL-IT	Osc	Passed	C/B	At rest	Not recommended
Pressurometer IV	Aus	Failed	C/D	At rest	Not recommended
Profilomat	Aus	Passed	B/A	At rest	Recommended]
	Aus	Passed	B/C	In pregnancy	Not recommended
Profilomat II	Osc	Failed	C/B	At rest	Not recommended
QuietTrak*[47–51]	Aus	Passed	B/B	At rest	Recommended
	Aus	Passed	B/B	At rest. Abstract	Questionable recommendation
	Aus	Failed	D/D	In preeclampsia	Not recommended
	Aus	Failed	B/B	In pregnancy	Not recommended
	Aus	Passed	A/A	At rest	Recommended
			A/A	During exercise	Recommended
			A/A	Different posture	Recommended
			A/A	In the elderly	Recommended
			A/A	In children	Recommended
			A/A	In pregnancy	Recommended
Save 33, Model 2	Osc	Passed	B/B	At rest	Recommended
Schiller BR-102	Aus	Passed	B/B	At rest	Recommended
	Osc	Failed	D/B	At rest	Not recommended
SpaceLabs 90202	Osc	Passed	B/B	At rest	Recommended
SpaceLabs 90207	Osc	Passed	B/B	At rest	Recommended
[64]	Osc	Passed	A/C	In pregnancy	Not recommended
[65]	Osc	Passed	B/B	In pregnancy	Recommended
[53]	Osc	Passed	B/C	In pregnancy	Not recommended
[57]	Osc	Failed	D/D	In pre-eclampsia	Not recommended
[66]	Osc	Passed	C/C	In pre-eclampsia	Not recommended
[67]	Osc	SBP pass	C	In children	Not recommended
		DBP fail	D	In children	Not recommended
[68]	Osc	Passed	A/B	Elderly standing and sitting SBP ≤ 160 mmHg	Recommended
[69]	Osc	Passed	A/D	Elderly supine over all pressures	Not recommended
	Osc	Passed	C/B	During hemodialyis	Not recommended
SpaceLabs 90217	Osc	Passed	A/A	At rest	Recommended
TM-2420/TM-2020	Osc	Failed	D/D	At rest	Not recommended
TM-2420 Model 6	Osc	Passed	B/B	At rest	Recommended
TM-2420 Model 7	Osc	Passed	B/B	At rest	Recommended
TM-2421	Osc	Passed	B/A	At rest	Recommended
Takeda 2421 [76]	Osc	n/a	C/C	In children and different posture	Not recommended
	Aus	n/a	A/B		Questionable recommendation [67]
Takeda 2430	Osc	Passed	A/A	At rest	Recommended

180   Osc = oscillometric, Aus = auscultatory, n/a = not applicable.

automated device for hospital and general practice, or put another way, manufacturers are becoming aware of the enormous potential market that will exist if mercury sphygmomanometers are phased out of use. There is an urgent need, therefore, for those involved in the management of hypertension to impress upon purchasing officers in the health services (whose responsibility it will be to order replacement automated devices for the traditional sphygmomanometer) that protocols are in existence for validating blood pressure devices, and that evidence of independent validation should be demanded from manufacturers. Again, soundings from hospital authorities suggest that there is presently a tendency to substitute aneroid for mercury sphygmomanometers without evidence as to the accuracy of these devices, especially after a period of time in use. Moreover, aneroid sphygmomanometry is prone to all the problems of the auscultatory technique, i.e., observer bias and terminal digit preference. Automated devices, by providing timed printouts of blood pressure, remove these sources of error and thereby improve the overall accuracy of measurement, provided, of course, that they themselves are accurate.

Of course, automation is not without problems. As already mentioned, automated devices have been notorious for their inaccuracy [9], and though accurate devices are now appearing on the market, they are not yet designed for hospital use, and their accuracy after a period of time in such use has not been established. Moreover, without the mercury standard against which to compare measurements generated by algorithmic interpretation of blood pressure, the clinician will become dependent on the consistency and accuracy of such algorithms. It will be necessary, therefore, to retain the mercury sphygmomanometer in certain laboratories as the gold standard against which algorithms may be checked from time to time.

What does the future hold?

At present automated blood pressure measuring devices rely, almost exclusively, on either auscultatory detection of Korotkoff sounds using one or more microphones, or oscillometric analysis of the pulse waveform. However, there has been such a significant shift from auscultatory to oscillometric devices in the last decade, it may be anticipated that in the near future, the microphonic recording of sounds will no longer be used [13]. What then of devices that utilize alternative measurement techniques to auscultation and oscillometry? The various methods of blood pressure measurement have been well reviewed by Ng and Small [13], to whom I am indebted for much of what follows. It may be anticipated that as technology develops, at least some of these innovative methodologies will be applied to the clinical detection of blood pressure. The majority of methods use a compressive cuff or bladder to fully, or partially, occlude an artery during the measurement process. All methods of measuring blood pressure can be further classified into intermittent or continuous measurement techniques. ECG gating techniques may be used to minimize artifact and thereby enhance accuracy.

Vascular unloading measurement

Also known as the volume-compensation, volume-clamp, and servo-plethysmomanometric method, this technique is based on the principle that if external pressure applied to an artery is equal to the arterial pressure at all times, the artery will be unloaded and cannot change in size. Usually a pneumatic finger cuff and plethysmographic transducer are used to detect changes in arterial volume. Using this technique of dynamic unloading of the finger arterial walls with an inflatable finger cuff incorporating a built-in photoelectric plethysmograph a continuous waveform of finger blood pressure can be obtained non-invasively over 24 or more hours. Known as the Finapres (FINger Arterial PRESsure), this device can be used to detect subtle changes in arterial pressure, which might be missed with intermittent pressure recording [14]. However, the transmission of the pressure pulse along the arm arteries causes distortion of the pulse waveform and depression of the mean blood pressure level, which results in poor comparative accuracy with the standard technique. The distorting effects of transmission on the pulse waveform may be reduced, and perhaps ultimately removed, by filtering techniques which are being developed at present. The unique value of the Finapres is attributable not to its accuracy when compared with traditional sphygmomanometry, but rather to the facility to assess beat-to-beat changes in blood pressure and the effect of various interventions and circumstances on blood pressure variability.

Applanation arterial tonometry measurement

Tonometry is based on the principle that if a superficial artery close to an underlying bone is partially flattened, or applanated with a fat rigid surface and kept in that state, the force exerted on the surface is nearly proportional to the pressure in the artery. This relationship can then be used to derive the relative arterial pressure waveform, which when calibrated against measurements made by a reference method (usually oscillometric pressure), yields absolute, continuous blood pressure measurement. The use of an array of sensors circumvents the practical difficulty of precisely positioning a single tonometer over the applanated artery [13].

Pulse-wave velocity (PWV) measurement

This method is based on the principle that the rate of propagation of pressure pulse waves along arteries – the pulse-wave velocity – increases with increasing arterial pressure. This relationship can be used to derive the relative arterial pressure waveform, which when calibrated against measurements made by the reference method, yields absolute, continuous blood pressure measurement. The PWV is usually computed from the pulse-transit time (PTT), which is the time it takes for a pulse wave to travel from one arterial site to another [13].

Infrasound measurement

This is a refinement of the auscultatory method in which the spectral energy of inaudible low-frequency Korotkoff vibrations is analyzed to detect blood pressure [13].

Ultrasound measurement

In this method, a piezoelectric transducer transmits ultrasound waves to an artery, while another transducer receives the reflected waves; blood pressure is determined from the frequency shift (Doppler effect) between the transmitted and reflected waves. The technique has been used extensively for measuring blood pressure in children [13].

Volume-oscillometric measurement

This method is similar to the oscillometric method except that it is based on arterial volume oscillations instead of cuff pressure oscillations [13].

Constant cuff oscillometric measurement

This method, developed by Cor Medical and sometimes called the COR method, is based on the principle that oscillometric pulses generated at a low, constant cuff pressure, give a complete waveform of oscillometric pulses, permitting continuous beat-to-beat arterial blood pressures to be measured, whereas the traditional oscillometric method is limited to a certain characteristic of the oscillometric pulses at different cuff pressures allowing only for intermittent measurement of blood pressure [13].

Pulse dynamic measurement

This method is based on oscillometry, but unlike traditional oscillometric techniques, in which calculations are dependent upon the amplitude and slope characteristics of the pulsation signal, the pulse dynamic method examines changes in the oscillometric signal. The pattern-recognition algorithm identifies the characteristic changes in phase which correspond to systolic, diastolic, and mean arterial pressures based on the dynamic effect of blood flow past the cuff (Bernoulli's effect) [14].

Sphygmooscillographic measurements

This method is also based on oscillometry; an algorithm derives the blood pressures from the amplitude and morphology of pulse waves recorded from a cuff transducer [15].

Pulse oximetry measurement

In this method the plethysmographic waveform derived from pulse oximetry measured on the finger is used to determine systolic blood pressure [16].

Arterial photoplethysmographic measurement

This method is based on photoplethysmographic signals derived from a large superficial artery during electrocardiographic-gated rapid removal of a previously applied occluding counterpressure [17].

Conclusion

We are moving into an age in which automated measurement of blood pressure will soon replace the conventional technique of sphygmomanometry. It may be anticipated that advances in computer technology will facilitate further the development of innovative measuring techniques. While welcoming these advances, clinical scientists must be prepared to examine such techniques critically and to ensure that accuracy does not fall victim to technological ingenuity.

References

1. O'Brien E. Ave atque vale: the centenary of clinical sphygmomanometry. *Lancet* 1996;**348**:1569–1570.
2. Blake E. Recent British researches on arterial tension. *Medical Times Gazette* 1895;**23**:29–30.
3. O'Brien E, Beevers G, Marshall D. *ABC of Hypertension*, 3rd edn, BMJ Publications, London, 1995, p. 4.
4. O'Brien E. Will mercury manometers soon be obsolete? *J Human Hypertension* 1995;**9**:933–934.
5. O'Brien E. Will the millimetre of mercury be replaced by the kilopascal? *J Hypertension* 1998;**16**:259–261.
6. O'Brien E. Automated blood pressure measurement: state of the market in 1998 and the need for an international validation protocol for blood pressure measuring devices. *Blood Pressure Monitor* 1998;**3**:205–211.
7. O'Brien E, Mee F, Atkins N, O'Malley K, Tan S. Training and assessment of observers for blood pressure measurement in hypertension research. *J Human Hypertension* 1991;**5**:7–10.
8. O'Brien E, Beevers G, Marshall D. *ABC of Hypertension*, 3rd edn, BMJ Publications, London, 1995, pp. 18–19.
9. O'Brien E, Mee F, Atkins N, O'Malley K. Inaccuracy of seven popular sphygmomanometers for home-measurement of blood pressure. *J Hypertension* 1990;**8**:621–634.
10. O'Brien E, Waeber B, Parati G, Staessen G, Myers MG, on behalf of the European Society of Hypertension Working Group on Blood Pressure Monitoring. Blood pressure measuring devices: recommendations of the European Society of Hypertension. *BMJ* 2001;**322**:531–536.
11. Association for the Advancement of Medical Instrumentation. American National Standard, Electronic or automated sphygmomanometers, ANSI/AAMI SP 10–1992, 3330 Washington Boulevard, Suite 400, Arlington, VA 22201–4598, p 40.
12. O'Brien E, Petrie J, Littler WA *et al*. The British Hypertension Society Protocol for the evaluation of blood pressure measuring devices. *J Hypertension* 1993;**1**(Suppl 2):S43–S63.
13. Ng K-G, Small CF. Survey of automated noninvasive blood pressure monitors. *J Clin Engin* 1994;**19**:452–475.
14. Brinton TJ, Walls ED, Yajnik AK, Chio S-S. Age-based differences between mercury sphygmomanometer and pulse dynamic blood pressure measurements. *Blood Pressure Monitor* 1998;**3**:125–129.
15. Sapinski A. Comparison of the sphygmooscillographic method with the direct and auscultatory methods of measuring blood pressure. *J Clin Monitor* 1994;**10**:373–376.
16. Talke PO. Measurement of systolic blood pressure using pulse oximetry during helicopter flight. *Crit Care Med* 1991;**19**:934–937.
17. Schnall RB, Gavriely N, Lewkowicz S, Palti Y. A rapid noninvasive blood pressure measurement method for discrete value and full waveform determination. *J Appl Physiol* 1996;**80**:307–314.

Section

4

Specific (secondary) causes of hypertension

Chapter

4.1

Renovascular hypertension

JEF Pohl

4

4

Introduction

It used to be customary to regard the classification of a patient presenting with hypertension as permanent and to be satisfied with attributing no particular cause in about 95% of cases. Renal causes identified on presentation were classified as either parenchymatous or renovascular. In the latter case, it provided the incentive of attempting a cure if a localized stenosis of a major renal artery is found and its effect eliminated. Unfortunately, in an aging population largely afflicted by progressive atheromatous disease, renal arterial obstruction by atheromatous plaques is likely to supervene with increasing probability with increasing years in patients initially classified as 'essential hypertension'. This chapter focuses on renovascular causes of hypertension at all ages but its slant is heavily influenced by the universality of progressive atheroma in our patient population which not only determines presentation and treatment of hypertension but also becomes a major prognostic factor because of cardiac and cerebrovascular mortality and morbidity.

Frequency of renovascular hypertension

Strictly speaking, the prevalence of renovascular hypertension is unknown and its incidence varies between less than 1% and 32% depending on whether at the lower bound of this estimate we are looking for new cases amongst primary care patients or whether our source is malignant hypertensives referred to a secondary center specializing in secondary hypertension[1]. Because of the possibility of reversal and the great severity of the hypertension in at least a proportion of the patients, the importance of renovascular hypertension is not open to doubt.

Etiology of renovascular hypertension

The critical feature of renovascular hypertension is the kidneys' hormonal response to the development of a critical stenosis in one or both renal arteries[2]. Atheroma is by far the commonest cause and may well complicate previously present essential hypertension. Particularly in young patients fibromuscular dysplasia, which is commonly bilateral, is the commonest cause and in some referral centres accounts for up to 25% of total cases. The much rarer causes listed in Table 4.1.1 have an incidence that is also subject to marked geographical variation.

The renin–angiotensin system

Goldblatt induced renal artery stenosis in dogs by clipping of the renal artery and thereby produced an important animal model of hypertension which, reinforced by the application of its methods to other animal species by countless other workers, has been used to explain the pathogenesis of human renovascular hypertension[4]. Table 4.1.2 sets out the animal models used and their presumed human counterparts.

Table 4.1.1 The causes of renovascular hypertension

Atheromatous disease (70–80%)
Fibromuscular dysplasia (20–25%)
Dissecting aortic aneurysm
Renal artery thrombosis or embolism
Abdominal trauma
Neurofibromatosis
Post-radiation fibrosis
Takayasu's arteritis [3]

Table 4.1.2 Comparison of animal and human models of renovascular hypertension

Parameter	Animal	Human
	Two-kidney, one-clip	Unilateral stenosis
Renin	High	High
Plasma volume	Normal	Normal
Response to ACE I	Blood pressure ↓	Blood pressure ↓
	One-kidney, one-clip	Bilateral stenosis
Renin	Normal	Normal/high
Plasma volume	High	High
Response to ACE I	Poor	Blood pressure (↓)

The marked elevation of the renin levels produced by the kidney supplied by the stenosed renal artery and the commonly seen suppression of renin secretion by the opposite kidney fit in well with the two-kidney one-clip animal model. The combination of high angiotensin II levels, escalating hypertension and the presence of a normally functioning unprotected kidney (albeit renin secretion suppressed) lead to a diminishing plasma volume thus further increasing renin activity and in extreme cases setting up a vicious circle of marked hypokalemia, marked hyponatremia and malignant hypertension. The supervention of renal failure with its obligatory plasma volume expansion terminates the operation of this vicious circle that at least in the predialysis and prerenal transplantation era culminated in the death of the patient. The fit of the animal models is less satisfactory in the case of bilateral renal artery stenosis or renal artery stenosis complicated by major renal impairment. This is due to the complex interaction between plasma volume expansion, a renin level moving from a high or very high value into the so-called 'normal range' but remaining at first inappropriately high and the blood pressure response of the human body to a combination of vasoconstriction and volume expansion. Figure 4.1.1 details the effect of the renal artery stenosis on the renin–angiotensin system.

A further reason for the discrepancy between the animal models and human renovascular hypertension is that bilateral disease in man often starts unilaterally and, as evidenced by the differences in renal size and renal vein renin, does not usually progress symmetrically. Goldblatt's work summarized in his 1934 paper took two decades before its influence on clinical practice was documented by Howard's series of six patients whose presumed renovascular hypertension was ameliorated by unilateral nephrectomy.

4.1

Pathology of renovascular
hypertension

Atherosclerosis

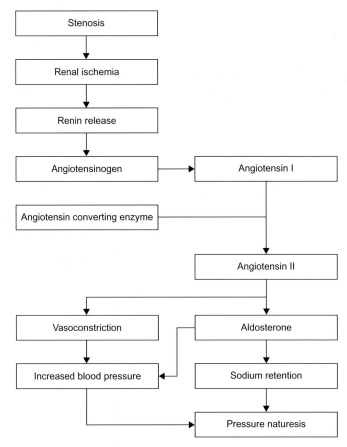

Fig. 4.1.1 The renin-angiotensin system.

Pathology of renovascular hypertension
Atherosclerosis

This is a systemic disorder affecting large and medium-sized arteries including the renal arteries in a patchy but seemingly random fashion. This implies that atheromatous renal artery stenosis is more likely to affect the main artery rather than its branches, that associated aortic involvement is highly probable and that symptoms and prognosis are likely to be affected by associated coronary or leg artery atheroma. If abdominal atheromatous lesions are severe, complicated ostial renal artery lesions may occur which are difficult to treat and may cause critical reductions in renal blood flow and hence function without the involvement of plaque rupture[5]. This complication of renal artery atheroma may lead to reduction in renal function by cholesterol embolism or a supervening thrombotic process may progress to renal artery occlusion[6]. In this context instrumentation of the renal vessels may be a decisive factor in precipitating irreversible changes leading to the loss of a kidney or the need for renal replacement therapy.

Fibromuscular dysplasia

This is the commonest cause of non-atheromatous renal artery stenosis, it is commonly bilateral and occurs more often in women[7]. The not infrequent occurrence of a number of cases in the same sibship suggests an important genetic predisposition which may amount to an autosomal dominant mode of transmission with incomplete penetrance in some family trees. It is unlikely that estrogens play a significant role because female gender predominance is incomplete and prepubertal onset does occur. Descriptively ischemia due to occlusion of vasa vasorum is documented and can experimentally induce fibrotic stenotic renal lesions in dogs but cause and effect cannot be easily separated.

The different histological appearances which have been described may not result from the same mechanism and the above-mentioned etiological hypotheses should not be regarded as mutually exclusive:

- *Medial fibroplasia*, which is rare in children, is the commonest at 65–70%. It gives rise to a classic beaded appearance on angiography due to areas of thickening of the media alternating with regions of aneurysmal dilatation. Complete occlusion is very rare.
- *Perimedial fibroplasia*, which occurs in 25% of cases, lacks the regions of aneurysmal dilatation and occasionally progresses to complete renal artery occlusion.
- *Dissection of the internal elastic membrane* gives rise to an appearance of fusiform enlargement of the renal artery.
- *Medial hyperplasia and intimal fibroplasia* are angiographically indistinguishable and may produce a single proximal stenosis akin to that produced by atheroma.
- *Takayasu's arteritis*[3], usually producing multiple stenotic lesions in the aorta and other main arteries, may of course also affect the renal arteries. It occurs almost exclusively in women but its extreme rarity in the West can no longer be relied upon to dismiss this possibility from the differential diagnosis because of increases in international migration and travel.

Clinical features of renovascular hypertension

If renovascular hypertension were a condition generally not amenable to therapy with hypotensive drugs and certainly curable by successful relief of renal artery stenosis by surgical means or angioplasty, the selection of patients for investigation on the basis of presentation and statistically corelated features would make sense. In fact features such as increasing age, cigarette smoking[8], peripheral vascular disease and diminishing renal function are all correlated with renovascular hypertension but the ultimate therapeutic returns of investigating larger numbers of patients on such non-specific indications are poor. Severe systolic hypertension in the elderly is an indication of loss of elastic recoil by the damaged large arteries primarily and this may of course, as part of the advanced atherosclerotic process, include stenotic renal artery plaques. Flash pulmonary edema, especially in a hypertensive

Table 4.1.3 Factors in the history distinguishing different causes of renovascular hypertension

Atherosclerosis	Fibromuscular dysplasia
Older male smoker	Young female non-smoker
Coexisting vascular disease	No family disease of essential hypertension
Malignant hypertension	
Loss of control in previously stable patient	Family history of fibromuscular dysplasia
Renal impairment	Features of renal artery dissection
Deterioration in renal function with ACE I	No evidence of end-organ damage
'Flash' pulmonary edema	

Table 4.1.4 Signs suggestive of renovascular hypertension

Severe grade III and IV hypertensive retinopathy
Abdominal bruits
Bruits elsewhere
Signs of peripheral vascular disease

patient with renal impairment is sufficiently rare to justify investigation for renal artery stenosis.

A better strategy is to base the decision to investigate on severity of hypertension[1] (especially whether the hypertension is accelerated) lack of responsiveness to treatment and particularly the emergence of resistance to medical therapy in a compliant patient previously well controlled for long periods. In this context, the distinction between a suspicion of fibromuscular dysplasia and atherosclerotic renal artery stenosis, summarized in Table 4.1.3, becomes relevant.

Physical signs which are listed in Table 4.1.4 are not usually helpful with the exception of the finding of a machinery type abdominal bruit which is continuous throughout systole and diasystole. Shorter abdominal bruits are increasingly common with advancing years beyond middle age and are too non-specific.

Sharp deterioration of renal function after treatment with an ACE I is usually due to volume depletion attributable to previous diuretic therapy or religious compliance with a severely sodium-restricted diet but if it persists after volume repletion, may well indicate renal artery stenosis particularly if the stenosis is bilateral.

Although normalization of the blood pressure in a patient with moderate-to-severe hypertension after treatment with an ACE I may raise suspicion, this is a cause for congratulation rather than renovascular investigation. Acute occlusion of a renal artery with loin pain, hematuria and hypertension is a justification for urgent investigation which may lead to successful remedial action.

Investigations in renovascular hypertension

Table 4.1.5 lists the investigations that should be performed routinely on patients with hypertension and this is followed by a section discussing screening investigations designed to reduce the proportion of patients suspected of renovascular hypertension that leads to renal angiography.

Table 4.1.5 Basic investigations for any hypertensive patient

Parameter	Technique
Urine	Dipstick for blood, protein, glucose
	24-hour urinary catecholamine excretion
	Microscopy
	Culture
Blood	Full blood count and erythrocyte sedimentation rate or plasma volume or
	C-reactive protein
	Urea, creatinine, and electrolytes
	Glucose, cholesterol, LDL, HDL, and triglycerides
Other	ECG
	Chest X-ray
	Echocardiogram

Screening investigations

Renal ultrasound [9]

This allows assessment of renal size and in particular disparity between the two sides which increases the suspicion of a renal cause. Duplex scanning to assess renal blood flow is operator and equipment dependent but if good tracings are obtained renal artery stenosis can be diagnosed or excluded with a high degree of probability[10,11].

Captopril challenge test

In centers which measure plasma renin routinely the change in peripheral vein plasma renin produced within 60 minutes of oral administration of 50 mg captopril can be used to diagnose significant renovascular disease[12]. Sensitivity and specificity can be traded off against each other and high values for both have been claimed.

Renal vein renin ratio

This invasive test which requires catheterization of both renal veins is subject to the vagaries of renal venous anatomy and imposes a requirement of simultaneous sampling from each renal vein and the inferior vena cava[13]. To reach the widely accepted minimum positive ratio of 1 : 5, a variety of methods to stress the renin–angiotensin system such as salt restriction, diuretic and ACE I administration have been employed[14]. Despite some claims to the contrary it has not proved possible to achieve acceptable sensitivity or specificity and the test is not recommended.

Isotope renography [15]

Although renography using ^{99m}Tc-diethylenetrianaminepentaacetic acid (DPTA), merceptacetyl triglycine (MAG3), or diatrizoate, is neither sufficiently sensitive nor specific to use as a screening test it can be used as a follow-up surveillance test after previous successful renal angioplasty[16]. The addition of a dose of oral captopril has improved particularly the DPTA test sufficiently for some centers to claim a respectable sensitivity of 90% and specificity of 95% for it.

BOX 4.1.1 Captopril renography

Glomerular filtration rate (GFR) is measured by DPTA uptake and renal blood is measured by ^{123}I-hippuran uptake before and 60 minutes after 25 mg of oral captopril. A positive test indicating a functionally significant renal artery stenosis is characterized by a fall in GFR and a delay in hippuran secretion. Functionally significant renal artery stenosis is defined as a hypotensive response to subsequent dilatation of the stenosis by angioplasty associated with the restoration of a normal renal angiogram. Although a 95% sensitivity and specificity is claimed for this procedure, the yield from unselected hypertensive patients is far too low to make this test suitable for general screening[12].

Renal angiography

This provides direct visualization of renal arterial lesions and will allow accurate localization, the detection of multiple, including branch, stenoses and will usually, particularly when coupled with intra-arterial digital-subtraction techniques, provide enough high-quality pictures to decide on anatomical suitability for angioplasty or reconstructive surgery[17]. The major limitation remains the linkage of the anatomical demonstration of renovascular disease with functional significance and clinical outcome. The remedy does not lie in measuring the pressure drop across candidate lesions which, although technically often feasible, is far from infallible but in the rigorous selection of patients who are subjected to renal angiography in the first place.

Incidental renal artery stenosis

It is not surprising that patients both with and without hypertension should develop atheromatous renal artery deposits as part of more generalized atheroma[18]. The occurrence of any degree of renal arterial stenosis, even to the point of producing complete occlusion, is therefore no guarantee that the stenosis is clinically relevant. In a Scandinavian series of 450 patients undergoing angiography for peripheral vascular disease, half had radiologically diagnosable severe renovascular disease and yet 20% of these patients were normotensive. It follows that unless a patient meets the criteria for renovascular investigation, usually hypertension of severe degree or resistant to determined medical therapy, any incidentally discovered renal artery lesion should be disregarded.

Spiral computed tomography

This technique, which is currently on trial in some centers to rival angiography as a gold standard, has the great advantage of producing good quality images non-invasively but shares the two major disadvantages of the latter, viz. the use of contrast medium and the lack of information about clinical significance of lesions shown.

4

BOX 4.1.2 Dangers of angiography!

This is an expensive invasive procedure which should not be used as a
screening test. Apart from the obvious risks of hemorrhage, infection and
arteriovenous fistual formation there are several mechanisms by which renal
function may deteriorate or the kidney be lost altogether. Dissection of the
arterial wall may lead to irreversible thrombotic occlusion of a renal artery
and dislodged plaque material may freely embolize distally into the kidney.
Contrast media are toxic to the kidney which is a particular problem in
diabetic nephropathy or if the patient is volume depleted or the kidney is
underperfused for some other reasons. The management of the procedure
should include stopping diuretics beforehand and enhanced
postangiography hydration to ensure a good urine flow. The estimate of an
overall mortality of 0.1% is probably not exaggerated.

Treatment of renovascular hypertension

Fortunately we are now in possession of overwhelming evidence that all
hypertensives should be treated and that the ultimate target must be
normalization of both the systolic and the diastolic blood pressures
preferably with the re-establishment of a normal diurnal pattern
including a satisfactory drop during deep sleep and the avoidance of
blood pressure escape during arousal in the early hours of the morning.
The phantom of the J-curve has been vanquished[19], the systolic blood
pressure has regained its deserved status and the final arbiter of blood
pressure control is the 24-hour ambulatory measurement.

It is customary in many centers to set an arbitrary limit of 75%
stenosis below which intervention is not attempted lest the benefits do
not balance the possible harm which results. Apart from the uncertainty
which attaches to the estimated degree of stenosis, the thinking
underlying this approach appears to be suspect. By analogy to the
coronary circulation, it is not the degree of obstruction produced by the
stenosis (calculated to be small at 75%)[20] but its potential for
deterioration and non-obstructive effects such as distal embolization
which determine the significance of the lesion. The Cleveland Series[21]
provides alarming information about the possible natural history of
progression of renal artery stenosis which must be seen in its historical
context, however. We now know that fibromuscular dysplasia behaves
on the whole more benignly than atheromatous stenosis. Moreover,
again using coronary arterial disease experience as an analogy,
determined therapy of lipid profiles with statins and dietary
modification (in that order) and acknowledging the absence of a
threshold, is already known to diminish the incidence of atheroma-
related events in other areas and can therefore be confidently expected
to do the same in renovascular disease. It must also be appreciated that
the definition of effective antihypertensive treatment has considerably
altered over the last two decades before one uses the Cleveland Series
(Table 4.1.6) as a justification for medical as opposed to surgical
therapeutic nihilism.

Table 4.1.6 Two-year progression of untreated renovascular disease: the Cleveland series

Patients (n)	Initial stenosis	Unchanged	Worse	Occluded
78	<50%	69%	26%	5%
30	50–75%	53%	37%	10%
18	75–99%	61%	0%	39%

Schreiber *et al. Urol Clin N Am* 1984;**11**:383–392.

Medical treatment strategy

The adequate control of hypertension utilizing the criteria enunciated above is almost certain to involve the use of a number of hypotensive drugs in parallel and not in series, having due regard to multiplying the number of drug action mechanisms employed simultaneously and to use the highest doses tolerable to the patient whose compliance must be buttressed by frequent personal contact with the patient. Only persistence in establishing and maintaining rapport with the patient will be rewarded by the level of compliance which masters the doubts created by the side effects of the drugs and perhaps equally importantly by learning to live with a blood pressure significantly lower than the patient is used to. Successful attention to the other aspects aggravating the atheromatous state such a hypolipidemic therapy, dietary modification and cessation of smoking is also dependent on being the patient's friend.

George Pickering's opinion (1968)[22], that the hypertension associated with renal artery stenosis should, in the first instance, be treated medically, still holds more than thirty years later. The number of hypotensive drugs available and our willingness to use multiple drugs simultaneously has increased, however. The definition of blood pressure control is being progressively sharpened and in particular the requirement of controlling the systolic blood pressure is now universally accepted. The current target of 130 mmHg systolic and 80 mmHg diastolic is particularly difficult to achieve in older patients who have sustained large and medium-size artery damage over years of previously accepted, nay encouraged, partial diastolic blood pressure control in parallel with almost uncontrolled systolic blood pressures. The safety of beta-blockers, alpha-blockers, calcium antagonists and low doses of diuretics has been well established. Direct acting vasodilators such as hydralazine, minoxidil and exceptionally diazoxide require high doses of loop diuretics to correct the fluid retention produced by the false signal of fluid depletion received by the kidneys. This raises the issue of avoiding fluid overload which jeopardizes blood pressure control on the one hand and over diurezing patients producing postural hypotension, transient impairment of renal function, hyponatremia and hypokalemia on the other hand. The management of fluid balance requires considerable skill in such patients and benefits from substantial hospital specialist input whenever this is available.

The use of older centrally-acting drugs such as methyldopa which has become obsolete in the treatment of milder or non-renovascular

4

hypertension still continues in renovascular hypertension because the need to achieve target blood pressure renders the greater side effects, provided they are minimized by skillful management, acceptable.

Although a trial of ACE inhibitors or angiotensin-receptor antagonists may help in the diagnosis of renal artery stenosis these drugs are not indicated in known cases of renal artery stenosis.

BOX 4.1.3 Dangers of ACE inhibitors

If activation of the renin–angiotensin system plays a major part in sustaining the raised blood pressure in renovascular hypertension, angiotensin-converting enzyme inhibitors are likely to lower the blood pressure but the risk to the patient is high. The risk has three major components.

- Firstly in the presence of major arterial stenotic lesions an abrupt fall of angiotensin II levels or antagonism of high and even rising angiotensin II levels will compromise the glomerular filtration rate at least in part by a reduction of renal blood flow.
- Secondly, renal function will worsen irrespective of whether the particular angiotensin-converting enzyme inhibitor administered is predominantly cleared by the kidneys. This reduction in renal function may be irreversible and a figure of 15% has been quoted in one series of patients.
- Thirdly, the capacity of such patients to withstand volume depletion whether caused by inability to drink excessive water and electrolyte loss by intercurrent gastrointestinal tract illness or by excessive use of diuretics is much reduced.

ACE I are best avoided in renovascular disease but in any case close attention to renal function and diligent measurements of lying and standing blood pressures are mandatory.

Surgical treatment

Nephrectomy by primary intention is only appropriate if the affected kidney has been identified as the probable cause of refractory hypertension and divided renal function studies suggest a contribution of less than 10% by the affected kidney to total renal function which is not significantly impaired. None of the large number of surgical techniques currently in use, which include endarterectomy, arterial resection and reanastomosis and autotransplantation of the kidney into the iliac fossa can rival percutaneous transluminal renal angioplasty[23,24].

Percutaneous renal angioplasty

Success is operator dependent and results can be excellent for carefully selected patients. The possible complications have been described above but the technique is considered relatively safe in skilled and experienced hands[21,25]. Technical success varies with type and location of stenosis and at 70–100% is always higher than clinical success which demands significant lowering of blood pressure without jeopardizing renal function. The best results are claimed for fibromuscular dysplasia whilst the technique is least suitable for ostial lesions which are commonest in atheromatous renal vascular disease. Restenosis, at least prior to the use of stents, was reported in over 20% of patients after two years. The results suffer either from antiquity or small numbers and must be taken as a baseline from which to progress rather than a secure predictor of future results.

BOX 4.1.4 Outcome data for angioplasty – Mayo Clinic 1995

According to Bonelli *et al. Mayo Clin Proc* 1995;**70**:1041–1052

- Retrospective analysis of 320 patients over 14 years
- All had at least one 70% stenosis of a renal artery
- Technical success (i.e. <30% residual stenosis) was achieved in 81% of patients with atherosclerosis and 89% of patients with fibromuscular dysplasia
- 70% of patients with atherosclerosis benefited (8.4% cured), 63% of patients with fibromuscular dysplasia benefited (22% cured). 'Cured' defined as blood pressure <140/80 mmHg off therapy
- Cure more common in younger patients and those with hypertension of short duration
- No beneficial effect on renal function
- 5.6% dissected, 1.6% perforated, 0.9% occluded, 5.6% had contrast nephropathy
- All causes 30-day mortality was 2.2%

According to Davidson *et al. Am J Kid Dis* 1996;**28**:334–338

- 23 patients with fibromuscular dysplasia: 100% technically good results
- 12 cured, 5 improved, 6 unchanged
- Younger patients and those with a shorter duration of hypertension benefited more or were more likely to be cured

---

The outcomes of angioplasty are less satisfactory than one might have predicted theoretically but there are a number of good reasons for this. Firstly, there is wide but variable heterogenity of the patient material. Young patients with fibromuscular dysplasia and/or a relatively short history of hypertension yield better results than individuals who are old and heavily laden with generalized atheroma. The latter are expected to have a high short-term mortality from coronary artery disease, strokes and other manifestations of atherosclerosis. Their hypertension will be irreversible because of its long duration and technically satisfactory results will be difficult to obtain on account of the frequently ostial location of a tight renal artery stenosis and the presence of multiple stenoses combined with reduced renal function at the time of the angioplasty. Secondly, complications often related to advanced complicated atheroma are quite common and may exceed 10%. Mortality figures of 3% have been reported by reputable institutions. Lastly, restenosis of successfully dilated lesions which may also at times be related to other complications at the time of angioplasty not uncommonly blights the outcome of the procedure. The use of metal stents which has led to sizeable improvements in the results of coronary angioplasty is becoming more widespread but it is too early to assess its impact on the problem of renal artery restenosis. The reported effect of angioplasty on renal function has at best been neutral and does not encourage undertaking the procedure primarily because of diminishing renal function.

BOX 4.1.5 Angioplasty complications

- Arterial puncture hemorrhage
- Arteriovenous fistula formation
- Renal artery dissection or occlusion
- Renal artery perforation
- Distal cholesterol embolization
- Contrast nephropathy

Prognosis in renovascular disease

Grouping all patients with renovascular disease together leads to a gloomy view of their outlook[26]. Owing to the widespread occurrence of the manifestation of atherosclerosis in the aging population it is only to be expected that the contribution of renovascular disease to end-stage renal failure, currently standing at 8–14% of all dialysis patients, will continue to increase. Nor is it surprising that the prognosis of patients with end-stage renal failure due to renal artery stenosis is very poor with a five-year survival of 10% or less[27].

It would be wrong, however, to allow these reflections to lead to therapeutic paralysis. Prevention of unnecessary renal failure by prohibiting the use of ACE I- and probably also angiotensin (ANG) II-receptor antagonists in established renal artery stenosis and careful attention to the response of the renal function to ACE I treatment in patients whose renal vascular anatomy has not been elucidated would go a small way to improve overall prognosis. The investigation of younger patients with severe or difficult-to-control hypertension would unearth many of the fibromuscular dysplasia cases whose treatment by angioplasty yields much better results. Finally, aggressive treatment of atherosclerosis which forms an important part of many state supported health-improvement programs is likely to help prevent the increasing prevalence of atheroma-related renovascular disease with increasing age, and if regression of lesions becomes a likely prospect in the future, the abysmal fate of those who have already reached end-stage renal failure will be ameliorated.

Summary

With the widespread occurrence of atherosclerosis in our aging population, renovascular hypertension is getting commoner. About one-third are caused by fibromuscular dysplasia which occurs in younger

4

patients, is less likely to lead to renal artery occlusion and has a better chance of responding to angioplasty. The initial management of all cases of renovascular hypertension consists of aggressive multidrug hypotensive therapy. Failure to respond and reach currently set targets for systolic and diastolic blood pressure is the best indication for confirming suspicion of renal artery stenosis by definitive tests of which renal angiography is still accepted as the gold standard. Malignant hypertension or severe hypertension in younger, fitter patients are also indications for screening tests. Diminishing renal function is not a good indication for a confirmatory investigation since the results of treatment by angioplasty are too poor. Angioplasty produces good results in fibromuscular dysplasia and intermediate results in atheromatous renal artery stenosis with relatively preserved renal function and no apparent atheromatous manifestations in other systems. A general case for aggressive management of atheromatosis is made to include cases with renal arterial involvement and it is hoped that success in that direction will eventually stem the tide of increasing prevalence of renovascular hypertension and renal function loss secondary to atherosclerosis.

References

1. Davis BA, Crook JE, Vestal RE *et al*. Prevalence of renovascular hypertension in patients with Grade II or IV hypertensive retinopathy. *N Engl J Med* 1979;**301**:1273.
2. Hall JE, Guyton AC, Jackson TE *et al*. Control of glomerular filtration rate by the renin angiotensin system. *Am J Physiol* 1977;**233**:F366–372.
3. Jain S, Kumari S, Ganguly NK, Sharma BK. Current status of Takayasu arteritis in India. *Int J Cardiol* 1996;**54**:S111–116.
4. Goldblatt H, Lynch J, Hanzal RF, Summerville WW. Studies on experimental hypertension. The production of persistent elevation of systolic blood pressure by means of renal ischaemia. *J Exp Med Sci* 1934;**59**:347–378.
5. Tollefson DFJ, Ernst CB. Natural history of atherosclerotic renal artery stenosis associated with aortic disease. *J Vasc Surg* 1991;**14**:327–331.
6. Rimmer JM, Gennari FJ. Atherosclerotic renovascular disease and progressive renal failure. *Ann Intern Med* 1993;**118**:712–719.
7. Stanley FC, Fry WJ. Pediatric renal artery occlusive disease and renovascular hypertension. Etiology diagnosis and operative treatment. *Arch Surg* 1981;**116**:669–676.
8. Nicholson JP, Teichman SL, Alderman NH *et al*. Cigarette smoking and renovascular hypertension. *Lancet* 1983;**ii**:765.
9. Hoffman V, Edwards JM, Carer S *et al*. Role of duplex scanning for the detection of atherosclerotic renal artery disease. *Kidney Int* 1991;**39**:1232–1239.
10. Olin JW, Piedmonte MR, Young JR *et al*. The utility of duplex ultrasound scanning of the renal arteries for diagnosing significant renal artery stenosis. *Ann Intern Med* 1995;**122**:833.
11. Zierler RE, Bergelin RO, Isaacson JA, Strandness DE. Natural history of renal artery stenosis. A prospective study with duplex ultrasonography. *J Vasc Surg* 1994;**19**:250–258.
12. Müller FB, Sealey JE, Case CB *et al*. The captopril test for identifying renovascular disease in hypertensive patients. *Am J Med* 1986;**80**:633–644.
13. Pickering TG, Sos TA, James GD *et al*. Comparison of renal vein renin activity in hypertensive patients with stenosis of one or both renal arteries. *J Hypertension* 1985;**3**:S291–293.
14. Vaughan ED Jr, Bühler FR, Laragh JH *et al*. Renovascular hypertension: renin measurement to indicate hypersecretion and contralateral suppression, estimate renal plasma flow and score for surgical correctability. *Am J Med* 1973;**55**:402.

15. Fommey E, Ghione S, Palla L *et al*. Renal scintigraphic captopril test in the diagnosis of renovascular hypertension. *Hypertension* 1987;**10**:212–220.

16. Dondi M, Monetti N, Fanti S *et al*. Use of ^{90m}Tc MAG$_3$ for renal scintigraphy after angiotensin converting enzyme inhibitor. *J Nucl Med* 1991;**32**:424–428.

17. Saint-Georges G, Aube M. Safety of outpatient angiography. A prospective study. *Am J Radiol* 1985;**144**:235–236.

18. Missouris CG, Buckenham T, Cappuchio FP, Macgregor GA. Renal artery stenosis: a common and important problem in patients with peripheral vascular disease. *Am J Med* 1994;**96**:10–14.

19. Result of HOT Study. *Lancet* 1998;**356**:1755–1762.

20. Shipley RE, Gregg DE. The effect of external constriction of a blood vessel on blood flow. *Am J Physiol* 1944;**141**:287.

21. Bonelli FS, McKusick MA, Textor FC *et al*. Renal artery angioplasty. Technical results and clinical outcome in 320 patients. *Mayo Clin Proc* 1995;**70**:1041–1052.

22. Pickering GW. *High Blood Pressure*, 2nd edn, p. 80. J&A Churchill: London, 1955.

23. Lawrie GM, Morris GC, Glaeser DH, DeBakey ME. Renovascular reconstruction: Factors affecting long term prognosis in 919 patients followed for 31 years. *Am J Cardiol* 1985;**63**:1085–1092.

24. Bartlett ST, Sugoni WE Jr, Ward RE. Improved results with surgical treatment of renovascular hypertension: an individualized approach. *J Cardiovasc Surg* 1990;**31**: 351–355.

25. Sos TA, Pickering TG, Sniderman K *et al*. Percutaneous transluminal renal angioplasty in renovascular hypertension due to atheroma or fibromuscular dysplasia. *N Engl J Med* 1983;**309**:274–279.

26. Plovin PF, Chatellir G, Darne B, Raynaud A. EMMA Study. *Hypertension* 1998;**31**: 823–829.

27. Mailloux LV, Belluci AG, Mossey RT *et al*. Predictors of survival in patients undergoing dialysis. *Am J Med* 1988;**84**:855–862.

Further reading

Textor SC, Smith-Powell L. Pathophysiology of renal failure in ischaemic renal disease. In: *Renovascular Disease* (eds Novick AC, Scoble J, Hamilton G), pp. 289–302. WB Saunders: Philadelphia, PA, 1996.

Brown AL, Wilkinson R. Clinical approach to hypertension. In: *Oxford Textbook of Nephrology* (eds Cameron JS, Davison AM, Gunfeld JP, Kern DNS, Ritz E), Oxford University Press: Oxford, 1996.

Ledingham JGG. Renal vascular disease. In: *Oxford Textbook of Medicine*, 2nd edn. (eds Weatherall DJ, Leddingham JGG, Warrell DA). Oxford University Press: Oxford, 1989.

Wilkinson R. Renal and renovascular hypertension. In: *Textbook of Hypertension* (ed. Swales JD), pp. 831–850. Blackwell Scientific Publications: Oxford, 1994.

References

Further reading

4

Chapter

4.2

4

Renal parenchymal hypertension

RA Preston and M Epstein

Introduction

Chronic renal disease and systemic hypertension may coexist in one of three distinct clinical settings. Firstly, it is well known that sustained, poorly controlled primary hypertension leading to hypertensive nephrosclerosis is an independent and important risk factor for development of chronic renal failure and end-stage renal disease[1–8]. Secondly, renal parenchymal disease is a well established cause of secondary hypertension[9–15]. Renal parenchymal disease is the most common cause of secondary hypertension, accounting for 2.5–5.0% of all cases of systemic hypertension. Moreover, hypertension may also accelerate the decline in renal function in patients with kidney disease if inadequately controlled. Therefore, hypertension may be either a cause or a consequence of renal disease, and it may often be difficult to distinguish clinically between these two separate situations. The third major circumstance in which hypertension and renal failure occur simultaneously is in ischemic renal disease[16]. This is generally secondary to arteriosclerotic renal artery disease causing bilateral renal artery stenosis or unilateral renal artery stenosis in a solitary functioning kidney. Ischemic renal disease is a recently recognized and increasingly common cause of hypertension and renal dysfunction leading to end-stage renal disease.

In this chapter we will focus our discussion on various aspects of the pathophysiology and management of renal parenchymal hypertension.

Pathophysiology of renal parenchymal hypertension

The precise mechanisms that produce hypertension in patients with kidney disease remain to be completely elucidated. Renal parenchymal hypertension most probably results from the combined interactions of many independent mechanisms: potential factors include sodium retention leading to volume expansion, increases in pressor activity, and decreases in endogenous vasodepressor compounds.

The importance of sodium balance in determining blood pressure control

Altered renal sodium handling is the most clinically important mechanism that leads to development of renal parenchymal hypertension[9–15,17]. Many patients with renal parenchymal hypertension have sodium-sensitive hypertension. Patients with renal failure have increased total exchangeable sodium (NaE) compared to normal controls or patients with essential hypertension, and blood pressure elevation in mild-to-moderate renal failure is correlated with both plasma volume and NaE. Changes in sodium intake directly influence blood pressure in patients with chronic renal failure, and this relationship seems stronger at lower levels of renal function. Increasing salt intake in patients with chronic renal failure increases extracellular fluid volume (ECFV) and blood pressure, and the increment in blood pressure for a given increase in ECFV tends to be greater in the patients

4

with more advanced renal failure. Of clinical importance is the observation that reduction of dietary sodium and other measures that reduce NaE and extracellular fluid volume will tend to lower blood pressure in many patients with chronic renal insufficiency.

The mechanisms that lead from sodium retention and ECFV expansion to an increased blood pressure are incompletely elucidated. Despite the importance of impaired sodium excretion and ECFV expansion in the genesis of renal parenchymal hypertension, the most consistently observed hemodynamic alteration is an elevation of peripheral vascular resistance rather than an increase in cardiac output. The mechanism(s) for this elevation in peripheral vascular resistance remain unclear: the relationship of ECFV expansion to pressure elevation appears to be complex and may involve diverse neural and hormonal pathways.

Endogenous digitalis-like factor (DLF)

There is a complex coupling between volume expansion and peripheral vascular resistance in patients with the salt-sensitive hypertension associated with chronic renal disease. Recent interest has been generated by the hypothesis that an endogenous, circulating, digitalis-like factor (DLF) may contribute to the pathogenesis of both the sodium-sensitive hypertension of chronic renal parenchymal disease, and the sodium-sensitive, low renin forms of essential hypertension[18]. The DLF is believed to be a steroid produced in the adrenal, the hypothalamus, or both, and that acts by inhibiting cellular $Na^+; K^+$-ATPase activity in a manner similar to digitalis.

The hypothesis posits that a DLF is normally released in response to ECFV expansion, and that the DLF decreases renal sodium reabsorption by inhibiting cellular $Na^+; K^+$-ATPase activity[18]. While this action of DLF enhances renal sodium excretion and tends to restore total body sodium to normal, there is a tradeoff: DLF also increases peripheral vascular resistance. Because DLF inhibits $Na^+; K^+$-ATPase in vascular smooth muscle, cytosolic sodium rises. The rise in cytosolic sodium inhibits calcium moving out of cells via sodium–calcium exchange, and therefore indirectly increases vascular smooth muscle calcium. The increase in smooth muscle calcium, in turn, favors increased vascular smooth muscle tone and elevated peripheral vascular resistance.

Regardless of the precise mechanism(s) leading from ECFV expansion to hypertension, sodium retention with associated ECFV expansion plays a central role in the pathogenesis of renal parenchymal hypertension and reduction of total body sodium is frequently very effective in lowering blood pressure. From a practical standpoint, control of blood pressure in patients with chronic renal disease may be difficult without therapeutic interventions that mobilize excess sodium.

Renin–angiotensin–aldosterone system

There is compelling evidence that the renin–angiotensin–aldosterone system is at least partly responsible for the hypertension associated with

4

4

renal parenchymal disease[9–11,19]. In hypertensive patients with mild-to-moderate renal insufficiency, plasma renin activity (PRA) and angiotensin II concentrations are frequently increased and tend to correlate with severity of hypertension. Both the systemic and renal vasculatures are especially sensitive to the vasoconstrictor action of angiotensin II. In addition, there is an abnormal relationship between exchangeable sodium and plasma renin activity or plasma angiotensin II. Normal levels of these hormones are inappropriately high in relation to the ECFV.

The precise role of the renin–angiotensin–aldosterone system in end-stage renal disease patients, however, remains the subject of controversy. The majority of patients receiving maintenance hemodialysis demonstrate sodium sensitivity and are able to achieve blood pressure control by sodium removal with dialysis therapy. In these patients, the PRA and angiotensin II levels are high with respect to the corresponding degree of volume overload. This sodium-sensitive form of hypertension has been termed 'volume-dependent' but is still characterized by inappropriately elevated PRA and angiotensin II levels.

A much smaller percentage of dialysis patients demonstrate poor control of blood pressure despite antihypertensive therapy and adequate control of volume with hemodialysis. These patients respond with a striking fall in blood pressure following bilateral nephrectomy. The hypertension in this patient group is designated 'renin-dependent' hypertension. These patients may have very high renin and angiotensin II levels despite apparent euvolemia.

Aldosterone

There is substantial animal data to suggest a role for aldosterone, independent of angiotensin II, in the microangiopathy seen in malignant nephrosclerosis[20–23]. Studies of stroke-prone spontaneously hypertensive rats (SHRSP) suggest a marked protective effect of spironolactone against the development of malignant nephrosclerotic and cerebrovascular lesions and are consistent with a major role for mineralocorticoids as hormonal mediators of vascular injury[20,21]. Rocha *et al.* [20,21]have suggested that mineralocorticoids, independent of the renin–angiotensin system, may play a pathophysiological role in the SHRSP. In addition, they studied whether a two-week infusion of aldosterone would reverse the renal vascular protective effects of captopril in SHRSP. Captopril treatment reduced plasma aldosterone levels concomitant with marked reductions in proteinuria and the absence of histologic lesions of malignant nephrosclerosis. Aldosterone substitution during captopril treatment resulted in the development of severe renal lesions and proteinuria comparable with that observed with either aldosterone or vehicle alone. These findings support a major role for aldosterone in the development of malignant nephrosclerosis in this model, independent of the effects of blood pressure. As noted in several recent reviews, several clinical trials are being conducted presently to corroborate this postulate[22,23].

Renal prostaglandins

Prostaglandins are important modulators of renal hemodynamics in patients with renal parenchymal disease. Their role in maintaining renal function assumes increasing importance in disorders characterized by contracted ECFV and impaired renal function[9–11,19]. Therefore, impaired production of the vasodilatory prostaglandins could play a role in the development of hypertension secondary to renal parenchymal disease.

Renal vasodilator prostaglandins (i.e. PGE_2 and PGI_2) exert diverse effects in the kidney, including renal vasodilation, mesangial cell relaxation, modulation of renal blood flow (RBF), glomerular filtration rate (GFR), sodium and water excretion. The renal prostaglandins are thought to counteract the vasoconstrictive effects of angiotensin II and other pressor compounds in renal parenchymal hypertension. Consequently, the support of RBF and GFR by PGI_2-induced vasodilation and mesangial cell relaxation would assume increasing importance in chronic renal insufficiency.

Interestingly, most studies have not been able to demonstrate a decrease in urinary prostaglandin excretion in patients with renal parenchymal hypertension. Urinary excretion of PGE_2 has been found to be normal or elevated. These observations are relevant in the management of patients with disorders characterized by diminished ECFV because administration of prostaglandin synthesis inhibitors (such as the non-steroidal anti-inflammatory agents) in patients with chronic renal failure may decrease GFR and simultaneously increase blood pressure. In summary, it is unlikely that a decreased production of renal vasodilatory prostaglandins plays an important role in hypertension secondary to renal parenchymal disease.

Sympathetic nervous system

Increased activity of the sympathetic nervous system may interact with other factors in the pathogenesis of sustained arterial hypertension in patients with essential hypertension. By analogy, increased activity of the sympathetic nervous system could also contribute to the hypertension of renal parenchymal disease[9–11]. Norepinephrine (noradrenaline) levels are normal or increased both in patients with mild-to-moderate chronic renal failure, and many patients with renal parenchymal hypertension (compared with normal controls or normotensive patients with renal disease). One study suggested a positive correlation between plasma norepinephrine and blood pressure in renal disease, but another was unable to confirm this observation. Plasma norepinephrine is cleared more slowly in patients with renal failure than in normals, and therefore plasma concentrations of norepinephrine may be poor indicators of sympathetic nervous system activity in chronic renal failure. Blood pressure declines more with sympathetic blockade in patients with end-stage renal disease than in normotensive dialysis patients or in normal subjects. Although these findings suggest that sympathetic nervous system hyperactivity may play a role in the pathogenesis of hypertension in end-stage renal disease, newer methodologies, including radiotracer norepinephrine kinetic techniques, are required to further clarify this possibility.

Endothelin

Endothelin-1 (ET-1) exerts a wide range of biologic effects in the kidney, including constriction of most renal vessels, mesangial cell contraction, inhibition of sodium and water reabsorption by the nephron, enhancement of glomerular cell proliferation, and stimulation of extracellular matrix accumulation[24]. Because ET-1 functions primarily as an autocrine or paracrine factor, its renal effects must be viewed in the context of its local production and actions. Numerous studies indicate that ET-1 is involved in the pathogenesis of a broad spectrum of renal diseases and deranged ET-1 production in the nephron may cause inappropriate sodium and water retention, thereby contributing to the development and/or maintenance of hypertension.

Based on these considerations, it has been postulated that ET could participate in the mechanisms leading to the elevation of blood pressure in patients with chronic renal disease. Although plasma ET levels and urinary ET excretion are increased in patients with combined hypertension and chronic renal failure, a correlation of plasma or urinary ET with blood pressure has not been clearly demonstrated. Furthermore, because ET is produced, and acts locally, the precise significance of plasma ET levels and urinary ET excretion is somewhat unclear.

Nitric oxide

Alterations in the metabolism of the endogenous vasodilator nitric oxide (NO) may be involved in the hypertension associated with renal parenchymal disease. During basal conditions, endothelial cells produce NO continuously to maintain a state of active vasodilation. Thus impaired NO synthesis could contribute to the hypertension in patients with renal parenchymal disease[25,26].

Factors that impair NO function also favor vasoconstriction. Methylated L-arginine derivatives that possess NO synthase inhibitor capabilities (e.g. N^G, N-dimethylarginine and N-monomethyl-L-arginine) are found in human plasma and urine. Patients with chronic uremia have impaired elimination of these compounds, and that circulating concentrations of these compounds may rise sufficiently to inhibit NO production. Thus, accumulation of endogenous NO synthase inhibitors might contribute to the hypertension of advanced renal failure. In addition, removal of these inhibitors by hemodialysis may partly explain the decrease in blood pressure observed in most end-stage renal disease patients when dialysis is initiated.

The potential roles of this endogenous vasodilator compound in hypertension secondary to renal parenchymal disease provide exciting new avenues for further investigation, but the precise contribution of altered NO metabolism in the pathophysiology of the hypertension of end-stage renal disease is not established.

Nephron number, hypertension and renal injury

Brenner *et al.*[27–29] have proposed that the number of functioning nephron units present at birth determines an individual's predisposition to the subsequent development of hypertension and renal damage. Brenner suggested that low birthweight may impair renal development, reduce the number of glomeruli, and/or decrease the filtration surface area. This decrease in filtration surface area would eventually lead to an increase in glomerular capillary hydraulic pressure (glomerular hypertension), with consequent development of glomerular sclerosis. Thus, the 'dose' of functioning nephrons present at birth may not only determine the risk of developing hypertension and renal disease later in life, but may even affect survival of renal transplants.

Specifically there may be a balance between nephron number and metabolic requirements imposed upon the transplanted (or nephron-deficient) kidney; consequently a 'nephron dose' below some critical value relative to the metabolic demands of the recipient (or chronic renal failure patient) may be inadequate for survival of the allograft (or nephron-deficient kidney). Thus, the number of functioning nephrons in the transplanted (or remnant) kidney may not suffice for the patient and the single nephron GFR may increase leading to intraglomerular hypertension, proteinuria and declining graft function. This hypothesis provides a construct for considering potential hemodynamic mechanisms that could contribute to progressive renal failure or to chronic allograft loss, in addition to the immunologically-mediated mechanisms of chronic allograft rejection.

Although the role of 'nephron dosing' in the pathogenesis of renal parenchymal hypertension has not been established, Brenner has proposed that the number of nephrons is related to the risk of developing hypertension in association with the progression of chronic renal disease. This formulation may provide a basis for future investigations to explore the pathogenesis of renal parenchymal hypertension.

Management of renal parenchymal hypertension

The most important component of the management of a patient with hypertension and renal disease is the control of blood pressure[1]. Hypertension is a powerful, and independent predictor of end-stage renal disease and long-term follow up of large numbers of male veterans in the Hypertension Screening and Treatment Program and of men screened for the Multiple Risk Factor Intervention Trial[2–4] provide strong evidence for a direct and graded connection between hypertension and end-stage renal disease. There is extensive evidence that hypertension accelerates deterioration of renal function and that appropriate antihypertensive therapy can retard the rate of progression of renal impairment and thereby delay the progression to end-stage renal disease. Therefore, preservation of renal function is a compelling reason for early diagnosis and vigorous treatment of hypertension.

Management of renal
parenchymal hypertension
Dietary sodium reduction

4

The Joint National Committee on Detection, Evaluation and Treatment of High Blood Pressure (JNC VI) recommendations for hypertensive patients with chronic renal failure are for a reduction to a target blood pressure of 130/85 mmHg – or to a lower value of 125/75 mmHg in patients with greater than 1 g proteinuria per day[1]. The management of hypertension in patients with chronic renal disease is a common and often perplexing problem confronting the clinician. The mechanisms that produce hypertension in the setting of renal parenchymal disease are different from those that cause primary hypertension. Accordingly, there are differences in therapeutic approaches between primary hypertension and hypertension associated with renal disease as well. The precise mechanisms that give rise to hypertension in patients with kidney disease are not completely elucidated, although sodium retention leading to volume expansion plays a central role.

Dietary sodium reduction

The JNC VI report recommends sodium reduction to less than that recommended for uncomplicated primary hypertension (< 100 mmol per day)[1]. To maintain even this modest level of sodium restriction intake requires dietary education and patient cooperation. For example, processed foods, such as canned vegetables and soups, prepared meat products, and most so-called 'fast foods', are extremely high in sodium content, as are most seasonings. The preparation of many processed foods adds a great deal of sodium. Repeated counseling and education by clinical dieticians along with diligent follow up is important. Patients should be cautioned about the use of salt substitutes: many contain potassium and should be avoided altogether in patients with renal impairment and diminished potassium excretory capacity.

Sodium intake must be individualized and each patient should be followed carefully for signs of ECFV depletion or worsening azotemia. Serial measurements of body weight and blood chemistries are often useful to identify an 'ideal' weight (ECFV) at which optimal blood pressure control is attained. In our clinical practice, we have found the daily weight to be the most useful indicator of changes in extracellular sodium. When done at the same time of day and on the same scale, the daily weight is quite helpful in determining net changes in sodium balance. An 'ideal' weight can often be established, at which the blood pressure becomes easier to manage. Measurements of 24-hour urinary excretion of sodium are somewhat time consuming and cumbersome, but may be useful for the evaluation of patient compliance with sodium restriction or suspected sodium wasting.

In clinical practice, attempts to lower blood pressure by dietary salt restriction alone are often not well tolerated by patients. This is particularly true in patients with advanced renal disease in view of the concomitant dietary restrictions often needed to manage renal failure (i.e. protein restriction, potassium restriction). Therefore, loop diuretics are required as a next step in most cases.

Diuretic therapy in chronic renal failure

An important difference between renal parenchymal hypertension and primary hypertension is the general lack of responsiveness of renal parenchymal hypertension to thiazide diuretics. Thiazide diuretics alone are not usually effective natriuretics in a patient with a serum creatinine above 2.0 mg/dl or a creatinine clearance below 30 ml/min, probably due to diminished delivery of the sodium load to the distal nephron and of the drug to its site of action. Therefore, the use of thiazide diuretics alone is not recommended at low levels of renal function.

The loop-acting diuretics (furosemide, ethacrynic acid, bumetanide, torasemide) are the agents of choice for the management of extracellular fluid volume and hypertension when the GFR falls below 30 ml/min[30–32]. Unlike the thiazides, the loop agents are effective natriuretics at GFRs well below 30 ml/min, even when used alone, although very high doses may be required as renal failure progresses. The loop diuretics act by inhibiting chloride (and sodium) reabsorption at the medullary thick ascending limb of the loop of Henle, which reabsorbs approximately 25–30% of the filtered sodium load. Because so much filtered sodium is reabsorbed in this nephron segment, it is understandable why these agents are such potent natriuretics.

Loop diuretics act from the luminal side and, therefore, they must enter the tubular lumen, both by glomerular filtration and by tubular secretion, before they can act. The dose–response curve of the loop diuretics is sigmoidal because the natriuretic response depends upon a threshold concentration of drug being delivered to its site of action. One approach to obtaining the optimal diuretic dose is to increase the dosage of diuretic carefully until the desired natriuresis occurs. This dosage would correspond to some point on the 'steep' part of the curve, where a small increase in diuretic delivery results in a large increase in natriuresis.

A common pitfall in the practical use of loop diuretics is increasing dose frequency rather than dose size: a dosage is tried which produces an insufficient natriuresis, but rather than increasing the dose, the clinician repeatedly administers the same dose (mistakenly expecting an additive response). The single dose size should be increased until a reasonable natriuresis is achieved. If still more natriuresis is desired, either the dose size or the dose frequency can be increased. Note that the dose–response curve flattens above a certain dose. Beyond this point there is no advantage to increasing the single dose. If further sodium excretion is required than is produced with the maximum single effective dose, then additional effective doses of the diuretic may be prescribed, but again, the risk of toxicity increases. In general, furosemide requires twice daily dosing whereas bumetanide is usually given once daily. Large doses of loop diuretics are usually needed. If the response is insufficient, single doses can be increased to a maximum of about 480 mg of furosemide. Larger single doses are unlikely to be more effective, and increase the risk of toxicity.

Dietary sodium restriction is important during diuretic therapy because compensatory sodium retention may occur between doses. This sodium retention may be sufficient to completely neutralize the natriuretic effects of the loop diuretics. On the other hand, care must be exercised to avoid overdiuresis, with consequent intravascular volume depletion and prerenal azotemia.

In patients with severe renal impairment who are refractory to loop diuretics, a combined regimen of furosemide and metolazone or thiazide can be effective, even with a creatinine clearance below 10 ml/min[31–33]. The combination works because proximally active diuretics increase distal delivery and the additional distal blockade results in greater natriuresis.

A minority of hypertensive patients with chronic renal failure are 'volume unresponsive'. This group is characterized by significant hypertension refractory to sodium restriction and diuretics, and will often require the addition of potent non-diuretic antihypertensive agents, such as calcium antagonists, angiotensin-converting enzyme inhibitors, or minoxidil. The calcium antagonists and the angiotensin-converting enzyme inhibitors are generally safe and effective agents in the setting of chronic renal failure and are sufficiently potent to treat severe arterial hypertension. They may also be used together to treat severe, resistant renal parenchymal hypertension. Because both the prevalence and the severity of hypertension increase as the glomerular filtration rate declines, it is important to continue close follow up and frequent reassessment of patients with hypertension and renal parenchymal disease, regardless of the initial therapeutic regimen employed.

Retarding the progression of renal failure – renoprotective effects of specific antihypertensives

Recently, increasing attention has focused on the importance of therapeutic interventions in addition to effective blood pressure control that may be renoprotective[34–39]. These measures focus on the preferential use of specific antihypertensive agents that may have renoprotective effects independent of their effects on blood pressure. The reader is referred to several recent reviews[39,40] for a discussion of this topic.

Summary

Renal parenchymal hypertension continues to constitute an important and common problem confronting the clinician. Hypertension complicating chronic renal disease is the major cause of secondary hypertension, and may result from diverse renal diseases. Unless properly treated, renal parenchymal hypertension can accelerate the progression of renal failure. The precise mechanisms which lead to hypertension in chronic renal failure have not been completely defined, but recent investigations have provided exciting new insights. The

4

traditional focus has been on volume-mediated mechanisms, the renin–angiotensin system and renal prostaglandins; recently, increasing attention has been given to other pressor and vasodilator systems, including endothelin and NO.

Consequently, our understanding of the pathogenesis of renal parenchymal hypertension has been rendered both more complex and more challenging. For example, the synthesis of NO by the vascular endothelium is responsible for the basal vasodilator tone essential for the downregulation of blood pressure. The description of a circulating inhibitor of the NO vasodilatory system which accumulates in renal failure provides a new potential mechanism by which chronic renal disease can produce hypertension. The endogenous production of a vasoconstrictor DLF which inhibits cellular Na^+, K^+-ATPase may likewise play a role. Additional insights into the pathogenesis of renal parenchymal hypertension await a more precise definition of the role of such mediators.

The mainstay of treating hypertension in renal parenchymal disease is the initiation of measures which will favor mobilization of sodium, such as dietary sodium restriction and the rational use of loop-acting diuretics. A practical knowledge of the difficulties of sodium restriction and the clinical pharmacology of loop diuretics is essential. In addition, preliminary data suggest that certain antihypertensive agents, such as the angiotensin-converting enzyme inhibitors and the calcium antagonists, may be important renoprotective agents.

In light of recent advances in our understanding of the pathogenesis and newer developments in pharmacologic management of hypertension secondary to renal parenchymal disease, we await studies that may yield additional information on its mechanisms and management.

References

1. Joint National Committee on Detection, Evaluation and Treatment of High Blood Pressure (JNC VI). The Sixth Report of the Joint National Committee on Detection, Evaluation and Treatment of High Blood Pressure (JNC VI). *Arch Intern Med* 1997;**157**:2413–2444.
2. Perry HM Jr, Miller JP, Fornoff JR *et al*. Early predictors of 15-year end-stage renal disease in hypertensive patients. *Hypertension* 1995;**25**:587–594.
3. Klag MJ, Whelton PK, Randall BL *et al*. Blood pressure and end-stage renal disease in men. *N Engl J Med* 1996;**334**:13–18.
4. Klag MJ, Whelton PK, Randall BL *et al*. End-stage renal disease in African-American and white men. 16 year MRFIT findings. *J Am Med Ass* 1997;**277**:1293–1298.
5. Perneger TV, Whelton PK, Klag MJ. History of hypertension in patients treated for end-stage renal disease. *J Hypertension* 1997;**15**:451–456.
6. Whelton PK, He J, Perneger TV, Klag MJ. Kidney damage in 'benign' essential hypertension. *Curr Opin Nephrol Hypertension* 1997;**6**:177–183.
7. Ruilope LM, Campo C, Rodriguez-Artalejo F *et al*. Blood pressure and renal function: therapeutic implications. *J Hypertension* 1996;**14**:1259–1263.
8. Maki DD, Ma JZ, Louis TA, Kasiske BL. Long-term effects of antihypertensive agents on proteinuria and renal function. *Arch Intern Med* 1995;**155**:1073–1080.
9. Preston RA, Singer I, Epstein M. Renal parenchymal hypertension: current concepts of pathogenesis and management. *Arch Intern Med* 1996;**154**:637–642.

References

10. Preston RA, Epstein M. Hypertension and renal parenchymal disease. *Semin Nephrol* 1995;**15**(2):138–151.

11. Smith MC, Dunn MJ. Hypertension associated with renal parenchymal disease. In: *Diseases of the Kidney* (eds Schrier RW, Gottschalk CW), pp 1333–1365. Little, Brown: Boston, MA, 1997.

12. Campese VM. Pathophysiology of renal parenchymal hypertension. In: *Hypertension Primer: The Essentials of High Blood Pressure* (eds Izzo Jr JL, Black HR), pp. 135–137. Lippincott Williams & Wilkins: Baltimore, MA, 1999.

13. Pohl MA. Management of hypertensive patients with chronic renal insufficiency. In: *Hypertension Primer: The Essentials of High Blood Pressure* (eds Izzo Jr JL, Black HR), pp. 407–409. Lippincott Williams & Wilkins: Baltimore, MA, 1999.

14. Kaplan N. Renal parenchymal hypertension. In: *Clinical Hypertension*, 7th edn. (ed Kaplan N), pp. 281–299. Williams & Wilkins: Baltimore, MA, 1998.

15. Walls MJ, Breyer JA. Hypertension in chronic renal failure, dialysis and transplantation. In: *Current Therapy in Nephrology and Hypertension*, 4th edn. (ed. Glassock RJ), pp. 335–351. Mosby Year-Book: St Louis, MO, 1998.

16. Preston RA, Epstein M. Ischemic renal disease: an emerging cause of chronic renal failure and end-stage renal disease. *J Hypertension* 1997;**15**:1365–1377.

17. Campese VM. Salt sensitivity in hypertension. Renal and cardiovascular implications. *Hypertension* 1994;**23**:531–550.

18. Haddy FJ, Buckalew VM. Endogenous digitalis-like factors in hypertension. In: *Hypertension: Pathophysiology, Diagnosis, and Management* (eds Laragh JH, Brenner BM), pp. 1055–1067. Raven Press: New York, 1995.

19. Lakkis FG, Nassar GM, Badr KF. Hormones and the kidney. In: *Disease of the Kidney*. (eds Schrier RW, Gottschalk CW), pp. 231–250. Little, Brown: Boston, MA, 1997.

20. Rocha R, Chander PN, Zuckerman A, Stier CT Jr. Role of aldosterone in renal vascular injury in stroke-prone hypertensive rats. *Hypertension* 1999;**33**(1 Pt 2):232–237.

21. Rocha R, Chander PN, Khanna K *et al.* Mineralocorticoid blockade reduces vascular injury in stroke-prone hypertensive rats. *Hypertension* 1998;**31**(1 Pt 2):451–458.

22. Epstein M. Aldosterone as a mediator of progressive renal disease: pathogenic and clinical implications. *Am J Kidney Dis* 2001;**37**:677–688.

23. Epstein M. Aldosterone and the hypertensive kidney: its emerging role as a mediator of progressive renal dysfunction: a paradigm shift. *J Hypertension* 2001;**19**:829–842.

24. Kohan DE. Endothelins in the normal and diseased kidney. *Am J Kidney Dis* 1997;**29**:2–26.

25. Kone BC. Biosynthesis and homeostatic roles of nitric oxide in the normal kidney. *Am J Physiol* 1997;**272**:F561–578.

26. Kone BC. Nitric oxide in renal health and disease. *Am J Kidney Dis* 1997;**30**:311–333.

27. Mackenzie HS, Brenner BM. Current strategies for retarding progression of renal disease. *Am J Kidney Dis* 1998;**31**:161–170.

28. Mackenzie HS, Garcia DL, Anderson S, Brenner BM. The renal abnormality in hypertension: a proposed defect in glomerular filtration surface area. In: *Hypertension: Pathophysiology, Diagnosis, and Management* (eds Laragh JH, Brenner BM), pp. 1539–1552. Raven Press: New York, 1995.

29. Anderson S, Brenner BM. The role of nephron mass and of intraglomerular pressure in initiation and progression of experimental hypertensive-renal disorders. In: *Hypertension: Pathophysiology, Diagnosis, and Management* (eds Laragh JH, Brenner BM), pp. 1539–1552. Raven Press, New York, 1995.

30. Brater DC. Diuretic therapy. *N Engl J Med* 1998;**339**:387–395.

31. Greger R, Dillingham MA, Schrier RW. Mechanism of diuretic action. In: *Diseases of the Kidney* (eds Schrier RW, Gottschalk CW), pp. 2321–2341. Little, Brown; Boston, MA, 1997.

32. Epstein M, Materson BJ. Furosemide. In: *Cardiovascular Drug Therapy* (ed. Messerli FH), pp. 318–336. WB Saunders: Philadelphia, PA, 1990.

33. Oster JR, Epstein M, Smoller S. Combined therapy with thiazide-type and loop diuretic agents for resistant sodium retention. *Ann Intern Med* 1983;**99**:405–406.

34. Striker GE, Klahr S. Clinical trials in the progression of renal failure. *Adv Intern Med* 1997;**42**:555–593.

35. Remuzzi G, Ruggenenti P, Benigni A. Understanding the nature of renal disease progression. *Kidney Int* 1997;**51**:2–15.
36. Gaansevoort RT, Navis GJ, Wapstra FH *et al*. Proteinuria and progression of renal disease: therapeutic implications. *Curr Opin Nephrol Hypertension* 1997;**6**:133–140.
37. El Nahas AM. Progression of renal scarring: a balancing act. *Adv Nephrol* 1998;**27**:67–84.
38. Preston RA. Renoprotective effects of antihypertensive drugs. *Am J Hypertension* 1999;**12**:19S–32S.
39. Epstein M. Angiotensin II receptor antagonist: current status. In: *Angiotensin II Receptor Antagonists* (eds Epstein M, Brunner HR), pp. 257–261. Hanley & Belfus: Philadelphia, PA, 2001.
40. Cooper M, Epstein M. Evolving role of angiotensin II receptor antagonists in diabetes mellitus. In: *Angiotensin II Receptor Antagonists* (eds Epstein M, Brunner HR), pp. 317–328. Hanley & Belfus: Philadelphia, PA, 2001.

References

4.3

Pheochromocytoma

G Grassi

4

Introduction

Pheochromocytoma represents one of the rare forms of secondary hypertension, accounting for 0.1–0.9% of all cases of hypertension. The large interindividual variability of its clinical manifestations, which are mainly related to the effects of high circulating levels of norepinephrine and epinephrine on the hemodynamic, metabolic and biochemical profiles, explains why this pathologic condition has received various definitions throughout the years, such as the 'great mimic' or the 'kaleidoscopic image'. Although uncommon, pheochromocytoma has major clinical relevance for at least three reasons. Firstly, it represents one of the few causes of hypertension that can be successfully cured. Secondly, its diagnosis and the therapeutic approach are not infrequently difficult and complex, often requiring a close interaction between different branches of clinical medicine, such as cardiology, neurology, endocrinology, anesthesiology, and surgery. Finally, pheochromocytoma still represents a unique model of adrenergic activation, which sheds light on several physiopathological aspects of the sympathetic function.

Frequency of pheochromocytoma

As mentioned above, pheochromocytoma accounts for a small fraction of all hypertensive cases. However, its true prevalence rate, is somewhat underestimated, because a considerable number of pheochromocytomas are only revealed at autopsy[1]. The fourth and fifth decades of age are usually those displaying the highest incidence, although the disease has also been diagnosed in newborns, children and in elderly individuals over 80 years of age, with no clearcut evidence of any gender predilection.

Location and etiology

Pheochromocytoma has been referred in the past as the 10% tumor, given the evidence that about 10% of cases are familial, 10% of malignant nature and 10% multiple or bilateral. According to recent reports, however, the rule of 10%, which also applies to its prevalence in children, does not apply to the extraadrenal location of the tumor, which appears to be detectable in about 20–30% of cases in very young individuals[2]. It is well established that the malignant nature of pheochromocytoma is peculiar to extraadrenal tumors[3] which usually display widespread metastases to several organs, such as the kidneys, the bones, the lungs and the lymphatic tissues. The tumor can be also sometimes found in patients affected by multiple endocrine neoplasias (MEN), medullary thyroid carcinoma, neurofibromatosis, von Hippel–Lindau disease and the so-called Carney syndrome, in which gastric and cartilaginous neoplasias may coexist with an extraadrenal pheochromocytoma.

As described in the following section, pheochromocytoma is a tumor of chromaffin cells anatomically located in the sympathoadrenal tissue which, by releasing large amounts of norepinephrine and epinephrine, accounts for the clinical picture of the disease.

4

The sympathetic nervous system

Catecholamines represent the biochemical transmitters through which the sympathetic nervous system regulates several cardiovascular and metabolic functions maintaining whole body homeostasis. Since the demonstration by Von Euler, more than 50 years ago, that norepinephrine represents the main neuroadrenergic neurotransmitter, much data have been gained on different aspects of catecholamine metabolism. It is now well established that, along with norepinephrine, there are two other adrenergic neurotransmitters, i.e. epinephrine and dopamine[4]. As shown in Figure 4.3.1, which schematically depicts the various pathways of biosynthesis and catabolism of catecholamines, dopamine represents a precursor of the other two compounds. Although all three adrenergic neurotransmitters are detectable in the blood stream as well as in urine, there are profound differences between various catecholamines regarding their sites of synthesis and their main physiological functions[4,5]. Epinephrine is mainly released from adrenal glands, a small fraction, usually not entering the circulation, being secreted from the central nervous system. Moreover, epinephrine can also be coreleased with norepinephrine from sympathetic nerve terminals particularly when the rate of nerve stimulation is markedly elevated[5]. Conversely, only a small fraction of norepinephrine entering the circulation is derived from the adrenal glands, the vast majority being directly released from peripheral sympathetic nerves. Dopamine, a precursor of both norepinephrine and epinephrine, is also an important adrenergic neurotransmitter in its own right in the central nervous system and, to a lesser extent, in some peripheral nerve terminals as well[5].

BOX 4.3.1 Differences between catecholamines

The differences between the various catecholamines are not limited to their chemical structures and sites of secretion. Table 4.3.1 shows that some cardiovascular and non-cardiovascular effects of norepinephrine and epinephrine are different each other and that these effects are mediated by stimulation of receptors which are specific for each compound. A classical example is represented by the vascular effects of catecholamines. While norepinephrine almost invariably induces vasoconstriction mediated by α_1-adrenoreceptor stimulation, both epinephrine and dopamine can elicit vasodilatation by acting on β_2-adrenoreceptors and dopaminergic receptors, respectively. In the case of epinephrine, however, this vasodilatation appears to occur selectively at the arteriolar level in the skeletal muscles. It should be underlined, however, that similar to what has been described in congestive heart failure state (also displaying high levels of circulating catecholamines), pheochromocytoma is characterized by a down regulation (i.e. a desensitization) of both alpha- and beta-adrenergic receptors which are thus less responsive to endogenous and exogenous adrenergic stimulation[6]. This adrenoreceptor downregulation may be responsible (or coresponsible) for the orthostatic hypotension not infrequently described in pheochromocytoma patients[7].

4

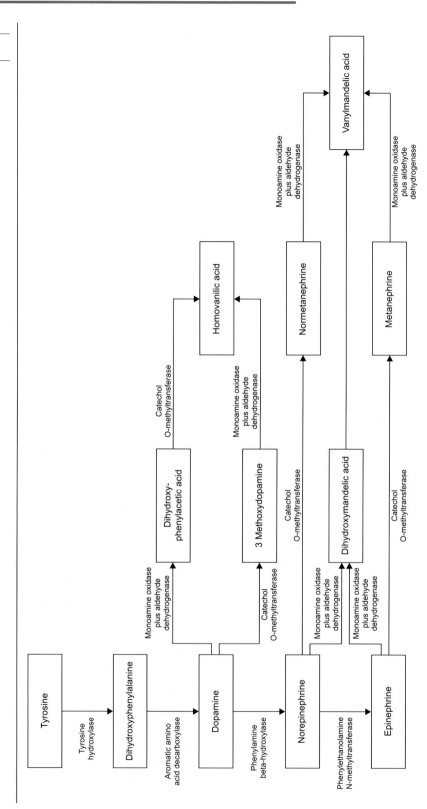

Fig. 4.3.1 Pathways of synthesis and metabolism of catecholamines with enzymes catalyzing various reactions

Table 4.3.1 Cardiovascular and metabolic effects of epinephrine and norepinephrine

Effect	Epinephrine	Norepinephrine
Cardiac		
Heart rate	+	–
Stroke volume	++	++
Cardiac output	+++	0, –
Arrhythmias	++++	++++
Coronary blood flow	++	++
Blood pressure (BP)		
Systolic BP	++	+++
Mean BP	+	++
Diastolic BP	+, 0, –	++
Mean pulmonary pressure	++	++
Peripheral circulation		
Total peripheral resistance	–	++
Cerebral blood flow	+	0, –
Muscle blood flow	+++	0, –
Skin blood flow	n/a	n/a
Renal blood flow	–	–
Splanchnic blood flow	+++	0, +
Metabolic effects		
Oxygen consumption	++	0, +
Blood glucose	+++	0, +
Blood lactic acid	+++	0, +

+: increase; –: reduction; 0: no change; n/a: not assessed.

Pathology of pheochromocytoma

The weight of pheochromocytoma is highly variable. In about 70% of cases, the weight is less than 100 g and their size less than 1–3 cm in diameter[2].

Tumors weighting more than 4 kg, have also been reported but in most cases most of this mass can be ascribed to the cystic and/or liquid nature of the masses. From a histological viewpoint chromaffin cells:

- are larger than those physiologically characterizing the normal tissue;
- show pleomorphism similar to that found in normal cells; and
- display a cytoplasmic compound characterized by eosinophilic and basophilic materials with multiple norepinephrine- and epinephrine-containing granules.

Usually the tumor is highly vascularized, and capsulated by a thin collagenous membrane and it may include a hemorrhagic or cystic core surrounded by chromaffin tissue frequently arranged in trabeculae or alveoli. The histologic features do not usually allow establishing of the malignant nature of a pheochromocytoma, which is generally determined by the invasivity of the tumor to adjacent tissues and/or organs and the presence of metastases. The prevalence of malignancy, however, is usually low (3–8% of cases according to data collected in different reports) and sometimes higher in extraadrenal pheochromocytoma. However, this should not be considered a general rule.

4

Biosynthesis and turnover of catecholamines in pheochromocytoma

The chromaffin tissue characterizing pheochromocytoma is capable of synthetizing both norepinephrine and epinephrine but not dopa and dopamine. However, frequently, but not invariably, tumors located in the adrenal glands preferentially secrete epinephrine, while extraadrenal pheochromocytomas store and secrete both types of catecholamines. In contrast to what happens in physiological conditions, the secretion of catecholamines from the tumor does not seem to be regulated by the central nervous system, presumably because pheochromocytoma tissues are not innervated[5]. A controversial issue is whether in pheochromocytoma central sympathetic neural activity is increased, thus contributing to the blood pressure elevation or rather suppressed by the inhibitory effects exerted by high levels of catecholamines on central adrenergic outflow[8]. Data collected by our group in a recent study[9], performed by directly measuring efferent postganglionic muscle sympathetic nerve traffic via the microneurographic technique, are in favour of the second hypothesis. This is because in patients with an adrenal pheochromocytoma sympathetic nerve traffic values (1) are markedly reduced when compared to those displayed by age-matched essential hypertensive patients characterized by a blood pressure elevation of similar magnitude and (2) undergo a clearcut increase following surgical removal of pheochromocytoma, and thus, normalization of plasma catecholamine profile (Figure 4.3.2). Therefore, it appears that the elevated values of plasma norepinephrine and epinephrine characterizing pheochromocytoma exert marked sympathoinhibitory effects on central sympathetic outflow.

Three other issues related to the secretion and metabolism of humoral agents by pheochromocytoma deserve to be mentioned. The first refers to the evidence that catecholamine secretion by the tumoral cells (1) does not occur by exocytosis, as physiologically happens, but via diffusion of amines through the cytoplasma and cellular wall and (2) is independent on the synthesis rate, in contrast to what usually occurs in normal states[8]. The second issue is related to the demonstration that catecholamine secretion process may be intermittent and sudden (usually due to tumor compression) or continuous[10]. Finally, several other neurohormonal substances, particularly of a peptidic nature with vasodilatatory or vasoconstrictive properties, may be released, in conjunction with catecholamines, by pheochromocytoma. They include the intestinal vasoactive peptide, enkephalins, β-endorphins, neuropeptide Y, atrial natriuretic factor, calcitonin, serotonin, and P substances[8,11].

Clinical features of pheochromocytoma

As mentioned above, the clinical symptoms of the disease are highly variable and this variability depends on how predominant is the

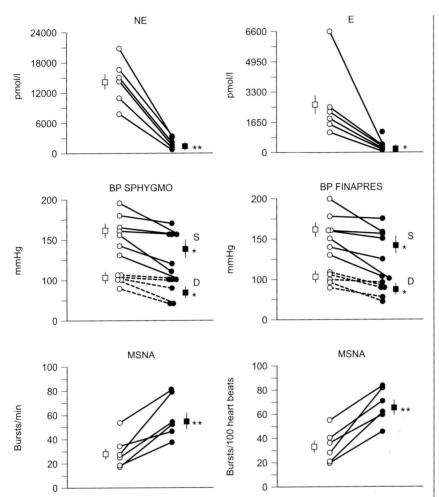

Fig. 4.3.2 Effects of surgical removal of pheochromocytoma on plasma norepinephrine (NE), plasma epinephrine (E), systolic (S) and diastolic (D) sphygmomanometric (sphygmo) and Finapres blood pressure (BP) values and muscle sympathetic nerve activity (MSNA). Data from six patients are shown. Values before intervention are depicted as empty symbols while closed symbols refer to the post-surgical condition. Modified from Grassi et al.[9].

secretion of norepinephrine or epinephrine, as well as the concomitant secretion of other neurohormones. It is also worth mentioning that the clinical picture, although dependent on the adverse effects of catecholamines on the hemodynamic and metabolic profile, is not related either to circulating levels of the adrenergic neurotransmitters or to the tumor size and weight[7,11]. In other words, it is possible to find patients displaying very few symptoms with a large tumor and vice versa a variegate clinical picture in subjects with small adrenal (or extra-adrenal) masses. Figure 4.3.3 illustrates the clinical signs and symptoms that can be found in pheochromocytoma patients listed according to the frequency of occurrence[12]. The 'classic triad' of

Clinical features of
pheochromocytoma

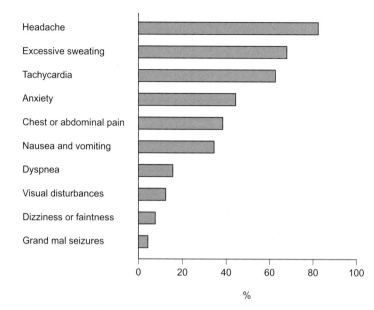

Fig. 4.3.3 Percentage incidence of symptoms in a series of 324 pheochromocytoma patients. After Ross and Griffith[12].

symptoms, which is highly suggestive for the presence of a pheochromocytoma, includes:

- hypertension,
- headache and
- excessive and generalized sweating.

Blood pressure elevation is almost always the rule, although pheochromocytoma patients with normal blood pressure and hypertensive crises have also been described. It is, therefore, possible to find different patterns of blood pressure behavior, i.e. (1) a stable and sustained hypertensive state, (2) a sustained hypertension with hypertensive crises and (3) a normotensive state with brief, sudden and marked blood pressure elevations. The hypertensive crises are usually asymptomatic but they can also be preceded by clinical manifestations, such as dizziness, flushing, visual disturbances, nausea, vomiting or an epileptic-like 'aura'. The episodic increases in blood pressure values do not display any clearcut relation to the period of the day, usually last a few minutes (in 80% of cases less than 2 minutes) and can be triggered by the mechanical compression of the tumor (sometimes occurring during the physical examination of the patient), exercise, postural changes, micturition, Valsalva manouver, eating and digestion. On some occasions the hypertensive crises can be so pronounced or complicated by cardiac rhythm disturbances as to cause cardiogenic shock, myocardial ischemia or infarction, pulmonary edema, cerebral ischemia and sudden death, mainly due to ventricular fibrillation.

4

BOX 4.3.2 signs and symptoms characterizing pheochromocytoma

These depend on the adverse cardiovascular and metabolic effects of high
circulating levels of norepinephrine and epinephrine:

- *Cardiovascular effects*
Tachycardia
Rhythm disturbances
Postural hypotension

- *Metabolic effect*
Elevated blood glucose
From a cardiovascular viewpoint this is, for example, the case for tachycardia
and cardiac rhythm disturbances, ascribable to the positive chronotropic and
proarrhythmogenic effects of catecholamines on the myocardial tissue[4].
From a metabolic viewpoint this is exemplified by the increased plasma
glycemic levels displayed by pheochromocytoma patients, which depend on
the stimulating effects of norepinephrine and epinephrine on glucogenesis
and gluconeogenesis and to a lesser extent on the anti-insulinemic effects
(e.g. insulin resistance) of catecholamines[4,5]. A sign which is present in
more than half of the patients is orthostatic hypotension, which has been
ascribed either to a reduced circulating blood volume or to a functional
impairment in reflexogenic areas involved in blood pressure control, such as
the arterial baroreceptors and the cardiopulmonary receptors, and/or in the
above-mentioned alpha- and beta-adrenoreceptor cardiovascular
regulation[7].

Differential diagnosis

A wide spectrum of cardiovascular, neurological, endocrinological,
psychiatric and systemic diseases can mimic the clinical picture of
pheochromocytoma, sometimes making the clinical diagnosis
particularly difficult to be performed. These include, in particular, all
forms of essential and secondary hypertension, hyperthyroidism,
myocardial infarction and angina, autonomic dysfunctions and
paroxysmal episodes of vasodilating headaches. It should also be
stressed that assumption of various drugs (amphetamines, ephedrine,
phenylephrine, isoproterenol, etc.) may cause clinical symptoms similar
to those found in pheochromocytoma.

Diagnosis of pheochromocytoma

Due to the diverse clinical manifestations of pheochromocytoma, it is
difficult to suggest guidelines for the diagnosis. There are, however, a
group of clinical conditions or manifestations suggestive for
pheochromocytoma and thus requiring further diagnostic examinations.
These conditions include:

- symptomatic hypertension, if the etiology is uncertain,
- severe hypertension,
- sustained and/or paroxysmal hypertension with recurrent attacks of
  symptoms suggestive for pheochromocytoma

- orthostatic hypotension,
- weight loss,
- hyperglycemia,
- paradoxic blood pressure rise during antihypertensive drug treatment and
- presence at X-ray of a suprarenal mass.

There are three steps that should be followed sequentially for the diagnosis of pheochromocytoma:

- Laboratory tests
- Pharmacological tests
- Anatomical localization

The first step is based on laboratory tests, i.e. biochemical assay:

- 24-hour urinary excretion of catecholamines, vanylmandelic acid and metanephrines, i.e. the metabolites of norepinephrine and epinephrine and
- circulating levels of the two adrenergic neurotransmitters.

Due to the evidence that several pheochromocytomas have only intermittent hypersecretion of norepinephrine and epinephrine, the assay of 24-hour urinary excretion of catecholamines and their metabolites is considered the best methodological approach for screening patients suspected for having the disease[70]. This is because the plasma norepinephrine and epinephrine assay, although it has improved technically in recent years with the availability of high-pressure liquid chromatography[13], still has some technical and physiological pitfalls. They include their suboptimal specificity and sensitivity and evidence that several factors (e.g. venepuncture, anxiety, posture, drugs and others) may affect plasma catecholamine values[4]. In addition, as previously mentioned, due to intermittency of secretion, some patients with pheochromocytoma may have normal plasma catecholamines values.

The second class of diagnostic tools are represented by the so-called pharmacological test, aimed at increasing or suppressing sympathetic activity and thus catecholamine secretion. As shown in Figure 4.3.4, which depicts a diagnostic flowchart for pheochromocytoma proposed by Bravo some years ago, these tests are indicated in patients displaying the clinical

---

BOX 4.3.3 The clonidine suppression test

The clonidine suppression test, which is based on evidence that this drug reduces plasma catecholamines in normal subjects but not in pheochromocytoma, is relatively safe[15]. A normal clonidine suppression test reduces plasma catecholamines to below 500 pg/ml, while in pheochromocytoma it does not affect circulating levels of adrenergic neurotransmitters. Sudden and marked blood pressure reductions sometimes may occur and this explains why this pharmacological test should not be performed without careful blood pressure monitoring.

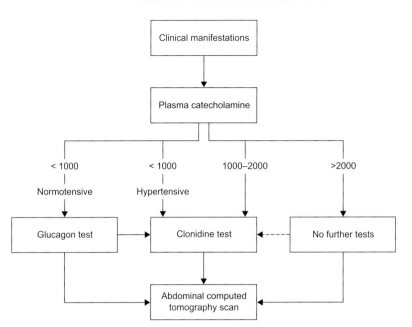

Fig. 4.3.4 Clinical flow-chart for pheochromocytoma proposed by Bravo[7]. Modified from
Bravo[7].

picture of pheochromocytoma, but with plasma catecholamine levels in
the so called 'borderline range' (below 1000 pg/ml). It should also be
noted that at present only suppressive tests (i.e. the clonidine test) can be
recommended, given the reports that provocative tests (glucagon and
others) are potentially dangerous, occasionally eliciting marked blood
pressure uses[14].

Ambulatory monitoring of 24-hour blood pressure values or
prolonged beat-to-beat blood pressure recordings may be useful, due to
the ability of these techniques to detect hypertensive crises (Figure
4.3.5)[16]. In addition, there is evidence that pheochromocytomas do not
display the physiological blood pressure fall occurring during sleep.
However, this finding does not seem to be peculiar to this secondary
form of hypertension, its occurrence being described also in
renovascular hypertension and in some patients with an essential
hypertensive state.

The final group of diagnostic tests are those aimed at defining the
anatomical localization of the mass. These imaging techniques include
computed tomographic (CT) scans, magnetic resonance imaging (MRI)
and meta-iodobenzylguanidine scintigraphic (MIBG) evaluation[17]. As
shown in Table 4.3.2, all these diagnostic procedures display advantages
and disadvantages but in general they can provide complementary
information[18]. Due to the increasing availability of CT scanning in
hospitals, this technique should be considered preferentially. However,
due to the reduced accuracy of a CT approach for extraadrenal tissues,
MRI is considered complementary. Most recently, Bravo[7] indicated
MRI as the procedure of choice. The MIBG scintigraphic approach

4

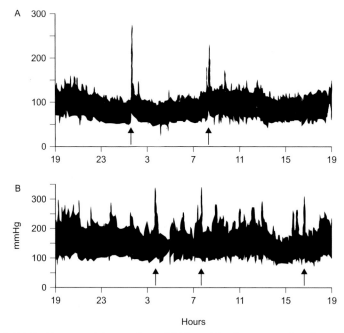

Fig. 4.3.5 Original intraarterial recordings of 24-hour blood pressure values in two patients (A: normotensive, B: hypertensive) with pheochromocytoma. Arrows indicate hypertensive crises. Figure modified from Mancia *et al.*[16].

Table 4.3.2 Pros and cons of different imaging techniques employed in pheochromocytoma diagnosis

Technique	Pros	Cons
Computed tomography	Good anatomic information	No functional information Radiation exposure Questionable in extraadrenal pheochromocytoma
Magnetic resonance imaging	No radiation exposure No contrast media Good anatomic information	Expensive No functional information
MIBG scintigraphy	Functional as well as structural data	Radiation exposure Poor anatomical information

should be reserved for a suspicion of malignant pheochromocytoma, due to the ability of the technique to detect metastases or multiple tumors. Positron emission tomographic examinations, although promising, require further evaluation.

Treatment of pheochromocytoma

Surgical treatment is, of course, the only effective therapeutic approach of pheochromocytoma, independently of the benign or malignant nature of the tumor. Antihypertensive drug treatment, however, is required in the preoperative phase, in order to avoid marked blood pressure oscillations and hypertensive crises during the anesthetic management and the surgical procedures[7]. The drugs commonly used are α_1-adrenergic antagonists (prazosin, doxazosin), drugs combining α_1- and β-adrenergic antagonistic properties (labetalol) and more recently beta-blockers with vasodilatory properties, such as carvedilol. Another therapeutic cornerstone in the preoperative phase is volume repletion in order to avoid postsurgical hypotensive episodes and to counterbalance the hypovolemia not infrequently detectable in pheochromocytoma[7]. The postoperative follow up requires a careful blood pressure monitoring particularly during the first 72 hours after surgery. In general, about 50% of surgically-treated patients display normal blood pressure values one year after pheochromocytoma removal, while plasma catecholamines return to control values usually within 10 weeks[19]. The reasons for this different time-course of the catecholamine and blood pressure reductions remain obscure.

References

1. Sutton M, Sheps SG, Lie JI. Prevalence of clinically unsuspected pheochromocytoma: review of 50 year autopsy series. *Mayo Clin Proc* 1981;**56**:354–360.
2. Samaan NA, Hickey RC, Shutts PE. Diagnosis, localization and management of pheochromocytoma. *Cancer* 1988;**62**:2451–2460.
3. Whalen RK, Althausen AF, Daniels GH. Extra-adrenal pheochromocytoma. *J Urol* 1992;**147**:1–10.
4. Kopin IJ. Catecholamine metabolism: basic aspects and clinical significance. *Pharmacol Rev* 1985;**40**:1534–1541.
5. Esler M, Jennings G, Lambert G *et al*. Overflow of catecholamine neurotransmitters to the circulation: source, fate and functions. *Physiol Rev* 1990; **70**(4):963–985.
6. Greenacre JK, Conolly ME. Desensitization of the beta-adrenoreceptor of lympocytes from normal subjects and patients with pheochromocytoma: studies *in vivo*. *Br J Clin Pharmacol* 1978;**5**:191–197.
7. Bravo EL. Evolving concepts in the pathophysiology, diagnosis and treatment of pheochromocytoma. *Endocrine Rev* 1994;**15**:356–368.
8. Bravo EL Pheochromocytoma: new concepts and future trends. *Kidney Int* 1991;**40**:544–556.
9. Grassi G, Seravalle G, Turri C, Mancia G. Sympathetic nerve traffic responses to surgical removal of pheochromocytoma. *Hypertension* 1999;**34**:461–465.
10. Bravo EL, Tarazi RC, Gifford RW, Stewart BH. Circulating and urinary catecholamines in pheochromocytoma. Diagnostic and pathophysiologic implications. *N Engl J Med* 1979; **301**:682–686.
11. Sheps SG, Jiang N, Klee GG. Recent development in the diagnosis and treatment of pheochromocytoma. *Mayo Clin Proc* 1990;**65**:88–95.
12. Ross ZJ, Griffith DN. The clinical presentation of pheochromocytoma. *Q J Med* 1989;**71**:485–494.
13. Hjemdahl P. Catecholamine measurements by high-performance liquid chromatography. *Am J Physiol* 1984;**247**:E13–E20.
14. Grossman E, Goldstein DS, Hoffman A, Keiser HR. Glucagon and clonidine testing in the diagnosis of pheochromocytoma. *Hypertension* 1991;**17**:733–741.
15. Bravo EL, Tarazi RC, Fouad FM *et al*. Clonidine-suppression test: a useful aid in the diagnosis of pheochromocytoma. *N Engl J Med* 1981;**305**:623–626.
16. Mancia G, Ferrari A, Gregorini L. *et al*. Prolonged intra-arterial blood-pressure recording in diagnosis of pheochromocytoma. *Lancet* 1979;**ii**:1193–1194.
17. Velcick MG, Alavi A, Kressel HY, Engelman K. Localization of pheochromocytoma: MIBG, CT and MRI correlation. *J Nucl Med* 1989;**30**:328–341.
18. Pommier RF, Brennan MF. Management of adrenal neoplasms. *Curr Probl Surg* 1991;**28**:657–669.

References
Further reading

19. Van Heerden JA, Roland CF, Carney JA *et al*. Long-term evaluation following resection of apparently benign pheochromocytoma(s)/paraganglioma(s). *World J Surg* 1990; **14**:325–329.

Further reading

Kebebew E, Duh Q. Benign and malignant pheochromocytoma. *Surg Oncol Clin N Am* 1998;**7**:765–789.

Manger WM, Gifford RW *Clinical and Experimental Pheochromocytoma*, 2nd edn. Blackwell Science: Cambridge, MA, 1996.

4

Chapter

4.4

Cortico-adrenal hypertension

JA Whitworth

4

Introduction

The adrenal glands were identified by Bartolommeo Eustachio in 1563 – the 'glandular renibus incumbentes'; their role in medicine was first recognized by Addison in 1855, and hypertension due to the adrenals has been recorded only this century.

Adrenocortical steroid hypertension has long been regarded as a rarity, but it may be much more common than previously realized. Although Cushing's syndrome remains uncommon it is now clear that relative or local cortisol excess may be responsible for hypertension in a variety of clinical situations including a proportion of patients with essential hypertension which will not be considered in this chapter. Similarly, although Conn suggested, many years ago, that primary aldosteronism may be a common condition, these notions were not confirmed by other workers until recently. Popularization of the aldosterone : renin ratio in the diagnosis of primary aldosteronism has led to increasing recognition of cases, so that in some centers primary aldosteronism is now the most common curable form of secondary hypertension.

This chapter considers both naturally occurring and iatrogenic adrenocortical hypertension. A working classification is shown in Table 4.4.1.

Table 4.4.1 A classification of cortico-adrenal hypertension

- *Mineralocorticoid excess*
  Primary aldosteronism (Conn's syndrome)
    Adrenal adenoma
    Bilateral adrenal hyperplasia
    Adrenal carcinoma
    Glucocorticoid-suppressible hyperaldosteronism (GSH; FH1)
  Congenital adrenal hyperplasia (CAH)
    11β-hydroxylase deficiency
    17α-hydroxylase deficiency
  Deoxycorticosterone-secreting adrenal tumors
  Apparent mineralocorticoid excess
  Iatrogenic mineralocorticoid excess
    9α-fluorinated steroids
    glycyrrhizinic acid (licorice)

- *Glucocorticoid excess (Cushing's syndrome)*
  ACTH excess
    Pituitary excess (Cushing's disease)
    Ectopic ACTH production
  Adrenal Cushing's syndrome
    Adenoma
    Carcinoma
    Hyperplasia
  Iatrogenic hypertension
    ACTH treatment
    Glucocorticoid therapy
    Alcohol induced (pseudo-Cushing's)

Mineralocorticoid excess

Forms of mineralocorticoid excess

Primary aldosteronism (Conn's syndrome)

The syndrome of excess secretion of aldosterone (Figure 4.4.1) with hypertension and hypokalemic alkalosis was first described by Jerome W. Conn, a US physician and endocrinologist[1]. The condition is frequently asymptomatic, but hypokalemia if severe may manifest with weakness, cramps, fatigue, parasthesiae or even periodic paralysis, and polyuria and polydipsia. Glucose intolerance is common, and hypertension may be severe, even malignant[2].

Primary aldosteronism usually leads to increased aldosterone secretion, raising plasma concentration and urinary excretion, leading to potassium depletion, hypokalemia and renal potassium wasting. There is also sodium retention with increased exchangeable sodium, often extracellular fluid and plasma volume expansion and mild hypernatremia; extracellular alkalosis with increased plasma bicarbonate concentration; and suppression of renin and hypertension which may be severe. Hypokalemia may be spontaneous or diuretic induced and is exacerbated by sodium loading. It is accompanied by evidence of urinary potassium leak (> 30 mmol/day). However, it is important to recognize that the condition may be present without the classical hypokalemia and may present as simple hypertension.

Adrenal adenoma

A solitary adrenal adenoma is the cause of Conn's syndrome in around 65% of cases[3] and is the classical form of the condition. The tumor is usually small (< 2 cm) with a yellow cut surface. It is more common in women than men and rare in children.

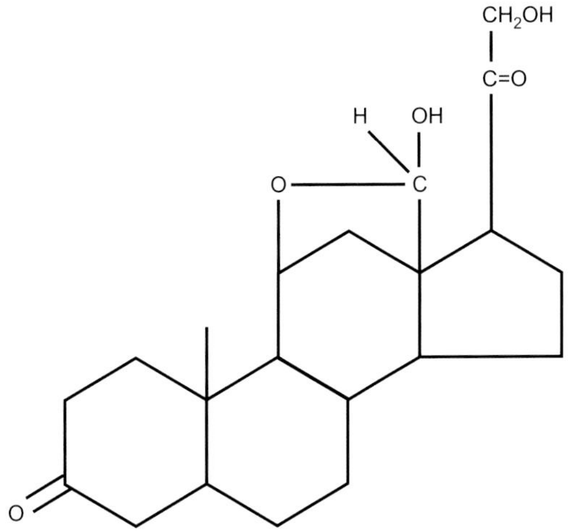

Fig. 4.4.1 Aldosterone: the very highly preferred 11,18 hemiketal form.

Bilateral adrenal hyperplasia

Bilateral hyperplasia, with or without discrete nodules, is found in around 25% of cases of primary aldosteronism and more commonly in men. Clinical features tend to be less marked than in adenoma. The distinction from adenoma is important in determining the need for medical versus surgical treatment.

Adrenal carcinoma

Adrenocortical cancer is a rare cause of hyperaldosteronism[4]. Adrenal cancers usually secrete excess glucocorticoids, androgens, and other mineralocorticoids as well as aldosterone, and are usually larger than aldosteronomas. Hyperaldosteronism has also been described with ovarian cancer[5].

Glucocorticoid-suppressible hyperaldosteronism (GSH) (FH1)

Glucocorticoid-suppressible hyperaldosteronism (GSH), also known as 'dexamethasone-suppressible hyperaldosteronism' (DSH), 'glucocorticoid remediable hyperaldosteronism' (GRA), or 'familial hyperaldosteronism type 1' (FH1) is a rare autosomal dominant form of primary aldosteronism (around 3%) in which aldosterone is under ACTH rather than renin–angiotensin control. It often presents in childhood.

BOX 4.4.1 Glucocorticoid-suppressible hyperaldosteronism

Although first described over 30 years ago[6], the key to understanding the genesis of GSH came from the delineation of the mutation whereby a chimaeric 11β-hydroxylase/aldosterone synthase gene is responsible for the observed biochemical and clinical features[7]. This hybrid gene on chromosome 8 has a 5′ region derived from the 11β-hydroxylase gene and a 3′ portion derived from the aldosterone synthase gene. It is thus regulated by ACTH but codes for aldosterone synthase, so that aldosterone secretion is regulated by ACTH rather than angiotensin. Patients have features of primary aldosteronism frequently associated with early onset hemorrhagic stroke and ruptured cerebral aneurysm[8]. Biochemically GSH is characterized by hyperaldosteronism, in which plasma aldosterone fails to rise normally or falls during upright posture or angiotensin infusion and is markedly and persistently suppressed by dexamethasone. There is associated excess production of 18-oxo- and 18-hydroxycortisol. The hybrid gene is detectable by Southern blotting or a long polymerase chain reaction method[9].

Gordon and colleagues have described a familial form of primary hyperaldosteronism which is not glucocorticoid-suppressible but associated with either adenoma formation or apparent bilateral hyperplasia, which they called familial hyperaldosteronism type 2 (FH2)[10], to distinguish it from FH1 (GSH) in which tumor formation has not been reported. They have suggested that hereditable genetic defects in FH2 predispose to bilateral adrenal hyperfunction, which sometimes progresses to tumor formation, analogous to multiple

4

endocrine neoplasia (MEN). FH2 differs from FH1 in a number of ways. Aldosterone secretion is not glucocorticoid-suppressible, some FH2 patients show aldosterone responsiveness to angiotensin and they do not have the hybrid gene[11].

Diagnosis and treatment

Diagnosis of primary aldosteronism until relatively recently was usually considered in the investigation of hypokalemic hypertension. It is now clear that this approach will miss many surgically remediable cases of normokalemic primary aldosteronism[12]. It is generally agreed that the best screening test is the aldosterone : renin ratio (normal <25–30) [13], as it is relatively independent of diet and therapy. A simplified schema for diagnosis of primary aldosteronism is shown in Figure 4.4.2.

In primary aldosteronism, urinary aldosterone excretion remains high despite sodium loading (either oral or intravenous) or exogenous mineralocorticoid administration.

The various types of primary aldosteronism also need to be distinguished because management differs. In normal subjects and

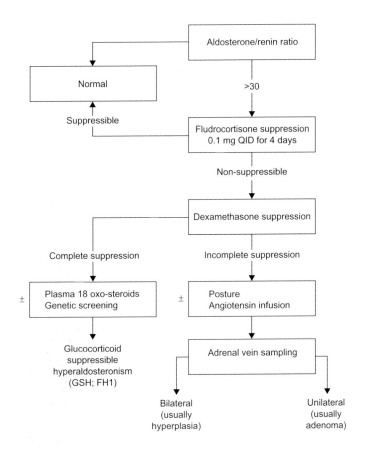

Fig. 4.4.2 A simplified scheme for diagnosis of primary aldosteronism.

adrenal hyperplasia, upright posture after overnight recumbency increases plasma aldosterone concentration, but in adenoma and GSH usually decreases or fails to increase, because of lack of response to angiotensin II. However, some 20% of adenomas are angiotensin responsive. GSH can be distinguished because of the profound fall in aldosterone and often blood pressure after dexamethasone. In adenoma, aldosterone often also falls following dexamethasone, but the fall is much less than in GSH. Increases in 18-hydroxycortisol and 18-hydroxycorticosterone are also seen in adenoma.

Localization of the adrenal abnormality is crucial prior to surgery. Carcinomas or larger adenomas are seen on CT scanning or MRI. Radionuclide scanning with radiolabelled iodocholesterol after dexamethosone suppression is also useful – tracer is accentuated in adenoma. The gold standard for localization is adrenal venous sampling with measurement of aldosterone : cortisol ratios in both adrenal veins and inferior vena cava.

Adrenal adenoma is best treated surgically, either in open or laparoscopic procedure. Infarction under radiologic control using a venous catheter has also been reported. In the majority of operated cases the hypertension is cured or improved. Medical therapy with spironolactone is usually effective in reversing the biochemical abnormalities of primary aldosteronism but additional antihypertensive medication may be required for blood pressure control. Spironolactone is also of value prior to surgery for blood pressure control and potassium repletion. Dosage may be limited by side effects as impotence, gynecomastia, and gut symptoms.

In GSH, glucocorticoid, usually dexamethasone, which suppresses ACTH and thus aldosterone, is used at the lowest dose compatible with appropriate biochemical and blood pressure control. Amiloride and spironolactone are also of value.

Congenital adrenal hyperplasia (CAH)

A simplified steroid biosynthetic pathway is shown in Figure 4.4.3.

Forms of CAH

11β-Hydroxylase deficiency

11β-hydroxylase deficiency comprises around 5–8% of cases of CAH, around 1 in 200 000 births[14]. A number of mutations have been described in the gene *CYP11B1* on chromosome 8q 21-q 22 in patients with classic defects. Deficiency of 11β-hydroxylase causes decreased conversion of 11-deoxycortisol to cortisol and 11-deoxycorticosterone to corticosterone, with consequent increases in ACTH secretion leading to overproduction of precursors proximal to the 11β-hydroxylase step. Deoxycorticosterone and/or 11-deoxycortisol concentrations in serum are increased, as are their tetrahydro metabolites in urine. The cause of the hypertension is unresolved.

Most patients have early-onset hypertension, but only a minority have features of mineralocorticoid excess. Signs of androgen excess are

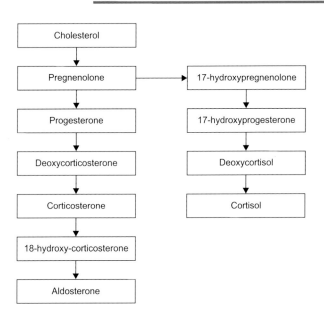

Fig. 4.4.3 Simplified steroid biosynthetic pathways.

common. Clinical features usually respond to glucocorticoid administration but antihypertensive therapy may also be required.

17α-Hydroxylase deficiency

A number of mutations have been described in coding regions of the *CYP17* gene on chromosome 10q 24–25, resulting usually in absent activity of a microsomal cytochrome P450. Cortisol cannot be synthesized and sex hormones are deficient. There is excessive secretion of deoxycorticosterone with corticosterone production adequate to prevent adrenal insufficiency. Hypertension occurs in most cases[14].

Deoxycorticosterone secreting tumors

Excess of deoxycorticosterone occurs rarely in adrenal adenomas and carcinomas and has also been reported in isolation[15].

Apparent mineralcorticoid excess (AME)

Apparent mineralcorticoid excess is an inherited autosomal recessive condition characterized by hypertension, hypokalemia and renin aldosterone suppression, first described in children[16] and later in an adult,[17]. The diagnosis relies on a characteristic urinary steroid profile with a rise in the ratio of cortisol metabolites (tetrahydrocortisol and allotetrahydrocortisol) to cortisone metabolites (tetrahydrocortisone). Plasma cortisol has a long half-life and low secretion rate with apparently normal plasma cortisol concentrations and intact circadian rhythm. Some but not all patients have raised urinary free cortisol levels. The hypertension and metabolic effects are at least in part reversed by administration of dexamethasone. The defect is a mutation in the gene for 11β-hydroxysteroid dehydrogenase 2 (*11BHSD2*), on chromosome 16q22, which leads to minimal or absent enzyme activity[18].

It is thought that the hypertension is a consequence of the deficiency of *11BHSD2* resulting in raised intra-renal glucocorticoid concentrations, which access the mineralocorticoid receptor. Renal transplantation cures the defect indicating that AME is a renal disorder[19] and compatible with the observation that the kidney is the major site for cortisone generation[20]. Although this explains the metabolic effects, whether the hypertension in this condition can be explained by the action of cortisol on the type I mineralocorticoid receptor is less clear. The blood pressure raising effects of cortisol in subjects with AME are quite rapid in onset, in contrast to the very gradual onset of hypertension seen with classical mineralocorticoid agonists as aldosterone. Further, the effects of the mineralocorticoid receptor antagonist spironolactone in the hypertension are incomplete and may be explained simply by the natriuretic effect of the drug seen also in non-steroid forms of hypertension[21].

In a few cases (the so-called type II form of AME) ratios of tetrahydrocortisol to tetrahydrocortisone are normal but as in type I, the ratio of free urinary cortisol to cortisone is high[22].

Iatrogenic mineralocorticoid excess

9α-Fluorinated steroids

Severe but reversible hypertension with hypokalemia and suppression of renin and aldosterone has been reported with both skin creams and nasal drops containing 9α-fluoroprednisolone[23].

Glycyrrhizinic acid (licorice)

It has been recognized for many years that a moderate-to-high licorice intake can produce hypertension with hypokalemia and renin suppression. Licorice is found not only as a confectionery or in chewing gum but also in health products, licorice root, chewing tobacco and alcoholic drinks[24]. The active metabolite is glycyrrhetinic acid, which inhibits *11BHSD2* in the kidney.

BOX 4.4.2 Glycyrrhizinic acid

Glycyrrhizinic acid or licorice (Figure 4.4.4) is known to ameliorate symptoms of Addison's disease (providing some adrenal function remains) and glycyrrhetinic acid binds weakly to type I mineralocorticoid receptors. However it is now recognized that the hypertension of licorice use or abuse is a consequence of inhibition of *11BHSD2* in the kidney leading to defects in cortisol metabolism with an increase in the urinary ratio of tetrahydrocortisol to tetrahydrocortisone, high urinary free cortisol concentrations and prolonged cortisol half-life[28]. The evidence of mineralocorticoid-type hypertension which is slow in onset is compatible with the notion that cortisol is exerting its effects through occupancy of type I mineralocorticoid receptors.

4

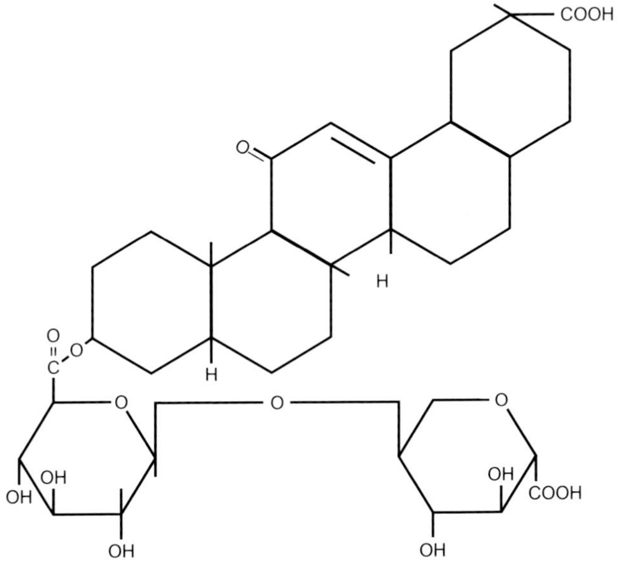

Fig. 4.4.4 Glycyrrhizinic acid.

The hypertension due to the antiulcer drug carbenoxolone (Fig. 4.4.5) is produced similarly. However carbenoxolone at a dose that induces mineralocorticoid effects in patients does not produce significant changes in the urinary cortisol to cortisone tetrahydro metabolite ratio. Rather carbenoxolone produces marked inhibition of ring A reduction of both cortisol and cortisone to tetrahydro metabolites. Urinary cortisol is unchanged but urinary cortisone is decreased and cortisol to cortisone ratio increased[26].

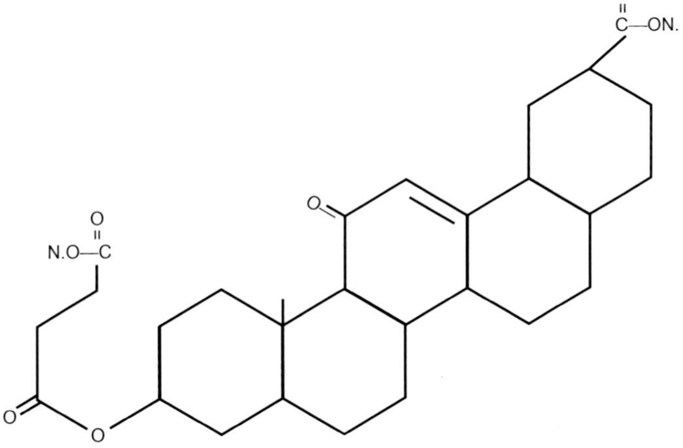

Fig. 4.4.5 Carbenoxolone.

4.4

4

Glucocorticoid excess (Cushing's syndrome)

Harvey Cushing (1869–1939) was a US neurosurgeon who first described the disorder that bears his name in a monograph entitled 'The pituitary body and its disorders' in 1912[1]. Cushing's syndrome is characterized by hypertension, susceptibility to infection, moon face with truncal obesity and abdominal striae, hirsutism, plethora, hyperglycemia, glucose intolerance, diabetes, cataracts, myopathy, osteoporosis, and renal calculi.

The most common cause of naturally occurring Cushing's syndrome is pituitary ACTH excess or Cushing's disease. Cushing's syndrome due to therapy with synthetic glucocorticoids is common and iatrogenic hypertension also complicates ACTH therapy, which is used in some uncommon neurological conditions.

There is good evidence that the hypertension of Cushing's syndrome can be explained by the excess cortisol secretion[27]. Prolonged cortisol excess is associated with hypertension, hypercholesterolemia, hypertriglyceridemia, impairment of glucose tolerance and accelerated atherosclerosis and in consequence cardiovascular morbidity and mortality is substantial.

Cushing's syndrome is a rare cause of clinical hypertension in that it affects less than 0.1% of the population but hypertension is a very common finding in Cushing's syndrome affecting some 80% of subjects[28].

The diagnosis of Cushing's syndrome can be difficult (Figure 4.4.6) but in patients with Cushing's syndrome who present with hypertension is usually obvious clinically. In practice the obese hypertensive patient with syndrome X may be difficult to distinguish.

ACTH excess

Pituitary ACTH excess (Cushing's disease)

Cushing's disease accounts for around two-thirds of cases with excess ACTH secretion and often elevated plasma ACTH concentrations leading to bilateral adrenal hyperplasia. Pituitary microadenomas are found in most cases but around 10% have discrete pituitary adenomas resulting in enlargement of the pituitary fossa, either chromophobe or basophil.

Ectopic ACTH production

ACTH secretion by primary extrapituitary tumors produces suppression of pituitary ACTH secretion and bilateral adrenal hyperplasia. Hypertension is less common in Cushing's syndrome secondary to ectopic ACTH production than in other forms. Ectopic ACTH classically affects men and produces severe hypokalemic alkalosis and often weakness and pigmentation. Ectopic corticotropin-releasing factor (CRF) production by non-hypothalamic tumors is an extremely rare cause of ACTH-dependent Cushing's syndrome.

If suspected (usually abnormal 24-hour urine free cortisol)
(2—3 24-hour urine free cortisol if elevated)

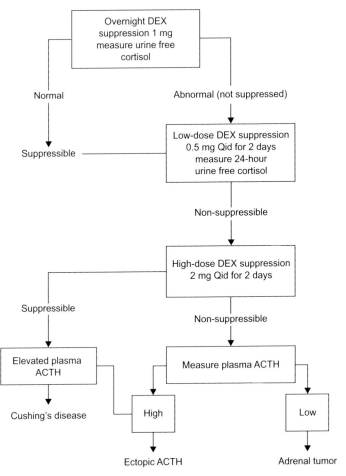

Fig. 4.4.6 A simplified scheme for diagnosis of Cushing's syndrome. DEX=dexamethasone.

Adrenal Cushing's syndrome

Adrenal adenoma

Adrenal adenoma (usually single) causes around 9% of Cushing's syndrome with atrophy of both ipsilateral normal adrenal tissue and the normal contralateral adrenal due to pituitary ACTH suppression.

Cushing's syndrome may also occur as part of other rare syndromes[29]. Carney's syndrome is an autosomal dominant with skin pigmentation and a variety of tumors (mesenchymal, peripheral nerve and endocrine) which can include the adrenals – pigmented multinodular adrenocortical dysplasia. It may result from ACTH receptor antibody stimulation. McCune–Albright syndrome comprises fibrous dysplasia, skin pigmentation and endocrine hyperfunction including the adrenal. The defect is in the stimulatory G-protein linked to adenyl cyclase[29].

241

4

Adrenal carcinoma

Adrenal carcinoma causes around 8% of cases often in early life with pronounced hypertension and electrolyte abnormalities.

Adrenal hyperplasia

Occasional patients have bilateral adrenal hyperplasia. Inappropriate adrenal sensitivity to gastric inhibitory polypeptide – food dependent Cushing's syndrome – is one cause.

Iatrogenic hypertension

ACTH treatment

ACTH administration was shown to cause hypertension when first used in clinical practice. It is still used for some neurological conditions, e.g. infantile spasms.

Glucocorticoid therapy

Since Hench showed, about 50 years ago, that cortisone could reverse features of rheumatoid arthritis, synthetic glucocorticoids have been used extensively in clinical practice. Both oral and topical administration may be associated with severe hypertension. Hypertension is a problem in around 20% of patients who receive exogenous glucocorticoid but synthetic glucocorticoids invariably increase pressure to at least some extent[30]. Intra-articular and intranasal steroids have also caused Cushing's syndrome.

Alcohol induced (pseudo-Cushing's syndrome)

Alcohol abuse can cause a reversible pseudo-Cushing's syndrome in which hypertension is prominent.

Diagnosis and treatment

Cushing's syndrome is characterized by oversecretion of cortisol with increase in 24-hour urinary free cortisol excretion. Plasma cortisol levels may be elevated and circadian rhythm disappears. The overnight dexamethasone suppression test, 1 mg of dexamethasone at bedtime with a plasma cortisol sample next morning, is a simple screening test (Figure 4.4.6).

Cushing's disease features increased plasma ACTH concentration (or at least upper-normal levels), enhanced ACTH stimulation of cortisol, and suppression of plasma cortisol by high-dose dexamethasone (2 mg 6-hourly). With ectopic ACTH, plasma ACTH concentration may be very high, ACTH-stimulated cortisol production is normal and plasma cortisol does not suppress with dexamethasone. In patients with adenoma, plasma ACTH concentration is usually normal, and there is little suppression of plasma cortisol following dexamethasone. Patients with carcinoma have elevated plasma cortisol concentrations, which do not increase following ACTH, and plasma ACTH is low.

Pituitary and adrenal imaging are important in localization of tumors and occasionally selective venous sampling is used.

The prognosis of untreated Cushing's syndrome is poor, with a 50% five-year survival. The preferred approach in Cushing's disease is selective excision of the pituitary adenoma by transspheroidal microsurgery. Response rate is high but around 5% relapse. Pituitary irradiation is often used following pituitary surgery to prevent recurrence, or following adrenal surgery to prevent development of Nelson's syndrome. Adrenal tumors are usually removed surgically, but adrenal malignancy carries a poor prognosis. Benign adrenal adenoma is treated by unilateral adrenalectomy with excellent results.

Medical management has included: metyrapone, which inhibits 11β-hydroxylase; cyproheptadine, which is a serotonin antagonist; bromocriptine and lisuride, which are dopaminergic agonists; aminoglutethimide, which inhibits the cytochrome P450 side-chain cleavage enzyme; reserpine, mitotane (*o, p*-DDD), which destroys fasciculata and reticularis; trilostane, which is an inhibitor of 3β-hydroxysteroid dehydrogenase; sodium valproate which inhibits GABA-transaminase; ketoconazole (which blocks steroid synthesis and itself may produce hypertension); and the glucocorticoid antagonist, RU486. Medical therapy has been used for extensive and inoperable disease.

Conclusion

Substantial advances have been made in our understanding of the molecular pathophysiology of various forms of steroid hypertension, paralleled by better recognition and treatment of these not so rare entities. The broader question of the potential role of steroids in hypertension previously regarded as essential is currently the subject of considerable interest.

Acknowledgements

Ms Laura Vitler prepared the manuscript.

References

1. Firkin BG, Whitworth JA. *Dictionary of Medical Eponyms*, 2nd edn. Parthenon; Parkridge, NJ, 1996.
2. Murphy BF, Whitworth JA, Kincaid-Smith P. Malignant hypertension due to aldosterone producing adrenal adenoma, *Clin Exp Hypertension* 1985;**7**:939–950.
3. Litchfield WR, Dluhy RG. Primary aldosteronism. *Endocrin Metab Clin N Am* 1995;**24**:593–611.
4. Filipecki S, Feltynowsi T, Poplawska W *et al*. Carcinoma of the adrenal cortex with hyperaldosteronism. *J Clin Endo Metab* 1972;**35**:225–229.
5. Mantero F, Todesco S, Armani D, Boscaro M. Primary aldosteronism due to an ovarian arrhenoblastoma: *in vivo* and *in vitro* studies. In: *Research in Steroids*, Vol. 6 (eds Breuer H *et al*.), pp. 409–419. North-Holland: Amsterdam, 1975.
6. Sutherland DJA, Ruse JL, Laidlaw JC. Hypertension, increased aldosterone secretion and low plasma renin activity relieved by dexamethasone. *Can Med Ass J* 1966;**95**:1109.
7. Lifton RP, Dluhy RG, Powers M *et al*. Chimaeric 11β-hydroxylase/aldosterone synthase gene causes glucocorticoid remediable aldosteronism and human hypertension. *Nature* 1992;**355**:362.

4.4

References

8. Litchfield WR, Anderson BF, Weiss RJ *et al.* Intracranial aneurysm and haemorrhagic stroke in glucocorticoid remediable hyperaldosteronism. *Hypertension* 1998;**31**:445–450.

9. Stowasser M, Bachaman AW, Jonsson JR *et al.* Clinical biochemical and genetic approaches to the detection of familial hyperaldosteronism type 1. *J Hypertension* 1995;**13**:1610–1613.

10. Gordon RD, Stowasser M, Tunny TJ *et al.* Clinical and pathological diversity of primary aldosteronism, including a new familial variety. *Clin Exp Pharmacol Physiol* 1991;**18**:283–286.

11. Gordon RD. Primary aldosteronism: a new understanding. *Clin Exp Hypertension* 1997;**19**:857–870.

12. Brown MA, Cramp HA, Zammit VC, Whitworth JA. Primary aldosteronism: a missed diagnosis in 'essential hypertensives'? *Aust NZ J Med* 1996;**26**:533–538.

13. Hiramatsu K, Yamada T, Yukimura Y *et al.* A screening test to identify aldosterone-producing adenoma by measuring plasma renin activity. *Arch Intern Med* 1981;**141**:1589–1593.

14. White PC. Inherited forms of mineralocorticoid hypertension. *Hypertension* 1996;**28**:927–936.

15. Brown JJ, Ferriss JB, Fraser R *et al.* Apparently isolated excess deoxycorticosterone in hypertension. *Lancet* 1972;**ii**:243–247.

16. Ulick S, Levine LS, Gunczler P *et al.* A syndrome of apparent mineralocorticoid excess associated with defects in the peripheral metabolism of cortisol. *J Clin Endocrinol Metab* 1979;**49**:757–644.

17. Stewart PM, Corrie JE, Shackleton CH, Edwards CR. Syndrome of apparent minerocorticoid excess. A defect in the cortisol–cortisone shuttle. *J Clin Invest* 1988;**82**:340–349.

18. Wilson RC, Krozowski ZS, Li K *et al.* A mutation in the *HSD11B2* gene in a family with apparent mineralocorticoid excess. *J Clin Endocrinol Metab* 1995;**80**:2263.

19. Palermo M, Cossu M, Shackleton CHL. Cure of apparent mineralocorticoid excess by kidney transplantation. *N Engl J Med* 1998;**339**:1787.

20. Whitworth JA, Stewart PM, Burt D *et al.* The kidney is the major site of cortisone production in men. *Clin Endocrinol* 1989;**31**:355–361.

21. Whitworth JA, Kelly JJ. Evidence that hydrocortisone induced sodium retention in man is not mediated by the mineralocorticoid receptor. *J Endocrinol Invest* 1995;**18**:586–591.

22. Ulick S, Tedde R, Mantero F. Pathogenesis of the type II variant of the syndrome of apparent mineralocorticoid excess. *J Clin Endocrinol Metab* 1990;**70**:200–206.

23. Bartorelli A, Rimondini A. Severe hypertension in childhood due to prolonged skin application of a mineralocorticoid ointment. *Hypertension* 1984;**6**:586–588.

24. deKlerk JG, Nieuwenhuis MG, Beutler JJ. Hypokalemia and hypertension associated with use of liquorice flavoured chewing gum. *Br Med J* 1997;**314**:731–732.

25. Stewart PM, Wallace AM, Valentino R *et al.* Mineralcorticoid activity of liquorice 11-beta-hydroxysteroid dehydrogenase deficiency comes of age, *Lancet* 1987;**ii**:821–824.

26. Ulick S, Wan JZ, Hanukoglu A, Rosler A. The effect of carbenoxolone on the peripheral metabolism of cortisol in human patients. *J Lab Clin Med* 1993;**122**:673–676.

27. Soszynski P, Sliwinska-Szednicka J, Casperlik-Zaluska A, Zgliczynski S. Endogenous natriuretic factors: atrial natriuretic hormone and digitalis-like substance in Cushing's syndrome. *J Endocrinol* 1991;**129**:453–458.

28. Whitworth JA. Cushing's syndrome and hypertension. In: *Textbook of Hypertension* (ed. Swales JD), pp. 893–903. Blackwell Scientific Publications: Oxford, 1994.

29. Edwards CRW, Adrenocortical diseases. In: *Oxford Textbook of Medicine*, 3rd edn. (eds Weatherall DJ, Ledingham JGG, Warrell DA), p. 1639. Oxford: Oxford Medical Publications, 1996.

30. Whitworth JA, Gordon D, Andrews J, Scoggins BA. The hypertensive effects of synthetic glucocorticoids in man: role of sodium and volume. *J Hypertension* 1989;**7**:537–549.

Further reading

Ganguly A. Primary aldosteronism. *N Engl J Med* 1996;**26**:533–538.

Litchfield WR, Dluhy RG. Primary aldosteronism. *Endocrinol Metab Clin N Am* 1995;**24**:593–611.

White PC. Inherited forms of mineralocorticoid hypertension. *Hypertension* 1996;**28**:927–936.

Whitworth JA. Cushing's syndrome and hypertension. In: *Textbook of Hypertension* (ed. Swales JD), pp. 893–903. Blackwell Scientific Publications: Oxford, 1994.

4

Chapter 4.5

Hypertension from exogenous substances

T Saruta

4

4.5

4

Introduction

Some drugs and poisons and a few foods may raise blood pressure leading to a hypertensive state. Although hypertension due to chemical substance or food is an infrequent occurrence, it is important to pay close attention to the medical and the lifestyle histories considering this important possibility in the evaluation of hypertensive patients, since such hypertension is almost always reversible. These chemical substances or foods elevate blood pressure by a variety of mechanisms including activation of the sympathetic nervous system, sodium and water retention, vascular constriction, and alteration of the hormonal factors. This chapter reviews the chemical substances and the foods that can cause hypertension and discusses the mechanisms involved (Table 4.5.1).

Drugs affecting the sympathetic nervous system

Drugs stimulating the sympathetic nervous system directly or indirectly occasionally elevate blood pressure.

Table 4.5.1

Substances	Mechanism of hypertension
Drugs activating the sympathetic nervous activity Phenylpropranolamine, epinephrine, Phenylephrine, caffeine, oxymetazoline. metoclopramide, monoamine oxidase inhibitors, antidepressants	Increased peripheral vascular resistance
Oral contraceptive pills and estrogen	Increased vascular resistance induced by angiotensin II Sodium and water retention
Glucocorticoids	Relative increase in angiotensin II Increased vascular angiotensin II receptors Reduced vasodepressor substances Increased pressor response
Glycyrrhetinic acid	Increased sodium and water retention due to inhibition of 11β-hydroxysteroid dehydrogenase
Erythropoietin	Increased vascular resistance due to increased blood viscosity or direct vascular effect of erythropoietin
Cyclosporin	Changes due to calcineurin inhibition: increased sympathetic nervous activity, increased tubular reabsorption of sodium and water, altered renin–angiotensin system and prostaglandin synthesis
Non-steroidal anti-inflammatory drugs	Inhibition of the synthesis of prostaglandins and other vasodilating substances
Vitamin D	Increased vascular resistance due to hypercalcemia
Heavy metals (lead)	Disturbed calcium metabolism and endothelial dysfunction
Alcohol	Increased sympathetic nervous activity Altered sodium transport across cell membrane Altered insulin sensitivity

Drugs affecting the sympathetic nervous system directly

When used in high dose, ophthalmic solutions, nasal decongestants, cough medicines and anorexics, containing phenylephrine, epinephrine, pseudoepinephrine, phenylpropranolamine, caffeine, or oxymetazoline, elevate blood pressure by increasing the peripheral vascular resistance. Blood pressure elevation by these drugs tends to be more prominent at supine than at standing. Concomitant use of sympathomimetic or beta-blocking agents may severely augment the rise of blood pressure by these agents due to unopposed alpha-adrenergic vasoconstriction.

Drugs affecting the sympathetic nervous system indirectly

Metoclopramide

Intravenous administration of metoclopramide to a patient with pheochromocytoma may induce a hypertensive crisis. The mechanism involved may not be the direct stimulation of catecholamine release from the tumor or sympathetic nerve endings. It is more likely that metoclopramide indirectly stimulates catecholamine release by its presynaptic dopaminergic blocking effect[1]. Sulpiride and droperidol are also known to induce pheochromocytoma crisis. Antiemetics, such as metoclopramide, alizapride and prochlorperazine, are also reported to increase blood pressure in some normotensive subjects being treated with cisplatin[2], although the precise mechanism involved remains unknown.

Cocaine

Cocaine abuse increases blood pressure and produces a variety of cerebrocardiovascular events due to adrenergic hyperactivity. Cocaine acts on vascular smooth muscles indirectly by blocking norepinephrine reuptake at the sympathetic nerve terminals, as well as directly by altering cellular calcium flux. Cocaine ingestion increases the risk of hypertension and abruption of the placenta in pregnant women. Furthermore, prenatal cocaine exposure may cause hypertension in the newborn by altering the developing sympathetic nervous system and elevating the circulatory catecholamine levels[3].

Monoamine oxidase inhibitors and other antidepressants

Monoamine oxidase inhibitors and other antidepressants are effective for the treatment of depression by delaying the metabolism of sympathomimetic amines and 5-hydroxytryptophan and by increasing the norepinephrine store in the postganglionic sympathetic neurons. When monoamine oxidase inhibitors are used with exogenous sympathomimetic amines, elevation of blood pressure will be exaggerated. There are many reports that foods containing tyramine, such as aged cheese, wine, avocado, chocolate and carrot, induce

4

hypertensive episodes in individuals receiving monoamine oxidase inhibitors. Other types of antidepressants, such as tricyclic antidepressants, serotonin receptor type-la agonist (busiprone), and selective serotonin reuptake inhibitor (fluoxetine), have been known to increase blood pressure and heart rate. Tricyclic antidepressants have cocaine-like sympathomimetic actions. Heart rate, cardiac contraction, and blood pressure may be increased by the administration of a small amount of these agents.

Oral contraceptives and estrogens

The incidence of hypertension induced by oral contraceptives is approximately 5% among the users of high dose pills that contain at least 50 µg of estrogen and 1–4 mg of progestogen[4]. However, the incidence of hypertension may be less with the present-day lower-dose formulas containing 30–35 µg of estrogen and new synthetic progestogens[5]. The risk of hypertension does not significantly depend on age, family history of hypertension, ethnic background, or body mass index. However, women with prior pre-eclampsia or pre-existing primary hypertension may be more susceptible.

BOX 4.5.1 Oral contraceptive-induced hypertension

The mechanism of this hypertension is still controversial. The most significant pathophysiological change in oral contraceptive pill users is the modified state of the renin–angiotensin system due to greatly increased angiotensinogen. This change in the renin–angiotensin system is observed in all oral contraceptive users regardless of whether hypertension develops or not. However, the following observations support the role of renin–angiotensin system in the development of oral contraceptive-induced hypertension[6].

- Angiotensin II antagonists readily reduce blood pressure in a significant number of such cases.
- Blood pressure declines a short time after stopping the oral contraceptives in parallel with normalization of the renin–angiotensin profile.

In addition to the change in the renin–angiotensin system, Woods *et al.*[7] suggested that direct sodium and water retention induced by oral contraceptive agent or intrarenal vascular lesions might contribute to the development of hypertension.

Postmenopausal estrogen replacement is associated with favorable changes in multiple cardiovascular risk factors. Recently, Akkad *et al.*[8] reported that increase in ambulatory 24-hour blood pressure was observed in almost one-third of the women given either oral or transdermal estrogen replacement. However, large prospective studies have shown no increase in office blood pressure in women given estrogen replacment, and even decrease in blood pressure has been documented in some instances. The difference in these results is possibly related to the different doses of estrogen administered and choice of progestogens used in combined preparations.

Glucocorticoids

Administration of a high dose of glucocorticoids induces hypertension in infants and adults. According to the report by Smets and Vanhaesebrouck[9], systolic blood pressure rose significantly in all of the 22 neonates with chronic lung disease treated with dexamethasone for four weeks. Blood pressure returned to the pretreatment level within two weeks after stopping dexamethasone. Administration of a high dose of cortisol (200 mg/day) also increased blood pressure significantly in normal male subjects. Moreover, ~70% of the subjects with iatrogenic Cushing's syndrome are hypertensive.

The following mechanisms are proposed for hypertension due to glucocorticoids[10]:

- Elevated angiotensin II level due to increased angiotensinogen production.
- Inhibition of vasodilating substances such as kallikrein, prostaglandins, and nitric oxide.
- Biological changes of the vascular smooth muscle cells and increased pressor response to norepinephrine and angiotensin II.
- Increased number of angiotensin II type I receptor.
- Enhanced angiotensin I-stimulated inositol triphosphate production.

Glycyrrhetinic acid

It has long been known that sodium retention, potassium wastage, and hypertension result from ingestion of glycyrrhetinic acid, the active ingredient of licorice extract, and carbenoxolone, a semisynthetic hemisuccinate derivative of glycyrrhetinic acid. Recent studies have revealed similarities between the syndrome induced by glycyrrhetinic acid and the syndrome of apparent mineralocorticoid excess. It has also been shown that glycyrrhetinic acid inhibits the renal 11 β-hydroxysteroid dehydrogenase type 2, which is deficient in the syndrome of apparent mineralocorticoid excess[11,12].

Sigurjonsdottir *et al.*[13] have reported that daily ingestion of relatively small amount (50–100 g) of confectionery licorice by normal subjects for four weeks resulted in sodium retention, potassium wastage, suppression of renin and aldosterone, and a rise in blood pressure. We showed[14] that administration of 225 mg of glycyrrhizin per day for seven days induced suppression of plasma renin activity, hypokalemia, and kaliuresis. And, this effect was comparable to that of 0.1 mg of 9α-fluorocortisol per day for seven days. During the administration of glycyrrhizin, urinary excretion of cortisol increased without change in its plasma concentration, while the plasma level and the urinary excretion of cortisone decreased. These results suggested that inhibition of 11 β-hydroxysteroid dehydrogenase type 2 is closely involved in the mineralocorticoid-like action of glycyrrhizin in men.

4

4

Erythropoietin

Recombinant human erythropoietin (rHuEPO) is now being widely used
to correct anemia of chronic renal failure. While rHuEPO has greatly
improved the quality of life in patients with end-stage renal failure,
hypertension has been a significant side effect being seen in
approximately one-third of those receiving the therapy.

BOX 4.5.2 Recombinant human EPO

Blood pressure increases in association with rise of hematocrit and blood
viscosity in most of the cases. Hemodynamically, rHuEPO elevates blood
pressure by markedly increasing the peripheral vascular resistance in
association with a mild decrease in cardiac output[15]. The increase in
peripheral vascular resistance may reflect the reversal of compensatory
hypoxic peripheral vasodilation. However, increase in blood pressure
induced by rHuEPO cannot be fully explained by the improvement of
anemia and the rise of blood viscosity alone. Ishimitsu *et al.*[16] followed the
blood pressure change in 53 patients treated with rHuEPO for 10 weeks.
Twenty-six of these 53 patients had positive family history of hypertension,
and the mean blood pressure increased significantly in this subgroup.
Meanwhile, the blood pressure remained unchanged in those who lacked
family history of hypertension. The two groups were similar in terms of the
total dose of rHuEPO, the extent of anemia improvement, and the basal
blood pressure. Thus, it was suggested that genetic predisposition was
involved in the development of hypertension. rHuEPO may also increase
intracellular calcium concentrations[17] raising the possibility that it exerts a
direct vasopressor effect on vascular smooth muscle cells in patients with
positive family history of hypertension.

To prevent the increase in blood pressure during treatment with
rHuEPO, close attention should be directed to maintain the appropriate
fluid volume control. Calcium-channel blockers are effective to reduce
the increased peripheral vascular resistance in this type of hypertension.

Cyclosporine and tacrolimus

Cyclosporine is a novel immunosuppressive agent that is highly useful
in human organ transplantation and in the treatment of many
autoimmune diseases. The major side effect of cyclosporine is
nephrotoxicity and hypertension.

The incidence of cyclosporine-associated hypertension varies with the
patient population under evaluation. Schorn *et al.*[18] studied the pre-
and post-transplantation incidences of hypertension in patients who
received renal transplantation and compared the effects of two
immunosuppressive treatments, azathioprine/prednisone and
cyclosporine/prednisone. In the group treated with
azathioprine/prednisone, the incidence of hypertension decreased
significantly at three months post-transplantation (68% before and 53%
after transplantation). Meanwhile, there was a significant increase in the

incidence of hypertension in the group treated with cyclosporine/prednisone (71% before and 85% after transplantation).

Blood pressure in the cardiac transplant recipients on cyclosporine was higher than those not receiving it (112 ± 3 mmHg vs. 96 ± 4 mmHg, $P < 0.05$). Furthermore, 2.7 times higher rate of sympathetic nerve firing was observed in those treated with cyclosporine[19]. The cumulative post-transplant prevalence of hypertension was 52% at one year and was 77% at four years in those who received cyclosporine as the major immunosuppressant. Post-transplant hypertension with cyclosporine was more common in older males and in those with positive family history of hypertension and/or major cardiovascular complications.

Dieterie *et al.*[20] reviewed the incidence of hypertension in patients with autoimmune diseases treated with cyclosporine for up to two years: 11% of the 321 patients developed hypertension during the treatment in this study.

BOX 4.5.3 Cyclosporine-induced hypertension

A number of abnormalities have been suggested for the cyclosporine-induced hypertension: increased sympathetic nervous activity, increased renal proximal tubular reabsorption, altered synthesis of vasodilating prostaglandins, change in the renin–angiotensin system, and direct vascular effect. Recent basic studies have revealed that cyclosporine binds to cytoplasmic receptors leading to inhibition of calcineurin, a calcium calmodulin-dependent protein phosphatase, and this intracellular action of cyclosporine is considered to account for its immunosuppressive effect on T-lymphocytes[21]. It is also likely that the same intracellular events taking place in a variety of other tissues including central nervous system, vascular smooth muscle, and kidney, are involved in the prohypertensive effect of cyclosporine.

Tacrolimus (FK-506) is a novel immunosuppressant isolated from a *Streptomyces*, which is approximately 100 times more potent than cyclosporin and can also induce hypertension.

Both calcium-channel blockers and angiotensin-converting enzyme inhibitors have been used to treat hypertension and nephrotoxicity due to cyclosporine or tacrolimus. Calcium-channel blockers interfere with the renal and vascular effects of cyclosporine and reverse vasoconstriction, and are proposed to be the drugs of choice for this condition. Early administration of verapamil or diltiazem may decrease the incidence of delayed graft function and rejection episodes and to improve the graft function. Angiotensin-converting enzyme inhibitors are probably not suitable to treat hypertension and nephrotoxicity due to cyclosporin or tacrolimus in view of the low-normal renin levels observed in these conditions and the risk of hyperkalemia and potential acute renal deterioration.

Non-steroidal anti-inflammatory drugs

Non-steroidal anti-inflammatory drugs (NSAIDs) may cause renal impairment and raise blood pressure. These side effects are mainly due

4

to inhibition of prostaglandin-induced vasodilation, although other factors such as altered responsiveness to pressor substances such as angiotensin II, sodium retention, and direct vasoconstrictive effect are also involved. According to the meta-analysis of the effects of NSAIDs on blood pressure by Pope *et al.*[22], indomethacin and naproxen were associated with the greatest increases in blood pressure with short-term use, while piroxicam, aspirin, ibuprofen and sulindac did not increase blood pressure significantly.

Vitamin D

Hypertension occasionally develops in patients with renal failure or osteoporosis being treated with vitamin D preparations. Hypertension due to vitamin D intoxication tends to parallel the degree of hypercalcemia. Direct vasoconstriction of the resistance vessels or hormonal changes induced by hypercalcemia is proposed to be involved in the development of hypertension.

Heavy metals

Several heavy metals including lead, copper, and cadmium are supposed to elevate blood pressure. There is sufficient evidence to support that chronic exposure to low level of lead causes renal impairment and hypertension. Several mechanisms have been proposed for lead-induced hypertension, including changes in calcium metabolism, inhibition of Na^+, K^+-ATPase, and alteration of humoral factors including endothelin and nitric oxide released from the endothelium.

In the experiment by Vaziri *et al.*[23], rats loaded with lead for 12 weeks developed hypertension in association with increased levels of lipid peroxidation products and a twofold reduction in excretion of nitric oxide metabolites. Administration of lazaroids, potent inhibitors of oxygen radical species, normalized blood pressure and urinary excretion of nitrates and nitrites. Therefore, increased reactive oxygen species production and decreased nitric oxide synthesis may play important roles in lead-induced hypertension.

Alcohol

Chronic alcohol intake of more than 2 ounces per day may raise blood pressure, and alcohol can be an important etiological agent for hypertension when consumed in excess. According to the review of 30 cross-sectional population studies on the relationship between alcohol consumption and blood pressure[24] the majority of the reports documented small but significant increase in blood pressure with alcohol consumption. Interestingly, in about 40% of studies, the blood pressure was higher in the non-drinkers than in those consuming one to two drinks per day. The proposed mechanisms by which alcohol induces hypertension include increased sympathetic nervous activity, altered cellular membrane sodium transport, increased cortisol secretion, and disturbed insulin sensitivity.

References

1. Abe M, Orita Y, Nakashima Y, Nakamura M. Hypertensive crisis induced by metoclopramide in a patient with pheochromocytoma. *Angiology* 1984;**35**:122–128.
2. Roche H, Hyman G, Hahas G. Hypertension and intravenous antidopaminergic drugs. *N Engl J Med* 1985;**312**:1125–1126.
3. Horn PT. Persistent hypertension after prenatal cocaine exposure. *J Pediatr* 1992;**121**:288–291.
4. Wilson ESB, Cruickshank J, McMaster M, Weir RJ. A prospective controlled study of the effect on blood pressure of contraceptive preparations containing different types and dosages of progestogen. *Br J Obstetr Gynecol* 1984;**91**:1254–1260.
5. Fuchs N, Dusterberg B, Weber-Diehl F, Muhe B. The effect of blood pressure of a monophasic oral contraceptive containing ethinylestradiol and gestogen. *Contraception* 1995;**51**:335–339.
6. Saruta T, Nakamura R, Nagahara S *et al*. Effects of angiotensin II analog on blood pressure, renin and aldosterone in women on oral contraceptives and toxemia. *Gynecol Obstetr Invest* 1981;**12**:11–20.
7. Woods JW. Oral contraceptives and hypertension. *Hypertension* 1988;**11**(suppl II): II-11–II-15.
8. Akkad A, Halligan A, Abrams K, Al-Azzawi F. Differing responses in blood pressure over 24 hours in normotensive women receiving oral or transdermal estrogen replacement therapy. *Obstet Gynecol* 1997;**89**:97–103.
9. Smets K, Vanhaesebrouck P. Dexamethasone associated systemic hypertension in low birth weight babies with chronic lung disease. *Eur J Pediatr* 1996;**155**:573–575.
10. Saruta T. Mechanism of glucocorticoid-induced hypertension. *Hypertension Res* 1996;**19**:1–8.
11. Stewart PM, Wallace AM, Atherden SM *et al*. Mineralocorticoid activity of carbenoxolone: contrasting effects of carbenoxolone and liquorice on 11-beta-hydroxysteroid dehydrogenase activity in man. *Clin Sci* 1990;**78**:49–51.
12. Stewart PM, Korozowski ZS, Gupta A *et al*. Hypertension in the syndrome of apparent mineralocorticoid excess due to mutation of the 11-beta-hydroxysteroid dehydrogenase type 2 gene. *Lancet* 1996;**347**:88–91.
13. Sigurjonsdottir HA, Ragnarsson J, Franzson L, Sigurdsson G. Is blood pressure commonly raised by moderate consumption of liquorice? *J Human Hypertension* 1995;**9**:345–348.
14. Kageyama Y, Suzuki H, Saruta T. Glycyrrhizin induces mineralocorticoid activity through alterations in cortisol metabolism in the human kidney. *J Endocrinol* 1992;**135**:147–152.
15. Verbeelen D, Bossuyt A, Smitz A *et al*. Hemodynamics of patients with renal failure treated with recombinant human erythropoietin. *Clin Nephrol* 1989;**31**:6–11.
16. Ishimitsu T, Tsukada H, Ogawa Y *et al*. Genetic predisposition to hypertension facilitates blood pressure elevation in hemodialysis patients treated with erythropoietin. *Am J Med* 1993;**94**:401–406.
17. Vogel V, Kramer HJ, Backer A *et al*. Effects of erythropoietin on endothelin-1 synthesis and the cellular calcium messenger system in vascular endothelial cells. *Am J Med* 1997;**10**:289–296.
18. Schorn T, Frei U, Brackman H *et al*. Cyclosporin associated post transplant hypertension: incidence and effect on renal transplant function. *Transplant Proceed* 1988;**20**(suppl 3):610–614.
19. Scherrer U, Vissing SF, Morgan BJ *et al*. Cyclosporine-induced sympathetic activation and hypertension after heart transplantation. *N Engl J Med* 1990;**323**:693–699.
20. Dieterie A, Abeymickrama K, Von-Griffenried B. Nephrotoxicity and hypertension in patients with autoimmune disease treated with cyclosporin. *Transplant Proc* 1988;**20**(suppl 4):349–355.
21. Jean-Louis A, Rostaing L. Cyclosporin nephrotoxicity: pathophysiology and comparison with FK-506. *Curr Opin Nephrol Hypertension* 1998;**7**:539–545.
22. Pope JE, Anderson JJ, Felson DT. A meta-analysis of the effects of nonsteroidal anti-inflammatory drugs on blood pressure. *Arch Intern Med* 1993;**153**:477–481.

4

References

23. Vaziri ND, Ding Y, Ni Z, Gonick HC. Altered nitric oxide metabolism and increased oxygen free radical activity in lead-induced hypertension: effect of lazaroid therapy. *Kidney Int* 1997;**52**:1042–1046.
24. MacMahon S. Alcohol consumption and hypertension. *Hypertension* 1997;**9**:111–121.

4

Essential hypertension

Chapter

5.1

Excluding secondary causes of hypertension

A Morganti

5

Introduction

Secondary forms of hypertension are relatively rare diseases, their overall prevalence being 10–15% of all the cases of hypertension. Moreover, the great majority of cases requires complex, expensive and sometimes risky investigations to be diagnosed. Thus, when dealing with hypertensive patients, the clinician should always wonder to what extent it is worthwhile to push forward with the diagnostic procedures to discover the few cases with an identifiable cause of hypertension. However, an aggressive diagnostic approach can identify a minority of patients who can be cured of a disease which would otherwise require a life-time pharmacological treatment which, in turn, implies a huge cost saving. On the other hand, an indiscriminate extension of the sophisticated investigations required to reach a diagnosis of secondary hypertension brings about an unsustainable economical burden. In addition, because of the low prevalence of these diseases, a relevant proportion of the diagnostic procedures, no matter how sensitive and specific, will turn out falsely positive leading the patient to take additional and often useless investigations. Thus, the clinician is left with the difficult task of excluding, first on a clinical basis and with the minimum work-up recommended for all the hypertensive patients (Table 5.1.1) and second with the more complex techniques, the various known causes of secondary hypertension; the specular counterpart of this process is obviously represented by the concomitant selection of the few patients with true secondary hypertension.

This chapter describes how one may proceed with this process of exclusion with respect to patients more likely to harbour a secondary form of hypertension (Table 5.1.2). Since the procedures needed to reach

Table 5.1.1 Routine laboratory tests recommended for all hypertensive patients

Obligatory	*Optional test*
Urine analysis	Creatinine clearance
Full blood count	Microalbuminuria
Blood sodium and potassium	24-hour urinary protein
Blood glucose	Triglycerides
Plasma creatinine	LDL-cholesterol
Total and HDL-cholesterol	Glycosylated hemoglobin
12-lead electrocardiogram	Thyrotropin
	Echocardiogram

After[1]

Table 5.1.2 Patients in whom identifiable causes of hypertension should be excluded.

- Patients whose age, history, physical examination, severity of hypertension or initial laboratory findings suggest a secondary form of hypertension.
- Patients whose blood pressure responds poorly to drug therapy.
- Patients with well-controlled hypertension whose blood pressure suddenly increases or becomes uncontrolled in spite of regular antihypertensive treatment.
- Patients with stage 3 hypertension.
- Patients with sudden onset of hypertension.

After[1].

these diagnoses have been extensively addressed in previous chapters, this chapter will discuss when and in which sequence these tests should be applied. The criteria proposed derive from the personal experience of the author.

How to exclude renal parenchymal hypertension

History and clinical examination of the patient are of little help in excluding this form of hypertension since even severe nephropathies may occur without overt clinical signs. Also, the absence of the symptoms listed in Table 5.1.3 makes less likely, but does not rule out, the possibility of renal parenchymal hypertension. Equally, a lack of alteration in renal function does not allow a firm conclusion as to the renal origin of hypertension since an elevation in blood pressure is often present when the glomerular filtration rate is still normal or only minimally reduced; with advancing renal insufficiency, hypertension occurs on average in 75–80% of the cases but this percentage may vary depending upon the underlying nephropathy (Table 5.1.4). Thus hypertension and renal diseases are often associated but not necessarily related.

Urine analysis is much more helpful in excluding renal parenchymal hypertension in that the presence in the urine of white and red blood cells, hyaline casts and protein more than 1 g/day are present in 90% of these patients while these anomalies are rarely observed in patients with other forms of hypertension unless in the severe or malignant stage. Whenever these urinary alterations occur an ultrasound or computed tomography (CT) scan of the kidneys is mandatory. These techniques, which have largely replaced the conventional urography, are particularly useful for ruling out glomerulonephritis, pyelonephritis, and obstructive nephropathies; in addition these procedures may disclose the presence of renal cysts or tumors. In such cases patients

Table 5.1.3 Clinical clues of renal parenchymal hypertension

- Family history of renal diseases
- History of previous nephropathies (glomerulonephritis; pyelonephritis, kidney stones)
- Abuse of analgesics (interstitial nephritis)
- Enlarged kidneys at abdominal examination (polycystic kidney disease)

Table 5.1.4 Prevalence of hypertension in renal-parenchymal disease

Disease	Prevalence
Focal glomerulosclerosis	75–80%
Membranoproliferative glomerulonephritis	65–70%
Diabetic nephropathy	65–70%
Membranous nephropathy	40–50%
IgA nephropathy	30%
Minimal change disease	15–20%
Polycystic kidney disease	50–60%
Chronic interstitial nephritis	30%

After[2–4].

should undergo a renal angiography which may visualize the stretching and divarication of the interlobar arteries confirming the diagnosis of polycystic disease. Aortography may also reveal the presence of an anomalous vessel compressing the pyeloureteral junction, a condition often associated with hypertension.

Renal biopsy is scarcely used for excluding renal parenchymal hypertension because of the variable relationship between the elevation in blood pressure and the underlying disease. In addition, in patients with serum creatinine above 2.5–3 mg/dl the histologic picture is essentially meaningless in that the great majority of the glomeruli is already sclerotic whatever the nature of the initial disease.

How to exclude renovascular hypertension

Renovascular hypertension (RVH) the most common curable form of secondary hypertension, has an increasing prevalence with advancing age (Table 5.1.5) and jeopardizes renal functional. For these reasons RVH must be excluded in all hypertensive patients with the clinical features listed in Table 5.1.6. Indeed, epidemiological studies carried out in large populations of hypertensive patients have shown that the probability of

Table 5.1.5 Prevalence of renovascular hypertension in relation to age

Hypertension	18–29	30–39	40–49	50–59	60–69	>70	Total
FD-RAS	1.1%	0.8%	0.4%	0%	0%	0%	0.4%
AS-RAS	0.1%	1.3%	2.1%	4.2%	5.7%	6.5%	2.7%
Total	1.2%	2.1%	2.5%	4.2%	5.7%	6.5%	3.1%

FD-RAS = fibrodysplasia of renal artery.
AS-RAS = atherosclerotic renal artery stenosis.
Data from[5].

Table 5.1.6 Clinical clues for renovascular hypertension

History
Negative family history of hypertension
Cigarette smoking
Onset of hypertension before age 30
Atherosclerotic disease
Diabetes
Sudden aggravation of a previously well-controlled hypertension
Unexplained deterioration of renal function during treatment with ACE inhibitors or angiotensin II receptor antagonists
Congestive heart failure of unexplained origin

Examination
Abdominal bruits
Bruits elsewhere suggestive of atherosclerotic disease
Severe end-organ damage

Laboratory
Hypokalemia
Proteinuria > 0.5 g/day
Recent unexplained rise in serum creatinine

having RVH increases up to nine times when one or more of these signs are present (hypokalemia and severe diastolic hypertension are particularly relevant). Yet none of these signs is *per se* sufficient to confirm or to refute with certainty the diagnosis of RVH. Indeed, even the most common, i.e. the systolic abdominal bruit is present only in 60% of patients with true RVH. If none of these clinical and laboratory signs is present and hypertension is not resistant to medical treatment, the probabilities of RVH are extremely low. Moreover, in such patients the renal artery stenosis, even if present, is unlikely to be hemodynamically significant and therefore responsible for the elevation in pressure. Thus, under these circumstances, we believe that there is no need for additional investigations for excluding RVH.

In contrast, whenever there is a clinical suspicion of RVH, patients should undergo several functional and morphological investigations starting from the least invasive and expensive. Among the biochemical tests, the measurement of plasma renin activity (PRA) under controlled conditions of sodium intake and posture and taking care of avoiding the interference of the many drugs which may affect renin release, is the one we prefer; according to classical studies it is abnormally elevated in 75% of patients with true RVH. One limitation of PRA evaluation is that is may produce a false positive result in about 15% of the essential hypertensives (usually young borderline hypertensives with a hyperkinetic circulation). A simple way for discriminating these patients from those with true RVH is by treating them with a short course of a beta-blocker. These compounds, because of the selective blockade of neurally-mediated renin release, cause a marked reduction in PRA in high renin essential hypertensives but lower it to a much lesser extent in patients with RVH in whom the secretion of the enzyme is mostly mediated through the intrarenal baroreceptors. A second limitation of PRA measurement is that it may be normal in about 30% of patients with RVH. In these subjects the RVH can be ruled out with a captopril test which, when positive (Table 5.1.7), has a sensitivity and specificity greater than 95%. The captopril test may be misleading in patients with essential hypertension and high renin in that both the reduction in blood pressure and the increments in PRA in response to the drug may be similar to those observed in patients with RVH.

Because of these limitations of PRA measurement we believe that to rule out RVH this test should be always combined with a morphological investigation. Among these we prefer the echo-Doppler technique

Table 5.1.7 Criteria for a positive captopril test

- Stimulated PRA of 12 ng/ml/h or more
- Absolute increase in PRA of 10 ng/ml/h or more
- Percent increase in PRA of 150% or more; or of 400% or more if baseline PRA is below 3 ng/ml/h.

A positive captopril test requires that all the criteria are satisfied. Values of PRA refer to blood samples collected from a peripheral vein with patients in the sitting position before and 60 minutes after the administration of 50 mg captopril. After[10].

5.1

Table 5.1.8 Accuracy of echo-Doppler velocimetric indices in diagnosing renal artery stenosis

Parameter	Pulsatility index	Resistive index	Acceleration	Acceleration time
Threshold	0.93	0.59	7.4 m/s^2	60 ms
Sensitivity	86%	82%	96%	94%
Specificity	73%	70%	89%	89%
Correct diagnosis	80%	77%	93%	92%

'Threshold' indicates cut-off values associated with the least false-positive and false-negative examinations having renal angiography as a reference standard. Data refer to 146, 124, 116 and 116 arteries examined respectively, with pulsatility index, resistive index, acceleration and acceleration time.
After[13].

associated with the determination of the velocimetric indices because these latter allow the evaluation of the hemodynamic effects of the renal artery stenosis. Among these indices those sampled at the renal hylum or at the interlobar arteries, i.e. the distal ones, are in our opinion particularly useful in that some of them (acceleration and acceleration time) have a diagnostic accuracy greater than 90% (Table 5.1.8). The way we proceed in patients with clinical suspicions of RVH according to the results of combined PRA and echo-Doppler velocimetric evaluation is summarized in Figure 5.1.1. If PRA and echo turn out positive we believe that the hypothesis of RVH is very likely and the patient should directly undergo a renal angiography; if this examination confirms the presence of the suspected renal artery stenosis patients should be treated in the same session with angioplasty or stent implantation because this intervention will be followed by cure or, at least, some improvement in blood pressure control in 85–90% of those in whom the procedure was

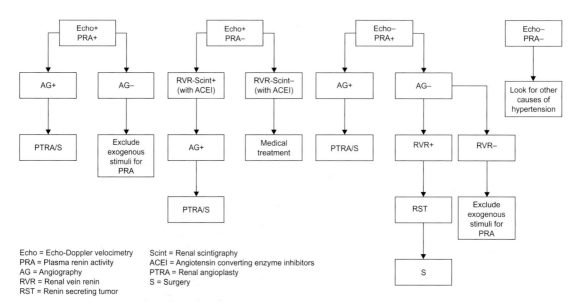

Echo = Echo-Doppler velocimetry
PRA = Plasma renin activity
AG = Angiography
RVR = Renal vein renin
RST = Renin secreting tumor

Scint = Renal scintigraphy
ACEI = Angiotensin converting enzyme inhibitors
PTRA = Renal angioplasty
S = Surgery

Fig. 5.1.1 Clinical suspicion of renovascular hypertension (off anti-HT treatment except for calcium-antagonists).

technically successful. If the renin profile is negative, while the echo Doppler velocimetric evaluation is positive, one may be dealing with one of those 30% of patients with 'normal' renin but still true RVH. To exclude this possibility it may be useful if the measurement of PRA in blood is collected from the renal veins (RVR). The lack of lateralization in renin secretion (i.e. a difference smaller than 50% between the levels of PRA found in blood collected from vein of the stenotic kidney and that of the contralateral one) indicates that the stenosis is not hemodynamically relevant and, therefore, not worth dilating for improving blood pressure control. The RVR test may be potentiated by captopril administration because of the selective increase in renin release from the stenotic side. In our experience the RVR test, when applied in combination with peripheral renin profile correctly predicts the effect of renal artery dilatation on blood pressure in 84% of the cases. As an alternative to RVR, renal scintigraphy can be used to exclude a true RVH; this technique which has the advantage of being less invasive, when combined with captopril test, has a sensivity and specificity of 95% and 90%, respectively.

If the echo-Doppler is negative and the renin profile is abnormally high we believe that patients should undergo a renal angiography in that the echo-Doppler study may have missed a hemodynamically relevant stenosis located in an accessory artery. If the renal artery stenosis is not confirmed by angiography, an RVR should be performed to exclude the rare possibility of a renin secreting tumor which can mimic the pattern of renin secretion observed in the true RVH.

Finally, if both renin profile and echo-Doppler velocimetric indices are negative we believe that, in spite of the clinical suspicion, the hypothesis of RVH can be reasonably dismissed.

How to exclude endocrine hypertension

Primary hyperaldosteronism

This form of hypertension is either due to an adrenal adenoma or to adrenal hyperplasia. While the former condition must be treated surgically, the latter should be treated pharmacologically; failure to establish this differential diagnosis may lead to needless adrenalectomies.

Patients suspected of having primary hyperaldosteronism should be evaluated with combined measurements of PRA and plasma aldosterone; the coexistence of suppressed values of PRA and high values of aldosterone strongly suggests primary hyperaldosteronism but does not discriminate between adenoma and hyperplasia. To do this we proceed according to the flow-chart shown in Figure 5.1.2. PRA and aldosterone should be measured again after applying several manouvers addressed at demonstrating the persistence of angiotensin II control on aldosterone secretion. The most common among these tests is represented by 1–2 hours of ambulation: a parallel increase in both PRA and aldosterone in response to this postural stimulus rules out primary hyperaldosteronism; lower than normal responses of renin suggest that

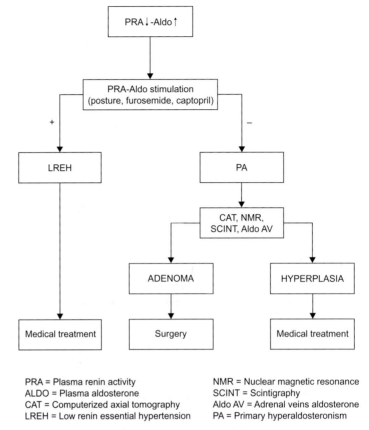

Fig. 5.1.2 Clinical suspicion of primary hyperaldosteronism.

PRA = Plasma renin activity
ALDO = Plasma aldosterone
CAT = Computerized axial tomography
LREH = Low renin essential hypertension

NMR = Nuclear magnetic resonance
SCINT = Scintigraphy
Aldo AV = Adrenal veins aldosterone
PA = Primary hyperaldosteronism

primary hyperaldosteronism is due to adrenal hyperplasia whereas persistently suppressed levels of renin with unchanged or increased levels of aldosterone indicate adrenal adenoma. Alternative methods for stimulating the renin–angiotensin–aldosterone system consists in the acute administration of furosemide or captopril; in both cases increments in renin in response to these two compounds indicate adrenal hyperplasia rather than adenoma. Another functional test for discriminating between these two forms of primary hyperaldosteronism consists in expanding plasma volume via an i.v. infusion of 2 liters of saline over 2 hours. A reduction of plasma aldosterone to less than 50% of the basal values strongly militates against primary hyperaldosteronism due to adrenal adenoma.

If none of these tests turns out positive the patient's most likely cause is low renin essential hypertension, a condition, according to many authors, somehow in between essential hypertension and adrenal hyperplasia. If these tests are positive, an ultrasound scan of the adrenals may be useful to reveal masses greater than 3 cm in diameter. Since the majority of the adrenal adenomas are smaller, a CT Scan is preferable to rule out this possibility given that the diagnostic accuracy of this technique is 80–85%. However, CT evaluation, by itself, is insufficient for diagnosing primary hyperaldosteronism because of the high prevalence of functionally inactive adrenal masses ('incidentalomas'). Adrenal scintigraphy potentiated by 5–7 days of treatment with 2 mg/day dexamethasone is the ultimate investigation for discriminating adenoma from hyperplasia; this pharmacological preparation by suppressing ACTH secretion inhibits the uptake of radiolabeled cholesterol from the normal and hyperplasic adrenals leaving it unaffected in the adenomas. Adrenal vein catheterization for selective measurement of plasma aldosterone is the last diagnostic resource, the concentration of the hormone being ≥10 times greater in the adenomatous side with respect to the contralateral normal one. However, this test may give a false-negative result because of the intermittent release of aldosterone. In addition, we rarely use it because of the risk of intra-adrenal bleeding or infarction.

Pheochromocytoma

This is another very rare disorder (less than 0.1% of all cases of hypertension) in which hypertension can be surgically cured except in 10% of the cases in whom essential hypertension coexists. The clinical signs suggestive of pheochromocytoma are all quite non-specific. We believe that whenever they are present patients should have a urinary measurement of catecholamines or their metabolites; if these are repeatedly normal, particularly if in specimens collected during or within few hours after a clear-cut elevation of blood pressure the diagnosis of pheochromocytoma is unlikely. Plasma catecholamines can be used as an alternative to urinary catecholamines but this measurement, besides being technically more complex, is frequently negative if blood samples are not collected during a hypertensive crisis.

If urinary catecholamines turn out slightly elevated it is important to exclude the 15–20% of essential hypertensives who are known to have some degree of sympathetic overactivity (an expression of which very often are the coexistence of high levels of plasma renin). In those patients who have stable hypertension, a clonidine-suppression test is indicated. This drug lowers both blood pressure and catecholamines in essential hypertensives but blood pressure only in those with pheochromocytoma (Figure 5.1.3). In patients with paroxysmal hypertension, the provocative tests with histamine, glucagon and metaclopramide are used less than in the past because of the high rate of false results; in addition these procedures may cause alarming rises in blood pressure.

Adrenal CT scan is a convenient investigation for localizing an adrenal mass up to the dimension of 1 cm in diameter with diagnostic accuracy of 90%. However, a negative CT does not rule out the diagnosis of pheochromocytoma because about 10% of these tumors lay out of the adrenals (7–8% intra-abdominal, 2–3% extra-abdominal). Thus, to exclude the possibility of an unusually located pheochromocytoma ^{131}I-metaiodiobenzylguanidine (MIBG) scintigraphy is used, which can reveal active masses of chromaffin tissue down to

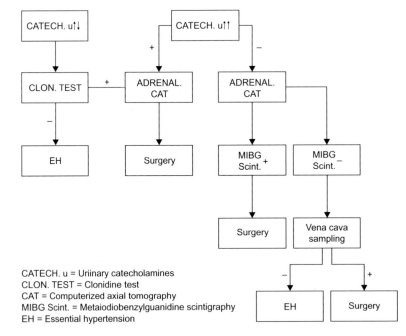

CATECH. u = Uriinary catecholamines
CLON. TEST = Clonidine test
CAT = Computerized axial tomography
MIBG Scint. = Metaiodiobenzylguanidine scintigraphy
EH = Essential hypertension

Fig. 5.1.3 Clinical suspicion of pheochromocytoma.

1–2 cm in diameter. An important limitation of this technique is that in 10–15% of the cases, it may result falsely positive because of the accumulation of the tracer either in the spleen or in the bladder. If MIBG scintigraphy fails, an alternative way to localize the tumor is to perform a venous catheterization for analyzing plasma catecholamines in samples collected at different levels of the vena cava; however, even this procedure may result falsely negative because of the intermittent release of catecholamines.

How to exclude hypertension from exogenous substances

Accurate collection of data on the patient's history is, by far, the most powerful tool in the hands of the clinician for diagnosing these forms of secondary hypertension. This may be a difficult task because patients tend not to mention substances which, in their opinion, are not related to the development of hypertension. Licorice ingestion is a classical example and specific questioning about this should always be posed, particularly in patients who have quitted smoking and those with apparently unexplained hypokalemia. Yet even with a collaborative patient, excluding exogenous substances as a possible cause of hypertension is difficult because the quantity and the duration of consumption needed to raise blood pressure is highly variable among individuals. As far as the ingestion of estrogens is concerned, which is one of the most common forms of secondary hypertension in premenopausal women, it is usually considered that estradiol needs to be assumed for several months at doses greater than 50 µg/day to cause clear-cut elevation in blood pressure. However, even shorter periods of time may be sufficient in susceptible individuals. The best way of excluding this cause of hypertension is to stop estrogen treatment for 3–6 months. If, after this time, hypertension persists it is very likely due to other causes (in most cases essential hypertension).

The pressor effect of sympathomimetic drugs such as local vasoconstrictors, salbutamol and isoproterenol, should last only for days or, at most, for a few weeks. Of similar duration usually are the elevations in pressure due to the abrupt withdrawal of clonidine and beta-adrenergic blockers. Some humoral measurements may be helpful for excluding these drug-related forms of hypertension. For example, in patients with hypertension and prolonged assumption of cortisone, a finding of suppressed PRA and aldosterone is confirmatory of the clinical suspicion. Moreover, the progressive normalization of these hormones matches that of serum potassium and blood pressure.

How to exclude coarctation of the aorta

This is the only form of secondary hypertension that can be excluded simply on the basis of the physical examination. Indeed, the absence of the systolic murmur over the spinous processes of the back as well as of a diminished and/or delayed pulsations in the femoral arteries makes the diagnosis very unlikely in adult hypertensives. In contrast, the finding in X-ray of the thorax of a dilated ascending aorta in a standard film or of the typical notching of the ribs, due to the erosion by dilated collateral vessel, raises the possibility of a coarctation requiring aortography to localize accurately the site and length of the obstruction. Measurement of PRA is useful to assess to what extent the aortic malformation reduces renal blood flow leading to a renin-dependent hypertension similar to RVH.

References

1. The Sixth Report of the Joint National Committee on Prevention, Detection, Evaluation and Treatment of High Blood Pressure. *Arch Intern Med* 1997;**157**:2413–2446.
2. Blythe WB. Natural history of hypertension in renal parenchymal disease. *Am J Kidney Dis* 1985;**5**:A50–A56.
3. Danielson H, Kornerup HJ, Olsen S, Posborg V. Arterial hypertension in chronic glomerulonephritis. An analysis of 310 cases. *Clin Nephrol* 1983;**19**:284–287.
4. Acosta JH. Hypertension in chronic renal disease. *Kidney Int* 1982;**22**:702–712.
5. Anderson GH, Blakeman N, Streeten DHP. The effect of age on prevalence of secondary forms of hypertension in 4429 consecutively referred patients. *J Hypertension* 1994;**12**:609–615.
6. Anderson GH, Blakeman N, Streeten DHP. Prediction of renovascular hypertension. Comparison with clinical diagnostic indices. *Am J Hypertension* 1988;**1**:301–304.
7. Vaughan ED Jr, Bühler FR, Laragh JH *et al*. Renovascular hypertension: renin measurement to indicate hypersecretion and contralateral suppression, estimate renal plasma flow and score for surgical curability. *Am J Med* 1973;**55**:402–414.
8. Sealey JE, Bühler FR, Laragh JH, Vaughan ED Jr. The physiology of renin secretion in essential hypertension: estimation of renin secretion rate and renal plasma flow from peripheral and renal vein renin. *Am J Med* 1973;**55**:391–401.

9. Laragh JH, Sealey JE, Bühler FR *et al*. The renin axis and vasoconstriction volume analysis for understanding and treating renovascular and renal hypertension. *Am J Med* 1975;**58**:4–13.

10. Muller FB, Sealey JE, Case CB *et al*. The captopril test for identifying renovascular disease in hypertensive patients. *Am J Med* 1986;**80**:633–644.

11. Pickering TG, Sos TA, Vaughan ED Jr *et al*. Predictive value and changes of renin secretion in hypertensive patients with unilateral renovascular disease undergoing successful renal angioplasty. *Am J Med* 1985;**76**:398–404.

12. Leonetti G, Mayer G, Morganti A *et al*. Hypotensive and renin suppressive activities of propranolol in hypertensive patients. *Clin Sci Mol Med* 1975;**48**:491–499.

13. Burdick L, Airoldi F, Marana I *et al*. Superiority of acceleration and acceleration time over pulsatility and resistance indices as screening tests for renal artery stenosis. *J Hypertension* 1996;**14**:1229–1235.

14. Fommei E, Ghione S, Palla L *et al*. Renal scintigraphic captopril test in the diagnosis of renovascular hypertension. *Hypertension* 1987;**10**:212–220.

15. Biglieri EG, Kater C, Mantero F. Adrenocortical forms of human hypertension. In: *Hypertension: Pathophysiology, Diagnosis and Management* (eds Laragh JH, Brenner BM), pp. 2145–2162. Raven Press: New York 1995.

16. Lim RC, Nakayama DK, Biglieri EG *et al*. Primary hyperaldosteronism: changing concepts in diagnosis and management. *Am J Surg* 1986;**152**:116–121.

17. Manger WM, Gifford RW. *Clinical and Experimental Pheochromocytoma*, pp. 205–331. Blackwell Science: Oxford, 1996.

18. Bravo EL, Tarazi RC, Fouad FM *et al*. Clonidine-suppression test: a useful aid in the diagnosis of pheochromocytoma. *N Engl J Med* 1981;**305**:623–626.

19. Sisson JC, Frager MS, Valk TW *et al*. Scintigraphic localization of pheochromocytoma. *N Engl J Med* 1981;**305**:12–17.

20. Task Force on Oral Contraceptives. The WHO Multicentre Trial of the vasopressor effects of combined oral contraceptives: Comparison with IUD. *Contraception* 1989;**40**:129–145.

21. Cairns V, Keil V, Doering A *et al*. Oral contraceptives use and blood pressure in a German metropolitan population. *Int J Epidemiol* 1985;**14**:389–395.

22. Farese RV, Biglieri EG, Schackleton CHL *et al*. Licorice induced hypermineralocorticoidism. *N Engl J Med* 1991;**325**:1223–1227.

23. Chua SS, Benrimoj SI. Non prescription sympathomimetic agents and hypertension. *Med Toxicol* 1988;**3**:387–417.

24. Sealy WC. Coarctation of the aorta and hypertension. *Ann Thorac Surg* 1967;**3**:15–28.

5

Chapter

5.2

Assessment of hypertensive organ damage

L Hansson

5

Introduction

The assessment of hypertensive organ damage is an important part of the clinical routine work-up of hypertensive patients, since the identification of such changes may affect the choice of therapy and the intensity of the antihypertensive treatment. For these reasons it is customary to evaluate a number of clinical chemistry variables such as creatinine, test the urine for proteinuria and to screen the electrocardiogram (ECG) for possible signs of left ventricular hypertrophy.

Another reason for assessing hypertensive organ damage in hypertension is to identify intermediate endpoints, sometimes referred to as 'surrogate endpoints', in hypertension intervention trials. Such endpoints appear to be of particular value in trials comprising patients with milder forms of hypertension, where few 'hard' endpoints such as cardiovascular death or non-fatal myocardial infarctions or stroke can be expected. In this situation more refined methodology may be called for than in the clinical routine management of patients.

Emphasis here will be on four major organs or organ systems that may all be affected by arterial hypertension: the blood vessels, the heart, the kidneys and the brain. More detailed information can be found in Hansson and Birkenhäger[1].

The vasculature

The hemodynamic 'hallmark' of hypertension is increased total peripheral resistance (TPR)[2] which increases with the duration of the disease[3]. Most hypertension in the elderly is associated with normal TPR. The increase in TPR is due mainly to structural changes in the precapillary arterioles (resistance vessels)[4,5], the term 'resistance vessels' usually referring to arterioles with a diameter < 300 μm[6].

Structural arteriolar changes can, in a simplified view, be seen as being particularly important in relation to TPR, the level of diastolic blood pressure and mean arterial pressure. Changes in the larger conduit arteries are also common in hypertension and affect compliance, pulse wave velocity and pulse wave reflection. This means that they play a relatively more important role for the systolic blood pressure and the pulse pressure.

The arterioles

Structural changes in the arterioles of hypertensive patients have been known for more than a hundred years. They were first reported in 1868 in patients with 'Bright's disease'[7]. This observation has been subsequently confirmed both in hypertensive animals[4] and in patients with essential hypertension[5]. These vessels are difficult to study in man for obvious reasons. They are small and their diameter can vary considerably depending on vasomotor nerve tone as well as a the influence of a number of vasoactive substances, released in response to the metabolic needs of the tissue that is being perfused. Some of the techniques used to assess arteriolar changes in hypertension will be discussed briefly here.

> **BOX 5.2.1 Classification of arterioles**
>
> The arterioles are sometimes divided into three different categories:
>
> 1. A1. First-order or feeding arterioles. These have a diameter of 70–150 μm and are the major feeding vessels that transport blood into the tissues.
> 2. A2. Second-order arterioles. Their diameter is 30–80 μm. They are the first branches of the A1 vessels.
> 3. A3–A4. Third- and fourth-order arterioles with diameters < 30 μm. They connect the A2 vessels with the capillaries. It is usually in this segment of the arteriolar tree that the major resistance to blood flow is executed. Thus, the term 'precapillary resistance vessels' is quite adequate.

Venous occlusion plethysmography

This method is suitable for certain vascular beds such as the forearm, the calf or the hand, i.e. vascular beds, in which it is possible to mechanically occlude venous drainage and thereby assess arterial flow by measuring the volume change of the organ over a short period of time.

In order to get a reliable assessment of structural vascular changes, the studies must be conducted at maximal vascular dilatation, i.e. the effect of all conceivable vasoconstrictor stimuli must be abolished. This is usually achieved by measuring postischemic flow. In such a situation flow resistance is determined solely by the anatomical structure of the vessels.

Studies both in hypertensive animals by Folkow *et al.*, and in hypertensive patients by Sivertsson, have found elevated vascular resistance at maximal vasodilatation in several different vascular beds[4,5], changes that can only be explained by a structural arteriolar abnormality.

Capillary flow

The assessment of capillary flow can be seen as a surrogate method for the evaluation of arteriolar changes. By using TV-connected microscopic techniques, certain skin vessel beds can be examined with a 'flying spot' technique[8], a frame-to-frame technique[9] and with videophotometric capilloscopy[10]. Fagrell *et al.* have refined the capillary flow examinations by introducing a computerized videophotometric technique to measure red blood cell velocity in skin capillaries[11]. With this technique it is possible to demonstrate a difference in response to mental stress between nutritional and thermoregulating skin capillaries[12]. Using laser Doppler flowmetry of capillary blood cell velocity values between 350 ± 90 μm/s[13] and 500 ± 390 μm/s[12] have been reported in normotensive subjects.

Using similar techniques in the conjunctiva, a rarefaction of arterioles has been described in hypertensive animals[14,15] as well as in patients with borderline hypertension[16] and patients with untreated essential hypertension[17].

Biopsy and postmortem examinations

Biopsy techniques, most frequently using skin or subcutaneous tissue, provide a way to obtain arterioles for microscopic examination[18,19]. The invasive nature of the biopsy methodology is an obvious drawback, and the technical difficulties are considerable (as briefly reviewed by Sivertsson[5]). Postmortem examinations obviously have little to offer in a clinical setting.

Increased wall-to-lumen ratio has been described in intestinal biopsy specimen taken from patients with severe hypertension[20]. Such observations are in agreement with the hemodynamic results obtained during maximal vasodilatation[4,5], although some investigators have not reported an increased wall : lumen ratio in skin arterioles with a diameter < 100 µm from patients with hypertension[21].

We have previously reviewed the reversibility of structural arteriolar changes in hypertensive patients, using the venous occlusion plethysmographic methodology at maximal vasodilatation, following long-term antihypertensive treatment with various therapies[22]. Although most therapies reduced the structural abnormality, a complete normalization was never achieved, possibly because antihypertensive therapy was started too late or because it did not reduce blood pressure sufficiently[22]. In later years, several studies, in particular by Schiffrin and coworkers, using microscopic examination of subcutaneous biopsies, have shown different degrees of reversibility of the structural arteriolar abnormality depending on the choice of antihypertensive agent, an angiotensin-converting enzyme inhibitor being more effective in this regard than, for example, a beta-blocker[23].

Retina examinations

The vessels of the retinas are of particular interest since they are readily visible using appropriate techniques, basically ophthalmoscopy, sometimes with the addition of photography. Indeed, in 1939 Keith, Wagener and Barker published their classic paper on the classification of the severity of hypertension based on the retinal vascular changes[24]. Long before them, in 1898, Gunn had described ophthalmoscopic hypertensive retinal vessel changes in patients[25] and nowadays this technique has been refined to allow quantification of vascular changes and their modification by antihypertensive therapy[26].

Conclusions

It can be concluded that the assessment of structural arteriolar changes in hypertensive patients is of great pathophysiologic interest. However, the clinical application is limited by either the tedious and time-consuming techniques (venous occlusion plethysmography at maximal vasodilation)[5] or by being invasive, requiring biopsies[18,19]. The studies of retinal vessels or capillary flow variables may find their use in special circumstances.

Arteries

The relationship between arterial pressure and degenerative arterial changes was first described by Gull and Sutton in the 1870s[27]. An up-to-date review of arteries in hypertension, with special emphasis on large arteries and how increased stiffness in these vessels affect systolic, diastolic, mean and pulse pressure was provided by O'Rourke in 1997[28]. It is well established that arteriosclerotic vascular changes in large arteries is associated with increased systolic blood pressure[29]. In recent years it has also been shown, in several large intervention trials comprising patients with isolated systolic hypertension, that antihypertensive treatment is highly effective in reducing cardiovascular morbidity in such patients[30–32].

An important consequence of increased arterial stiffness is its impact on pulse wave velocity, which is increased, and the retrograde pulse wave reflection, which appears earlier[28,33]. For reasons such as these the assessment of arterial changes in hypertension have several important clinical implications[34]. It should be noted, however, that increased aortic stiffness and reduced arterial compliance are found not only in hypertension but also in a number of other conditions, many of which may be linked to hypertension. Aortic compliance is markedly decreased with aging and this contributes to the reduction in diastolic blood pressure seen in the elderly[35]. Decreased arterial compliance is also commonly found in patients with coronary heart disease[35]. Diabetes mellitus and tobacco smoking will also lead to reduced arterial compliance, mainly due to acceleration of the arteriosclerotic process.

In this context it is of interest to note that Franklin and Weber took a novel approach when linking clinical and epidemiologic observations in the Framingham Heart Study to the hemodynamic alterations at hand[34].

There are several methods for the evaluation of arterial changes in hypertension, such as applanation tonometry for the assessment of pulse pressure at various sites of the arterial tree[35–38]. The ratio between ankle and brachial systolic pressure is also a useful indicator of arterial stiffness[39] as is the determination of pulse wave velocity[40].

Although the determination of arterial changes is of great interest in hypertension, both from a pathophysiologic aspect and from a clinical and epidemiologic viewpoint, it must be concluded that a more elaborate or refined assessment of arterial changes in the routine care of hypertensive patients is not a realistic undertaking. On the other hand, in intervention trials such examinations could provide valuable information and findings could easily be seen to constitute intermediary endpoints.

The heart

Left ventricular hypertrophy (LVH) is a common finding in hypertensive patients[41]. Even when assessing LVH with the less specific ECG method, marked increments in cardiovascular risk in the

Table 5.2.1 Risk increments in the Framingham Heart Study in the presence of electrocardiographically diagnosed left ventricular hypertrophy

Event	Risk increase
Coronary heart disease	3–5 times
Myocardial infarction	2–5 times
Angina pectoris	1–6 times
Stroke	6–10 times
Congestive heart failure	6–17 times
Cardiovascular disease	4–8 times

Modified after Levy[42].

presence of LVH have been reported from the Framingham Heart Study (Table 5.2.1)[42]. By using the more sensitive method of echocardiography the Framingham Heart Study investigators reported that LVH constitutes the most powerful risk indicator for cardiovascular morbidity in that study[43].

Several different forms of LVH can be distinguished[44]. It is of some interest that impaired left ventricular diastolic function usually is the first result of LVH[45]. The increased thickness and stiffness of the left ventricle, even in the presence of left atrial enlargement and thickening, results in suboptimal filling of the left ventricle during diastole. Only in later stages is the systolic function compromised, the end result being left ventricular failure.

From a therapeutic point of view, a large number of trials have been conducted with the aim of assessing the impact of various antihypertensive therapies on LVH. Many of these trials have been analyzed together in meta-analyses[46–49]. It appears that angiotensin-converting enzyme (ACE) inhibitors, as well as calcium antagonists, are more effective in reducing left ventricular mass even when expressed in relation to the magnitude of blood pressure reduction[46,47,49]. More important is the observation that a reduction in LV mass, or a prevention of an increase in left ventricular mass, thanks to long-term antihypertensive therapy positively affects cardiovascular morbidity[50].

It can be concluded that the assessment of cardiac performance and status, usually by echocardiographic technique, is an important and valuable part of the initial work-up in most patients with hypertension. It is conceivable that newer techniques, such as magnetic resonance imaging may offer certain advantages, but by and large they are still not available to such an extent that they provide a realistic alternative to echocardiography. Myocardial scintigraphy, usually with radioactive thallium as the tracer, provides useful information on myocardial perfusion, especially when conducted during physical exercise, but it has no place in the routine assessment of uncomplicated hypertensive patients.

The kidney

The role of the kidney in the pathogenesis, as opposed to being a victim of hypertension, has always been a challenging problem. It can be, and over the years has been, debated whether observed changes in the

The heart

The brain

kidneys of patients with essential hypertension are the cause of the disease or the consequences of long-term blood pressure elevation[51]. It is worth noting that nephrosclerosis, the most common endpoint of chronic hypertension, currently accounts for 10–20% of all new patients needing dialysis in Europe[52] with even higher numbers being reported from the USA.

Glomerular filtration rate

In addition to creatinine and urea, which are frequently used in the clinical assessment of glomerular function, more sensitive techniques are available, in particular clearance techniques using markers such as inulin or ^{51}Cr-EDTA[53] that are released into the urine solely via glomerular filtration and not by renal tubular excretion.

From a practical point of view, glomerular filtration rate (GFR) in patients with essential hypertension, as assessed with ^{51}Cr-EDTA clearance, has been shown to be better preserved during long-term treatment with an ACE inhibitor than with a beta-blocker[54,55]. Such results are in agreement with observations in patients with renal forms of hypertension[56].

Microalbuminuria

The determination of microalbuminuria in hypertensive patients has become increasingly applied in recent years. Microalbuminuria is seen as a marker of renal involvement in hypertension[57] and the term is usually applied if protein excretion is in the range 30–300 mg/24 hours. Microalbuminuria was first used in 1982 to define slightly elevated excretion of protein in the urine that did not qualify for the accepted term 'albuminuria'[58]. In non-diabetic individuals microalbuminuria is found in 5–10% of a non-selected population, higher rates being reported in diabetics and in hypertensive patients[57]. To what extent microalbuminuria is a prognostic marker in hypertension or just a reflection of the level of blood pressure remains somewhat controversial. If it only reflects the level of blood pressure it is obviously easier and less costly to just measure the blood pressure.

It can be concluded that the kidney is an important organ in hypertension. To what extent it should be seen as culprit or victim can be debated. In the routine care of hypertensive patients it is rarely necessary to conduct refined measurements of GFR, the exception being patients with various renal forms of hypertension in whom the determination of the rate of progression towards uremia may be of vital importance.

The brain

The brain, like the kidneys, can be seen both as an important culprit and victim in hypertension. Much of the dysregulation of hemodynamics in hypertension obviously have a central nervous origin and the brain is also the victim of one of the most dreaded complications of hypertension - stroke.

Stroke

Stroke is strongly linked to arterial hypertension. In many countries in Europe and in the United States there is fortunately a decreasing incidence of stroke, and although the treatment of hypertension can be assumed to play an important role in this development, it is not obvious that this is the only cause of the declining rate[59]. Indeed, it is quite clear that the falling stroke incidence was observed even before the introduction of antihypertensive therapies[60]. Undoubtedly virtually every major hypertension intervention trial has demonstrated significant reductions in stroke morbidity as an effect of antihypertensive treatment[30–32,61–63], the only exception being the relatively small ($n = 840$) European Working Party against High blood pressure in the Elderly (EWPHE) trial[64].

In this context, the regulation of cerebral blood flow is of great interest[65]. Cerebral blood flow is autoregulated over a wide range of blood pressures. Below a certain blood pressure, the level of cerebral blood flow cannot be maintained and as a consequence brain hypoxia occurs with symptoms such as dizziness, vertigo, somnolence and ultimately unconsciousness and death.

At the other end of the autoregulation of cerebral blood flow, a breakthrough of autoregulation will occur if blood pressure rises above a certain level. This will be accompanied by symptoms such as headache, convulsions, unconsciousness and ultimately death.

When assessing a patient with stroke it is essential to differentiate between a hemorrhagic stroke and a thromboembolic one. Computed tomography scanning (CT scan) is the method of choice, whereas assessment of carotid artery status by sonography and echocardiographic examination of the heart may be of value in selected cases.

Dementia and reduced cognitive function

The relationship between blood pressure and dementia was reviewed by Skoog in 1997[66]. It is interesting to note that Skoog *et al.* clearly demonstrated that elevated blood pressure preceded the onset of Alzheimer's disease in elderly individuals in a population-based long-term survey[67]. The link between vascular dementia and hypertension is obviously better established[68].

In a series of 999 men from a population survey in Uppsala, we were able to demonstrate significant relationships between blood pressure at age 50 and cognitive function at age 70: the lower the blood pressure the better the cognitive function twenty years later[69]. Thus, contrary to popular belief, low blood pressure seems to be a consequence of dementia of the Alzheimer type, rather than its cause.

That antihypertensive therapy may prevent or delay the onset of dementia was suggested by a subgroup analysis of the Systolic Hypertension in Europe (SYST-EUR) trial[70]. This interesting possibility is now being assessed in the ongoing Study on Cognition and Prognosis in Elderly (SCOPE) trial, in which 4964 elderly hypertensive patients have been randomized to either active antihypertensive treatment with candesartan, cilexetil or placebo[71]. In the SCOPE study, the Mini Mental State Examination (MMSE) test is used as the basic assessment of cognitive function[71].

It can be concluded that a brain CT scan and the determination of cerebral blood flow rarely, if ever, is indicated in the routine assessment of hypertensive patients. If a stroke has occurred, on the other hand, a CT scan should be seen as a routine examination. The assessment of cognitive function in hypertensive patients, using for example the MMSE test, is still in its early stages of evaluation. The test is simple to conduct and has been validated in many languages. It may become more widely used if studies such as SCOPE demonstrate that cognitive function may be preserved thanks to antihypertensive treatment.

Conclusions

Numerous investigations, in addition to the routinely performed clinical chemistry tests and ECG, are available for the assessment of hypertensive organ damage. To what extent such investigations should be performed is related to the purpose of the investigation, whether it be for the clinical management of a patient or for the evaluation of intermediary endpoints in a trial, as well as to the expenditure that can be used.

References

1. Hansson L, Birkenhäger WH (eds) *Handbook of Hypertension*, Vol. 18. *Assessment of Hypertensive Organ Damage*. Elsevier: Amsterdam, 1997.
2. Freis ED. Hemodynamics in hypertension. *Physiol Rev* 1960;**40**:27–54.
3. Lund-Johansen P. Hemodynamics trends in untreated essential hypertension. Preliminary report on a 10-year follow-up study. *Acta Med Scand* 1977; Suppl.**602**:68–75.
4. Folkow B, Grimby G, Thulesius O. Adaptive structural changes in the vascular walls in hypertension and their relation to the control of peripheral resistance. *Acta Physiol Scand* 1958;**44**:255–272.
5. Sivertsson R. The hemodynamic importance of structural vascular changes in essential hypertension. *Acta Physiol Scand* 1970, Suppl. 343.
6. Clement DL, De Buyzere M, Duprez D. (Pre)capillary patterns in hypertension. In: *Handbook of Hypertension*, Vol. 18. *Assessment of Hypertensive Organ Damage* (eds Hansson L, Birkenhäger WH), pp. 85–104. Elsevier: Amsterdam, 1997.
7. Johnson G. On certain points in the anatomy of Bright's disease of the kidney. *Trans R Med Chir Soc* 1868;**51**:57–58.
8. Brånemark PI, Johnsson P. Determination of the velocity of corpuscles in blood capillaries. *Biorheology* 1963;**1**:143–146.
9. Bollinger A, Botti P, Barras JP *et al*. Red blood cell velocity in nail fold capillaries in man measured by a television microscopy. *Microvasc Res* 1974;**7**:61–72.
10. Fagrell B, Fronek A, Intaglietta M. A microscope television system for studying flow velocity in human skin capillaries. *Am J Physiol* 1977;**233**:H318–H321.
11. Fagrell B, Rosén L, Eriksson SE. Comparison between a new computerized and an analogue videophotometric cross-correlation technique for measuring skin capillary blood cell velocity in humans. *Int J Microcirc* 1994;**11**:133–138.
12. Lemne C, De Faire U, Fagrell B. Mental stress induces different reaction in nutritional and thermoregulatory human skin microcirculation: a study in borderline hypertensives and normotensives. *J Hum Hypertension* 1994;**8**:559–563.

5.2

References

13. Östergren J, Kahan T, Hjemdahl P *et al*. Effects of sympatho-adrenal activation on finger circulation in mild hypertension. *J Hum Hypertension* 1992;**6**:169–173.

14. Prewitt R, Chen I, Dowell RF. Microvascular alterations in the one-kidney, one-clip renal hypertensive rat. *Am J Physiol* 1984;**246**:H728–H732.

15. Hutchins P, Darnell A. Observations of a decreased number of small arterioles in spontaneously hypertensive rats. *Circulation Res* 1974;**34**(Suppl. 1):161–165.

16. Sullivan J, Russel M, Josephs J. Attenuation of the microcirculation in young patients with high output borderline hypertension. *Hypertension* 1982;**5**:844–851.

17. Harper RN, Moore MA, Marr ML *et al*. Arteriolar rarefaction in the conjunctiva of human essential hypertension. *Microvasc Res* 1978;**16**:369–372.

18. Mulvany MJ, Alkjær C. Structure and function of small arteries. *Physiol Rev* 1990;**70**:921–961.

19. Heagarty AM, Alkjær C, Bund SJ *et al*. Small artery structure in hypertension: dual process of remodelling and growth. *Hypertension* 1993;**21**:391–397.

20. Giaconi S, Levanti C, Frommei E *et al*. Microalbuminuria and casual blood pressure and ambulatory blood pressure monitoring in normotensives and in patients with borderline and mild hypertension. *Am J Hypertension* 1989;**2**:259–261.

21. Redon J, Gomez-Sanches MA, Baldo E *et al*. Micro-albuminuria is correlated with left ventricular hypertrophy in male hypertensive patients. *J Hypertension* 1991;**9**(Suppl. 6):S148–S149.

22. Hansson L, Sivertsson R. Regression of structural cardiovascular changes by antihypertensive treatment. *Hypertension* 1984;**6**(Suppl. III):147–149.

23. Schiffrin EL, Deng LY, Larochelle P. Progressive improvement in the structure of resistance arteries of hypertensive patients after two years of treatment with an angiotensin I converting enzyme inhibitor. Comparison with effects of a beta-blocker. *Am J Hypertension* 1995;**8**:229–236.

24. Keith NM, Wagener HP, Barker MW. Some different types of essential hypertension: their course and prognosis. *Am J Med Sci* 1939;**197**:332–343.

25. Gunn M. On ophthalmoscopic evidence of general arterial disease. *Trans Ophthalmol Soc UK* 1898;356–381.

26. Dahlöf B, Stenkula S, Hansson L. Hypertensive retinal vascular changes: Relationship to left ventricular hypertrophy and arteriolar changes before and after treatment. *Blood Press* 1992;**1**:35–44.

27. Gull WW. Chronic Bright's disease with contracted kidney (arterio-capillary fibrosis). *Br Med J* 1872;**ii**:692.

28. O'Rourke M. Relative importance of blood pressure components on cardiovascular integrity: systolic, diastolic, mean or pulse pressure. In: *Handbook of Hypertension*, Vol. 18. *Assessment of Hypertensive Organ Damage* (eds Hansson L, Birkenhäger WH), pp. 1–27. Elsevier: Amsterdam, 1997.

29. Safar ME, Totomoukouo JJ, Asmar RA, Laurent SM. Increased pulse pressure in patients with arteriosclerosis obliterans of the lower limbs. *Arteriosclerosis* 1987;**7**:232–237.

30. SHEP Cooperative Research Group. Prevention of stroke by hypertensive drug therapy in older persons with isolated systolic hypertension: Final results of the Systolic Hypertension in the Elderly Program. *J Am Med Ass* 1991;**265**:3255–3264.

31. Staessen JA, Fagard R, Thijs L *et al*. for the Systolic Hypertension in Europe (SYST-EUR) Trial Investigators. Randomised double-blind comparison of placebo and active treatment for older patients with isolated systolic hypertension. *Lancet* 1997;**350**:757–764.

32. Liu L, Wang JG, Gong L *et al*. for the Systolic Hypertension in China (SYST-CHINA) Collaborative Group. Comparison of active treatment and placebo for older Chinese patients with isolated systolic hypertension. *J Hypertension* 1998;**16**:1823–1829.

33. O'Rourke M. Arterial stiffness, systolic blood pressure, and logical treatment of arterial hypertension. *Hypertension* 1990;**15**:339–347.

34. Franklin SS, Gustin IVW, Wong ND *et al*. Hemodynamic patterns of age-related changes in blood pressure. The Framingham Heart Study. *Circulation* 1997;**96**:308–315.

35. Safar ME, London G. Assessment of arterial damage in clinical hypertension: basic concepts and clinical implications. In: *Handbook of Hypertension*, Vol. 18. *Assessment of*

Hypertensive Organ Damage (eds Hansson L, Birkenhäger WH), pp. 43–64. Elsevier: Amsterdam, 1997.

36. Murgo JP, Westerhof N, Giolma SA. Aortic input impedance in normal man: relationship to pressure shapes. *Circulation* 1980;**62**:105–116.

37. Stefanidis C, Wooley CF, Bush CA *et al.* Aortic distensibility abnormalities in coronary artery disease. *Am J Cardiol* 1987;**59**:1300–1304.

38. Benetos A, Laurent S, Hoek SAP *et al.* Arterial wave reflections and increased systolic and pulse pressure in chronic uremia: study using noninvasive carotid pulse waveform registration. *Hypertension* 1993;**20**:10–19.

39. Hugue CJ, Safar ME, Alifierakis MC *et al.* The ratio between ankle and brachial systolic pressure in patients with sustained uncomplicated essential hypertension. *Clin Sci* 1988;**74**:179–182.

40. O'Rourke MF, Kelly R, Avolio A. *The Arterial Pulse*. Lee & Febiger: Philadelphia, PA, 1992.

41. Strauer BE. Ventricular function and coronary hemodynamics in hypertensive heart disease. *Am J Cardiol* 1979;**44**:999–1006.

42. Levy D. Left ventricular hypertrophy. Epidemiological insights from the Framingham Heart Study. *Drugs* 1988;**35**(Suppl. 5):1–5.

43. Levy D, Garrison RJ, Sagae DD *et al.* Prognostic implications of echocardiographically determined left ventricular mass in the Framingham Heart Study. *N Engl J Med* 1990;**322**:1561–1566.

44. Tomanek RJ, Wangler RD, Bauer CA. Prevention of coronary vasodilator reserve decrement in spontaneously hypertensive rats. *Hypertension* 1985;**7**:533–540.

45. Gudbrandsson T, Sivertsson R, Herlitz H, Hansson L. Cardiac involvement in hypertension. A non-invasive study of patients with previous malignant hypertension and 'benign' hypertension. *Eur Heart J* 1983;**3**:246–254.

46. Dahlöf B, Pennert K, Hansson L. Reversal of left ventricular hypertrophy in hypertensive patients. A metaanalysis of 109 treatment studies. *Am J Hypertension* 1992;**5**:95–110.

47. Jennings GL, Wong J. Reversibility of left ventricular hypertrophy and malfunction by antihypertensive treatment. In: *Handbook of Hypertension*, Vol. 18. *Assessment of Hypertensive Organ Damage* (eds Hansson L, Birkenhäger WH), pp. 184–223. Elsevier: Amsterdam, 1997.

48. Schmieder RE, Martus P, Klingbeil A. Reversal of left ventricular hypertrophy in essential hypertension. A meta-analysis of randomized double-blind studies. *J Am Med Ass* 1996;**275**:1507–1513.

49. Schmieder RE, Schlaich MP, Klingbeil AU, Martus P. Update on reversal of left ventricular hypertrophy in essential hypertension (a meta-analysis of all randomized double-blind studies until December 1996). *Nephrol Dial Transplant* 1998;**13**:564–569.

50. Muiesan ML, Salvetti M, Rizzoni D *et al.* Association of change in left ventricular mass with prognosis during long-term antihypertensive treatment. *J Hypertension* 1995;**13**:1091–1095.

51. de Leeuw PW, Birkenhäger WH. Renal hemodynamics and glomerular filtration in essential hypertension; effects of treatment. In: *Handbook of Hypertension*, Vol. 18. *Assessment of Hypertensive Organ Damage* (eds Hansson L, Birkenhäger WH), pp. 345–363. Elsevier: Amsterdam, 1997.

52. Brunner FP, Selwood NH on behalf of the EDTA Registration Committee. Profile of patients on RRT in Europe and death rates due to major causes of death groups. *Kidney Int* 1992;**42**(Suppl. 38):S4–S15.

53. Granérus G, Aurell M. Reference values for ^{51}Cr-EDTA clearance as a measure of glomerular filtration rate. *Scand J Clin Lab Invest* 1981;**41**:611–616.

54. Himmelmann A, Hansson L, Hansson B-G *et al.* ACE inhibition preserves renal function better than β-blockade in the treatment of essential hypertension. *Blood press* 1995;**4**:85–90.

55. Himmelmann A, Hansson L, Hansson B-G *et al.* Long-term renal preservation in essential hypertension. ACE inhibition superior to β-blockade. *Am J Hypertension* 1996;**9**:850–853.

56. Björck S, Mulec H, Johnsen SA *et al.* Renal protective effects of enalapril in diabetic nephropathy. *Br Med J* 1992;**304**:339–343.

5

References

57. Ruilope LM, Suarez C. Clinical significance of microalbuminuria. In: *Handbook of Hypertension*, Vol. 18. *Assessment of Hypertensive Organ Damage* (eds Hansson L, Brikenhäger WH), pp. 332–344. Elsevier: Amsterdam, 1997.

58. Viberti CC, Mackintosh B, Bilous RW *et al*. Proteinuria in diabetes mellitus: role of spontaneous and experimental variations of glycemia. *Kidney Int* 1982;**21**:714–720.

59. Bonita R, Beaglehole R. Cerebrovascular disease. Explaining stroke mortality trends. *Lancet* 1993;**341**:1510–1511.

60. Donnan GA, You RX, Dewey HM *et al*. Important issues in stroke today. In: *Handbook of Hypertension*, Vol. 18. *Assessment of Hypertensive Organ Damage*, (eds Hansson L, Birkenhäger WH), pp. 269–281. Elsevier: Amsterdam, 1997.

61. Collins R, Peto R, MacMahon S *et al*. Blood pressure, stroke, and coronary heart disease. Part 2. Short-term reductions in blood pressure: over-view of randomised drug trials in their epidemiological context. *Lancet* 1990;**335**:827–838.

62. Dahlöf B, Lindholm LH, Hansson L *et al*. Morbidity and mortality in the Swedish Trial in Old Patients with Hypertension (STOP-Hypertension). *Lancet* 1991;**338**:1281–1285.

63. MRC Working Party. Medical Research Council trial of treatment of hypertension in older adults: principal results. *Brit Med J* 1992;**304**:405–412.

64. Amery A, Birkenhäger W, Brixko P *et al*. Mortality and morbidity results from the European Working Party on High Blood Pressure in the elderly trial. *Lancet* 1985;**i**:1351–1354.

65. Edvinsson L. Physiological control of the cerebral circulation. In: *Handbook of Hypertension*, Vol. 18. *Assessment of Hypertensive organ damage* (eds Hansson L, Birkenhäger WH), pp. 224–248. Elsevier: Amsterdam, 1997.

66. Skoog I. Blood pressure and dementia. In: *Handbook of Hypertension*, Vol. 18. *Assessment of Hypertensive Organ Damage* (eds Hansson L, Birkenhäger WH), pp. 303–331. Elsevier: Amsterdam, 1997.

67. Skoog I, Lernfelt B, Landahl S *et al*. 15-year longitudinal study of blood pressure and dementia. *Lancet* 1996;**347**:1141–1145.

68. Johansson BB. Pathogenesis of vascular dementia: the possible role of hypertension. *Dementia* 1994;**5**:519–521.

69. Kilander L, Nyman H, Boberg M *et al*. Hypertension is related to cognitive impairment. A 20-year follow-up of 999 men. *Hypertension* 1998;**31**:780–786.

70. Forette F, Seux M-L, Staessen JA *et al*. on behalf of the SYST-EUR Investigators. Prevention of dementia in randomised double-blind placebo-controlled Systolic Hypertension in Europe (SYST-EUR) trial. *Lancet* 1998;**352**:1347–1351.

71. Hansson L, Lithell H, Skoog I *et al*. for the SCOPE Investigators. Study on cognition and prognosis in the elderly (SCOPE). *Blood Press* 1999 (accepted for publication).

5

5.3

Special measures of end-organ damage

K Kario and TG Pickering

5

Introduction

The measurement of target organ damage is becoming increasingly important in the evaluation of hypertensive patients, and may add substantially to the assessment of cardiovascular risk and hence the need for treatment. The morbidity resulting from hypertension is the end result of target organ damage, which can be divided into two sorts: clinically manifest disease (such as stroke or coronary heart disease) and subclinical or silent target organ damage. The importance of the latter type, on which this review will focus, is that its detection offers the theoretical possibility of preventing progression to clinically manifest disease. The presence of target organ damage may reflect the cumulative effects of blood pressure over time, but also the effects of other risk factors. Several markers of target organ damage have been shown to predict cardiovascular morbidity independently of blood pressure. Many of these abnormalities are reversible by antihypertensive treatment, and an active area of research is whether this will also reduce the risk of morbidity. Figure 5.3.1 shows the significance of the major types of silent target organ damage. In Table 5.3.1 we summarize the specific non-invasive methods for the precise assessment of damage of the major target organs – the heart, kidneys, brain, eyes, and arteries. Emphasis is given to methods which are not yet part of the routine clinical work-up, but which have the potential for widespread clinical application.

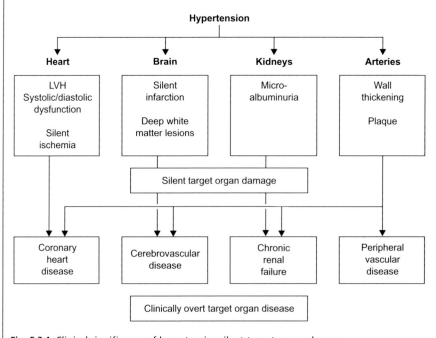

Fig. 5.3.1 Clinical significance of hypertensive silent target organ damage.

Table 5.3.1 Evaluation of target organ damage

Organ	Technique	Evaluation	Feasibility/cost	Prognostic significance
Heart	ECG (digitized)	LVH	High/low	Yes
		QT dispersion	High/low	?
	ECG (ambulatory)	Silent ischemia	High/low	Yes
	Echocardiography	LVH	Moderate/high	Yes
		Systolic/diastolic function	Moderate/high	Yes
	MRI	LVH systolic/diastolic function	Low/high	?
	Blood biochemical markers	BNP	High/low	?
Brain	MRI		Low/high	Yes
Eye	Fundal photography	Quantitative retinopathy	Low/high	?
Kidneys	Urine collection	Microalbuminuria	High/low	Yes
Arteries	Ultrasonography	IMT/plaque	Moderate/high	Yes
		Compliance	Moderate/high	Yes
	Pulse wave velocity	Compliance	Moderate/high	?
	Echocardiography	Compliance (SV/PP)	Moderate/high	Yes
	Blood biochemical markers	Various	High/low	?

Target organ damage and risk stratification

The two leading guidelines for the evaluation and treatment of the hypertensive patient (the Sixth Report of the Joint National Committee on Prevention, Detection, and Treatment of high blood pressure, or JNC VI [1], and the World Health Organization–International Society of Hypertension recommendations [2]) both include the assessment of target organ damage as an integral part of the work-up of the hypertensive patient. JNC VI identifies three risk groups: group A has no major risk factors other than blood pressure, and no target organ damage or clinical cardiovascular disease (TOD/CCD), group B has at least one risk factor, but also no TOD/CCD, while group C, at highest risk, has evidence of TOD/CCD. The cardiac elements of TOD/CCD that are identified include left ventricular hypertrophy (LVH), angina or prior myocardial infarction, coronary revascularization, or heart failure. Other measures include stroke or transient ischemic attack, nephropathy, peripheral arterial disease, and retinopathy.

WHO-ISH adopts a similar approach, but treats TOD and CCD separately. It too identifies three risk groups (Figure 5.3.2). The markers of TOD are defined as LVH (identified by ECG, echocardiogram, or chest X-ray), proteinuria, ultrasound or radiologic evidence of atherosclerotic plaque, and retinopathy. Treatment is guided by the level of risk.

The heart

Left ventricular hypertrophy is the most frequently studied marker of hypertensive target organ damage. Even in asymptomatic hypertensive patients, those will LVH have a worse cardiovascular prognosis than those without LVH [3], so the diagnosis of LVH is important in clinical

Target organ damage and risk stratification

The heart

285

5.3

Blood pressure mmHg

Other risk factors and disease history	Grade 1 140–159/90–99	Grade 2 160–179/100–109	Grade 3 >180/>110
I No other risk factors	LOW RISK	MED RISK	HIGH RISK
II 1-2 risk factors	MED RISK	MED RISK	V. HIGH RISK
III 3 or more risk factors TOD or diabetes	HIGH RISK	HIGH RISK	V. HIGH RISK
IV ACC	V. HIGH RISK	V. HIGH RISK	V. HIGH RISK

Fig. 5.3.2 Classification of risk according to blood pressure, other risk factors, and target organ damage. Adapted from WHO ISH recommendations.

practice. Patients with LVH are more likely to develop congestive heart failure, sudden cardiac death from arrhythmia, or coronary artery disease [4]. LVH has customarily been evaluated from the ECG, despite its acknowledged inaccuracy when used in the traditional way. However, the introduction of digital ECG recording has given the technique a new lease of life.

Echocardiography is now the clinical 'gold standard' for assessing LVH, although it is not yet accepted as being part of the routine work-up for every patient. MRI is potentially more accurate, but is still an investigative procedure.

Another potential marker of target organ damage is silent myocardial ischemia, which can be detected in about 20–30% of patients, and may be a risk factor for coronary artery disease and sudden death. Finally, there are biochemical markers of target organ damage which also have clinical promise.

Resting ECG

The standard 12-lead ECG remains the most widely used initial diagnostic test in the screening process for LVH and myocardial ischemia. There are several traditional voltage criteria based on the measured QRS amplitude, of which the most popular are the Sokolow–Lyon voltage criteria ($S_{v1} + R_{v5}$ or R_{v6}) [5] and the Romhilt–Estes score [6]. However, all have relatively poor sensitivity (levels of 20–50%), although the specificity often exceeds 90%, limiting the clinical utility and cost-effectiveness of the ECG for the detection of LVH. More recently, the Cornell criteria have been developed ($S_{v3} + R_{aVL}$ >2.8 mV in men, and >2.0 mV in women), with improved specificity [7]. Finally, Schillaci *et al.* [8] used a combination of the Cornell voltage criteria, the Romhilt–Estes score, and a left ventricular strain pattern in

V_5 and V_6 the sensitivity increased to 34%, with a specificity of 93%. Further, for the detection of LVH by ECG, gender-specific criteria improve the sensitivity in both the conventional voltage method (Cornell voltage criteria: $S_{v3} + R_{v1}$ 20 mm in women and 28 mm in men) and time–voltage area of the QRS method.

A major step forward in the ECG analysis for the detection of LVH has been provided by the analysis of digitized signals, based on the observations that relate increased LV mass to increases in the time–voltage area of the QRS complex. The simple product of QRS voltage and duration, as an approximation of the time–voltage area of the QRS, can improve the ECG identification of LVH as defined at autopsy and echocardiography. Using the gender-specific criteria of time–voltage area of the QRS method, at the level of 98% detection specificity, the sensitivity is improved to 71% for men and 81% for women [9].

A related measure which can be evaluated using digitized ECGs is QT dispersion, which is an index of increased regional heterogeneity of repolarization that may be a non-invasive marker of susceptibility to malignant ventricular arrhythmias and sudden death [10]. It is associated with the presence of concentric hypertrophy on the echocardiogram, and may be normalized when LVH regresses [10]. QT dispersion is more pronounced in non-dippers (whose blood pressure remains high during the night) than in dippers, which would be consistent with the poorer prognosis in non-dippers [11].

Silent ischemia

Not uncommonly, asymptomatic hypertensive patients demonstrate ECG changes of myocardial ischemia, either on stress testing or during ambulatory ECG monitoring, which can now be combined with ambulatory blood pressure monitoring. In a population study of 341 elderly Swedish men without any history of coronary heart disease, 23% had at least one episode of silent ischemia during a 24-hour monitoring period [12]. Silent ischemia was most common in men with poorly controlled hypertension, and was also a predictor of morbid events. The presence of silent ischemia does not necessarily imply that there is coronary artery disease, and it may be the result of changes in ventricular geometry and function resulting from the hypertension [13,14].

Echocardiography

Determination of left ventricular mass (LVM) by echocardiography is the most commonly used non-invasive clinical method of detecting LVH. However, it is not yet recommended for routine use on every patient by JNC VI on the grounds that it is too expensive. WHO-ISH recommends echocardiography 'whenever the clinical assessment reveals the presence of target organ damage or suggests the possibility of left ventricular hypertrophy'.

5

BOX 5.3.1 Echocardiography

The precise measurement technique and derived parameters are described in a previous review [2,15]. Usually, M-mode echocardiography is recommended, and three primary measurements (the interventricular septal wall thickness (IVS), posterior wall thickness (PWT) and left ventricular internal dimensions (LVID) at the end-diastolic phase are used to calculate the LVM as follows: [16]

$$LVM = 1.04 [(LVID + PWT + ISV)^3 - LVID^3] - 13.6 \text{ g}.$$

To compensate for the effect of body size, LVM index is calculated by dividing LVM by body surface area. Relative wall thickness (RWT) is calculated as follows:

$$RWT = 2PWT/LVID.$$

Abnormal values are shown in Table 5.3.2. In contrast to the 3–8% of patients with mild-to-moderate essential hypertension who have ECG-LVG, echocardiographic LVM is increased in 12–30% of relatively unselected hypertensive patients, and in 20–60% of patients with uncomplicated hypertension seen in referral centers [17].

Table 5.3.2 Abnormal values of LVM and left ventricular geometry using M-mode echocardiography

Left ventricular Mass (Penn method)
Men: >134 g/m²; women: >110 g/m²*
Men: >131 g/m²; women: >100 g/m²†
Relative wall thickness >0.45

*(Derived from apparently healthy Framingham population)
† (Derived from racially mixed normotensive population)

In addition to LVM, echocardiography can detect the different geometric patterns of left ventricular hypertrophy (concentric or eccentric), which are also important [3]. Concentric hypertrophy refers to a ventricle with thick walls relative to its cavity volume, and may be regarded as a response to a pressure load, while eccentric hypertrophy refers to a ventricle with an expanded cavity volume in proportion to wall thickness, and occurs in response to a volume load, such as occurs in endurance athletes. In concentric LVH, the ratio of ventricular wall thickness to radius – the relative wall thickness (RWT) – is increased to >0.45, while this ratio is decreased in eccentric hypertrophy. The prognosis of concentric hypertrophy is the worst of these different geometric patterns in hypertensive patients (Figure 5.3.3).

Usually, systolic left ventricular function, which is assessed by ejection fraction or systolic fractional shortening, is preserved in hypertensive patients even with LVH, while diastolic function is frequently impaired. The compliance curve of the stiff left ventricle is shifted to the left and is steeper in hypertensive patients with LVH, which results in an increase of diastolic pressure and eventually to diastolic heart failure. This leftward shift of the compliance curve is also strongly affected by aging. Thus, elderly hypertensives with LVH are a high-risk group for congestive heart failure (diastolic). To assess diastolic

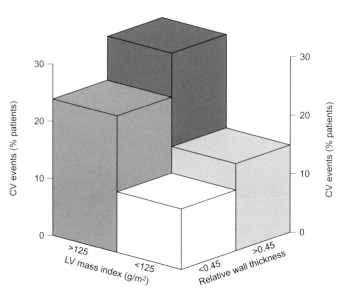

Fig. 5.3.3 Cardiovascular events and left ventricular remodelling in 253 hypertensive patients: (reproduced with permission from [11]). CV event = cardiovascular events. Solid column is concentric hypertrophy, lined column is eccentric hypertrophy, stippled column is concentric remodelling, and open column is normal ventricular geometry.

left ventricular function, the ratio of the peak velocity of early left ventricular filling (E) to the peak velocity of late left ventricular filling resulting from atrial contraction (A) – the E:A ratio – can be used with Doppler interrogation of the left ventricular inflow tract at the mitral valve. The E:A ratio is the most popular measure of diastolic dysfunction, and is thought to reflect changes in the diastolic compliance of the ventricle. Unlike left ventricular mass, however, its value is load dependent, and will vary according to factors such as the heart rate at the time of measurement. It is diminished in hypertensive patients, and interestingly, does not appear to recover after prolonged antihypertensive treatment, despite a reduction of left ventricular mass [18]. Although it has been claimed that changes in diastolic function may precede the development of structural changes, the most comprehensive study to date found that in young adults with mild hypertension changes of left ventricular mass and geometry were more consistently seen than changes in diastolic function [19].

Cardiac MRI

MRI of the heart has the ability to provide the most precise and objective non-invasive information about LVH, left ventricular geometry and cardiac function, even when compared with echocardiography [20]. Its chief advantage is that it can give a truly three-dimensional image of the heart. In addition, there is no radiation exposure and no need of contrast injection which may be of concern to the patient's renal function. The disadvantages of this technique are:

- the patient is required to remain still for a prolonged time;

- it cannot be performed at the bedside;
- it is contraindicated in patients who have metallic implants in the region of the heart, e.g. pacemakers;
- it has high cost; and
- experience with it is relatively limited.

It has been claimed that m-mode echocardiography overestimates left ventricular mass in comparison with MRI [21], although this has been disputed [22,23].

Biochemical markers

The human heart has the characteristics of an endocrine organ, in that it secretes atrial natriuretic peptide (ANP) and brain natriuretic peptide (BNP) [24,25]. These cardiac hormones have diuretic, natriuretic, and vasodilator actions; ANP is mainly secreted from the atria, and BNP from the ventricles [26]. The plasma levels of these hormones have been reported to be increased in various pathological conditions including acute myocardial infarction, heart failure, and renal disease [26]. In patients with hypertension defined by the office blood pressure, the plasma levels of ANP and BNP have been reported to be increased mildly compared with those in normotensive subjects, and those levels were more correlated with 24-hour ambulatory blood pressure levels than office blood pressure[27–29]. However, in hypertensive patients, BNP levels are correlated positively with left ventricular mass [27]. In addition, its BNP concentration also reflects left ventricular geometry [28], and highest levels are found in the presence of concentric hypertrophy. BNP levels also reflect the left ventricular end-diastolic pressure, and when antihypertensive successfully decreases systemic blood pressure level, BNP levels decrease before the left ventricular mass decreases.

The brain

The most precise technique for detecting chronic cerebral ischemic lesions is brain MRI, although brain computed tomography (CT) can detect cerebral hemorrhage better than MRI [30]. Recently, following advances in these non-invasive techniques, several studies have detected silent cerebral disease in asymptomatic hypertensive patients.

Brain MRI

Brain MRI can detect the following disease subtypes of hypertensive cerebrovascular lesions which may be associated with future clinical disease: (1) cerebral infarction (usually lacunar infarction), and (2) advanced deep white matter T2-weighted high-intensity lesions. Silent lacunar infarction can be detected by brain MRI in approximately 30–50% of asymptomatic elderly hypertensives (Figure 5.3.4) [31,32]. A recent prospective study disclosed that silent lacunar infarction is a strong predictor of clinically overt stroke (approximately ten times higher incidence of stroke compared with those without silent lesions) (Figure 5.3.5) [13,14,33]. A lacunar infarct is defined as a low signal intensity area

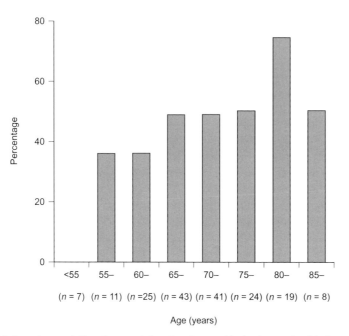

Fig. 5.3.4 Prevalence of silent lacunar infarction detected by brain MRI in elderly hypertensive patients.

(less than 1 cm) seen on a T1-weighted image which is also visible as a hyperintense lesion on a T2-weighted image (Figure 5.3.6). The lacunae as defined may include lesions other than true infarcts, such as enlargement of periventricular (Virchow–Robin) spaces, especially when their size is small (i.e. less than 5 mm). The FLAIR (fluid attenuated inversion recovery) technique may be helpful for distinguishing lacunar infarcts from enlargement of the periventricular spaces. Figure 5.3.7 shows the degree of periventricular hyperintensity (PVH) depicted on T2-weighted images (without T1-weighted low-intense lesion, which is classified into four grades) [32].

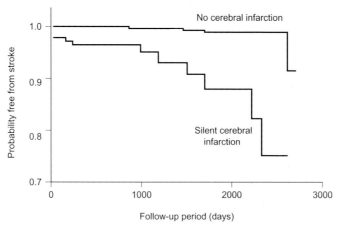

Fig. 5.3.5 Prognosis of silent cerebral infarction (adapted from [33]).

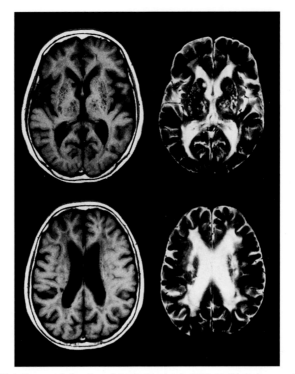

Fig. 5.3.6 Multiple lacunar infarction detected by brain MRI. Multiple lacunar infarcts defined as low signal intensity areas (less than 1 cm) on T1-weighted images (left) also visible as hyperintense lesion on T2-weighted (right) are detected in basal ganglia (upper) and deep white matter (lower).

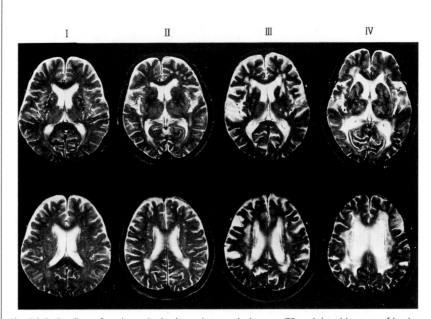

Fig. 5.3.7 Grading of periventricular hyperintense lesions on T2-weighted images of brain MRI. Grade III or IV lesions are considered as advanced deep white matter lesions corresponding to pathological significance.

BOX 5.3.2 Periventricular hyperintensity

- Grade I PVH is defined as no abnormality or minimal periventricular signal hyperintensities in the form of caps confined exclusively to the anterior horns or rims lining the ventricle.
- Grade II is defined as caps in both the anterior and posterior horns of the lateral ventricles, or periventricular unifocal patches.
- Grade III is defined as multiple periventricular hyperintense punctate lesions and their early confluent stages.
- Grade IV is defined as multiple areas of high signal intensity that reach confluency in the periventricular region.

The PVH of grade III or IV is considered to be advanced deep white matter lesions of pathological significance. The pathology of these T2-weighted high-intensity lesions is recognized as infarcts, enlarged periventricular space, gliosis, and demyelination. Some researchers consider that such lesions are associated with impairment of cognitive function and depression in the elderly. The dementia showing the most advanced lesions (grade IV) in Figure 5.3.7 is called Binswanger type of dementia, one subtype of vascular dementia. These advanced T2-weighted high-intensity lesions can also be detected in hypertensive encephalopathy.

The major determinants of silent lacunar infarction are aging and hypertension. A high level of ambulatory blood pressure may be the most important determinant of silent lacunar infarction, for patients with sustained hypertension have more advanced silent cerebral infarction and deep white matter T2-weighted high-intensity lesions than those with white coat hypertension (as well as more of other types of target organ damage such as LVH detected by ECG and microalbuminuria) (Table 5.3.3) [32]. In addition, not only blood pressure levels per se but also an abnormal diurnal blood pressure

Table 5.3.3 Silent target organ damage in white coat hypertension and sustained hypertension

Parameter	White coat hypertension (n = 31)	Sutained hypertension (n = 100)
Lacunar infarct (*n*/person)	0.58 (0.13–1.0)	2.0 (1.5–2.5)**
Lacunar infarction (%)	26	52*
Advance DWM (%)	19	34
ECG-LVH (%)	16	32
UAE (g/min)	13 (10–18)	23 (19–27)**
Microalbuminuria (%)	26	66***

Prevalence (percentage) are shown except lacunar (*n*/person) and UAE, which are expressed as the mean (95% confidence interval). *$P < 0.02$, **$P < 0.01$, ***$P < 0.001$. Advanced DWM = advanced deep white matter hyperintense lesion on T2-weighted images by magnetic resonance imaging; ECG-LVH = left ventricular hypertrophy diagnosed by electrocardiography; UAE = urinary albumin excretion rate. White coat hypertension is defined as those with mean 24-hour systolic blood pressure/24-hour diastolic blood pressure <135/80 mmHg and sustained hypertension, mean 24-hour systolic blood pressure ≥135 mmHg and/or 24-hour diastolic blood pressure ≥80 mmHg.

pattern are related to silent lacunar infarction [32]. In elderly hypertensive patients non-dippers (with a diminished nocturnal blood pressure fall) and also extreme-dippers (with a marked nocturnal blood pressure fall) have more advanced silent cerebrovascular disease (both lacunar infarction and advanced deep white matter lesions) when compared with dippers, who have an appropriate nocturnal blood pressure fall. In addition, elderly hypertensives with abnormal diurnal blood pressure patterns are a high-risk group for stroke. To prevent a subsequent clinically manifest stroke in these patients with silent cerebrovascular disease, non-dippers might require stronger antihypertensive therapy throughout the day and night, while extreme dippers may require more careful therapy without an additional nocturnal blood pressure fall to avoid the markedly decreased cerebral blood flow.

The eye

The description of hypertensive retinopathy in the evaluation of the hypertensive patient is hallowed by time, but notoriously inaccurate. A series of attempts have been made in the past few years to make it more objective, and to detect the subtle changes that are present in the early stages of hypertension. The basis of these is the use of quantitative analysis of photographs taken with a fundal camera. A number of measures have been used, including assessment of the diameter of the arterioles and venules, the overall vascularity [34], the relative diameter of proximal and distal branches [35], and the angle of bifurcation of branch vessels [35,36]. While these measures have shown minor differences between normotensive and hypertensive subjects, the overlap is usually substantial. A more promising measure is the length: diameter ratio of the retinal arterioles, which in a preliminary report has been found to be twice as great in hypertensives as in normotensives [37]. This is calculated by examining between nine and twenty arterial microvascular segments and bifurcations, and measuring the length and diameter of each segment. While this procedure holds great promise, it will need to be automated if it is to be widely used.

The kidneys

Renal disease is at the same time one of the most important consequences and causes of hypertension, and a variety of tests are available for evaluating both factors. These are not, however, recommended for the routine work-up, and the only test that is currently suitable for this purpose is the detection of microalbuminuria.

Microalbuminuria

Microalbuminuria is most widely used to monitor subclinical diabetic nephropathy. However, in both non-diabetic and diabetic patients it is one of the predictors of both renal and cardiovascular prognosis. It is listed as an optional test in the JNC VI recommendations.

Microalbuminuria is defined as a urinary albumin excretion ratio of 20–200 µg/min (30–200 mg/liter) [38]. It is usually measured by radioimmunoassay from 24-hour urine collections, but more recently can be detected using a semiquantitative dipstick test [39].

Microalbuminuria is thought to reflect the glomerular capillary leak which is a consequence of endothelial cell dysfunction and increased intraglomerular pressure, both of which are partly determined by the systemic blood pressure level. Microalbuminuria is considered not only to be an early marker of non-specific kidney disease but also an indicator of increased systemic capillary permeability, because it can be detected in systemic inflammatory diseases such as acute pancreatitis and bacterial meningitis. The 24-hour ambulatory blood pressure level is more closely related to microalbuminuria than office casual blood pressure, thus white-coat hypertensive patients are less likely to have microalbuminuria than patients with sustained hypertension (Table 5.3.3). In a survey of 779 never-treated hypertensive patients ambulatory systolic pressure was the only predictor of microalbuminuria; clinic pressure was not related to it [40]. Microalbuminuria is also more common in non-dippers (with diminished nocturnal blood pressure fall) than in the normal dippers (Figure 5.3.8) [32]. Cerasola *et al.* [41] studied 383 hypertensive patients and found microalbuminuria in 30%; it was correlated both with ambulatory blood pressure levels and with creatinine clearance. There were also associations between microalbuminuria, left ventricular mass index, and retinopathy, indicating that it is a valid marker of target-organ damage. However, Agewall *et al.* found that it was more closely related to indices of the insulin resistance syndrome than to markers of target organ damage [42]. Microalbuminuria has been found to be an independent predictor

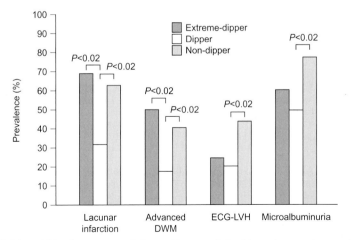

Fig. 5.3.8 Diurnal blood pressure variation patterns and silent target organ damage in elderly sustained hypertensive patients. Abnormal diurnal blood pressure variation patterns are extreme dippers with marked nocturnal blood pressure fall and non-dippers with diminished nocturnal blood pressure fall, compared with dippers with appropriate nocturnal blood pressure fall. Advanced DWM = advanced deep white matter T2 high intense lesion (graded as III and IV in Figure 5.3.7) detected by brain MRI.

of morbidity in the elderly [43], in hypertensive patients, and also to predict progression of renal disease [44].

Another interesting association of microalbuminuria is with race. In the Bogalusa Heart Study, microalbuminuria was more prevalent in young Blacks than in Whites, even after allowing for the higher blood pressures in the Blacks [45]. Blacks tend to have flatter diurnal profiles of blood pressure than whites, i.e. they are more likely to be non-dippers [46,47], and patients with microalbuminuria, whether diabetic or not, are also more likely to be non-dippers [48]. It is thus possible that the higher blood pressure during the night predisposes Blacks to renal damage, of which the first manifestation is microalbuminuria.

Hypertensive patients with microalbuminuria have increased plasma levels of endothelial cell-derived markers (von Willebrand factor and thrombomodulin) and activation markers of coagulation (activated factor VII and prothrombin fragment 1 + 2 (Table 5.3.4)). These levels in hypertensive patients with normoalbuminuria are not significantly different from those seen in normotensives, indicating that endothelial cell dysfunction and hypercoagulable state (which lead to cardiovascular disease) are detected in hypertensive patients only when accompanied by microalbuminuria [49]. On the other hand, these markers of endothelial cell dysfunction and hypercoagulability are found in normoalbuminuric diabetic patients and are augmented with the increase in the urinary albumin excretion ratio [50]. It has been postulated that insulin resistance may be one of the causal links between microalbumin and cardiovascular disease (Figure 5.3.9). The aggregations of these abnormalities may partly explain the linkage between microalbuminuria and cardiovascular disease in diabetic and non-diabetic subjects.

Table 5.3.4 Plasma levels of coagulation factor VII and endothelial cell-derived molecular markers in the sustained hypertensive patients with or without microalbuminuria and the normotensive controls

| Parameter | Normotensive (n = 25) | Sustained hypertensive patients | |
		Normoalbuminuria (UAE <15 mg/min) (n = 19)	Microalbuminuria (UAE=15–300 mg/ml) (n = 30)
Factor VIIa (ng/ml)	3.0 (2.6–3.3)	3.2 (2.8–3.7)	4.0 (3.6–4.4)**†
Factor VIIc (%)	115 (108–122)	116 (109–124)	117 (109–125)
Factor VIIag (%)	135 (122–149)	144 (129–160)	143 (130–156)
FVIIa : FVIIag ratio	1.04 (0.96–1.19)	1.07 (0.93–1.23)	1.33 (1.19–1.50)*†
Fibrinogen (mg/dl)	260 (241–280)	278 (235–303)	276 (247–304)
Von Willebrand factor (%)	144 (129–160)	163 (147–181)	188 (165–214)*
Thrombomodulin (ng/ml)	9.3 (8.5–10.3)	10.0 (8.6–11.5)	11.7 (10.3–13.3)*

The values are expressed as the mean (95% confidence interval). *$P < 0.01$, **$P < 0.001$, vs normotensive controls;
†$P < 0.05$ vs normoalbuminuric hypertensive group.
UAE = urinary albumin excretion ratio; factor VIIa = activated factor VII; factor VIIc = factor VII coagulant activity; Factor VIIag = factor VII antigen. For the calculation of the FVIIa: FVIIag ratio, the mean factor VIIa value of the healthy young subjects (2.1 ng/ml) was considered as 100%.

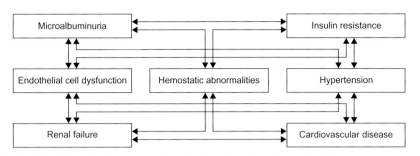

Fig. 5.3.9 Relationships between microalbuminuria and cardiovascular disease.

Treatment of hypertension reverses microalbuminuria [51], and there is some evidence, in both diabetics and non-diabetics [52], that ACE inhibitors may cause a greater reversal than other drugs.

Other biochemical markers

As listed in Table 5.3.5, other plasma proteins have been identified in normal urine. Excretion of all these lower molecular weight proteins is enhanced by any factors which increase the load filtered by the glomerulus, either by saturating tubular reabsorptive capacity, or simply as a result of increased tubular volume and flow rate. Thus, increased excretion rate of these proteins would result from any situation of increased renal blood flow and glomerular filtration rates and/or increased intraglomerular pressure and permeability.

The arteries

The arteries bear the brunt of the damage resulting from hypertension, and show major changes in their structure and function, which help to maintain the hypertension, but also set in motion the processes that lead to its adverse consequences. Routine evaluation of the arterial system in hypertensive patients is only now beginning to be incorporated into clinical practice, but is likely to play an increasingly important role, particularly as a result of the wider adoption of ultrasound techniques which permit direct visualization of the arteries for the first time. Nevertheless, another non-invasive method that has been available for

Table 5.3.5 Plasma proteins identified in normal subjects

Protein (mg/min)	Molecular weight (daltons)	Charge	Urinary excretion rate
Albumin	67 000	negative	0.1–15
β_2-microglobulin	21 000	neutral	0.01–0.3
IgG	160 000	neutral	1.0–1.7
Transferrin	90 000	neutral	0.1–0.5
α_1-microglobulin	30 000	neutral	1.0–5.0
α_1-acid glycoprotein	44 000	neutral	0.1–0.5
α_1-antitrypsin	45 000	neutral	0.1–0.5
Haptoglobin	85 000	negative	0.0–0.5
Ceruloplasmin	160 000	negative	0.01–0.05

5

many years, and which has not got the attention it deserves, is the ankle:
arm index. Magnetic resonance angiography can also evaluate arterial
stenoses non-invasively even in regions such as the intracranial carotid
artery and aorta where ultrasonographic visualization is incomplete.
However, it cannot assess the status of the intimal surface (irregularity,
thrombus attachment, etc.) or structural characteristics (such as
increased fatty component or calcification) of atherosclerotic lesions.
Arterial compliance is a functional measure of increasing relevance, and
is a major determinant of blood pressure changes associated with aging.
It can be assessed by ultrasonography, but also by techniques such as
the measurement of peripheral pulse wave velocity and the stroke
volume : pulse pressure ratio. Finally, the arteries are not merely passive
conduit vessels, but are also a physiologically active organ, and there is
a great potential for the identification of biochemical markers of vascular
damage to be incorporated into clinical practice.

The ankle:arm index (AAI)

The ankle:arm index (also called the ankle : brachial ratio) is one of the
few tests that can be performed in a physician's office, and the only
equipment that is required is a Doppler probe that can accurately detect
systolic pressure. It is particularly valuable in older patients. It is
measured while the patient is supine, and involves the measurement of
systolic pressure in the right brachial artery and the posterior tibial
arteries using a standard mercury sphygmomanometer and a Doppler
stethoscope. As a result of wave reflection, the systolic pressure is
normally higher at the ankle than in the forearm, but if there is
peripheral arterial disease it will be reduced. A ratio of less than 0.9 is
considered abnormal. Its importance lies in the fact that it may be
considered a marker of subclinical atherosclerosis. A low AAI has been
found to be an independent predictor of cardiovascular morbidity and
mortality in patients over the age of 65 [53]. Abnormalities are rare in
younger patients, so that it is less useful as a screening test for early
disease than as a specific test for more advanced disease. In the
Cardiovascular Heath Study, a community-based survey of elderly
people, it was found to have a sensitivity and specificity of 30% and 91%
for predicting cardiovascular mortality [53], which compares favorably
for the corresponding values for echo LVH of 43% and 70% [54].

Ultrasound evaluation of the arteries

Without doubt, ultrasonography is currently the optimal non-invasive
tool for evaluating the arterial system. Although it is not yet widely
used in clinical practice, vascular ultrasonography is recommended by
WHO-ISH whenever the presence of arterial disease is suspected in the
aorta, carotid, or peripheral arteries. Both structural and functional
changes can be detected. The former include the detection of
atherosclerotic lesions (distribution of plaques and degree of arterial
stenosis), and vascular hypertrophy (intima–media thickness, see Figure
5.3.10). The latter is exemplified by the measurement of arterial

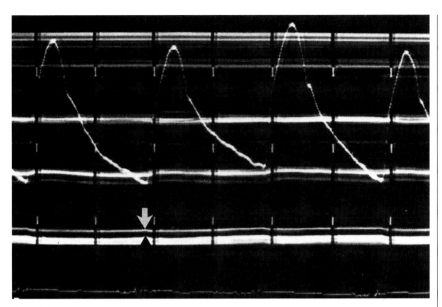

Fig. 5.3.10 M-mode tracing of common carotid artery with superimposed pressure
waveform. The intimal–medial thickness is indicated between the two arrows at end diastole
in a 71-year-old hypertensive man. Reproduced with permission from *Circulation* [74].

distensibility (derived when ultrasonography is combined with
measurement of pulse pressure). The most accessible and widely studied
vessels are the common carotid artery, the external carotid artery, and
the internal carotid artery within several centimeters of the carotid
bifurcation. The intracranial portion of the internal carotid artery cannot
be adequately visualized with this technique.

The most widely used non-invasive measure of atherosclerosis has
been the ultrasound estimate of intimal–media thickness (IMT) of the
carotid arteries. However, it has also been used as a measure of the
effects of hypertension on the arteries. In support of its use as a measure
of atherosclerosis, it has been shown that reduction of blood lipids with
fluvastatin causes a regression of IMT over a one-year period [55].
Since both atherosclerosis and hypertension increase the thickness of
the arterial wall, it probably reflects both processes. Thus the ARIC
study, a population survey of 15 587 men and women [56], found the
following odds ratios for IMT: smoking 3.9; hypertension 2.9; cholesterol
>240 mg/dl 2.9; HDL <35 mg/dl 1.7; triglycerides >170 1.7. In another
ARIC report, systolic hypertension was associated with subclinical
atherosclerosis in White men and women, Black women, but not Black
men [57]. In all groups there was a linear relationship between blood
pressure and IMT. In ARIC, the relation with diastolic pressure was
negative or J-shaped. This would be consistent with the concept that it is
the pulse pressure which is responsible for the vascular damage [57].
Whatever the relative contributions of atherosclerosis and hypertension
to IMT, it certainly has prognostic significance. Measures made at a
single point in time have been shown to predict myocardial infarction
[58], and more impressively, the progression of IMT over a two-year

5

period has also been shown to be predictive [59]. Hypertension has also been shown to predict the progression of atherosclerosis in a longitudinal study: 170 patients with renal artery stenosis were evaluated with duplex ultrasound scans over a three-year period [60]. The strongest predictor of progression was systolic pressure, which appeared to mediate the effects of age on progression.

Measures of arterial compliance

As well as delivering blood to the tissues of the body, the major arteries buffer the intermittent output of the heart to produce continuous flow. This capability is a function of the arterial compliance, which can be defined as the change in volume produced by a given change of pressure $(dV/V/dP)$. The accurate measurement of arterial volume is impractical, so surrogate measures such as the cross-sectional area of the artery are used. It is important to note that compliance is pressure-dependent, so that, ideally, measures of compliance should be normalized for pressure. While ultrasound is the most widely used method to measure it, other techniques include the measurement of pulse wave velocity and the stroke volume : pulse pressure ratio.

The changes of arterial compliance associated with hypertension vary according to the size of the artery. In the proximal conduit vessels, such as the carotid arteries, compliance is reduced. Compared with normotensive controls, mild hypertensives have the same arterial diameters but increased thickness, measured by ultrasound as the ratio of the intima–media thickness to lumen diameter [61]. These changes are paralleled by increases in left ventricular mass [62]. But in the radial artery compliance is increased in association with hypertension [63]. In contrast, arterial compliance and distensibility are reduced in both proximal and distal arteries in subjects with an elevated serum cholesterol or coronary heart disease. In subjects who are both hypercholesterolemic and hypertensive, the effects of cholesterol prevail, and compliance is reduced [63].

One of the simpler measures of overall arterial compliance is the stroke volume to pulse pressure (SV : PP) ratio. The former can be determined from echocardiography, and the latter from the conventional mercury sphygmomanometry. The SV : PP ratio decreases both with age and hypertension, and has been shown to be a predictor of cardiovascular risk independently of age and LVMI [64].

Arterial compliance is of particular relevance in isolated systolic hypertension, where it is generally thought to play a causal role [65]. Compliance is lower than in patients with diastolic hypertension, and is related to an increased left ventricular mass [66]. The greater pulse wave velocity that is observed in this condition has been held responsible for accelerated wave reflection, which results in a coincidence of the incident and reflected pressure wave, with a corresponding increase of systolic pressure and a reduction of diastolic pressure. It has been estimated that a 50% reduction of compliance results in an increase of 15% in systolic pressure and a 20% decrease in diastolic [67].

There is increasing recognition that pulse pressure may be the most important measure of blood pressure in the prediction of risk [68,69]. The two major determinants of pulse pressure are the peripheral resistance and the arterial compliance [70].

Biochemical markers

Table 5.3.6 shows some of the potential biochemical markers of target organ damage produced by the endothelium. Some are secreted from endothelial cells, and some are detectable in the blood. In hypertensive patients, increased plasma levels of von Willebrand factor (vWF), soluble forms of intercellular adhesion molecule (ICAM), vascular cell adhesion molecule (VCAM) and E-selectin have all been reported [71]. vWF levels were further increased in the extreme stress following an earthquake [72]. Further, one report disclosed that the soluble ICAM is a predictor of coronary artery disease in healthy men [73]. The plasma levels of these factors and their metabolites could be partly used to assess endothelial cell status (dysfunction or activation).

References

1. Anonymous. The Sixth Report of the Joint National Committee on Prevention, Detection, Evaluation, and Treatment of High Blood Pressure. *Arch Intern Med* 1997;**157**:2413–2446.
2. Anonymous. 1999 World Health Organization–International Society of Hypertension Guidelines for the Management of Hypertension. *J Hypertension* 1999;**17**:151–183.
3. Koren MJ, Devereux RB, Casale PN *et al*. Relation of left ventricular mass and geometry to morbidity and mortality in uncomplicated essential hypertension. *Ann Intern Med* 1991;**114**:345–352.
4. Levy D, Garrison RJ, Savage DD *et al*. Prognostic implications of echocardiographically determined left ventricular mass in the Framingham Heart Study [see comments]. *N Engl J Med* 1990;**322**:1561–1566.
5. Sokolow M, Lyon TP. The ventricular complex in left ventricular hypertrophy as obtained by unipolar precordial and limb leads. *Am Heart J* 1949;**37**:161–186.
6. Romhilt DW, Estes EH. *Am Heart J* 1968;**75**:752–759.
7. Casale PN, Devereux RB, Alonso DR *et al*. Improved sex-specific criteria of left ventricular hypertrophy for clinical and computer interpretation of electrocardiograms: validation with autopsy findings. *Circulation* 1987;**75**:565–572.
8. Schillaci G, Verdecchia P, Borgioni C *et al*. Improved electrocardiographic diagnosis of left ventricular hypertrophy. *Am J Cardiol* 1994;**74**:714–719.
9. Okin PM, Roman MJ, Devereux RB, Kligfield P. Time–voltage area of the QRS for the identification of left ventricular hypertrophy. *Hypertension* 1996;**27**:251–258.
10. Tomiyama H, Doba N, Fu Y *et al*. Left ventricular geometric patterns and QT dispersion in borderline and mild hypertension: their evolution and regression. *Am J Hypertension* 1998;**11**:286–292.
11. Kohno I, Takusagawa M, Yin D *et al*. QT dispersion in dipper- and nondipper-type hypertension. *Am J Hypertension* 1998;**11**:280–285.
12. Hedblad B, Janzon L. Hypertension and ST segment depression during ambulatory electrocardiographic recording. Results from the prospective population study 'men born in 1914' from Malmö, Sweden. *Hypertension* 1992;**20**:32–37.
13. Houghton JL, Carr AA, Prisant LM *et al*. Morphologic, hemodynamic and coronary perfusion characteristics in severe left ventricular hypertrophy secondary to systemic hypertension and evidence for nonatherosclerotic myocardial ischemia. *Am J Cardiol* 1992;**69**:219–224.

5

14. Yurenev AP, De Q, V, Dubov PB *et al*. Silent myocardial ischemia in patients with essential hypertension. *Am J Hypertension* 1992;**5**:169S–174S.

15. Devereux RB, Wallerson DC, de Simone G *et al*. Evaluation of left ventricular hypertrophy by M-mode echocardiography in patients and experimental animals. *Am J Card Imaging* 1994;**8**:291–304.

16. Devereux RB, Reichek N. Echocardiographic determination of left ventricular mass in man. Anatomic validation of the method. *Circulation* 1977;**55**:613–618.

17. Devereux RB, Roman MJ. Ultrasonic techniques for the evaluation of hypertension. *Curr Opin Nephrol Hypertension* 1994;**3**:644–651.

18. Gosse P, Jullien V, Jarnier P *et al*. Left ventricular filling in the hypertensive patient: long-term course and influence of treatment. *Clin Cardiol* 1999;**22**:472–476.

19. Palatini P, Visentin P, Mormino P *et al*. Structural abnormalities and not diastolic dysfunction are the earliest left ventricular changes in hypertension. HARVEST Study Group. *Am J Hypertension* 1998;**11**:147–154.

20. Bottini PB, Carr AA, Prisant LM *et al*. Magnetic resonance imaging compared to echocardiography to assess left ventricular mass in the hypertensive patient. *Am J Hypertension* 1995;**8**:221–228.

21. Missouris CG, Forbat SM, Singer DR *et al*. Echocardiography overestimates left ventricular mass: a comparative study with magnetic resonance imaging in patients with hypertension [see comments]. *J Hypertension* 1996;**14**:1005–1010.

22. Missouris CG, Underwood R, Forbat SM *et al*. Measurement of left ventricular mass in man [letter; comment]. *J Hypertension* 1998;**16**:257–258.

23. Devereux RB, Pini R, Aurigemma GP, Roman MJ. Measurement of left ventricular mass: methodology and expertise [editorial] [see comments]. *J Hypertension* 1997;**15**:801–809.

24. de Bold AJ. Atrial natriuretic factor: a hormone produced by the heart. *Science* 1985;**230**:767–770.

25. Sudoh T, Kangawa K, Minamino N, Matsuo H. A new natriuretic peptide in porcine brain. *Nature* 1988;**332**:78–81.

26. Bonow RO. New insights into the cardiac natriuretic peptides [editorial; comment]. *Circulation* 1996;**93**:1946–1950.

27. Kohno M, Horio T, Yokokawa K *et al*. Brain natriuretic peptide as a cardiac hormone in essential hypertension. *Am J Med* 1992;**92**:29–34.

28. Nishikimi T, Yoshihara F, Morimoto A *et al*. Relationship between left ventricular geometry and natriuretic peptide levels in essential hypertension. *Hypertension* 1996;**28**:22–30.

29. Kario K, Nishikimi T, Yoshihara F *et al*. Plasma levels of natriuretic peptides and adrenomedullin in elderly hypertensive patients: relationships to 24 h blood pressure. *J Hypertension* 1998;**16**:1253–1259.

30. Becker H. Imaging the aging brain. In: *Principles of Neural Aging* (eds Dani SU, Hori A, Walter GF), pp. 375–395. Elsevier: Amsterdam, 1997.

31. Kario K, Matsuo T, Kobayashi H *et al*. 'Silent' cerebral infarction is associated with hypercoagulability, endothelial cell damage, and high Lp(a) levels in elderly Japanese. *Arterioscler Thromb Vasc Biol* 1996;**16**:734–741.

32. Kario K, Matsuo T, Kobayashi H *et al*. Nocturnal fall of blood pressure and silent cerebrovascular damage in elderly hypertensive patients. Advanced silent cerebrovascular damage in extreme dippers. *Hypertension* 1996;**27**:130–135.

33. Kobayashi S, Okada K, Koide H *et al*. Subcortical silent brain infarction as a risk factor for clinical stroke. *Stroke* 1997;**28**:1932–1939.

34. Stanton AV, Mullaney P, Mee F *et al*. A method of quantifying retinal microvascular alterations associated with blood pressure and age. *J Hypertension* 1995;**13**:41–48.

35. Stanton AV, Wasan B, Cerutti A *et al*. Vascular network changes in the retina with age and hypertension. *J Hypertension* 1995;**13**:1724–1728.

36. Houben AJ, Canoy MC, Paling HA *et al*. Quantitative analysis of retinal vascular changes in essential and renovascular hypertension. *J Hypertension* 1995;**13**:1729–1733.

37. King LA, Stanton AV, Sever PS *et al*. Arteriolar length-diameter (L : D) ratio: a geometric parameter of the retinal vasculature diagnostic of hypertension. *J Hum Hypertension* 1996;**10**:417–418.

38. Pedrinelli R. Microalbuminuria in hypertension [editorial]. *Nephron* 1996;**73**:499–505.

39. Gerber LM, Johnston K, Alderman MH. Assessment of a new dipstick test in screening for microalbuminuria in patients with hypertension. *Am J Hypertension* 1998;**11**:1321–1327.

40. Palatini P, Graniero GR, Canali C *et al*. Relationship between albumin excretion rate, ambulatory blood pressure and left ventricular hypertrophy in mild hypertension. *J Hypertension* 1995;**13**:1796–1800.

41. Cerasola G, Cottone S, Mule G *et al*. Microalbuminuria, renal dysfunction and cardiovascular complication in essential hypertension. *J Hypertension* 1996;**14**:915–920.

42. Agewall S, Persson B, Samuelsson O *et al*. Microalbuminuria in treated hypertensive men at high risk of coronary disease. The Risk Factor Intervention Study Group. *J Hypertension* 1993;**11**:461–469.

43. Damsgaard EM, Froland A, Jorgensen OD, Mogensen CE. Microalbuminuria as predictor of increased mortality in elderly people. *Br Med J* 1990;**300**:297–300.

44. Bigazzi R, Bianchi S, Baldari D, Campese VM. Microalbuminuria predicts cardiovascular events and renal insufficiency in patients with essential hypertension. *J Hypertension* 1998;**16**:1325–1333.

45. Jiang X, Srinivasan SR, Radhakrishnamurthy B *et al*. Microalbuminuria in young adults related to blood pressure in a biracial (Black–White) population. The Bogalusa Heart Study. *Am J Hypertension* 1994;**7**:794–800.

46. Harshfield GA, Pulliam DA, Somes GW, Albert BS. Ambulatory blood pressure patterns in youth. *Am J Hypertension* 1993;**6**:968–973.

47. Yamasaki F, Schwartz JE, Gerber LM *et al*. Impact of shift work and race/ethnicity on the diurnal rhythm of blood pressure and catecholamines. *Hypertension* 1998;**32**:417–423.

48. Lindsay RS, Stewart MJ, Nairn IM *et al*. Reduced diurnal variation of blood pressure in non-insulin-dependent diabetic patients with microalbuminuria. *J Hum Hypertension* 1995;**9**:223–227.

49. Kario K, Matsuo T, Kobayashi H *et al*. Factor VII hyperactivity and endothelial cell damage are found in elderly hypertensives only when concomitant with microalbuminuria. *Arterioscler Thromb Vasc Biol* 1996;**16**:455–461.

50. Kario K, Matsuo T, Kobayashi H *et al*. Activation of tissue factor-induced coagulation and endothelial cell dysfunction in non-insulin-dependent diabetic patients with microalbuminuria. *Arterioscler Thromb Vasc Biol* 1995;**15**:1114–1120.

51. Agrawal B, Wolf K, Berger A, Luft FC. Effect of antihypertensive treatment on qualitative estimates of microalbuminuria. *J Hum Hypertension* 1996;**10**:551–555.

52. Alli C, Lombardo M, Zanni D *et al*. Albuminuria and transferrinuria in essential hypertension. Effects of antihypertensive therapy. *Am J Hypertension* 1996;**9**:1068–1076.

53. Newman AB, Shemanski L, Manolio TA *et al*. Ankle–arm index as a predictor of cardiovascular disease and mortality in the Cardiovascular Health Study. The Cardiovascular Health Study Group. *Arterioscler Thromb Vasc Biol* 1999;**19**:538–545.

54. Newman AB, Siscovick DS, Manolio TA *et al*. Ankle–arm index as a marker of atherosclerosis in the Cardiovascular Health Study. Cardiovascular Heart Study (CHS) Collaborative Research Group. *Circulation* 1993;**88**:837–845.

55. Forbat SM, Naoumova RP, Sidhu PS *et al*. The effect of cholesterol reduction with fluvastatin on aortic compliance, coronary calcification and carotid intimal–medial thickness: a pilot study. *J Cardiovasc Risk* 1998;**5**:1–10.

56. Heiss G, Sharrett AR, Barnes R *et al*. Carotid atherosclerosis measured by B-mode ultrasound in populations: associations with cardiovascular risk factors in the ARIC study. *Am J Epidemiol* 1991;**134**:250–256.

57. Arnett DK, Tyroler HA, Burke G *et al*. Hypertension and subclinical carotid artery atherosclerosis in Blacks and Whites. The Atherosclerosis Risk in Communities Study. ARIC Investigators [see comments]. *Arch Intern Med* 1996;**156**:1983–1989.

58. Salonen JT, Salonen R. Ultrasonographically assessed carotid morphology and the risk of coronary heart disease. *Arterioscler Thromb* 1991;**11**:1245–1249.

59. Hodis HN, Mack WJ, LA Bree L *et al*. The role of carotid arterial intima–media thickness in predicting clinical coronary events. *Ann Intern Med* 1998;**128**:262–269.

60. Caps MT, Perissinotto C, Zierler RE *et al*. Prospective study of atherosclerotic disease progression in the renal artery. *Circulation* 1998;**98**:2866–2872.

5

References

61. Gariepy J, Massonneau M, Levenson J *et al*. Evidence for *in vivo* carotid and femoral wall thickening in human hypertension. Groupe de Prévention Cardio-vasculaire en Médecine du Travail. *Hypertension* 1993;**22**:111–118.

62. Roman MJ, Pickering TG, Schwartz JE *et al*. Association of carotid atherosclerosis and left ventricular hypertrophy. *J Am Coll Cardiol* 1995;**25**:83–90.

63. Giannattasio C, Mangoni AA, Failla M *et al*. Combined effects of hypertension and hypercholesterolemia on radial artery function. *Hypertension* 1997;**29**:583–586.

64. de Simone G, Roman MJ, Koren MJ *et al*. Stroke volume/pulse pressure ratio and cardiovascular risk in arterial hypertension. *Hypertension* 1999;**33**:800–805.

65. Smulyan H, Vardan S, Griffiths A, Gribbin B. Forearm arterial distensibility in systolic hypertension. *J Am Coll Cardiol* 1984;**3**:387–393.

66. Dart A, Silagy C, Dewar E *et al*. Aortic distensibility and left ventricular structure and function in isolated systolic hypertension [see comments]. *Eur Heart J* 1993;**14**:1465–1470.

67. Glasser SP, Arnett DK, McVeigh GE *et al*. Vascular compliance and cardiovascular disease: a risk factor or a marker? *Am J Hypertens* 1997;**10**:1175–1189.

68. Benetos A, Safar M, Rudnichi A *et al*. Pulse pressure: a predictor of long-term cardiovascular mortality in a French male population. *Hypertension* 1997;**30**:1410–1415.

69. Madhavan S, Ooi WL, Cohen H, Alderman MH. Relation of pulse pressure and blood pressure reduction to the incidence of myocardial infarction [see comments]. *Hypertension* 1994;**23**:395–401.

70. Stergiopulos N, Westerhof N. Determinants of pulse pressure. *Hypertension* 1998;**32**:556–559.

71. Buemi M, Allegra A, Aloisi C *et al*. Cold pressor test raises serum concentrations of ICAM-1, VCAM-1, and E-selectin in normotensive and hypertensive patients. *Hypertension* 1997;**30**:845–847.

72. Kario K, Matsuo T, Kobayashi H *et al*. Earthquake-induced potentiation of acute risk factors in hypertensive elderly patients: possible triggering of cardiovascular events after a major earthquake. *J Am Coll Cardiol* 1997;**29**:926–933.

73. Ridker PM, Hennekens CH, Roitman-Johnson B *et al*. Plasma concentration of soluble intracellular adhesion molecule 1 and risks of future myocardial infarction in apparently healthy men. *Lancet* 1998;**351**:88–91.

74. Roman MJ, Saba PS, Pini R *et al*. Parallel cardiac and vascular adaptation in hypertension. *Circulation* 1992;**86**:1909–1918.

5

Section

6

Antihypertensive drugs

6

Chapter

6.1

Diuretics

K Paizis and PA Phillips

6

Classification and mechanism of action

Diuretics are classified into four groups according to their site of action in the kidney (Figure 6.1.1 and Table 6.1.1) All diuretics have a natriuretic action that leads to a decrease in body sodium and increase in sodium excretion [1]. The most potent diuretic action is seen with the loop diuretics, which remain effective in patients with impaired renal function. In contrast the diuretic effect of thiazides and indapamide is limited when the glomerular filtration rate (GFR) falls below 40 ml/min (creatinine >200 μmol) although metolazone is still active down to a GFR of 20 ml/min.

Table 6.1.1 Site of action of diuretics

Site of action	Diuretic
Proximal tubule	Carbonic anhydrase inhibitors
Thick ascending loop of Henle	Loop diuretics Frusemide, bumetanide, ethacrynic acid
Distal convoluted tubule	Thiazides, metolazone, indapamide
Collecting ducts	Potassium-sparing diuretics Triamterene, amiloride, spironolactone

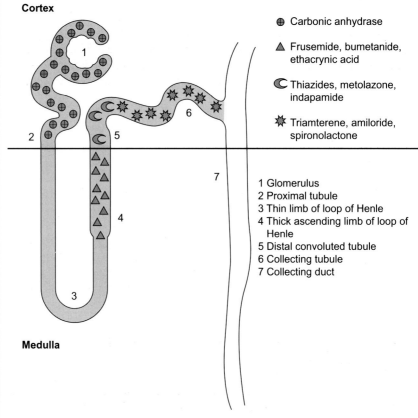

Fig. 6.1.1 Schematic representation of the site of action of diuretics in the nephron.

Antihypertensive action of diuretics

The precise mechanism by which diuretics – in particular thiazides – lower blood pressure is still controversial. The initial reduction in blood pressure appears to be related to natriuresis leading to a reduction in plasma volume and cardiac output. These effects are apparent in the first week, but as a result of compensatory mechanisms, in particular the renin–angiotensin–aldosterone pathway, the natriuretic effect is blunted. Long-term diuretic use is associated with a return of the initial hemodynamic changes towards the baseline level, but systemic vascular resistance remains low [2]. Diuretics have extrarenal antihypertensive activity that is most likely secondary to vasorelaxation and resultant decrease in peripheral vascular resistance. The proposed mechanisms of this action are (1) increase in synthesis of vasodilator prostaglandins and prostacyclines (not proven), (2) decrease vessel contractility due to a reduction in intracellular calcium in vascular smooth muscle cells, and (3) decrease in vascular reactivity to pressor stimuli (seen with indapamide).

When renal function is normal the thiazides and indapamide exhibit a greater antihypertensive effect than the more powerful loop diuretics [3]. This may be due to the short action of loop diuretics (less than 6 hours), but a more plausible explanation is one of calcium balance. Loop diuretics promote urinary calcium loss; slight reductions in plasma calcium have been shown to lead to elevated blood pressure levels [4]. It is possible, but not proven, that the antihypertensive effect of loop diuretics is ameliorated by this negative calcium balance. The situation is different in renal failure where hypertension is volume dependent and loop diuretics are important in maintaining optimal volume status.

Drugs and dosage

There is mounting evidence for *low-dose, combination therapy*. Low-dose diuretic therapy is safe and associated with significantly fewer side effects [5,6]. The dose–response relation for blood pressure is flat, whereas the risk of side effects both subjective and biochemical is dose-dependent. Treatment regimens using low-dose thiazides and related compounds have been shown to be effective in preventing strokes, coronary events, heart failure and renal failure in hypertensive groups. Combination therapy with angiotenson-converting enzyme inhibitors, beta-blockers and calcium-channel blockers is recommended when optimal control of blood pressure is not achieved [7]. It is advisable to avoid the use of diuretics where there is a significant problem of gout.

Mechanism of diuretic action in the kidney
Proximal tubule

The glomerular filtrate enters the proximal tubule; at this site, 60–65% of the total filtered sodium and water are reabsorbed. The uptake of sodium is an active process and as a result water and other filtered

Mechanism of diuretic
action in the kidney

Proximal tubule

Thick ascending loop of
Henle

Table 6.1.2 Drugs and dosages

Thiazides and related compounds	Minimum–maximum dosage/day	Frequency
Bendrofluazide	2.5–10 mg/day	Once daily
Chlorothiazide	250 mg1 gm	Once daily
Chlorthalidone	12.5–50 mg	Once daily
Hydrochlorothiazide	12.5–100 mg	Once daily
Indapamide	1.25–5 mg	Once daily
Metolazone	0.5–5 mg	Once daily
Loop diuretics		
Bumetanide	0.5–5 mg	Once or twice daily
Ethacrynic acid	25–200 mg	Once or twice daily
Frusemide	20–500 mg	Once or twice daily
Potassium-sparing diuretics		
Amiloride	5–10 mg	One to three times daily
Spironolactone	25–100 mg	Once or twice daily
Triamterene	50–150 mg	Once daily

solutes follow. At this site there is also secretion of hydrogen ions, organic anions and cations.

Carbonic anhydrase inhibitors inhibit the reabsorption of bicarbonate that is a requirement for sodium reabsorption in this segment. This results in a decrease in sodium absorption. The diuretic action of carbonic anhydrase inhibitors is minimal and is limited by (1) incomplete inhibition of the carbonic anhydrase enzyme and (2) distal tubule compensation.

Thick ascending loop of Henle

Between 40 and 50% of the filtrate that is not absorbed by the proximal tubule enters the loop of Henle. The majority of sodium in this filtrate is reabsorbed in the thick ascending loop of Henle. This structure is unique because it has the ability to absorb sodium, but is impermeable to water. Sodium absorption is an active process and entry into the tubular cells is via an electroneutral $Na^+–K^+–2Cl^-$ carrier found in the luminal membrane of the tubular cells. For sodium to be absorbed both potassium and chloride need to be present. The availability of chloride in the filtrate is usually the rate-limiting step in sodium absorption at this level. Absorption of sodium and the exclusion of water allow the development of a high interstitial osmolarity that gives rise to the countercurrent system. Absorption of calcium and magnesium also occur at this site.

Frusemide and bumetanide inhibit the action of the $Na^+–K^+–2Cl^-$ cotransporter; ethacrynic acid interferes with the metabolism of the cells of the thick ascending loop of Henle (Figure 6.1.2). Loop diuretics are powerful diuretics because the decrease in sodium absorption at this level results in increased delivery of sodium to the downstream nephron segments and more importantly a decrease in concentrating ability of the collecting tubules due to collapse of the countercurrent concentrating system.

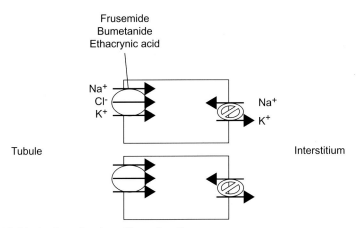

Fig. 6.1.2 Mechanism of action of loop diuretics.

Distal tubule

At this site, 5–10% of the filtered sodium is reabsorbed. There is little
reabsorption of water and the net effect is the production of very dilute
urine. The mechanism of sodium absorption is via Na^+–Cl^- cotransporter
found in the luminal membrane of these cells. Regulation of calcium
excretion also takes place at this site. Thiazides, indapamide and
metolazone inhibit the Na^+–Cl^- cotransporter thereby inhibiting
absorption of sodium and increasing sodium excretion (Figure 6.1.3).

Collecting tubule

At this site 5–7% of the filtered sodium and up to 20% of water is
reabsorbed. The tubular cells are unique in that sodium and water
absorption are two independent processes. Selective sodium channels

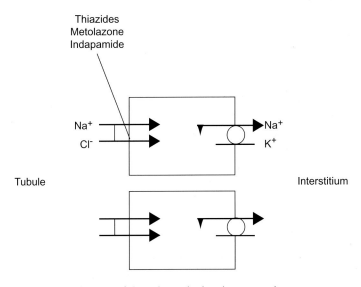

Fig. 6.1.3 Mechanism of action of thiazides and related compounds.

6

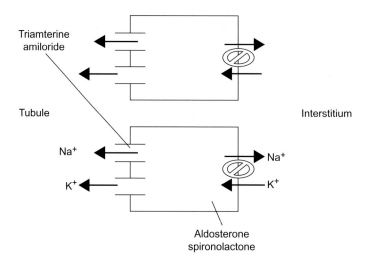

Fig. 6.1.4 Mechanism of action of potassium-sparing diuretics.

found in the luminal membrane allow sodium entry into the cells along an electrochemical gradient. Potassium is excreted in exchange for sodium to maintain this gradient. Aldosterone increases the number of sodium channels in the luminal membrane while atrial natriuretic peptide (ANP) closes these channels. Water absorption is via water channels that are also found in the luminal membrane, these are under the control of antidiuretic hormone (ADH). ADH increases the permeability of these cells to water giving rise to concentrated urine.

The potassium-sparing diuretics (spironolactone, triamterene and amiloride) exert their diuretic effect by closing sodium channels. Amiloride and triamterene have a direct effect on these channels, while spironolactone indirectly affects sodium transport by antagonizing the action of aldosterone (Figure 6.1.4).

Summary

Diuretics primarily act on one single nephron segment. This leads to changes to the composition of the filtrate that is delivered to the downstream nephron segments. The filtration process is complex and dynamic and has a great potential to cope with large fluctuations in concentration of solutes especially sodium, which has to be taken into account when considering the action of diuretics.

Adverse effects of diuretics (Table 6.1.3)

Specific side effects

Hypokalemia

This is commonly seen with the loop diuretics and to a lesser extent with thiazides and related compounds. Mild hypokalemia is well tolerated and not associated with increased risk of cardiac arrhythmias

Table 6.1.3 Adverse effects of diuretics

Carbonic anhydrase inhibitors
    Metabolic acidosis
Loop diuretics
  Fluid and electrolyte
    Volume depletion
    Hypernatremia (increased water loss)
    Hypokalemia
    Hypomagnesemia
    Hypocalcemia
  Metabolic
    Hyperuricemia
    Impaired glucose tolerance
    Hypercholesterolemia
    Hypertriglyceridemia
  Other
    Ototoxicity (high dose)
    Hypersensitivity
    Impotence
Thiazides, indapamide, metolazone
  Fluid and electrolyte
    Volume depletion (mild)
    Hyponatremia (sodium loss greater than water)
    Hypokalemia
    Hypercalcemia
    Hypomagnesemia
    Metabolic alkalosis
  Metabolic
    Hyperuricemia
    Impaired glucose tolerance
    Hypercholesterolemia
    Hypertriglyceridemia
  Other
    Impotence
    Nausea
    Constipation
Potassium-sparing diuretics
    Hyperkalemia – caution in elderly, renal failure,
    diabetics and when used in combination with ACE
    inhibitors, and non-steroidal anti-inflammatory drugs.
  Spironolactone
    Gynecomastia
    Mastodynia
    Decreased libido
    Menstrual irregularities

[8]. Depletion of total body potassium stores has been associated with decrease in glucose tolerance, hypercholesterolemia and may in fact increase the risk of hypertension and stroke [9]. Adequate potassium replacement is recommended during long-term diuretic use.

Hyperglycemia

Many studies have implicated long-term thiazide and related compound use with the development of hyperglycemia [10]. This effect is also seen with loop diuretics, but to a lesser degree. No effect on glucose metabolism has been observed with potassium-sparing diuretics. The effect was dose-dependent; bendrofluazide, 10 mg altered blood glucose significantly (7%) whereas a dose of 1.25 mg had no effect on blood glucose but reduced blood pressure to a similar degree as a higher dose. Several hypotheses have been put forward to explain this diuretic-induced glucose intolerance. These include (1) decreased pancreatic insulin secretion, (2) increased resistance to insulin peripherally, (3) increased insulin depletion in the prediabetic state, and (4) alteration of the enteropancreatic insulin axis. Although there is a theoretical increased risk of coronary heart disease as a result of these metabolic changes, several clinical trials have not borne this out especially when low doses are used. [11]

Hyperuricemia

This is a common complication of diuretic therapy with thiazides and related compound as well as loop diuretics. It has been estimated that ~75% of patients develop episodes of gout on diuretic therapy [12]. The mechanism by which diuretics lead to hyperuricemia include (1) competition between uric acid and diuretics for the same secreting pathway and (2) increased renal urate reabsorption due to plasma volume contraction.

Conclusion

Diuretics, in particular thiazides, indapamide and metolazone, are safe and effective in the management of hypertension in patients with normal renal function. There is no place for the use of high-dose diuretics in this population because of the increased incidence of adverse effects in particular hyperglycemia, hyperlipidemia, and gout. If blood pressure control is not achieved then it is best to combine the use of diuretics with other antihypertensive agents.

References

1. Johnston CI. The place of diuretics in the treatment of hypertension in 1993: can we do better? *Clin Exp Hypertension* 1993;**15**:1239–1255.
2. Shah S, Khatri I, Freis ED. Mechanism of antihypertensive effect of thiazide diuretics. *Am Heart J* 1978;**95**:611.
3. Ram CV, Garrett BN, Kaplan NM. Moderate sodium restriction and various diuretics in the treatment of hypertension. Effects on potassium wastage and blood pressure control. *Arch Int Med* 1981;**141**:1015.
4. Cutler JA, Brittain E. Calcium and blood pressure. An epidemiologic perspective. *Am J Hypertension* 1990;**3**(Pt2):137S.
5. Weir MR, Flack JM, Applegate WB. Tolerability, safety, and quality of life and hypertensive therapy: the case for low-dose diuretics. *Am J Med* 1996;**30**;101(3A):83S–92S.
6. Neutel JM. Metabolic manifestations of low-dose diuretics. *Am J Med* 1996;**30**;101(3A):71S–82S.
7. Plat F, Saini R. Management of hypertension: the role of combination therapy. *Am J Hypertension* 1997;**10**(Pt2):262S–271S.
8. Psaty BM, Heckbert SR, Koepsell TD *et al*. The risk of myocardial infarction associated with antihypertensive drug therapies. *J Am Med Ass* 1995;**274**:620–625.
9. Kaplan NM, Carnegie A, Raskin P *et al*. Potassium supplementation in hypertensive patients with diuretic-induced hypokalemia. *N Engl J Med* 1985;**312**:746–749.

6

10. Ramsay LE, Yeo WW, Jackson PR. Diabetes, impaired glucose tolerance and insulin resistance with diuretics. *Eur Heart J* 1992;**13**(Suppl G):68–71.
11. Collins R, Peto R, MacMahon S. Blood pressure, stroke and coronary heart disease. Short-term reduction in blood pressure. Overview of randomised trials in their epidemiological context. *Lancet* 1990;**335**:827–838.
12. Scott JT. Drug-induced gout. *Baillière's Clin Rheumatol* 1991;**5**:39–60.

References

6

Chapter

6.2

Beta blockade in hypertension

BNC Prichard and JM Cruickshank

6

Introduction

The first reports of the use of beta-blockers in hypertension was in 1964. Initially there was considerable resistance to their use as there was a reluctance to using drugs for hypertension that led to a fall in cardiac output and a rise in peripheral resistance and whose mode of action was not understood. Additionally, there was concern about the membrane-stabilizing (local anesthetic) effect of the then available beta-blocker, propranolol, although action has been subsequently found to be irrelevant [1,2].

Adrenergic receptors

The adrenergic receptors consist of two broad categories designated alpha and beta. The actions of epinephrine (adrenaline) at the alpha-receptors include vasoconstriction, and at the beta site, cardiac stimulation. The alpha-receptors have been divided into α_1- and α_2-receptors and they in turn can be further divided into subtypes. The beta-receptors consist of three discrete subtypes: β_1, β_2 and β_3 (Table 6.2.1).

Table 6.2.1 Distribution and responses mediated by adrenoceptors

Organ	Predominant receptor	Mediator of action	Physiological effect
Myocardium	$\beta_1 > \beta_2$	Cyclic AMP ↑	Stimulation of contractility and heart rate
Blood vessel smooth muscle	α_1	Ca^{2+} ↑	Vasoconstriction
	α_2	Cyclic AMP ↓	Vasoconstriction
	β_1	–	Vasodilatation coronary vessels
	β_2	Cyclic AMP ↑	Vasodilatation
Kidney	β_1	Cyclic AMP ↑	Renin release
Sympathetic terminals	α_2	Cyclic AMP ↓	Inhibition of norepirephrine release
	β_2	Cyclic AMP ↑	Stimulation of norepinephrine release
CNS	β_1/β_2 (ratio varies)	–	? Raise blood pressure
	α_2	–	Lower blood pressure
Eye	β_2	Cyclic AMP ↑	Increase intraocular pressure
Smooth muscle of bronchi	β_2	Cyclic AMP ↑	Bronchodilatation
Genitourinary tract smooth muscle	α_1	Ca^{2+} ↑	Muscle contraction
	β_2	Cyclic AMP ↑	Muscle relaxation
Fat tissue	α_2	Cyclic AMP ↓	Inhibition of lipolysis
	$\beta_2 > \beta_1$ (2:1)	Cyclic AMP ↑	Stimulation of lipolysis
Platelets	α_2	Cyclic AMP ↓	Aggregation
Liver	α_2	Ca^{2+} ↑	Glycogenolysis
	β_2	Cyclic AMP ↑	Glycogenolysis
			Glucogenolysis
Pancreas	α_2	Cyclic AMP ↓	Inhibition of insulin release
	β_2	Cyclic AMP ↑	Stimulation of insulin release
Skeletal muscle	β_2	Cyclic AMP ↑	Glycogenolysis
			Tremor
			Stimulation Na$^+$ – K$^+$ pump hypokalemia
Red blood cells	$\beta_2 > \beta_1$ (2:1)	Cyclic AMP ↑	? Stimulation Na$^+$ – K$^+$ pump hypokalemia
Lymphocytes	β_2	Cyclic AMP ↑	? Modulate immune function

6

Classification of beta-blocking drugs

The receptor-occupancy properties of beta-adrenoceptor blocking drugs can be used as a basis for classification. Beta-blockers can be selective or not for the subtypes or they may have an additional vasodilator action. The term 'cardioselective' should now be avoided as it is now known that both β_1- and β_2-receptors exist in the heart. The presence or absence of some stimulatory effect at the beta-receptor, i.e. intrinsic sympathomimetic activity (ISA) or partial agonist (stimulant) activity is a further basis for division as is finally the presence or absence of a membrane-stabilizing activity (MSA) or local anesthetic action. Beta-blockers which have been developed with peripheral vasodilator properties can achieve this by several different mechanisms. This may be by α_1-blocking activity, e.g. labetalol or carvedilol; another mechanism is seen with nebivolol which is a β_1-selective agent which has a nitric oxide-dependent vasodilator action.

All known beta-blocking drugs are competitive antagonists (Table 6.2.2) [1].

Hemodynamic effect of beta-blockers

Beta-blocking drugs without ISA reduce heart rate even when sympathetic tone is low, such as at rest in the supine position. When sympathetic activity is high, such as during exercise, all beta-blockers reduce the exercising heart rate. The acute intravenous administration of propanolol was shown to reduce heart rate and cardiac output at rest, reflexly increase peripheral resistance while resting blood pressure was not initially affected. With oral administration, heart rate and cardiac output remain reduced but there is also a decline in peripheral resistance and blood pressure falls. The fall in heart rate and cardiac output for non-ISA drugs are similar whether they are non-selective or β_1-selective [3,4].

6

Table 6.2.2 Examples of non-selective and β_1-selective (cardioselective) beta-blockers with and without ISA

No ISA	With intrinsic sympathomimetic activity	Vasodilating/alpha-blocking properties
Non-selective		
Nadolol	Alprenalol†	Bucindolol
Propranolol†	Bopindolol†	Carvedilol
Sotalol	Bufuralol†	Labetalol†
Timolol	Carteolol†	
	Mepindolol†	
	Oxprenolol†	
	Penbutolol†	
	Pindolol	
β_1-selective		
Atenolol	Acebutolol†	Bevantolol
Betaxolol	Epanolol	Celiprolol
Bisoprolol	Esmolol	Nebivolol
Metoprolol†		

† Membrane activity.

319

6.2

Hemodynamic effect of
beta-blockers

Those beta-blocking drugs that have ISA, e.g. pindolol, reduce heart rate to a lesser extent than non-ISA drugs. Some have no effect on resting heart rate. At modest levels of exercise, heart rates may not be very different for both ISA and non-ISA drugs, while at high levels of exercise drugs with ISA give less of a reduction of exercise tachycardia. The increase in exercise heart rate remaining after full doses of non-ISA drug is a result of the withdrawal of vagal inhibition. The increase in heart rate may be similar with exercise with an ISA-possessing beta-blocker but the actual heart rate is higher, as the result of the modest sympathetic stimulus from the ISA of the beta-blocker, present throughout at rest and on exercise [3,5].

The alteration of cardiac output after the administration of beta-blocking drugs usually follows the change of heart rate. It can be shown that at low levels of sympathetic activity (e.g. rest), drugs that possess ISA induce less reduction in cardiac output. Rises in peripheral resistance are small and can even fall. The rise in the systolic blood pressure during dynamic exercise is reduced by beta blockade. [4,5,6]. The increase in blood pressure with isometric exercise is not greatly modified by beta-blocking drugs, although the final pressure reached may be less because of lower baseline values.

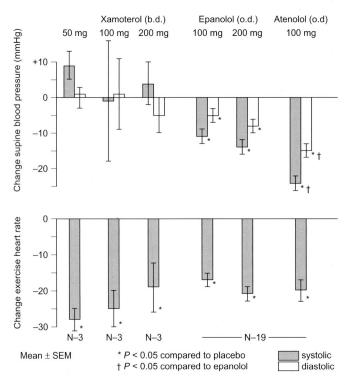

Fig. 6.2.1 Change in resting blood pressure and exercise heart rate compared to placebo from xamoterol for 5 days, epanolol for 15 days, and atenolol for 15 days. Measurements were made 2 hours post dose (after Leonetti et al [17]).

Many of the drugs that were used to treat hypertension before the introduction of propanolol interfered with the function of sympathetic nerves that elicited vasoconstriction mediated via alpha receptors. A postural fall in blood pressure not infrequently occurred with the use of adrenergic neuron inhibitory drugs, guanethidine and bethanidine and, to a lesser degree, the centrally acting inhibitor of vasoconstrictor tone methyldopa. A postural effect is unusual from beta-blockers as the vasoconstrictor mechanisms that are called into play from the effect of gravity in the erect posture are not inhibited, as vasoconstriction is mediated through alpha receptors [2,7].

Beta selectivity

When doses are given to result in equivalent inhibition of exercise tachycardia, far less antagonism of the cardiac effects of isoproterenol is seen with the β_1-selective drugs than with the non-selective agents with or without ISA. This is due to the presence of cardiac β_2-receptors in addition to β_1-receptors which are stimulated by isoproterenol in the right atrium (about 35%) and left ventricle (about 20%) while exercise tachycardia is mediated via β_1-receptors.

Airway resistance is less effected with β_1-blockade than with non-selective blockade, as would be expected from the predominance of β_2-bronchodilator receptors. This is the most important difference of the β_1-selective agents form the non-selective drugs. However, even the β_1-selective drugs must be regarded as hazardous in asthmatic subjects [8].

β_1-selectivity also confers important metabolic differences. They result in a lower increase in low-density lipoproteins (LDL) and a lower decrease in high-density lipoproteins (HDL) than non-selective agents. The β_1-selective agents, unlike non-selective drugs, do not appear to prolong the action of insulin or oral hypoglycemic drugs. Lastly, β_1-selective agents do not impair the metabolic changes in muscles that occur with exercise as much as non-selective beta-blocking drugs. This leads to better exercise tolerance with β_1-selective block compared to non-selective block [9] (see below).

Intrinsic sympathomimetic activity (ISA) or partial agonism

In patients with asthma, any beneficial β_2-stimulant action is more than offset by the blockade. Asthmatics are very susceptible to any receptor blockade, worsening their asthma. There is evidence that drugs with ISA do not interfere as much in metabolic processes, notably lipid metabolism or the liver metabolism of other drugs [9]. Finally, when a beta-blocker with considerable ISA such as pindolol is abruptly stopped, there is no post-beta blockade sympathetic hypersensitivity (see below).

6

Combination of beta and alpha blockade or vasodilator activity

The first combined non-selective beta-blocker and alpha-receptor blocking drug was labetalol. Carvedilol is also a non-selective beta-blocker with alpha-blocking properties, somewhat less of the latter compared to its beta-blocking action than labetalol. Celiprolol has β_1-blocking properties and a vasodilator action which seems to arise from a combination of β_2-stimulation and direct vasodilation.

Pharmacokinetics

There are two broad groups of beta-blocking drugs in terms of pharmocokinetics: the lipid-soluble drugs that undergo extensive first-pass metabolism in the liver and readily penetrate the brain and the water-soluble drugs which have low brain penetration and are excreted unchanged in the urine.

Pindolol and bisoprolol have moderate lipid solubility, but only about 50% is metabolized in the liver, first-pass effects are therefore less important while 50% is excreted by the kidney unchanged.

Unlike in lipid-soluble drugs, the water-soluble drugs are excreted in the urine unchanged (e.g. atenolol and sotalol) or as active metabolites. Not surprisingly the excretion is reduced and half-life increased with renal insufficiency with urinary excreted drugs.

Mode of action

It is now over thirty-five years since the use of beta blockade in hypertension was first reported. However, it is still not clear how they lower the blood pressure, although it is clear that it is a function of β_1 blockade and the presence of partial agonistic effect in a β_1-selective agent reduces the blood pressure-lowering activity as discussed below (Figure 6.2.1). The presence of β_2 blockade does not add to the antihypertensive effect, as noted above. Whatever the actual mechanism it seems clear that the β_1-selective drugs lower the blood pressure to a greater degree than non-selective agents.

There have been a number of proposals to account for the antihypertensive effect of beta adrenergic blocking drugs.

- Most beta-blockers reduce cardiac output at rest except those with marked partial agonist activity, but all reduce cardiac output and heart rate on exercise.
- Baroreceptor resetting, secondary to attenuation of pressor stimuli from the reduction in cardiac activity consequent to beta blockade.
- An antirenin activity.
- A direct action on the CNS.
- The blocking of adrenergic neurons.
- An increase in vasodilator prostaglandin concentrations.

Prominent have been attempts to correlate the antihypertensive effects of beta-blockers with renin levels, best responses being obtained

6

in patients with high renin levels. There are difficulties with this and other explanations and the mode of action remains unclear. It is possible that the mechanism may not be the same in all patients, or with all the beta-blocking drugs [1,10].

Use of beta-blockers combined with other drugs

Diuretics

Beta-blockers have been used in combination with thiazide diuretics since the earliest studies and many fixed beta-blocker–diuretic combination preparations are now available. Low-dose diuretic (e.g. hydrochlorothiazide 6.25 mg) in combination with beta blockade is a particularly useful approach [11] (Table 6.2.3).

ACE inhibitors

As both act (at least in part) through the renin–angiotensin system, the combination of beta blockade and ACE inhibition has in general given modest results but some studies have reported a useful additional antihypertensive effect [1].

Calcium-channel blockers

The dihydropropyridine calcium antagonists, with their peripheral vasodilator action, combine well with the beta blockade, resulting in additive antihypertensive action. The vasodilator-induced side effects such as headache and flushing are frequently reduced by the addition of beta blockade. The combination is hazardous with intravenous administration and if they are used together orally verapamil (or diltiazem) with their cardioinhibitory actions, should be avoided with beta-blockers in patients with coexistent left ventricular dysfunction or atrioventricular nodal disease [1].

6

Table 6.2.3 Mean change ± standard error from baseline sitting blood pressure (mmHg) and response rate at weeks 3–4 ($n = 509$)

	Mean change (response rate)			
Blood pressure	**Placebo** ($n = 75$)	**Bisoprolol 5 mg** ($n = 151$)	**Bisoprolol 5 mg/ Hydrochlorothiazide 6.25 mg** ($n = 150$)	**Hydrochlorothiazide 25 mg** ($n = 133$)
Systolic blood pressure				
< 60 years	−3.2 ± 1.4	−9.6 ± 1.1	−14.8 ± 1.0	−8.3 ± 0.9
≥ 60 years	−2.3 ± 2.2	−10.6 ± 1.6	−17.8 ± 1.5	−13.1 ± 1.3
Diastolic blood pressure				
< 60 years	−3.9 ± 1.0 (27)	−10.1 ± 0.6 (66)	−12.1 ± 0.6 (69)	−7.3 ± 0.8 (37)
≥ 60 years	−4.1 ± 1.2 (26)	−11.3 ± 0.8 (70)	−13.4 ± 0.8 (81)	−10.5 ± 0.8 (63)

Reproduced from Frishman *et al.* with permission [11].

Alpha-blockers

Alpha-1 blocking drugs which also reduce peripheral resistance can be given in combination with a beta-blocker give an additional hypertensive effect. It is important however, to be cautious at the initiation of therapy as the 'first-dose' postural hypertension that has been reported with prazosin. In particular, may be increased by pre-administered beta blockade [1].

Other drugs

Other drugs such as peripheral vasodilators (hydralazine, minoxidil) or methyldopa can be usefully combined with beta-blocking drugs. The combination of beta blockade and clonidine should be avoided as there have been reports of an enhanced overshoot of blood pressure when clonidine has been abruptly stopped, even with a case of fatal cerebral hemorrhage [1].

Beta blockade and the control of hypertension

After a rather slow start, beta-blockers have now become widely accepted in the treatment of hypertension and recommended as first-line treatment. The reduction in blood pressure following beta blockade has usually been observed to be proportional to the initial blood pressure. Large absolute falls of blood pressure occur in those patients with high initial levels, as is seen with other antihypertensive drugs. A study employing ambulatory blood pressure measurement reported falls of blood pressure of 18/12 mmHg with atenolol 50 mg. Considerably larger falls may be seen in patients with severe hypertension. Control is maintained over a 24-hour period with a once daily administration of a long acting beta-blocker like atenolol or bisoprolol. Overall beta blockers are similar in efficacy to lower the blood pressure to other major classes of antihypertensive drugs [12–15].

Ancillary properties and the control of hypertension

There is now evidence to indicate that β_1-selective blockers possess slightly greater antihypertensive effect some 2–3 mmHg greater than non-selective agents, i.e. it appears that β_2 blockade detracts from the antihypertensive effect of β_1 blockade. Large clinical trials have demonstrated that the β_1-selective blockers, atenolol or acebutolol are similar in antihypertensive efficacy to examples form the major classes of hypertensive drugs [12–15] (Figure 6.2.2). Similarly, in a recent large survey of Veterans hypertension clinics the achieved blood pressure with beta-blockers was similar to other agents, with or without the co-administration of a diuretic [16].

Beta-2 partial agonist activity (PAA) mediated peripheral vasodilator effect will lead to a fall in peripheral resistance and would be expected to contribute to the antihypertensive action. However, a β_1-selective beta-blocker with partial agonist effect, this at the β_1-receptor, will result

Beta blockade in hypertension

Beta blockade and the
control of hypertension

Ancillary properties and
the control of
hypertension

Peripheral vasodilator
action

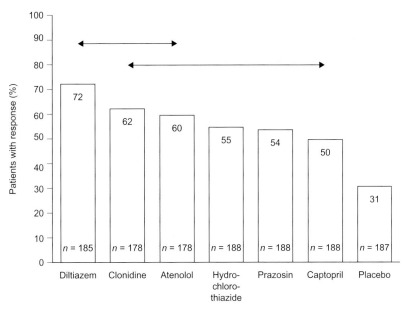

Fig. 6.2.2 A response was defined as a diastolic blood pressure of less than 90 mmHg at the end of the titration period and less than 95 mmHg at the end of one year of treatment. The horizontal arrows group drugs which were not significantly different from one another, but that were significantly different from the drugs not included under the arrow [12,13].

in less fall in cardiac output due to the partial β_1 cardiac stimulation, and there is no offsetting peripheral β_2 vasodilation giving a hypotensive influence. In one series of experiments it was found that the β_1 selective drug, atenolol, without PAA, lowered resting supine blood pressure by 24/15 mmHg, whereas epanolol, which is also β_1 selective but has PAA, lowered blood pressure by 14/8 mmHg while xamoterol, with a high degree of β_1 PAA did not show significant antihypertensive action [17] (Figure 6.2.1).

Pindolol possesses β_2-receptor partial agonist activity. This leads to a higher resting cardiac output mediated partly via cardiac β_2-receptors (a negative effect in the context of lowering blood pressure), and a reduction in peripheral resistance mediated by β_2-mediated peripheral vasodilator activity which helps to reduce blood pressure but also maintain cardiac output. The difference between β_1 and β_2 PAA was shown in an investigation where epanolol with its β_1 PAA which has shown to have considerably less antihypertensive effect than pindolol. The overall antihypertensive effect of pindolol is of the same order as the non-selective propranolol [18].

Peripheral vasodilator action

The first drug described with beta-blocking properties and also additional alpha-blocking action was labetalol. Carvedilol also has alpha-blocking activity, although less than labetalol in relation to its beta-blocking activity [19]. Carvedilol has been shown to have similar antihypertensive efficacy to propranolol, atenolol, metoprolol and enalapril. Celiprolol possesses β_1-blocking activity with β_2-mediated PAA. Its antihypertensive activity is also similar to other beta-blockers.

Effect of age

It has been perceived in the past that the response in the elderly is less favorable from beta blockade, than with a diuretic, a view based on studies with non-selective beta-blockers. Several studies have found similar falls of blood pressure in elderly subjects from diuretics and β_1-selective beta-blocking drugs, Materson *et al.* [12,13] reported a parallel group study, where elderly (over 60 years) White patients responded satisfactorily to atenolol ($n = 56$) with 72.4% achieving a diastolic blood pressure of less than 90 mmHg at the end of dose titration and less than 95 mmHg after one year. The corresponding figures were 71.7% with diltiazem ($n = 52$) 68.3% with hydrochlorothiazide ($n = 52$) and 61.8% with captopril ($n = 55$). Younger Whites had 64.9% response rate with atenolol (Figure 6.2.3). However, in elderly Blacks there was reduced response rate with atenolol (Figure 6.2.4) (44.7%).

Effect of race

A number of studies in African Americans published between 1988 and 1993, have suggested that there is less fall of blood pressure with ACE inhibitors and beta-blockers compared to calcium-channel blockers and diuretics [20]. However, useful reductions in blood pressure can be seen with β_1-selective agents in some patients. In the large multidrug study of Materson *et al.*[12,13] Blacks under 60 had a 51% response rate to atenolol. This was second only to diltiazem in this age group. However, while 45% of atenolol patients responded in the over-60s Blacks, better responses were obtained with diltiazem 85%, hydrochlorothiazide 64%, clonidine 58% and prazosin 49% (Figure 6.2.4).

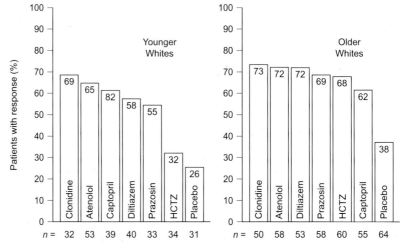

Fig. 6.2.3 A response was defined as a diastolic blood pressure of less than 90 mmHg at the end of the titration period and less than 95 mmHg at the end of one year of treatment [12,13].

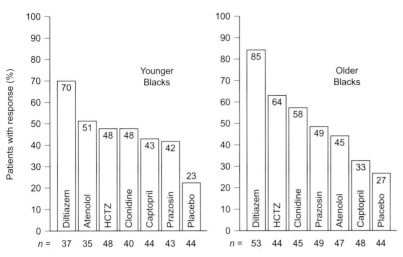

Fig. 6.2.4 A response was defined as a diastolic blood pressure of less than 90 mmHg at the end of the titration period and less than 95 mmHg at the end of one year of treatment [12,13].

Other investigations with the highly β_1-selective agent bisoprolol suggest that the difference in response between Black and non-Black patients may virtually disappear [11,21].

Hypertension in pregnancy

Beta blockade has been used to treat women with hypertension in the third trimester of pregnancy, with few adverse events [22]. The onset of maternal proteinuria is significantly less with the beta-blocker treatment. Although birthweights and placental weights tended to be slightly less in the atenolol group [22]. Because of this effect on birthweight, beta-blockers are generally avoided early in pregnancy, although the combined alpha- and beta-blocker labetalol is employed as an alternative to the usually preferred drug, methyldopa.

Coexistent disease

Recent evidence in important areas has led to a reappraisal of the use of beta-blockers in patients with certain coexistent diseases, some of which have previously been regarded as relative contraindications to the use of beta-blockers.

Ischemic heart disease

In a vast survey of postinfarction beta blockade usage in 201 752 patients, reported in the *New England Journal of Medicine* by Gottlieb and colleagues 1998 [23], it was found that survival benefit from beta blockade was seen regardless of systolic blood pressure, age, or ejection fraction. Perhaps most notably in patients who also had chronic obstructive pulmonary disease (COPD), which is commonly regarded as a contraindication to beta blockade, there was a reduction in the risk of death two years postinfarction with those who received a beta-blocker. Provided caution is

6

exercised, i.e. a β_1-selective agent is used, in low doses initially, and avoided in patients with a beta-responsive component to bronchodilators to their airways obstruction, beta-blockers can be used in COPD patients where there is a special indication for their use.

Heart failure

Heart failure has been regarded as an important contraindication to beta blockade. However, it has now been demonstrated that provided doses are very small and dose is titrated carefully beta blockade improves prognosis in patients with heart failure when added to a regimen including diuretics and ACE inhibitors. This was clearly shown with the combined non-selective agent with alpha-blocking action, carvedilol, but more recently also demonstrated with the β_1-selective agents, bisoprolol and metoprolol [24,25].

The coexistence of heart failure with hypertension should now be regarded as an indication for the use of beta blockade, although it would be recommended to first control the blood pressure by other means as has been our practice for many years. The large study of Gottlieb and colleagues [23] included postinfarction patients with reduced ejection fractions who benefitted from beta blockade and who had systolic blood pressures over 140 mmHg, although how many had both features is not indicated.

Diabetes mellitus

Diabetes mellitus in patients with hypertension has been considered as a relative contraindication for beta blockade (Table 6.2.4) [26]. However, a number of studies have reported that mortality and reinfarction rates in diabetic survivors of myocardial infarction also benefit from beta blockade at least to a similar degree as non-diabetics. The problems of risk of hypoglycemic reactions with beta-blockers seem to be more of a theoretical risk than real as with β_1-selective agents there is no unusual risk.

The UKPDS 38 study on middle-aged hypertensive type II diabetics in 1998 [27] compared tight control of the blood pressure with either atenolol or captopril aiming for less than 150/85 mmHg but achieving an average blood pressure of 144/82 mmHg ($n = 758$) with rather less

Table 6.2.4 Previous negative image of beta-blockers in diabetes

- A typical beta-blocker tends to increase triglyceride and lower HDL levels.
- A typical beta-blocker tends to increase fasting blood sugar, HbA1c and insulin resistance.
- A non-selective beta-blocker can prolong insulin-induced hypoglycemia and mask hypoglycemic signs.
- In the MRC Mild Hypertension study there was a trend to increase withdrawals on propranolol (versus placebo), due to impaired glucose tolerance.
- Beta-blockers cause patients to increase weight by 1–2 kg.
- In the postmyocardial infarction BHAT study, significantly more oral hypoglycemic agents were required in the propranolol, versus placebo, group.

Reproduced from Cruickshank with permission [26].

than tight control with other drugs aiming for less than 180/105 mmHg. The tight control group achieved an average blood pressure of 154/87 mmHg ($n = 390$) and a fall in deaths related to diabetes by 32% ($P = 0.019$), microvascular disease by 37% ($P = 0.0092$), stroke by 44% ($P = 0.013$), while any related diabetic related endpoint fell by 24% ($P = 0.0046$). All cause mortality and myocardial infarction showed a favorable, but non-significant, trend for tight control.

There was also a 50% reduction in the incidence of heart failure, in worsening retinopathy 34%, in loss of visual activity 47% and in the risk of urinary albumin excretion over 50 mg/liter of 29% (all with P values better than <0.01). A companion study, UKPDS 39 [28], found that tight control with atenolol 50 or 100 mg, i.e. 143/82 mmHg ($n = 358$) compared to captopril 25 or 50 mg b.d., i.e. 144/83 mmHg ($n = 400$) showed a non-significant trend in favor of atenolol in all the endpoints mentioned above. There was a higher glycated hemoglobin for the first four years with atenolol but not for the last five years. Notably incidence of hypoglycemic problems did not differ. Compliance was similar for the first four years but then it was 80% for captopril, 74% for atenolol in terms of patients years follow-up ($P = 0.0001$). Bronchospasm (6%) and claudication or cold feet (4%) on atenolol offset in some degree by cough (4%) on captopril appeared to be responsible for the compliance difference.

Left ventricular hypertrophy (LVH)

While left ventricular hypertrophy is compensatory to high blood pressure it is also an important indicator of poor prognosis. Some meta-analyses have suggested that ACE inhibitors have a greater effect in reversing LVH than other drugs. However in a study of treatment for at least a year, captopril, atenolol and hydrochlorothiazide reduced left ventricular mass unlike clonidine, diltiazem and prazosin which did not [29].

Primary prevention in hypertension

There have been indications from retrospective studies in hypertension that beta blockade reduces the incidence of fatal and non-fatal heart and cerebrovascular disease. There have been several prospective trials which have demonstrated that diuretics and beta-blockers reduce the development of complications of hypertension most clearly seen with stroke and heart failure, but less clear with beta blockade in coronary heart disease [30,31].

In a meta-analysis of four large studies, beta blockade significantly reduced the risk of stroke by 29% and the risk of the development of congestive heart failure by 42%. The reduction in coronary artery disease, cardiovascular and total mortality was not significant [30].

Some individual studies have shown a reduction in coronary events and mortality from beta blockade. The MRC study reported in 1985 [32] and 1988 [33] found a reduced incidence of myocardial infarction in non-smoking men with propranolol treatment. The MRC study and the IPPSH

6

study with oxprenolol were combined and analyzed by Wikstrand [34] and considered against diuretic therapy. There were 18% fewer total deaths, a reduction of 27% in fatal coronary disease, 28% less cardiovascular mortality and 21% less non-fatal infarction from beta blockade. The HAPPHY study reported by Wilhelmson *et al.* [35] comparing atenolol and metoprolol with a diuretic reported no difference in coronary artery disease and mortality while fatal strokes were less with beta blockade, smoking did not influence the difference. A 14-month extension of the study with these patients studied with metoprolol, described by Wikstrand and colleagues in 1988 (the MAPHY study) [36], reported a reduction in coronary mortality with metoprolol compared to diuretic over a five-year follow-up. This was most marked in smokers but also benefit was obtained in non-smokers. The difference in results of the HAPPHY Study and the MAPHY extension appeared to be due to the higher incidence of coronary mortality in the later study on diuretic treatment.

As discussed above, tight control of the blood pressure by beta-selective blockade with atenolol improves outcome in non-insulin-dependent diabetics, being at least as effective as ACE inhibition in preventing cardiovascular endpoints [27].

Primary prevention in the elderly

However, in the elderly there is evidence that diuretics may be superior to beta-blockers in primary prevention in hypertension for both coronary events and cardiovascular disease. This is based on the MRC trial in the elderly published in 1992 [37,38], in which patients treated with a diuretic showed a significant reduction in stroke and myocardial infarction, but beta blockade did not differ significantly from placebo.

BOX 6.2.1 Possible reasons for the beta-blocker/diuretic differences in young, middle-aged and elderly hypertensives

Younger, middle-aged hypertensives tend to have a high sympathetic drive, high plasma renin/angiotensin activity and relatively good arterial compliance. Such a background is not ideally suited to diuretic therapy (which tends to increase sympathetic activity and plasma renin/angiotensin levels). In contrast, beta-blockers, particularly β_1-selective agents, are suited to such an environment (they antagonize β_1 stimulatory activity and suppress plasma renin/angiotensin activity). This is particularly evident in hypertensive Type 2 diabetics (with high norepinephrine levels stemming from high plasma insulin concentration) where β_1-selective blockade is at least as effective as ACE inhibition.

Elderly hypertensives, in contrast, are essentially a low renin/low sympathetic activity group, with poor arterial compliance. Poor arterial compliance is associated with a more rapid reflected pulse wave velocity, giving rise to increased central systolic hypertension and left ventricular hypertrophy and diminished coronary filling during diastole. Such an environment is well suited to diuretics and unsuited to beta blockade. Diuretics, but not classic beta-blockers, improve arterial compliance and slow the velocity of the reflected wave, so as to reduce central systolic hypertension and supplement diastolic filling of the coronary arteries.

6

Adverse reactions [1]

Quality of life

It has been found that the non-selective propranolol has a less favorable effect on quality of life than captopril. However several studies with β_1-selective agents such as acebutolol, atenolol, and bisoprolol have indicated a similar effect on various measures of quality of life to ACE inhibitors [38,39,40] (Figure 6.2.5).

Bronchoconstriction

While it is potentially life threatening, provided patient selection is appropriate, bronchoconstriction is not usually a problem with beta blockade. A history of asthma should always be sought as its presence represent an absolute contraindication. While both non-selective and β_1-selective agents are contraindicated, the situation would be much worse if a non-selective agent, with or without partial agonist activity is used. Beta-2 blockade from a non-selective drug will more effectively block the action of β_2 stimulants such as salbutamol, while with a β_1-selective agent there is evidence that an increase in dosage of a β_2 stimulant will give clinically useful bronchodilatation.

Heart failure

Sympathetic stimulation represents an important compensatory mechanism to maintain cardiac output when ventricular function is poor. Blocking the cardiac sympathetic readily can precipitate acute heart failure. However, as discussed above, the careful introduction of small doses of the beta-blockers has now been shown to be valuable treatment for heart failure.

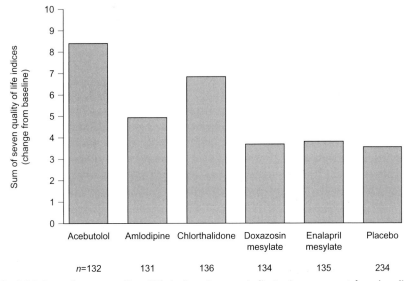

Fig. 6.2.5 Sum of seven quality of life indices. Increase indicates improvement from baseline [40].

Fatigue and lethargy

Fatigue and lethargy are the most frequent adverse reactions from β_1-selective and non-selective blockers. While inhibition of the increase in the cardiac output on exercise is important, impairment of exercise tolerance and training effect are also probably related to peripheral β_2 blockade that affects the muscle sodium–potassium pump and muscle metabolism. There is thus a low postexercise blood sugar and β_2 blockade also impairs muscle heat loss and sweating. This means that greater effect is seen with non-selective rather than β_1-selective agents.

CNS side effects

Placebo-controlled studies indicate that depression is not induced by beta blockade. Memory is not effected by beta blockade but that sleep disturbance, dreaming and hallucinations are more common with lipid-soluble beta-blockers.

Cardiovascular side effects

Primarily due to reflex vasoconstriction in response to a decreased cardiac output, cold peripheries are a common problem from both β_1-selective and non-selective beta-blockers. There may be less effect with β_1-selective agents as they do not block vasodilator β_2-receptors in arterial supply to muscles. Beta-blockers with moderate-to-high β_2 ISA or beta-blockers with peripheral vasodilator action also result in less reduction in peripheral flow.

Heart block, second or third degree, is very rare after oral beta-blockers in hypertensive patients. Asymptomatic sinus bradycardia is not unusual and is no reason to stop the beta-blocker but dosage can be reduced. Sometimes a very small dose may be sufficient to reduce heart rate. Hypertensive reactions have rarely been reported. Sotalol can cause proarrhythmias due to its Class III antiarrhythmic activity particularly at high dosage or in the presence of hypokalemia.

Impotence

Impotence on β_1-selective blockers appears similar to the incidence on placebo. The Treatment of Mild Hypertension Study (TOMHS) in 1997 [41] reported that the incidence of erectile problems on acebutolol was not different from placebo in up to four years of observation. Earlier studies with the non-selective lipid-soluble propranolol did find a greater incidence of impotence compared to placebo.

Gastrointestinal effects

Indigestion, nausea and diarrhea or constipation occasionally occur with beta-blockers, less commonly with β_1-selective agents. A weight gain of about 1 kg. may occur with beta blockade. Liver necrosis is a rare occurrence with labetalol and a few fatalities have occurred.

Metabolic effects

Lipids

Beta-blockers increase triglycerides and very low-density lipoproteins and lower high-density lipoprotein levels. The effect is greatest with non-selective agents, least with beta-blockers with ISA or high β_1 selectivity. Notwithstanding these unfavorable effects on lipid profile, non-selective agents like propranolol and timolol give significant reductions in mortality and reinfarction post-myocardial infarct and in animal models, the development of coronary atheroma is reduced.

Blood sugar and insulin

The non-selective beta-blockers, e.g. propranolol, to a greater degree than with β_1-selective agents, have been reported to impair glucose tolerance and increase blood sugar. Resting insulin levels tend to be unaffected but beta blockade reduces peripheral insulin sensitivity. The availability of glucose from liver and muscle is also influenced by β_2-receptors. Glycogenolysis is impaired, and β_2 blockade can result in hypoglycemia, e.g. with fasting or hemodialysis. Insulin-induced hypoglycemia may be prolonged by propranolol but not by β_1-receptor blocking drugs. Insulin-induced hypoglycemia is accompanied by increased epinephrine secretion; non-selective agents can induce a marked hypertensive response under such conditions, by inhibiting the β_2-dilator action of epinephrine leaving the alpha-constrictor action of epinephrine unopposed. Beta-1-selective agents do not effect glucose metabolism in a clinically important manner or induce a hypertensive response to insulin hypoglycemia. It appears that, in spite of any possible theoretical considerations, the β_1-selective agent atenolol is at least as beneficial in Type 2 diabetes as captopril (see above).

Serum potassium

A rise in serum potassium occurs from the non-selective beta-blockers but to a lesser degree from β_1-selective drugs. This is probably due to aldosterone suppression and inhibition of the predominantly β_2-linked Na^+–K^+ membrane transport in skeletal muscle with non-selective agents. Drugs which possess ISA have less effect.

Musculature

Beta-blockers which are non-selective and with moderate to high ISA, e.g. pindolol, can cause muscle cramps which is associated with raised serum creatine phosphokinase levels. Beta blockade has been reported to worsen myasthenia gravis and myotonia.

Skin rashes, hypersensitivity and folate reactions

In the MRC Mild Hypertension Study, skin rashes were more frequent in patients taking propranolol than diuretics, occasionally leading to

6

withdrawal. Beta-blockers have been reported to aggravate psoriasis. Very rarely skin necrosis occurs, mainly in the tips of the fingers. Scalp tingling is an occasional effect with labetalol. A hypersensitivity response to penicillin can occur, as well as to stings from bees, wasps, and ants; desensitization to pollens has been reported to be exacerbated. Deaths have occurred with patients taking a beta-blocker, a problem most likely to occur in patients with ectopy.

BOX 6.2.2 'Practolol' syndrome

A unique effect of practolol, a β_1-selective agent with ISA, was the 'practolol' or oculumucocutaneous syndrome. There was a psoriasiform rash with hyperkeratotic palms and soles, keratoconjunctivitis sicca and (more rarely) bilateral secretory otitis media. Sclerosing peritonitis causing bowel obstruction and occasional death, bilateral sclerosing pleuritis, and pericarditis were reported. The mechanism of this adverse reaction, which led to the drug being withdrawn from sale, remains unknown, although an immunological basis seems likely. Besides oculomucocutaneous syndrome, practolol caused positive serum ANF titres and LE cells with the occasional development of the lupus syndrome. This has been reported with acebutolol, and other beta-blockers have occasionally been implicated.

It has been suggested beta-blockers caused retroperitoneal fibrosis and Peyronie's disease. Larger series of patients, however, have eliminated a possible role of beta-blockers as a cause of these conditions.

Eyes

The β_2-receptors control tear secretion. Timolol eye drops cause dry eyes in about 10% of patients. This phenomenon can also occur after oral therapy. Probably as a result of a fall in intraocular pressure, blurred vision may result from beta-blockers.

BOX 6.2.3 Rebound after stopping beta-blockers

The administration of beta-blockers without ISA leads to beta-receptor upregulation. If beta-blockers are suddenly stopped these receptors are exposed to uninhibited catecholamines, thus palpitations and anxiety starting 12–72 hours after stopping the beta-blocker may occur and can last for several days. If a patient has ischemic heart disease, an increased incidence of myocardial ischemic events, including death, may occur in the few days following abrupt beta-blocker withdrawal. When possible, beta-blockers should be tailed off rather than stopped abruptly, with the final small dose given for two weeks before the drug is completely stopped. Alternatively, bed rest by reducing likelihood of sympathetic stimuli, will lessen the problem if beta blockade is suddenly stopped.

A beta-blocker which possesses moderate to high ISA, such as pindolol, is unlikely to exhibit rebound phenomenon as there is no upregulation of cardiac beta-receptors. In contrast, beta-receptors are downregulated by pindolol and a reduced catecholamine sensitivity is seen after pindolol is stopped [42].

Conclusions

The reason to treat hypertension is to prevent cardiovascular complications, i.e. myocardial infarction, sudden death, stroke and heart failure, as the condition itself is asymptomatic. A series of large, prospective, controlled studies have thrown a good deal of light upon the choice of antihypertensive agent. For middle-aged hypertensives, certainly men, the MRC Mild Hypertension study, the IPPPSH study and the MAPHY study suggest that benefit might best be obtained from beta-blockers, with β_1-selective blockers being preferable for smokers. The CAPP study [43] and HOT study [44] indicate that ACE inhibitors and calcium antagonists may be alternative choices for the middle-aged. Middle-aged hypertensives with Type 2 diabetes (UKPDS study) responded at least as well to β_1-selective blockade as ACE inhibition.

For the elderly, the SHEP study [45], the MRC Elderly study, the EWPHE study [46], the SYSTEUR study [47], the STOP study [48], the NORDIL study [49] and the INSIGHT study [50] indicate that low-dose diuretics ± a beta-blocker, calcium antagonists and ACE inhibitors are all effective agents, though meta-analyses [51,52] indicate that calcium antagonists may be less effective in preventing myocardial infarction and heart failure.

References

1. Cruickshank JM, Prichard BNC. *Beta-blockers in Clinical Practice*, 2nd edn, pp. 1204. Churchill Livingstone: London, 1994.
2. Gillam PMS, Prichard BNC. Discovery of the hypotensive effect of propranolol. *Postgrad Med J* 1976;**52** (Suppl. 4):70–75.
3. McDevitt DG, Brown CH, Carruthers SG, Shanks RG. Influence of intrinsic sympathomimetic activity and cardioselectivity on beta-adrenoceptor blockade. *Clin Pharmacol Ther* 1997;**21**:556–566.
4. Man in't Veld AJ, Schalekamp MA. How intrinsic sympathomimetic activity modulates the haemodynamic responses to beta-adrenoceptor antagonists. A clue to the nature of their antihypertensive mechanism. *Br J Clin Pharmacol* 1982;**13**(Suppl. 2):245S–257S.
5. Man in't Veld AJ, Schalekamp MA. Effects of 10 different beta-adrenoceptor antagonists on hemodynamics, plasma renin activity, and plasma norepinephrine in hypertension: the key role of vascular resistance changes in relation to partial agonist activity. *J Cardiovasc. Pharmacol* 1983;**5**:S30–S45.
6. Franz I-W, Behr U, Ketelhut R. Resting and exercise blood pressure with atenolol, enalapril and a low-dose combination. *J Hypertension* 1987;**5**(Suppl. 3):S37–S41.
7. Prichard BNC, Boakes AJ, Graham BR. A within-patient comparison of bethanidine, methyldopa and propanolol in the treatment of hypertension. *Clin Sci and Mol Med* 1976;**51**:567–570.
8. McDevitt DG. Pharmacologic aspects of cardioselectivity in a beta-blocking drug. *Am J Cardiol* 1987;**59**:10F–12F.
9. Kendall MJ. Impact of beta-1 selectivity and intrinsic sympathomimetic activity on potential unwanted noncardiovascular effects of beta blockers. *Am J Cardiol* 1987;**59**:44F–47F.
10. Prichard BNC, Owens CWI. β-adrenoceptor blocking drugs. In: *Handbook of Hypertension*, Vol. II. *Clinical Pharmacology of Antihypertensive Drugs*, (ed. Doyle AE; series eds Birkenhäger WH, Reid JL), pp. 187–243. Elsevier: Amsterdam, 1988.
11. Frishman WH, Burris JF, Mroczek WJ *et al*. First-line therapy option with low-dose bisoprolol fumarate and low-dose hydrochlorothiazide in patients with stage I and stage II systemic hypertension. *J Clin Pharmacol* 1995;**35**:182–188.

References

12. Materson BJ, Reda DJ, Cushman WC *et al*. Single-drug therapy for hypertension in men. A comparison of six antihypertensive agents with placebo. The Department of Veterans Affairs Cooperative Study Group on Antihypertensive Agents. *N Engl J Med* 1993;**328**(13):914–921.

13. Materson BJ, Reda DJ, Cushman WC *et al*. for the Department of Veterans Affairs Cooperative Study Group on Antihypertensive Agents. Department of Veteran Affairs Single-drug Therapy of Hypertension Study: revised figures and new data. *Am J Hypertension* 1995;**8**:189–192.

14. Philipp T, Anlauf M, Distler A *et al*. Randomised, double blind, multicentre comparison of hydrochlorothiazide, atenolol, nitrendipine, and enalapril in antihypertensive treatment: results of the HANE study. HANE Trial Research Group. *Br Med J* 1997;**315**:154–159.

15. Neaton JD, Grimm RH, Prineas RJ *et al*. for the Treatment of Mild Hypertension Study Research Group. Treatment of Mild Hypertension Study: final results. *J Am Med Ass* 1993;**270**:713–724.

16. Perry HM, Bingham S, Horney A *et al*. for the Department of Veterans Affairs Cooperative Study Group on Antihypertensive Agents. Antihypertensive efficacy of treatment regimens used in Veterans Administration hypertension clinics. *Hypertension* **31**:771–779.

17. Leonetti G, Sampieri L, Cuspidi C *et al*. Does β_1-selective agonist activity interfere with the antihypertensive efficacy of β_1-selective blocking Agents? *J Hypertension* 1985;**3**(Suppl. 3):s243–s245.

18. Floras JS, Jones JV, Hassan MO, Sleight P. Ambulatory blood pressure during once-daily randomized double-blind administration of atenolol, metoprolol, pindolol and slow release propranolol. *Br Med J* 1982;**285**:1387.

19. McTavish D, Campoli-Richards D, Sorkin EM. Carvedilol: A review of its Pharmacodynamic and pharmacokinetic properties, and therapeutic efficacy. *Drugs* 1993;**45**(2):232–258.

20. Jamerson K, DeQuattro V. The impact of ethnicity on response to antihypertensive therapy. *Am J Med* 1996;**101**(Suppl. 3A):22s–32s.

21. Frishman WH, Bryzinski BS, Coulson LR *et al*. A multifactorial trial design to assess combination therapy in hypertension. *Arch Intern Med* 1994;**154**:1461–1468.

22. Rubin PC, Butters L, Clark DM *et al*. Placebo-controlled trial of atenolol in treatment of pregnancy-associated hypertension. *Lancet* 1983;**i**:431–434.

23. Gottlieb SS, McCarter RJ, Vogel RA. Effect of beta-blockade on mortality among high-risk and low-risk patients after myocardial infarction. *N Engl J Med* 1998;**339**:489–497.

24. Lechat P, Packer M, Chalon S *et al*. Clinical effects of β-adrenergic blockade in chronic heart failure. A meta-analysis of double-blind, placebo-controlled, randomized trials. *Circulation* 1998;**98**:1184–1191.

25. CIBIS-II Investigators and Committees. The cardiac insufficiency bisoprolol study II (CIBIS-11): a randomised trial. *Lancet* 1999;**353**:9–13.

26. Cruickshank JM. Beta blockers continue to surprise us. *Eur Heart J* 2000;**21**:359–364.

27. UKPDS 38. Tight blood pressure control and risk of macrovascular and microvascular complications in Type 2 diabetes: UKPDS 38. UK Prospective Diabetes Study Group. *Br Med J* 1998;**317**:703–713.

28. UKPDS 39. Efficacy of atenolol and captopril in reducing risk of macrovascular and microvascular complications in Type 2 diabetes: UKPDS 39. UK Prospective Diabetes Study Group. *Br Med J* 1998;**317**:713–720.

29. Gottdiener JS, Reda DJ, Massie BM *et al*. Effect of single-drug therapy on reduction of left ventricular mass in mild to moderate hypertension: comparison of six antihypertensive agents. The Department of Veterans Affairs Cooperative Study Group on Antihypertensive Agents. *Circulation* 1997;**95**(8):2007–2014.

30. Psaty BM, Smith NL, Siscovick DS *et al*. Health outcomes associated with antihypertensive therapies used as first-line agents: a systematic review and meta-analysis. *J Am Med Ass* 1997;**277**:739–745.

31. Staesson JA, Wang JG, Birkenhäger WH, Fagard R. Treatment with beta-blockers for the primary prevention of the cardiovascular complications of hypertension. *Eur Heart J* 1999;**20**:11–25.

32. Medical Research Council Working Party. MRC trial of treatment of hypertension; principal results. *Br Med J* 1985;**291**:97–104.

33. Medical Research Council Working Party. Stroke and coronary heart disease in mild hypertension: risk factors and the value of treatment. *Br Med J* 1988;**296**:1565–1570.

34. Wikstrand J. Beta-blockers and cardioprotection – is there any good news from the recent trials? *J Clin Pharm Ther* 1987;**12**:347–350.

35. Wilhelmsen L, Berglund C, Elmfeldt D *et al*. Beta-blockers versus diuretics in hypertensive men: main results from the HAPPHY trial. *J Hypertension* 1987;**5**:561–572.

36. Wikstrand J, Warnold I, Olsson G *et al*. Primary prevention with metoprolol in patients with hypertension. Mortality results from the MAPHY study. *J Am Med Ass* 1988;**259**:1976–1982.

37. Messerli FH, Grossman E, Goldbourt U. Are β-blockers efficacious as first-line therapy for hypertension in the elderly? A systematic review. *J Am Med Ass* 1998;**279**:1903–1907.

38. Medical Research Council Working Party. MRC trial of treatment of hypertension in older adults: principal results. *Br Med J* 1992;**304**:405–412.

39. Weir MR, Bolli P, Prichard BNC, Weber MA. Bisoprolol. In: *Cardiovascular Drug Therapy* 2nd edn. (ed. Messerli FH), pp. 557–568. WB Saunders: Philadelphia PA, 1996.

40. Grimm RH Jr, Grandits GA, Cutler JA *et al*. Relationships of quality-of-life measures to long-term lifestyle and drug treatment in the Treatment of Mild Hypertension Study. *Arch Intern Med* 1997;**157**(6):638–648.

41. Grimm RH Jr, Grandits GA, Prineas RJ *et al*. Long-term effects on sexual function of five antihypertensive drugs and nutritional hygienic treatment in hypertensive men and women. Treatment of Mild Hypertension Study (TOMHS). *Hypertension* 1997;**29**(1 Pt 1):8–14.

42. Prichard BNC, Walden RJ, Tomlinson B, Liu J-B. The cardiovascular effect of withdrawal of beta-adrenoceptor blocking drugs. *Curr Opin Cardiol* 1988;**3**(Suppl. 2):s19–s29.

43. Hansson L, Lindholme LH, Niskanan *et al*. Effect of ACE-inhibition compared to conventional therapy on cardiovascular morbidity and mortality in hypertension: the Captopril Prevention Project (CAPP) randomised trial. *Lancet* 1999;**353**:611–616.

44. Hansson L, Zancetti A, Carruthers SG *et al*. Effects of intensive blood pressure lowering and low dose aspirin in patients with hypertension: principle results of the HOT randomised trial. *Lancet* 1998;**351**:1753–1762.

45. SHEP Cooperative Group. Prevention of stroke by antihypertensive drug treatment in older persons with isolated systolic hypertension. *JAMA* 1991;**265**:3255–3264.

46. Amery A, Birkenhager W, Briko P et al. Mortality and morbidity results from the European Working Party on High Blood Pressure in the Elderly trial. *Lancet* 1985;**I**:1359–1354.

47. Staessen JA, Fagard R, Thijs L. Randomised double-blind comparison of placebo and active treatment for old patients with isolated systolic hypertension. *Lancet* 1997;**350**:757–764.

48. Hansson L, Lindholm L, Ekbom T *et al*. Randomised trial of old and new antihypertensive drugs in elderly patients: cardiovascular mortality and morbidity in the Swedish Trial in Old Patients with Hypertension-2 study. *Lancet* 1999;**354**:1751–1756.

49. Hansson L, Hedner T, Lund-Johansen P *et al*. Randomised trial of effects of calcium antagonists compared with diuretics and beta-blockers on cardiovascular morbidity and mortality in hypertension: the Nordic Diltiazem (NORDIL) study. *Lancet* 2000;**356**:359–365.

50. Brown MJ, Palmer CR, Castainge A *et al*. Morbidity and mortality in patients randomised to double-blind treatment with long acting calcium-channel blocker or diuretic in the International Nifedipine GITS study: Intervention as a Goal in Hypertension Treatment (INSIGHT). *Lancet* 2000;**356**:366–372.

51. Pahor M, Psaty BM, Alderman MH et al. Health outcomes associated with calcium antagonists compared with other first line antihypertensive therapies: a meta-analysis of randomised controlled trials. *Lancet* 2000;**355**:1949–1954.

52. Blood Pressure Lowering Treatment Trialists' Collaboration. Effects of ACE inhibitors, calcium antagonists, and other blood pressure lowering drugs: results of prospectively designed overviews of randomised trials. *Lancet* 2000;**355**:1955–1964.

6

6.3

Calcium antagonists

PA Meredith

6

Introduction

When verapamil was first synthesized in 1962 it signaled the era of an important new class of drugs. Initially, it was thought that verapamil was a beta-adrenoceptor antagonist (beta-blocker) and it was not until the early 1970s that the true mechanism of action of this class of drugs was clearly established. Fleckenstein [1] and colleagues demonstrated that the negative inotropic effect on myocardial cells and the vasodilating properties in vascular smooth muscle were due to inhibition of calcium transport and, consequently, of the excitation–contraction coupling mechanism. This led to the term 'calcium antagonists' which characterizes the principal mode of action of these drugs. While verapamil itself was initially used for the treatment of angina pectoris and supraventricular arrhythmias, the range of calcium antagonist drugs comprises a heterogeneous group with wide applicability in the management of patients with a broad spectrum of cardiovascular and other disorders [2,3]. Calcium antagonists were described as one of the most important developments related to cardiovascular disease in the latter half of the twentieth century [4] and whilst this does not suggest that these drugs are a universal panacea, it does reflect the fundamental role of calcium ions as messengers in cardiovascular tissue and in the initiation of vascular smooth muscle and cardiac muscle contraction.

BOX 6.3.1 Calcium and calcium channels

Calcium has many critical effects in cellular communication and regulation [5]. For example, changes in intracellular calcium ion concentration are essential for the release of neurotransmitters and hormones, as well as for the cellular responses to these compounds and for cell division. In the cardiovascular system, increased intracellular calcium triggers the actin–myosin interaction and the subsequent contraction of the myocardium and vascular muscles. Calcium is also necessary for the pacemaker activity of sinus node cells and conduction through the atrioventricular node.
The concentration of intracellular calcium is controlled by three pathways involving different proteins located in the cell membrane [6]:

- The calcium–sodium exchange mechanism which transports one calcium ion out of the cell in exchange for three sodium ions.
- The ATP-dependent 'calcium pump' carries calcium out of the cell with the conversion of ATP to ADP. Both this process and the above one maintain a resting intracellular calcium concentration that is far lower than extracellular concentrations.
- Voltage-operated and receptor-operated channels which when open allow extracellular calcium to flow in to the cell. Receptor-operated channels are linked to pharmacological receptors via messengers, which include inositol, triphosphate or are integral components of pharmacological receptors. The voltage-operated channels form a large family of channel and belong to a 'super' family of voltage-gated ion channels, including those for sodium and potassium, which have many functional and structural properties in common. The voltage-operated calcium channels are of particular importance for the control of the cardiovascular system.

BOX 6.3.1 *Continued*

In recent years at least six different types of voltage-operated calcium channels have been identified in mammalian cells [6]. However, of these only the long-lasting L-type and the transient T-type channels contribute to the function of the cardiovascular system. The L- and T-type channels are present in the heart and vascular smooth muscle where they exhibit a differential distribution (Table 6.3.1). This differential distribution combined with the differing gating thresholds suggests that the L- and T-type channels have different physiological roles.

Table 6.3.1 The distribution of L- and T-type calcium channels in cardiovascular cells

Cell type	Primary role of calcium flux	T-type	L-type
Vascular smooth muscle cells	Smooth muscle contraction	+	++
Sinus node cells	Pacemaker function	+++	+
Myocardial cells	Heart contraction	+/−	+++

Classification

It is often considered that the development of an appropriate classification system might usefully serve as a guide to rational prescribing. Unfortunately, most classification systems have been created in a somewhat *ad hoc* fashion, usually to encompass the development of a new agent. At least eight different schemes have been proposed but three appear to have gained greatest credibility based upon their clinical applicability.

Structural classification

The most widely used classification is based upon the structural differences among the original prototype agents: diltiazem, nifedipine and verapamil. The listing in Table 6.3.2, which is not exhaustive, clearly demonstrates that the largest groups of calcium antagonists are the dihydropyridines, of which nifedipine is the prototype, while verapamil is a phenylalkylamine derivative and diltiazem is a benzothiazepine derivative. Mibefradil was the most recently developed prototype calcium antagonist and has been classified on the base of its structure as a tetralol derivative. Unlike all the other prototype calcium antagonists which are relatively selective L-type calcium channel blockers mibefradil was the first selective, but not specific, T-type channel blocker. Other drugs with calcium antagonist properties have different structures and a range of additional pharmacological properties but are not widely used in current clinical practice and as such will not be considered further in this chapter (Table 6.3.2).

Physicochemical classification

Physicochemical properties of calcium antagonists have been used as a criteria for classification (Table 6.3.3). This has resulted in somewhat

6

Table 6.3.2 Classification of calcium antagonists by structure

Dihydropyridines	Phenylalkyamines
Amlodipine Aranidipine Barnidipine Benidipine Cilnidipine Clevidipine Efonidipine Elgodipine Felodipine Isradipine Lacidipine Lemildipine Lercandipine Manidipine Nifedipine Niludipine Nimodipine Nisoldipine Nitrendipine Nivaldipine Pranidipine Ryosidine	Anipamil Gallopamil Riapamil Tiapamil Verapamil
	Benzothizepines Clentiazem Diltiazem
	Tetratol derivative Mibefradil
	Others Bepridil Cinnarizine Flunarizine Lidoflazine Perhexiline

Table 6.3.3 Physicochemical classification of calcium antagonists

Reference	Verapamil	Diltiazem	Dihydropyridines	Cinnarizine/ flunarizine
Glossman and Ferry [8]	II	III	1A	1B
Spedding [7]	B	B	A	C
Fleckenstein [1]	A	A	A	B

diverse classifications. The applicability of these is limited in a number of respects. Firstly, no account is made of tissue selectivity. Secondly, whilst classification according to receptor affinity highlights the potential pharmacodynamic differences among different agents, the approach is limited by the lack of definitive information regarding the molecular pharmacology of all the calcium antagonist binding sites.

Clinical pharmacological classification

Of all of the classification systems proposed perhaps the most clinically relevant and applicable are those based upon clinical pharmacological characteristics. The first proposal was based upon classifying calcium antagonists on the basis of their cardiac and peripheral activity [9]. Whilst this approach has its merits it has not been widely used and alternative more practical classification schemes have tended to be adopted. Of these perhaps the most practically useful was that of Toyo-Oka and Naylor [10] which was subsequently updated by Lüscher and Cosentino [11]. The classification scheme proposed three groups or 'generations' (Table 6.3.4) in which the focus is not only on the clinical effects of the drug as determined by receptor-binding properties, tissue cell activity and pharmacokinetic profiles. It is apparent from Table 6.3.4 that the original formulations of verapamil, diltiazem, nifedipine and mibefradil as prototypes are the first-generation drugs, whilst the second-generation agents include compounds developed with an

6

Table 6.3.4 Clinical pharmacological classification of calcium antagonists

| Group (tissue selectivity) | First generation | Second generation | | Third generation |
		Novel formulations (IIa)	New chemical entities (IIb)	
Dihydropyridine (artery > cardiac)	Nifedipine Nicardipine	Nifedipine SR/GITS Felodipine ER Nicardipine SR	Benidipine Nimodipine Isradipine Nisoldipine Manidipine Nitrendipine Nilvadipine	Amlodipine Lacidipine Lercanidipine
Benzothiazepine (artery = cardiac) Phenylalkylamine (artery ≤ cardiac) Phenylalkylamine/benzimidazolyl (artery > cardiac)	Diltiazem Verapamil Mibefradil	Diltiazem SR Verapamil SR Gallopamil		

improved pharmacokinetic profile and/or increased vascular selectivity. These agents are then further subdivided into slow-release formulations (IIa) and agents with novel chemical structure (IIb) The third-generation agents are exemplified by amlodipine and the lipophilic agents which are characterized by their intrinsically long duration of action and by slow onset and offset of hemodynamic effects.

Pharmacokinetics of calcium antagonists
Pharmacokinetics of the prototype agents

In contrast to their structural and pharmacological diversity, the galenic or instant-release formulations of the original prototype agents have remarkably similar characteristics. Diltiazem, nifedipine and verapamil are all highly cleared drugs which are subject to extensive first-pass hepatic metabolism [12] (Table 6.3.5). As a consequence of the extensive first-pass metabolism, the oral bioavailability of these compounds is comparatively low and in addition the apparent oral clearance is subject to wide inter- and intrapatient variability. All have comparatively short-term elimination half-lives and thus must be administered at least twice a day to achieve any consistency in their steady-state plasma concentration profiles. Mibefradil was not only chemically distinct from

Classification
Clinical pharmacological classification
Pharmacokinetics of calcium antagonists
Pharmacokinetics of the prototype agents

Table 6.3.5 Comparative pharmacokinetics of calcium antagonists

Parameter	Nifedipine	Verapamil	Diltiazem	Mibefradil	Felodipine	Isradipine	Nicardipine	Amlodipine	Nisoldipine	Lacidipine
Oral absorption (%)	>90	>90	>90	>90	>90	>90	>90	>90	>90	>90
Bio-availability (%)	30–60	10–30	30–60	70–90	10–25	20	35	60–65	5–15	5–15
Protein binding (%)	>90	>90	>90	>90	>90	>90	>90	>90	>90	>90
Elimination half-life (h)	3–5	3–7	3–6	17–30	2–8	6–9	3–8	35–50	4–10	3–15
Hepatic metabolism	+++	+++	+++	+++	+++	+++	+++	+++	+++	+++
Active metabolites	? Yes	Yes	Yes	No	No	No	No	No	No	No

343

the original prototype agents but the disposition characteristics were quite disparate. The oral bioavailability at steady state was high with an intrinsically long elimination half-life [13]. Unfortunately, mibefradil and one of its major metabolites were potent inhibitors of cytochrome P-450 3A4 and 2D6. This ultimately led to well-documented significant and clinically relevant drug interactions which resulted in the withdrawal of the drug from worldwide markets.

Pharmacokinetics of other calcium antagonists

The development of new calcium antagonists has largely focussed upon the synthesis of alternative dihydropyridine derivatives (Table 6.3.5). Whilst many of these agents share common pharmacokinetic characteristics with nifedipine, there are important differences within the class such that, for example, amlodipine has a relatively high oral bioavailability, slow absorption and prolong-term elimination half-life whilst in contrast lacidipine is subject to extensive presystemic hepatic metabolism, has low oral bioavailability and a relatively short-term elimination half-life. Lacidipine in common with other 'lipophilic' calcium antagonists such as lercanidipine and barnidipine, does have a high volume of distribution which has been attributed to a high membrane partition coefficient and a unique membrane-binding property which allows the agent to be administered once daily with sustained blood pressure control in the treatment of hypertension.

Modified release formulations

Many attempts have been made to prolong duration of action by sustaining circulating drug concentration profiles with the development of a wide range of modified pharmaceutical formulations. The success of this approach has been inconsistent and not all modified release formulations produce ideal steady-state plasma concentration profiles when administered once daily. However, two formulations are worthy of note. Firstly, the gastrointestinal therapeutic system (GITS) or osmotic pump formulation which has been utilized with nifedipine to produce plasma drug concentrations which are relatively smooth and consistent over a 24-hour period and secondly the controlled onset extended release (COER) formulation of verapamil which also utilizes an osmotic pump formulation but with further encapsulation designed to produce relatively low plasma drug concentrations during the night time period but sustained and consistent drug levels throughout the rest of the day.

BOX 6.3.2 Factors influencing the pharmacokinetics of calcium antagonists

Age

In general there is a tendency for increased plasma concentrations in the elderly which is attributed to a reduced rate of hepatic metabolism. Such findings are relatively consistent among calcium antagonists and independent of formulation, although increases in steady-state concentration in the elderly do not attain statistical significance in all studies.

BOX 6.3.2 *Continued*

Hepatic disease

The principal site of biotransformation for calcium antagonists is the liver and so hepatic disease results in a consistent pattern of reduced drug clearance higher drug concentrations in augmented pharmacodynamic response. Although detailed data exists for only some of the agent, it seems prudent to reduce the dose of all calcium antagonists in patients with advanced liver impairment.

Renal impairment

In contrast to the evidence relating to hepatic impairment, studies examining the effect of renal impairment on the disposition of calcium antagonists are less consistent and in part this is a direct reflection of the smaller number of studies performed. As a general rule, the disposition of most calcium antagonists does not appear to change to a clinically significant extent in patients with mild-to-moderate renal impairment and, on that basis, dosage adjustments are probably unnecessary.

Drug interactions

A number of studies have been performed with the aim of documenting potential drug interactions with calcium antagonists. It would seem prudent to focus on those which are either associated with other cardiovascular drugs or where a clinically relevant interaction is possible [14]. Perhaps the most notable interaction is that observed with digoxin which has been observed to a greater or lesser extent with all three of the prototype L-type calcium antagonists. Although the precise mechanism of this interaction is still a matter for discussion it is apparent that digoxin clearance, both renal and extrarenal, and the volume of distribution are decreased resulting in significant increases in plasma levels of digoxin. Pharmacokinetic interactions have also been documented between all of the prototype calcium antagonists and quinidine, this being most pronounced and of potential clinical relevance with verapamil and diltiazem. Significant kinetic interactions have also been reported for both diltiazem and verapamil when combined with propranolol. The antihypertensive consequences of combined alpha-blockade and calcium antagonism can be construed as being either particularly effective or potentially harmful. It has been suggested that this combination has an exaggerated first-dose response that places patients at risk for hypotension. In part, this may be associated with an interaction which is entirely pharmacodynamically mediated; however, a significant pharmacokinetic interaction between verapamil and prazosin has been well documented.

A number of interactions with calcium and non-cardiovascular drugs have been described, of these perhaps the interactions of greatest clinical interest and relevance are associated with the increased plasma levels of cyclosporine and theophylline when used in combination with the non-dihydropyridine calcium antagonists. Cimetidine appears to inhibit the metabolism of many of the available calcium antagonists resulting in an increase in circulating plasma levels of the drugs, a phenomenon which has also been documented for a number of dihydropyridine agents when they are ingested along with grapefruit juice, a known inhibitor of cytochrome P-450.

6

Concentration–effect relationships

The focus of development on calcium antagonists which have been reformulated to modify their plasma pharmacokinetics or agents with prolonged half-lives is a reflection of the direct relationship between the concentration–time profile and the elicited antihypertensive response for many of these compounds. Although some early studies with calcium antagonists failed to identify a clear relationship between plasma drug level and measured effects, more recently reports have repeatedly confirmed a close direct relationship between the two. This relationship is particularly apparent when individual patients are studied and when the measured response makes allowance for both placebo effects and circadian variability [13,15]. The concentration–effect relationships have been established for most calcium antagonists, and overall a considerable volume of evidence indicates that the antihypertensive effect (and other pharmacological responses) correlates directly with the concentration–time profile in terms of both magnitude and duration. However, it is clear that this principle is not universally applicable to all calcium antagonists, particularly the lipophilic agents which offer high tissue affinity. In this instance, it appears that these agents, despite having relatively short plasma elimination half-lives, do achieve consistent and sustained blood pressure control most likely due to their high lipophilicity and partitioning into the lipid bilayer of cell membranes and a consequent slow diffusion to the receptor-binding site[16].

Calcium antagonists in the management of hypertension

The antihypertensive effects of calcium antagonists are related to their ability to induce systemic arterial vasodilation. In isolated human blood vessels the dihydropyridines produce concentration-dependent relaxation of norepinephrine and epinephrine-preconstricted arteries and veins. In man, the partial venodilator effects of nifedipine are usually overcome by sympathetic reflex activity, resulting in arterial dilatation as the predominant vascular effect. In contrast, verapamil produces little change in heart rate or cardiac output and, like the dihydropyridines the principal antihypertensive effect is mediated by peripheral vasodilatation with reduction in peripheral vascular resistance. However, with both verapamil and diltiazem reflex sympathetic stimulation is blunted due to concomitant negative inotropic and negative chronatropic effects.

Calcium antagonists as antihypertensive agents

Despite their structural diversity, and their differential pharmacokinetic characteristics, all calcium antagonists have been shown to be effective antihypertensive agents relatively devoid of serious adverse effects, although concerns have been expressed about the long-term safety of calcium antagonists and this will be discussed later in this chapter. The

6

effective reduction of elevated blood pressure by calcium antagonists has been described in numerous communication and review papers and the role of the calcium antagonist in the treatment of hypertension has become established largely as there are relatively few patients in whom calcium antagonist therapy should be avoided. Partly as a consequence of this characteristic, calcium antagonists are recommended as a possible first line agent in a number of major guidelines including those of the World Health Organization/International Society of Hypertension (WHO/ISH). Thus, calcium antagonists as antihypertensives are effective in patients with essential hypertension, patients with renovascular hypertension, Black patients with hypertension (in whom responses to ACE inhibitors and other drugs may be modest) and patients with both hypertension and diabetes mellitus. However, due to a relative paucity of data calcium antagonists are not recommended for the treatment of hypertension in pregnancy.

Influence of demographic factors

It is clear from many studies that no single agent as monotherapy is capable of controlling blood pressure in all hypertensive patients. However, there is a degree of consistency in the two trials which have compared all the major classes of antihypertensive drugs in a single study design [17,18]. In both the TOMHS [17] and VA [18] studies the blood pressure control rates achieved were numerically higher with the calcium antagonists than they were with all the other classes of agents. However, the VA study [18] may be of particular importance with respect to identifying differential responses in patients with differing demographic features. The received wisdom has been that unlike beta-adrenergic antagonists which tend to show a decrease in efficacy in older patients, calcium antagonists are either equally effective in all age groups or potentially superior in older patients [19]. The suggestion has been made that the antihypertensive effect of calcium antagonists may be inversely proportional to the underlying baseline plasma renin activity [19]. Whilst undoubtedly the elderly tend to have lower plasma renin activity they also tend to have higher underlying baseline blood pressure which is also a determinant of the absolute antihypertensive response [20]. The findings of the VA study [18] support the contention that plasma renin activity and its interaction with age and race may be an important contributory factor with respect to antihypertensive response. Whilst there was relatively little differential between the major classes of antihypertensive in younger and older White patients, in the younger Black population the calcium antagonist offered statistical benefit compared to the other agents and this became even more pronounced in older Black patients [18]. Finally, the evidence suggests that calcium antagonists are equally effective in both men and women.

Use of calcium antagonists in patients with concomitant disease

As calcium antagonists were not originally introduced as antihypertensive agents, it is not surprising that much of the initial experience with these agents was accumulated in patients with coexisting problems. In particular calcium antagonists, especially diltiazem and verapamil, may be effectively used in patients with hypertension and ischemic heart disease particularly where beta-adrenergic antagonists are contraindicated.

A limited number of studies have addressed the issue as to whether calcium antagonists provide secondary protection in patients who have suffered an acute coronary syndrome. Increased survival and lower infarction rate were found in the DAVIT II trial in patients treated for 12–18 months after a myocardial infarction [21]. In a smaller postmyocardial infarction trial (MDPIT), a favorable trend was observed in patients without pulmonary congestion who were treated with diltiazem [22]. The available evidence suggests that dihydropyridine calcium antagonists have no benefit in postmyocardial infarction patients or in those with unstable angina and indeed may have a deleterious effect.

As suggested earlier, all classes of calcium antagonists have to a greater or lesser extent negative chronotropic or inotropic effects. As such it would be considered that these agents would be unlikely to be a benefit in patients with congestive heart failure. However, despite evidence that treatment with some dihydropyridine calcium antagonists in long-term studies results in hemodynamic deterioration in patients with chronic heart failure, there is evidence to suggest that the longer-acting agent amlodipine is neutral and may have some limited benefit in the treatment of heart failure [23].

Because of their essentially neutral metabolic profile, calcium antagonists are potentially an attractive option for the treatment of hypertension associated with diabetes mellitus. Studies on the effect of calcium antagonists on proteinuria and progression of nephropathy in diabetic patients suggest that calcium antagonists, particularly verapamil and diltiazem, may have a beneficial effect but the magnitude of the beneficial effect was not as great as that seen with ACE inhibitors. However subgroup analysis of the major outcome trials (see below) suggests that dihydropyridine calcium antagonists are effective in decreasing morbidity and mortality in diabetic hypertensive patients.

Calcium antagonists may also have desirable characteristics in other settings, they are unlikely to worsen symptomatic peripheral vascular disease and they certainly do not have a deleterious effect in patients with bronchospastic pulmonary disease.

Metabolic effects of calcium antagonists

Hypertension is often associated with impaired glucose tolerance, insulin resistance, Type 2 diabetes mellitus and dyslipidemia. As a consequence the potential metabolic effects of antihypertensive agents and their impact upon cardiovascular risk reduction are important areas of concern. The evidence clearly indicates that, unlike antihypertensive therapy with diuretics and beta-blockers, where hypocalcemia, hypercalcemia and hyperuricemia may be of concern, calcium antagonists are essentially metabolically neutral.

Side-effect profiles of calcium antagonists

The short-term adverse effects of calcium antagonists appear to differ with regard to the structural class of calcium antagonist involved. Thus, it is well recognized that with verapamil and related drugs and to a lesser extent with diltiazem constipation, impaired atrioventricular conduction, vasodilatation, flushing, headache and reduced cardiac contractile force may be of concern. In contrast with the dihydropyridines, the most common side effects are ankle edema, headache, flushing and palpitations associated with reflex tachycardia induced by vasodilatation. The newer dihydropyridine calcium antagonists appear to have a more favorable side-effect profile than short-acting nifedipine but the evidence suggests that ankle edema is class effect associated with the dihydropyridine calcium antagonist.

Combination therapy

Calcium antagonists can be combined with several types of antihypertensives usually with at least an additive antihypertensive effect and in some instances a synergistic effect. In particular, the combination of a beta-blocker and a dihydropyridine calcium antagonist is an effective and logical combination in that the reflex tachycardia often associated with the calcium antagonist is counteracted by the beta-blocker. Such a combination with verapamil or diltiazem can certainly be effective but caution should be exercised due to the potentially additive impairment of atrioventricular conduction and the risk of atrioventricular block. Calcium antagonists have also effectively been combined with α_1-adrenoceptor blockers and ACE inhibitors, indeed fixed-dose combinations of calcium antagonists and ACE inhibitors have proved to be particularly effective. Based largely on first principles, it has been suggested that the combination of diuretics and calcium antagonists is not logical; however, in certain instances, this combination may provide a useful additive antihypertensive effect.

Ancillary properties of calcium antagonists

It is widely acknowledged that calcium antagonists are effective antihypertensive agents but attention has focused upon their potential additional ancillary properties over and above the effects associated with blood-pressure lowering.

Calcium antagonists and atherosclerosis

In vitro and *in vivo* studies in experimental models of atherosclerosis have strongly suggested that calcium antagonists may have anti-atherosclerotic properties and prevent the development of atherosclerotic legions. This appears to be particularly the case when drugs are administered prior to the development of vascular lesions and that the lipophilic dihydropyridine calcium antagonists may be particularly effective in this setting.

Despite promising evidence from experimental studies, the evidence of anti-atherogenic effects of calcium antagonists in humans has been somewhat disappointing. Both the INTACT and Montreal Heart Study appeared to demonstrate some benefit associated with dihydropyridine therapy with regard to preventing the development of new lesions and reducing the progression of existing atherosclerotic lesions [24]. However, these positive benefits were outweighed by an apparent increase in cardiovascular events. Inconclusive results were derived from the MIDAS study and once again there appeared to be higher incidence of adverse events in patients treated with isradipine compared to those receiving hydrochlorothiazide [24]. In contrast the VHAS study [25] suggested that verapamil was more effective than chlorthalidone in the regression of carotid lesions and that these potentially beneficial changes were paralleled by a lower incidence or cardiovascular events with verapamil. The recently published PREVENT trial indicated that amlodipine had no demonstrable effect on angiographic progression of coronary atherosclerosis in patients with coronary artery disease [26]. There was also no significant effect on major cardiovascular events but amlodipine was associated with fewer hospitalizations for unstable angina and revascularization.

Thus to date, the evidence of the potential beneficial effect of calcium antagonists in atherosclerosis are somewhat equivocal and the results of the ELSA study with lacidipine is awaited with considerable interest [27].

Calcium antagonists and left ventricular hypertrophy

Left ventricular hypertrophy (LVH) is an important independent risk factor in hypertensive patients. Attention has, therefore, focused upon whether there may be differential benefit associated with one or other particular class of antihypertensive agent with respect to reversal of hypertensive LVH. A number of studies have suggested that different classes of antihypertensive do not have the same effect in reducing LVH but this has often been confounded by different blood pressure-lowering effects. A meta-analysis concluded that ACE inhibitors might be particularly effective in regression of LVH [28]. However, a more comprehensive analysis [29] has suggested that the major determinants of LVH regression are the fall in blood pressure associated with treatment combined with the initial left ventricular mass and that both ACE inhibitors and calcium antagonists are superior to beta-blockers or diuretic in their ability to regress LVH.

The effect of calcium antagonists on endothelial function and vascular protection

Numerous experimental studies have indicated that calcium antagonists and ACE inhibitors may exert vascular protective effects, partly by regressing vascular remodeling and, in addition, by correcting endothelial dysfunction. Calcium antagonists, particularly the dihydropyridine derivatives, can reverse impaired endothelium-dependent vasodilatation in different vascular beds including the subcutaneous, epicardial, renal and forearm circulation [30]. Furthermore, in hypertensive patients in whom blood pressure is controlled to a similar extent, treatment with long-acting calcium antagonists produced a regression of the structural and functional alterations in small arteries, a pattern that was not observed in patients treated with beta-blockers [31].

Outcome studies and the long-term safety of calcium antagonists as antihypertensive agents

Calcium antagonists effectively reduce blood pressure in many patients, often with lower incidents of side effects than are associated with thiazides and beta-blockers. For these and other reasons in many countries calcium antagonists are the most widely prescribed antihypertensive agent. Despite their high frequency of use, data on the benefit : risk ratio for calcium antagonists on clinically relevant outcomes when compared to alternative therapies have not, until comparatively recently, been available.

Outcome studies with calcium antagonists

A series of placebo-controlled and comparative trials utilizing calcium antagonists have been performed and a number are ongoing and these are summarized in Table 6.3.6.

STONE was a single-blind study of nifedipine versus placebo in Chinese hypertensives. In the active treatment arm of the study, nifedipine significantly reduced the overall risk of cardiovascular events by almost 60% [32]. The study has been subject to some criticism due to the sequential randomization schedule and, because of a low incidence, it was not possible to draw any conclusions regarding effects on myocardial infarction.

The SYST-EUR study was performed in 4695 patients aged 60 years and over with isolated systolic hypertension [33]. The study was stopped prematurely after two years of follow up because the active treatment with nitrendipine proved clearly beneficial when compared with placebo. In particular, the incidence of stroke was significantly and substantially reduced (by 42%) by treatment with nitrendipine and although there was a beneficial effect on myocardial infarction, this did not achieve statistical significance due to the premature termination of the trial.

The SYST-CHINA trial was similar in design to SYST-EUR and was performed in 2394 elderly Chinese patients with isolated systolic hypertension[34]. The intention-to-treat analysis demonstrated that active treatment reduced the incidence of total mortality, fatal and non-fatal stroke and all cardiovascular endpoints.

It is worthy of note that all three of these placebo-controlled trials are consistent, with respect to stroke reduction, with other outcome trials which utilized conventional antihypertensive treatment. This is

6

Table 6.3.6 Major trials in hypertension utilizing calcium antagonists

Trial	Sample Size	Study design	Result or year of completion
STONE [32]	1632	Nifedipine-based treatment regimen versus placebo in Chinese hypertensives	60% reduction in cardiovascular events (mainly stroke)
SYST-EUR [33]	4695	Nitrendipine-based treatment regimen versus placebo in treatment of isolated systolic hypertension	Terminated prematurely due to positive findings – 42% reduction in stroke
SYST-CHINA [34]	2394	Nitrendipine-based treatment regimen versus placebo in treatment of isolated systolic hypertension in a Chinese population	Active treatment significantly reduced the incidence of total mortality, fatal and non-fatal stroke and all cardiovascular endpoints
HOT [35]	19196	Assessing optimum target for diastolic blood pressure control (using a felodipine-based treatment regimen) also determining the benefit of low-dose aspirin in essential hypertensives	Intensive lowering of blood pressure in essential hypertensives was associated with a low rate of cardiovascular events
STOP-2 [36]	6628	Comparison of newer (calcium antagonist/ ACE inhibitor) and older (beta-blocker/diuretic) drugs	Old and new drugs were similar in prevention of cardiovascular mortality and major events
INSIGHT [38]	6321	Comparison of nifedipine GITS-based treatment regimen with diuretic-based regimen in essential hypertensives	The two regimens were comparable with respect to cardiovascular and cerebrovascular endpoints
NORDIL [37]	10881	Comparison of diltiazem-based treatment regimen with diuretic/beta-blocker based regimen in essential hypertensives	The two regimens were comparable with respect to cardiovascular and cerebrovascular endpoints
ALLHAT [39]	42448	Comparison of newer agents calcium antagonist (amlodipine), ACE inhibitor (lisinopril) and alpha-blocker (doxazosin) with chlorthalidone in high-risk hypertensives	2001/2002 (doxazosin arm terminated early in 2000)
ASCOT [40]	18000	Comparison of conventional antihypertensive treatment regimen (beta-blocker/diuretic) and contemporary drug treatment regimen based on amlodipine and perindopril (plus a prospective assessment of statin-based lipid lowering)	2004
CONVINCE [41]	15000	Comparison of conventional antihypertensive treatment regimen (beta-blocker/diuretic) and verapamil COER in mild/moderate essential hypertensives	2002

Outcome studies and the long-term safety of calcium antagonists as antihypertensive agents

Outcome studies with calcium antagonists

illustrated in Figure 6.3.1 where it is clear that the major determinant of the absolute benefit for stroke reduction is associated with the risk in the placebo group and that essentially a linear relationship is apparent between absolute benefit and risk.

For ethical reasons, all other outcome trials have focused upon comparisons of alternative active treatments. In the HOT trial, 18 790 patients all receive felodipine as initial therapy followed by additional drugs to achieve alternative blood pressure targets [35]. The trial achieved substantially greater reduction rates of cardiovascular events than expected from previous trials using alternative treatments.

The STOP-2 trial where 'newer' treatments were compared to 'older' treatments there was no significant difference in cardiovascular events between groups treated with beta-blockers/diuretics and those treated with ACE inhibitors and calcium antagonists. Although blood pressure reductions were comparable, when an analysis was undertaken

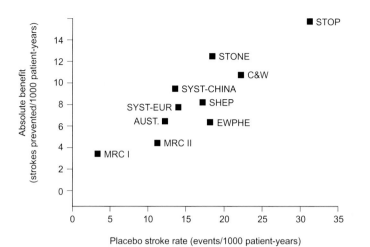

Fig 6.3.1 The relationship between absolute benefit of treatment and the incidence of stroke (fatal and non-fatal combined) in 10 major placebo-controlled outcome trials. MRCI and MRCII are Medical Research Council trials I and II respectively; AUST the Australian Study; SHEP the Systolic Hypertension in the Elderly Programme; EWPHE the European Working Party on High Blood Pressure in the Elderly trial; C&W – Coope and Warrender; STOP the Swedish Trial in Old Patients with Hypertension; SYST-EUR the Systolic Hypertension in Europe Trial; STONE the Shanghai Trial of Nifedipine in the Elderly; SYST-CHINA the Systolic Hypertension in China Trial.

comparing outcomes with ACE inhibitors and calcium antagonists the ACE inhibitors were found to have statistically fewer myocardial infarctions and congestive heart failure episodes [36].

Recently, the INSIGHT and NORDIL trials have reported the comparative outcomes among patients assigned to treatment with regimens based upon calcium antagonists (nifedipine, GITS and diltiazem, respectively) and among patients assigned a diuretic-based or beta-blocker-based regimen [37,38]. Neither study found clear evidence of any difference in the frequencies of the prespecified primary outcomes (combinations of major cardiovascular events), although both studies observed some differences in cause specific outcomes. In NORDIL there was a marginally lower risk of stroke with diltiazem-based therapy (despite a lesser reduction in blood pressure), but there was no clear evidence of a difference in stroke risk in INSIGHT. Conversely, in INSIGHT there was a marginally significant excess of heart failure with nifedipine-based treatment, but in NORDIL there was no clear evidence of a difference in heart failure risk. Furthermore, although fatal myocardial infarctions were commoner with nifedipine-based treatment than with diuretic-based treatment in INSIGHT, in neither study was there a clear difference in total number of major coronary heart disease events.

The essentially neutral findings of these outcome studies with calcium antagonists are in contrast to the findings of two small-scale studies in which calcium antagonists were compared to ACE inhibitors in diabetic patients. In both FACET [42] and the ABCD trial [43] treatment with the calcium antagonist appeared to be associated with significantly higher incidence of cardiovascular events when compared to the ACE inhibitor groups. However, considerable caution must be exercised in interpreting these very small-scale studies and perhaps greater attention should be focused on the findings of the subgroups of diabetic patients in the major outcome control trials which suggest that calcium antagonists may offer preferential benefit in older diabetic patients with isolated systolic hypertension [44].

Observational epidemiological studies with calcium antagonists

Despite the accumulating evidence of the potential benefits of calcium antagonists derived from major outcome trials, there remains a concern regarding the safety of long-term treatment with calcium antagonists. These concerns have largely been based upon observational epidemiological studies both case–control and cohort, in which patients prescribed calcium antagonists for hypertension appeared to be at greater risk for cardiovascular disease, cancer and bleeding than those prescribed other antihypertensive medications [45]. Not only are these studies subject to all the limitations of retrospective observational analysis but they are also contradictory in nature. This has resulted in an emotional, unconvincing and often biased debate as to the long-term safety of calcium antagonists in the treatment of hypertension. The individual outcome trials cannot refute the possibility of modest (10–15%) proportional differences between alternative treatment regimens in their effects on cause specific outcomes such as stroke or coronary heart disease. Whilst these differences are modest they could have important consequences especially for individuals at high risk. However, the detection of these differences requires studies that record very large numbers of events and it has been pointed out that to demonstrate reliably a 15% difference in the risk of myocardial infarction between different treatment regimens, requires evidence from randomized comparisons involving at least 1000 of such events [46]. This is unlikely to be achieved in any one trial and, therefore, a collaborative meta-analysis of 35 studies of regimens based upon calcium antagonists, ACE inhibitors, angiotensin II antagonists and diuretics or beta-blockers is currently being undertaken [46]. This analysis should include a total of more than 20 000 major cardiovascular events and more than 1000 cause-specific events in each of several prespecified comparisons. Any evidence of real differences between drug treatment regimens that emerges from this or other sources should go some way to enabling physicians to match antihypertensive treatments to the particular risks in individual patients.

Conclusions

Calcium antagonists are effective, well tolerated and widely used drugs in the treatment of hypertension, and compare well in their blood pressure-lowering effect with all the other major classes of antihypertensives. They may therefore be considered as established first-line agents and indeed are acknowledged as such by many of the major guidelines for the treatment of hypertension. They can be widely utilized in patients with concomitant disease and may offer ancillary properties over and above their blood pressure-lowering effects.

The proven antihypertensive efficacy of calcium antagonists has been supplemented by the evidence of proven benefit for cardiovascular outcomes in the randomized trials. However, some questions remain unanswered and it is not possible at present to exclude the possibility that compared to conventional treatments calcium antagonists may offer preferential benefit with respect to stroke reduction whilst at the same time being slightly inferior with regard to reducing coronary heart disease events. These questions can only be addressed by ongoing outcome trials and major meta-analyses.

References

1. Fleckenstein A. History of calcium antagonists. *Circ Res* 1983;**52**(Suppl. 1):113–116.
2. Nayler WE. In: *Calcium Antagonists*, pp. 1–298. Academic Press: London, 1988.
3. Opie LH. *Clinical use of Calcium Channel Antagonist Drugs*, 2nd edn., pp. 1–286. Kluwer Academic Press: Boston, 1990.
4. Braunwald E. Introduction to 'A symposium: calcium antagonists – emerging clinical opportunities'. *Am J Cardiol* 1987;**59**(3):1B–3B.
5. Katz A. Calcium channel diversity in the cardiovascular system. *J Am Coll Cardiol* 1996;**28**:522–529.
6. Triggle D. Mechanism of action of calcium antagonists. In: *Calcium Antagonists in Clinical Medicine*, 2nd edn. (ed. Epstein M), pp. 1–26. Hanley and Belfus: Philadelphia, 1998.
7. Spedding M. Changing surface charge with salicylate differentiates between sub-groups of calcium antagonists. *Br J Pharmacol* 1984;**83**:211–220.
8. Glossman H, Ferry DR. Solubilisation and partial purification of putative calcium channels labelled with 'H-nimodipine'. *Naunyn Schmiedebergs Arch Pharmacol* 1983;**323**:279–291.
9. Singh B. The mechanism of action of calcium antagonists relative to their clinical applications. *Br J Clin Pharmacol* 1986;**21**(Suppl):109–121.
10. Toyo-Oka T, Naylor WG. Third generation calcium entry blockers. *Blood Pressure* 1996;**5**:206–208.
11. Lüscher TF, Cosentino F. The classification of calcium antagonists and their selection in the treatment of hypertension. A reappraisal. *Drugs* 1998;**55**(4):509–517.
12. Echizen E, Brecht T, Niedergesess S *et al*. The effects of dextro, levo and racemic verapamil in atrioventricular conduction in humans. *Am Heart J* 1985;**109**:210–217.
13. Meredith PA. Clinical relevance of optimal pharmacokinetics in the treatment of hypertension. *J Hypertension* 1997;**15** (Suppl. 5):S27–S31.
14. Elliott HL, Meredith PA, Reid JL. Pharmacokinetics of calcium antagonists: implications for therapy. In: *Calcium Antagonists in Clinical Medicine*, 2nd edn. (ed. Epstein M), pp. 35–56. Hanley and Belfus: Philadelphia, 1998.
15. Donnelly R, Elliott HL, Meredith PA. Concentration–effect analysis of antihypertensive drug response: focus on calcium antagonists. *Clin Pharmacokinet* 1994;**26**(6):472–485.
16. Meredith PA. Lercanidipine: a novel lipophilic dihydropyridine calcium antagonist with long duration of action and high vascular selectivity. *Exp Opin Invest Drugs* 1999;**8**(7):1043–1062.
17. Liebson PR, Grandits GA, Dianzumba S *et al*. for the Treatment of Hypertension Study Research Group. Comparison of five antihypertensive monotherapies and placebo for change in left ventricular mass in patients receiving nutritional–hygienic therapy in the Treatment of Mild Hypertension Study (TOMHS). *Circulation* 1995;**91**:698–706.

6

18. Materson BJ, Reda DJ, Cushman WC for the Department of Veterans Affairs Cooperative Study Group of Antihypertensive Agents. Department of Veterans Affairs single-drug therapy of hypertension study. *Am J Hypertension* 1995;**8**:189–192.

19. Buhler FR. Antihypertensive treatment according to age, plasma renin and race. *Drugs* 1988;**35**(5):495–503.

20. Meredith PA, Elliott HL, Ahmed JF, Reid JL. Age and the antihypertensive efficacy of verapamil: an integrated pharmacodynamic–pharmacokinetic approach. *J Hypertension* 1987;**5**(Suppl. 5):S219–S221.

21. Danish Study Group on Verapamil in Myocardial Infarction. Effect of verapamil on mortality and major events after acute myocardial infarction (The Danish Verapamil Infarction Trial II-DAVIT II). *Am J Cardiol* 1990;**66**:779–785.

22. Multicentre Diltiazem Postinfarction Trial Research Group. The effect of diltiazem on mortality and reinfarction after myocardial infarction. *N Engl J Med* 1988;**319**:385–392.

23. Packer M, O'Connor M, Ghali JK *et al*. Effect of amlodipine on morbidity and mortality in severe chronic heart failure. *N Engl J Med* 1996;**335**:1107–1114.

24. Zannad F. Effects of calcium antagonists on the progression of atherosclerosis and intima media thickness. *Drugs* 2000;**59**(Spec. Iss. 2):39–46.

25. Zanchetti A, Rosei EA, Palu CD *et al*. for the Verapamil in Hypertension and Atherosclerosis Study (VHAS) investigators. *J Hypertension* 1998;**16**: 1667–1676.

26. Pitt B, Byington RP, Furberg CD *et al*. for the PREVENT Investigators. Effect of amlodipine on the progression of atherosclerosis and the occurrence of clinical events. *Circulation* 2000;**102**:1503–1510.

27. Zanchetti A, Bond MG, Hennig M *et al*. Risk factors associated with alterations in carotid intima-media thickness in hypertension: baseline data from the European Lacidipine study on atherosclerosis. *J Hypertension*. 1998;**16**(7):949–961.

28. Dahlof B, Pennert K, Hansson L. Reversal of left ventricular hypertrophy in hypertensive patients. A meta-analysis of 109 treatment studies. *Am J Hypertension* 1992;**5**(2):95–110.

29. Schlaich MP, Schmieder RE. Left ventricular hypertrophy and its regression: Pathophysiology and therapeutic approach: focus on treatment by antihypertensive agents. *Am J Hypertension* 1998;**11**(111):1394–1404.

30. Virdis A, Ghiadoni L, Sudano I *et al*. Effect of antihypertensive drugs on endothelial function in humans. *J Hypertension* 1998;**16**(Suppl. 8): S103–S110.

31. Schiffrin EL. Vascular protection with newer antihypertensive agents. *J Hypertension* 1998;**16**(Suppl. 5):S25–S29.

32. Gong L, Zhang W, Zhu Y *et al*. Shanghai trial of nifedipine in the elderly (STONE). *J Hypertension* 1996;**14**:1237–1345.

33. Staessen JA, Fagard R, Thijs L *et al*. for the Systolic Hypertension in Europe (SYST-EUR) Trial Investigators. *Lancet* 1997;**350**(9080):757–764.

34. Wang JG, Staessen JA, Gong L, Lisheng L for the Systolic Hypertension in China (SYST-CHINA) Collaborative Group. Chinese trial on isolated systolic hypertension in the elderly (original investigation). *Arch Intern Med* 2000;**160**(2):211–220.

35. Hansson L, Zanchetti A, Carruthers SG *et al*. for the HOT Study Group. Effects of intensive blood pressure lowering and low-dose aspirin in patients with hypertension: principal results of the Hypertension Optimal Treatment (HOT) randomised trial. *Lancet* 1998;**351**:1755–1762.

36. Hansson L, Lindholm LH, Ekbom T *et al*. Randomised trial of old and new antihypertensive drugs in elderly patients: cardiovascular mortality and morbidity the Swedish Trial in Old Patients with Hypertension-2 study. *Lancet* 1999;**354**:1751–1756.

37. Hansson L, Hedner T, Lund-Johansen P *et al*. for the NORDIL Study Group. Randomised trial of effects of calcium antagonists compared with diuretics and β-blockers on cardiovascular morbidity and mortality in hypertension: the Nordic Diltiazem (NORDIL) study. *Lancet* 2000;**356**:359–365.

38. Brown MJ, Palmer CR, Castaigne A *et al*. Morbidity and mortality in patients randomised to double-blind treatment with a long-acting calcium-channel blocker or diuretic in the International Nifedipine GITS study: Intervention as a Goal in Hypertension Treatment (INSIGHT). *Lancet* 2000; **356**:366–372.

39. Davis BR, Cutler JA, Gordon DJ *et al*. Rationale and design for the antihypertensive and lipid lowering treatment to prevent heart attack trial (ALLHAT). *Am J Hypertension* 1996;**9**(41):342–360.

6

40. Oparil S. Long-term morbidity and mortality trials with amlodipine. *J Cardiovasc Pharmacol* 1999;**33**(Suppl. 2):S1–S6.
41. Black HR, Elliott WJ, Neaton JD *et al*. Rationale and design for the Controlled ONset Verapamil Investigation of Cardiovascular Endpoints (CONVINCE) trial. *Controlled Clin Trials* 1998;**19**(4):370–390.
42. Tatti P, Pahor M, Byington RB *et al*. Outcome results of the Fosinopril versus Amlodipine Cardiovascular Events Randomised Trial (FACET) in patients with hypertension and NIDDM. *Diabetes Care* 1998;**21**:597–603.
43. Estacio RO, Jeffers BW, Hiatt WR *et al*. The effect of nisoldipine as compared with enalapril on cardiovascular outcomes in patients with non-insulin-dependent diabetes and hypertension. *N Engl J Med* 1998;**338**:645–652.
44. Staessen JA, Birkenhäger WH, Fagard RH. Dihydropyridine calcium-channel blockers for the treatment of hypertensive diabetic patients. *Eur Heart J* 2000;**21**: 2–7.
45. Buring JE, Glynn RJ, Hennekens CH. Calcium channel blockers in the treatment of hypertension. In: *Hypertension. A Companion to Brenner and Rector's The Kidney* (eds Oparil S, Weber MA), pp 389–397. 2000.
46. MacMahon S, Neal B. Differences between blood-pressure-lowering drugs. *Lancet* 2000;**356**:352–353.

References

Chapter

6.4

ACE inhibitors

DL Clement

6

History of ACE inhibitors

The history of angiotensin-converting enzyme (ACE) inhibition started in the mid-1960s. It was well appreciated in those days that renin secretion could exert a pressor effect, if angiotensin I (a non-vasoconstrictive decapeptide) was converted by a 'converting enzyme' to a pressor-active octapeptide hormone angiotensin II. Ferreira [1], in searching for a bradykinin-potentiating factor in snake venom (*Bothrops jararaca*), found components that inhibited the converting enzyme. In fact, the new idea was born that inhibition of this enzyme could offer an opportunity to block the renin–angiotensin cascade, which could be of use in the treatment of essential hypertension.

By the early 1970s, the chemical structure of the ACE inhibitors in the venom had been unravelled and the inhibitor was synthetized in the laboratory. About twenty-five years ago, Gavras *et al.* [2] described their experience with ACE inhibition (parenteral administration of the nonapeptide teprotide) to treat vasoconstriction and hypertension. In 1977, Ondetti *et al.* [3] summarized the work of the Squibb Institute at Princeton, where the first *orally* active ACE inhibitor was developed. A new class of orally active antihypertensive agents was thus born[4,5].

Many ACE inhibitors have been synthesized and pharmacologically and clinically tested in both animal and human studies (Table 6.4.1) since then. About 15 have been launched (some have lasted a long time) onto the market[6]. In the early days, captopril and enalapril were the most extensively studied ACE inhibitors.

Indications for ACE inhibition in essential hypertension

Since the early 1980s, overwhelming evidence has been built up indicating that ACE inhibitors significantly reduce blood pressure in

Table 6.4.1 Commonly used or clinically tested ACE inhibitors in hypertension

Drug	Usual dose (mg)	Freqency/day	Prodrug
Alacepril	25–75	1	+
Benazepril. HCl	5–40	1–2	+
Captopril	12.5–50	2–3	–
	25–150		
Ceranapril	–	–	–
Cilazapril	2.5–5	1–2	+
Delapril	7.5–60	1–2	+
Enalapril maleate	5–40	1–2	+
Fosinopril sodium	10–40	1–2	+
Lisinopril	5–40	1	–
Moexipril	7.5–15	2	+
Perindopril	4–8	1–2	+
Quinapril. HCl	5–80	1–2	+
Ramipril	1.25–20	1–2	+
Spirapril	12.5–50	1	+
Temocapril	–	–	+
Trandolapril	1–4	1	+
Zofenopril	30–60	1–2	+

6

mild-to-moderate essential hypertension, and that the spectrum of side effects is acceptable[7]. If ACE inhibitors in recommended doses are administered to mild-to-moderate hypertensive patients, most tolerate the drugs quite well, provided the problem of coughing does not occur. From these early studies, it was obvious that there was also a potential for ACE inhibition in a number of specific conditions sometimes associated with essential hypertension[8].

Numerous studies[9–11] have shown favorable results in comorbid conditions in hypertensive patients, including Type 1 and 2 diabetes mellitus with proteinuria (with significant reduction of the proteinuria), myocardial infarction and heart failure (with improvement of systolic dysfunction and influence on survival), and in renal insufficiency (creatinine < 3 mg/dl) not caused by renovascular hypertension. Table 6.4.2 summarizes the indications for antihypertensive drug therapy *with ACE inhibitors*, as given by the Sixth Report of the Joint National Committee (JNC VI) on prevention, detection, evolution, and treatment of high blood pressure[12]. The compelling indications for diabetes mellitus Type 1 with proteinuria, heart failure and post-acute myocardial infarct systolic dysfunction are all supported by evidence from randomized controlled trials.

Notwithstanding the beneficial effects of ACE inhibitors on blood pressure management and rapid reduction of left ventricular mass[13] (left ventricular hypertrophy is a well-accepted prognostic factor in essential hypertension), and the favorable results in diabetes mellitus, heart failure and mild-to-moderate renal insufficiency, the JNC VI report still hesitated in recommending the unrestricted use of ACE inhibitors as a first-line initial drug choice, in hypertensive patients without diabetes or renal disease.

Thus, the initial drug choice (if not contraindicated) for ACE inhibitors was restricted by JNC VI to the indications mentioned in Table 6.4.2; otherwise for *uncomplicated* hypertension, the first-line drug recommendations remained diuretics and beta-blockers, based on randomized controlled trials and cost-benefit and health economics considerations[14,15].

The CAPPP study (Captopril Prevention Project) conducted in Sweden and Finland randomized 10 985 hypertensive patients (≥ 100 mmHg

Table 6.4.2 Specific indications and contraindications for ACE inhibitors in hypertensive patients with comorbidity

*Compelling indications**
Type 1 diabetes mellitus with proteinuria
Chronic heart failure
Post-acute myocardial infarction with systolic dysfunction

Potentially favorable effects
Type 2 diabetes mellitus with proteinuria
Renal insufficiency (beware renovascular disease and creatinine > 3 mg/dl)

Unfavorable effects
Pregnancy (fetal abnormalities including fetal death)
Renovascular disease

* Based on randomized controlled trials.

6

diastolic blood pressure), to either ACE inhibitor, beta-blocker or diuretics[16]. The results demonstrated comparable incidences of fatal and non-fatal cardiovascular endpoints (the primary aim of the study) after a mean follow-up period of six years. Therefore ACE inhibitors may be considered a first-line drug choice in the treatment of essential hypertension, even in cases without diabetes or renal disease.

Concerning target organ damage, it has been advocated that ACE inhibitors are particularly suited for rapid reduction of left ventricular hypertrophy[14]. Indeed, some studies indicate that treatment with an ACE inhibitor alone, or combined with a diuretic, is more effective in the short-term reduction of left ventricular mass, and even for regressing left ventricular hypertrophy up to one year. Perhaps ACE inhibitors may reduce left ventricular hypertrophy somewhat more rapidly than other drug classes, due to their effect on limiting growth-promoting properties of angiotensin II on myocardial muscle tissue, besides their blood pressure-reducing capacity[17,18].

Antihypertensive mechanisms of ACE inhibitors in essential hypertension (Table 6.4.3)

ACE inhibition and angiotensin II

Early studies indicated that ACE inhibitors were effective in reducing circulating angiotensin II levels at doses that exerted vasodilatory and antihypertensive effects. However, the same studies indicated that for a given level of circulating angiotensin II there may be different degrees of blood vessel contractions and that total body sodium is also an interfering factor[19]. In several studies of short-term treatment with ACE inhibitors, the magnitude of initial blood pressure reduction, was correlated with initial plasma renin activity and angiotensin II. Nonetheless, in the long run, correlations became increasingly weaker. Therefore, circulating angiotensin II or renin are now thought to be of limited value in predicting good responders to ACE inhibition. During the 1990s, the *tissue* ACE-inhibition theory became more and more popular[20,21].

All the components of the renin–angiotensin system have now been discovered in vascular tissue; thus angiotensin II can be locally formed and exerts local vasoconstriction. The ACE enzyme formed in the endothelium, in part extends into the vascular lumen. Consequently,

Table 6.4.3 Summary of the most accepted mechanisms by which ACE inhibitors may lower blood pressure

- Inhibition of the renin–angiotensin II system (RAS)
    circulating RAS
    tissue (vascular) RAS
- Inhibition of release of norepinephrine from terminal neurons
- Potentiation of bradykinin by reduced degradation
- Potentiation of vasodilatory prostaglandins
- Reduced secretion of aldosterone leading to reduced volume and sodium retention
- Increase of renal blood flow
- Reduction of total peripheral vascular resistance and increase of venous capacitance

angiotensin II accounts for both the autocrine (effects on the same cell) and paracrine (i.e. effects on neighboring cells) effects. Thus, theoretically, ACE enzymes should not even penetrate tissues to generate angiotensin II, which acts directly in the tissues.

In animal experiments, chronic ACE inhibition nearly completely inhibits tissular-bound ACE at the endothelium in kidney, aorta, adrenals and also, probably in the heart, whilst the activity of circulating ACE is increased by a compensatory induction mechanism.

Most investigators now believe that the fall in blood pressure induced by ACE inhibitors is better correlated with the degree of inhibition of the tissue renin–angiotensin system rather than with the circulating system.

ACE inhibition and the sympathetic nervous system

For decades, the sympathetic nervous system has been thought to be involved in the pathophysiology of essential hypertension, and it was not unexpected that in the mid-1980s, interactions between the sympathetic and renin–angiotensin systems were described [22]; activation of one of the systems clearly amplifies the other. It remains a matter of debate as to whether ACE inhibition in the brain can interfere with sympathetic nervous function. The question is, do all ACE inhibitors pass the blood–brain barriers? On the other hand in peripheral sites, interactions between angiotensin II and the sympathetic nervous system have been described at pre- and postjunctional receptors (angiotensin II inhibiting the reuptake of catecholamines) and particularly enhancement of norepinephrine release by terminal nerve endings, and potentiation of the postjunctional effects of norepinephrine. Moreover, angiotensin II might mediate epinephrine release from the adrenal medulla.

If all these mechanisms hold true, there is a large potential for ACE inhibitors to interfere with the deleterious interplay between the sympathetic nervous system and the renin–angiotensin system. Experimental sympathetic nerve and α-adrenoceptor stimulation by exogenous norepinephrine which induce blood pressure rises, were blunted by administration of captopril. In both normotensive, but particularly in hypertensive subjects the pressor effect of norepinephrine is strongly reduced by captopril.

On the other hand, experiments on potentiation, resetting or increased sensitivity of the baroreflex sensitivity by ACE inhibitors, could not demonstrate a clear interaction with the baroreceptor system. Nevertheless, downregulation of baroreflexes has been described. ACE inhibitors do not functionally influence the role of the sympathetic nervous system; there is no consistent change in levels of circulating catecholamines and there is no important increase in heart rate. Some authors have described a parasympathomimetic effect of ACE inhibitors; acute and long-term treatment with ACE inhibitors increased parasympathetic activity in both normo- and hypertensive subjects (stimulation of the vagal activity by captopril). Perhaps, the interaction between the renin–angiotensin system and the autonomic nervous system should be discussed in terms of sympathicovagal balance.

ACE inhibition and the kallikrein–kinin system

In the early 1990s, studies on the mechanism underlying the antihypertensive properties of ACE inhibitors started to focus on the interactions with the kallikrein–kinin system. Since then, bradykinin has been recognized as an effective mediator in cardiovascular control mechanisms. Bradykinin is generated from kininogen by the action of an enzyme kallikrein (the active form of prekallikrein). Bradykinin is degraded by kininases, one of them (kininase II) identical to the ACE enzyme.

Thus, local inhibition by ACE inhibitors should lead to potentiation of the local action of bradykinin by inhibition of degradation. Generation of bradykinin is mainly confined to the endothelium and major determinants of bradykinin production comprise increased sheer forces by increased blood flow (for instance during exercise) and inflammation or endothelial damage, where factor XII activation induces the kallikrein cascade.

Through the action of receptors, bradykinin induces its vasodilatory properties. The mechanism is based on several pathways such as nitric oxide (NO) formation, increased production of PGE_2 or prostacyclin (PGI_2). There is now more compelling evidence that ACE inhibitors are effective in the prevention of the degradation of bradykinin, leading to their vasodilatory properties.

Another interesting aspect is the interaction between the renal kallikrein–kinin system and sodium metabolism. It is still unclear whether ACE inhibition facilitates natriuresis through the renal kallikrein–kinin system. A good correlation has been described between urinary kinin excretion and the blood pressure reduction by acute ACE inhibition, in contrast to a poor correlation with plasma bradykinin. Other investigations, on long-term ACE inhibition have failed to confirm these observations. An important factor, which will be discussed below, could be the fact that ACE inhibitors also decrease aldosterone, which might strongly influence urinary kallikrein.

ACE inhibition and prostaglandins [23]

The effect of ACE inhibitors on the increased local formation of the vasodilatory prostaglandins PGI_2 (prostacyclin) and PGE_2 is related (as mentioned above) to the increased local synthesis of the nonapeptide bradykinin in the kidney. The fact that pretreatment with indomethacin, which inhibits cyclooxygenase, reduces the hypotensive effect of ACE inhibitors is an argument in favor; nevertheless, it should be realized that indomethacin also affects plasma renin activity. Results with enalapril are much more conflicting. Whether the sulfhydryl group is responsible for this also remains unclear.

However, what is clear is that prostaglandins are involved in the blood pressure-lowering processes by drugs other than ACE inhibitors. Thus, many different mechanisms may contribute. Renal prostaglandins promote water and sodium excretion, regulate renal perfusion and intrarenal distribution of blood flow, antagonize angiotensin II in the

6

glomeruli and antidiuretic hormone (ADH) in the tubuli. There are many possibilities for ACE inhibitors to interact pathophysiologically with renal prostaglandins. The observation that in hypertensive patients, urinary PGE_2 and sodium excretion were positively correlated lends support to an active function of renal vasodilatory prostaglandins in the mechanism of ACE inhibition.

ACE inhibition, endothelin and atrial natriuretic peptides

The endothelium not only releases NO, angiotensins I and II, prostacyclin, and thromboxane but also endothelin. Endothelin is a potent vasoconstrictor. Angiotensin II is a major stimulus for the production of endothelin. In this way, ACE inhibitors might have the potential to reduce formation of endothelin. In turn, endothelin has been suggested as a stimulus for the release of atrial natriuretic peptide (ANP), which is a powerful driving force for sodium loss while the renin–angiotensin II system is a powerful driving force for sodium retention. Recently, a new group of molecules has been introduced which inhibit the degradation of ANP. Some also inhibit the ACE enzyme. They belong to the so-called group of vasopeptidase inhibitors. Clinical studies are ongoing to test the efficacy of this subgroup of molecules with ACE inhibiting properties, e.g. omapatrilat (a vasopeptidase inhibitor).

ACE inhibition in the inhibition of aldosterone secretion and increased renal blood flow

Angiotensin II is a potent stimulator for the formation of aldosterone, which is essentially a sodium-retaining and circulatory volume-controlling hormone. ACE inhibitors block, although *in vivo* only in part, the production of aldosterone. In several studies in hypertensive patients, total body sodium was reduced when blood pressure was lowered by ACE inhibitors. Unfortunately, the degree of aldosterone blocking seems to diminish during prolonged ACE inhibition ('the escape phenomenon'). After only months of therapy, aldosterone levels significantly increase. This late rise, resistant to ACE inhibitors, might be induced by counteracting mechanisms to excess natriuresis or reflect the rebound formation of circulating angiotensin II.

Renin release from the juxtaglomerular system is inhibited by angiotensin II. Thus, ACE inhibition may counteract this mechanism and increase renal blood flow. Long-term ACE inhibition raises plasma renin activity. Renin, by forming angiotensin II, maintains efferent arteriolar vasoconstriction (and intraglomerular pressure), which helps to preserve renal function.

ACE inhibition and hemodynamic actions

Volume change induced by reduction of aldosterone is one of the specific cornerstones of the action of ACE inhibitors (see above). Next to,

6

and associated with, the control of circulatory volume, another hallmark of ACE inhibition is the effect of ACE inhibitors on total peripheral vascular resistance (TPVR). Short-term blood pressure lowering by ACE inhibitors does not influence heart rate and cardiac output significantly. A large fall in systemic vascular resistance has been well documented. For instance, it has been demonstrated [24] that treatment with enalapril in moderate essential hypertension provokes arterial vasodilatation in calf and finger arteries, both at rest and during reactive hyperemia. Moreover, enalapril increased venous capacity in upper and lower limbs. This leads to an important reduction of TPVR by ACE inhibition. These observations point to a relaxant effect of ACE inhibitors on capacitance blood vessels.

Pharmacodynamic studies with ACE inhibitors
Early studies

After the initial studies with parenteral administration of the ACE inhibitor teprotide and the research work at the Squibb Institute, the first clinical studies (safety, feasibility) with the orally active molecule captopril started. As mentioned above, after the initial experience with captopril, it became obvious that at very high doses, the incidence of adverse effects was unacceptably high. Dose reduction, which was the general trend during the first half of the 1980s, clearly reduced the most severe adverse effects (see below). By 1985, many experts in the field of treatment of hypertension accepted oral treatment with captopril or enalapril, and even combination with a diuretic as an acceptable measure to treat hypertensives who did not respond to diuretics and beta-blocking agents or who exhibited adverse reactions to these first-line treatment options. For instance, Bergstrand *et al.* [25] demonstrated that blood pressure could be safely reduced in mild-to-moderate hypertension with enalapril at 2.5–40 mg/day.

From analysis of these early studies, it was clear that although the mechanisms of ACE inhibition were already largely known at that time and thought to be universal, not every patient responded positively to the new therapy, given as monotherapy. Good responders to the monotherapy were reported on the basis of percentage, from as little as 30% up to 70% and above. Confounding factors were salt intake and race. When interpreting the results from clinical studies, a difference should be made by the mean reduction of blood pressure for the group as a whole, which is highly significant in most of the studies, and the percentage of excellent, good and poor responders, which may vary considerably in the different studies.

Studies with ACE inhibitors versus placebo [26–28]

For most currently used commercialized ACE inhibitors (captopril, enalapril, fosinopril, lisinopril, perindopril, ramipril etc.) double-blind, randomized studies with a duration of at least 4–12 weeks have been undertaken versus placebo treatment. Endpoint in most of these studies was a reduction of diastolic blood pressure in responders. Many studies used a dose-ranging approach. The result was that blood pressure dropped significantly for a wide range of doses used. In hypertensive patients, for most ACE inhibitors, starting from a certain effective dose, the dose–response curves tended to be rather flat for diastolic blood pressure (e.g. data for captopril 37.5–100 mg/day, enalapril 10–40 mg/day, fosinopril 20–80 mg/day, lisinopril 20–80 mg/day, perindopril 4–16 mg/day, ramipril 2.5–10 mg/day). In these studies diastolic blood pressure reduction with ACE inhibitors varied from 5 to 15 mmHg; placebo correction reduced the main effect in most studies to less than 10 mmHg diastolic blood pressure. Confounding factors in the interpretation were also salt intake, race and posture during blood pressure measurements.

Ambulatory blood pressure recording has shown that although ACE inhibitors produced statistically significant blood pressure reductions the magnitude of the diastolic blood pressure responses, even in responders, is not very high.

Intercomparison of blood pressure-lowering capacity between ACE inhibitors

Since the early 1990s about 15 ACE inhibitors have been available on the market. The question arose whether all ACE inhibitors in 'equipotent' doses equally reduced blood pressure or whether some individual molecules had a better blood pressure-lowering capacity than others. Extensive comparative studies (double blind, randomized parallel or crossover, using office and ambulatory blood pressure measurements) have been published between captopril versus enalapril ramipril, and perindopril, between enalapril versus ramipril, lisinopril or peridopril, between lisinopril and ramipril etc.

Although results with office blood pressure and 24-hour ambulatory blood pressure are not identical and in some studies one ACE inhibitor performs somewhat better than another, it is generally accepted that at equipotency, blood pressure reductions among ACE inhibitors are largely comparable. Perhaps the longer-acting agents (Table 6.4.1) offer better 24-hour blood pressure control on ambulatory blood pressure and better trough : peak ratios. The clinical significance of this may be limited or even controversial.

Comparison of ACE inhibitors with other antihypertensive drugs

As diuretics and beta-blockers have been generally accepted for two decades as first-line drugs in the treatment of essential hypertension, it is not surprising that at least 50 studies have been published on direct comparisons between an ACE inhibitor and a diuretic or beta-blocker on the endpoint of blood pressure lowering, response rate or left ventricular hypertrophy (see below) however, studies are not available on long-term outcome variables.

6

Pharmacodynamic studies
with ACE inhibitors

Comparison of ACE
inhibitors with other
antihypertensive drugs

BOX 6.4.1 Blood pressure lowering with ACE inhibitors – comparison with other antihypertensive drugs

The number of studies on direct comparison of ACE inhibitors with diuretics is relatively restricted because by the mid-1980s there was compelling evidence that blood pressure reduction induced by an ACE inhibitor may not only be ameliorated under concomitant salt restriction but also under concomitant treatment with a diuretic [29–31].

In comparisons of ACE inhibitors with beta-blocking agents, it was clear from early studies that there was no great evidence that combinations with this class of drug would offer more benefits (also the recent JNC VI report does not recommend any combination of ACE inhibitor and beta-blocking agent for hypertension; the discussion of ACE inhibition and beta-blocking in concomitant heart failure is beyond the scope of this chapter). Direct comparisons have been made between short-term blood pressure reduction with ACE inhibition versus beta-blocking agents.

ACE inhibition versus beta-blockade therapy
At least thirty studies have been conducted directly comparing the antihypertensive blood pressure response by office or ambulatory blood pressure, and/or percentage response in randomized, double-blind parallel trial designs with durations varying from 2 to 24 weeks and comparing an ACE inhibitor with a beta-blocking drug. Examples of comparisons are enalapril versus propranolol, atenolol, metoprolol, and celiprolol, lisinopril versus atenolol and metoprolol. What conclusion can be derived from these comparisons? In most studies, ACE-inhibitor monotherapy was comparable with beta-blocker monotherapy as concerned reduction of diastolic blood pressure; in some studies, ACE inhibitor monotherapy performed even better in reducing systolic blood pressure. Incidence of side effects during the studies was also comparable, although, of course, very different in nature (see below). A number of studies also addressed a comparison of quality of life scores between the two drug classes. ACE inhibitors had a comparable spectrum of quality of life scores to atenolol or metoprolol.

ACE inhibition versus calcium antagonists
Calcium antagonists are not usually considered as first-line antihypertensive drugs. Nonetheless, most ACE inhibitors have been quite extensively compared with them in double-blind placebo-controlled parallel studies with durations ranging from 1 to 24 weeks on blood pressure reducing capacity. Most studies, however, were done on a limited number of patients. Comparisons made include captopril versus nifedipine (retard) and nitrendipine, enalapril versus isradipine, nifedipine retard, and lisinopril, and perindopril versus nifedipine retard.

What general conclusions can be derived from all these studies? ACE inhibitors have turned out to be equieffective drugs as concerns blood pressure lowering, although it should be admitted that in a number of single studies, calcium antagonists better reduce blood pressure. ACE inhibitors are more likely to be effective for reducing an already-lowered blood pressure. Optimal blood pressure control with ACE inhibitors requires a low sodium diet, and sometimes addition of a diuretic. In studies on Black patients, ACE inhibitors are clearly less effective.

Combined antihypertensive therapy which includes an ACE inhibitor [32]

Table 6.4.4 summarizes examples of fixed drug combinations (available on the market) of an ACE inhibitor with a calcium antagonist (e.g. enalapril + felodipine) or an ACE inhibitor with a diuretic (e.g. captopril + hydrochlorothiazide) derived from the JNC VI report. Data are taken from the American market; however, the principles underlying the choices can easily be extended to the European situation.

Combination of an ACE inhibitor with calcium antagonists

As mentioned above, at first glance it might not be logical to combine two drugs that are not considered first-line choices in the treatment of essential hypertension. What are the expected advantages of combining an ACE inhibitor and a calcium antagonist? The JNC VI report mentions two. Combination of a dihydropyridine calcium antagonist with an ACE inhibitor reduces pedal edema and low-dose combinations of a non-dihydropyridine calcium antagonist with an ACE inhibitor may reduce proteinuria more than either drug alone. It is increasingly accepted by experts in the field that combinations of low doses of two agents from different classes provide additional antihypertensive efficacy with a minimum likelihood of dose-dependent adverse effects.

Another theoretical premise on which to combine both drug classes is that they have no negative effect on the lipid or metabolic profile (K^+, uric acid), while that having a beneficial effect on renal function. Yet another important advantage may be that both classes act on the peripheral hemodynamics (vasodilation), without important central nervous system actions.

However, there may also be negative points to be balanced against the advantages. There are only limited and small studies available which support these theoretical advantages, and there are no data on mortality or morbidity. Besides, costs, for instance by combining an ACE inhibitor with a dihydropyridine long-acting calcium antagonist, are considerable.

Table 6.4.4 Examples of fixed combination drugs with ACE inhibitors

Fixed combinations with calcium antagonists	
ACE inhibitor +	Calcium antagonist
Enalapril maleate 5 mg +	Felodipine 5 mg
Enalapril maleate 5 mg +	Diltiazem. HCl 180 mg
Benazepril. HCl 10–20 mg +	Amlodipine besylate 2.5–5 mg
Trandolapril 1,2–4 mg +	Verapamil. HCl (*ER*) 180–240 mg
Fixed combinations with diuretics	
ACE inhibitor +	Diuretics
Captopril 25–50 mg +	Hydrochlorothiazide 15–25 mg
Enalapril maleate 5–10 mg +	Hydrochlorothiazide 12.5–25 mg
Lisinopril 10–20 mg +	Hydrochlorothiazide 12.5–25 mg
Benazepril. HCl 5, 10–20 mg +	Hydrochlorothiazide 6.25, 12.5–25 mg

6

Pharmacodynamic studies with ACE inhibitors

Combined antihypertensive therapy which includes an ACE inhibitor

Adverse effects, contraindications and drug interactions

Combination of an ACE inhibitor with a diuretic

Two conditions were identified, very soon after the introduction of ACE inhibitors, to potentiate their effect on blood pressure reduction: low sodium intake and addition of a diuretic. Numerous studies have demonstrated that in the presence of concurrent diuretics ACE inhibition becomes much more effective, as evidenced by much more (20–25% of mild-to-moderate hypertensives) good responders. For instance, addition of a dose of hydrochlorothiazide as low as 6.25 mg to a standard dose of an ACE inhibitor enhanced the efficacy of the ACE inhibitor much more than raising the dose of the ACE inhibitor! Typically, combinations of a relatively low dose of ACE inhibitor (25–50 mg captopril, 5–10 mg enalapril, 10–20 mg lisinopril) combined with 12.5–25 mg hydrochlorothiazide have been recommended. Without doubt, there is still an additive hypotensive effect if the combination ACE inhibitor + diuretic can be combined with a low dietary sodium intake. The reason for the relative success of the combination can be pathophysiologically explained: volume depletion and less reabsorbed sodium by treatment with a diuretic, induced or reactive increase of release of renin by juxtaglomerular cells. ACE inhibition may then reduce the production of angiotensin II and thus vasoconstriction. In other words, the reactive rise of angiotensin II which usually occurs under diuretics, and opposes the antihypertensive effect of diuretics, is counteracted by addition of an ACE inhibitor.

An additional advantage might be offered for the treatment of Black hypertensive patients; ACE inhibition + diuretic gives better responses than ACE inhibitor alone in Blacks. As for the combination ACE inhibitor + calcium antagonist, large trials with definite endpoints are lacking to prove any benefit; this is counterbalanced by more studies on blood pressure, more plausible mechanisms and lower costs.

Adverse effects, contraindications and drug interactions

In the early 1980s with high doses of ACE inhibition, many severe dose-related side effects were observed (neutropenia, renal disease with proteinuria, skin rash, ageusia, angioedema) but dose reduction reduced the incidence of side effects and ACE inhibitors were by the end of the 1990s considered as relatively safe drugs in the treatment of hypertension[33]. Nowadays, the most prominent adverse effect is coughing.

Table 6.4.5 Contraindications for ACE inhibitors

Absolute
  Pregnancy
  Bilateral renal artery stenosis
  Unilateral renal artery stenosis in a solitary kidney

Relative or administration under close supervision
  Severe renal insufficiency
  Aortic stenosis and obstructive cardiomyopathy (specific indications)

6

Table 6.4.6 Side effects with ACE inhibitors

Frequent
First-dose hypotension
Dry, hacking, non-productive cough
Blunting of normal compensatory responses to volume depletion
Plasma K^+ increase

Nonspecific
Headache, dizziness, fatigue, diarrhea, nausea...

Rare
Angioedema
Anaphylactoid reactions
Non-allergic, pruritic maculopapular eruptions
Leukopenia (high doses)
Taste disturbances (high doses)
Renal insufficiency (high doses)

Interactions with ACE inhibitors

Table 6.4.7 summarizes the major interactions between ACE inhibitors and other drugs. One of the best known and investigated drug interactions is that of non-steroidal anti-inflammatory (NSAIDs) and ACE inhibitors; NSAIDs decrease the efficacy of ACE inhibitors. The same holds true for antacids. In contrast, chlorpromazine (or clozapine) increases the efficacy of ACE inhibitors. ACE inhibitors also have effects on other drugs; they increase serum lithium concentrations and exacerbate the hyperkalemic effect of potassium-sparing diuretics. Food intake does not disturb the pharmacokinetic or pharmacodynamic action of ACE inhibitors. An exception is the decreased absorption of moexipril.

Table 6.4.7 Drugs interacting with ACE inhibitors

Action	Drug
Potentiation	Chlorpromazine
	Clozapine
Decrease	NSAIDs
	Antacids
Food	Decreased absorption of moexipril
Others	Increased serum lithium
	Hyperkalemic effect of potassium-sparing diuretics

References

1. Ferreira SH. A bradykinin-potentiating factor (BPF) present in the venom of *Bothrops jararaca. Br J Pharmacol Chemother* 1965;**24**:163.
2. Gavras H, Brunner HR, Laragh JH *et al.* An angiotensin converting enzyme inhibitor to identify and to treat vasoconstrictor and volume factors in hypertensive patients. *N Engl J Med* 1974;**291**:817.
3. Ondetti MA, Rubin B, Cushman DW. Design of specific inhibitors of angiotensin converting enzyme: new class of orally acting active antihypertensive agents. *Science* 1977;**196**:441.
4. Case DB, Wallace JM, Keim HT *et al.* Possible role of renin in hypertension suggested by renin-sodium profiling and inhibition of converting enzyme. *N Engl J Med* 1977;**296**:641–646.

6

6.4

6

5. Mimran A, Targhetta R, Laroche B. The antihypertensive effect of captopril in essential hypertension. *Hypertension* 1980;**2**:732–737.
6. Opie LH (ed.) Angiotensin Converting Enzyme Inhibitors: Scientific Basis for Clinical Use, 2nd edn, Wiley-Liss and Authors' Publishing House: New York, 1992.
7. Thind GS, Mahaptra R, Johnson A, Coleman RD. Low-dose captopril titration in patients with moderate-to-severe hypertension treated with diuretics. *Circulation* 1983;**67**:1340–1346.
8. Unger T, Gohlke P. Converting enzyme inhibitors in cardiovascular therapy: current status and future potential. *Cardiovasc Res* 1994;**28**:146–158.
9. Lewis EJ, Hunsicker LG, Bain RP, Rohde RD for the Collaborative Study Group. The effect of angiotensin-converting enzyme inhibition on diabetic nephropathy. *N Engl J Med* 1993;**329**:1456–1462.
10. Ravid M, Lang R, Rachmani R, Lishner M. Long-term renoprotective effect of angiotensin-converting enzyme inhibition in non-insulin dependent diabetes mellitus: a 7-year follow-up study. *Arch Int Med* 1996;**156**:286–289.
11. Giatras I, Lau J, Levey AS for the Angiotensin-converting Enzyme Inhibition and Progressive Renal Disease Study Group. Effect of angiotensin-converting enzyme inhibitors on the progression of nondiabetic renal disease: a meta-analysis of randomized trials. *Ann Intern Med* 1997;**127**: 337–345.
12. Joint National Committee on Detection, Evaluation and Treatment of High Blood Pressure. The Sixth Report of the Joint National Committee on Prevention, Detection and Treatment of High Blood Pressure (JNC VI). *Arch Intern Med* 1997;**157**:2413–2446.
13. Devereux RB. Do antihypertensive drugs differ in their ability to regress left ventricular hypertrophy? *Circulation* 1997;**95**:1983–1985.
14. Psaty BM, Smith NL, Siscovick DS *et al.* Health outcomes associated with antihypertensive therapies used as first-line agents: a systematic review and meta-analysis. *JAMA* 1997;**277**:739–745.
15. Garg R, Yusuf S for the Collaborative Group on ACE-Inhibitor Trials. Overview of randomized trials of angiotensin-converting enzyme inhibitors on mortality and morbidity in patients with heart failure. *JAMA* 1995;**273**:1450–1456.
16. Hansson L, Lindholm LH, Niskanen L *et al.* for the Captopril Prevention Project (CAPPP) Study Group. Effect of angiotensin-converting-enzyme inhibition compared with conventional therapy on cardiovascular morbidity and mortality in hypertension: the Captopril Prevention Project (CAPPP) randomised trial. *Lancet* 1999;**353**:611–616.
17. Schmieder RE, Martus P, Klingbeil A. Reversal of left ventricular hypertrophy in essential hypertension: a meta-analysis of randomized double-blind studies. *JAMA* 1996;**275**:1507–1513.
18. Gottdiener JS, Reda DJ, Massie BM, Materson BJ, Williams DW, Anderson RJ for the VA Cooperative Study Group on Antihypertensive Agents. Effects of single-drug therapy on reduction of left ventricular mass in mild to moderate hypertension: comparison of six antihypertensive agents: the Department of Veteran Affairs Cooperative Study Group on Antihypertensive Agents. *Circulation* 1998;**95**:2007–2014.
19. Hollenberg NK, Meggs LG, Williams GH *et al.* Sodium intake and renal responses to captopril in normal man and in essential hypertension. *Kidney Int* 1981;**20**:240–245.
20. Campbell DJ. Circulating and tissue angiotensin systems. *J Clin Investig* 1987;**79**:1–6.
21. Johnston CI. Tissue angiotensin-converting enzyme in cardiac and vascular hypertrophy, repair and remodeling. *Hypertension* 1994;**23**:258–263.
22. Zimmerman BG, Sybertz EJ, Wong PC. Interaction between sympathetic and renin–angiotensin system. *J Hypertens* 1984;**2**:581.
23. Moore TJ, Crantz FR, Hollenberg NK *et al.* Contribution of prostaglandins to the antihypertensive action of captopril in essential hypertension. *Hypertension* 1981;**3**:168–173.
24. Duprez D, Clement DL. Vasodilator effects of enalapril in patients with arterial hypertension. *Acta Cardiologica* 1986;**5**:359–364.
25. Bergstrand R, Herlitz M, Johansson S *et al.* Effective dose range of enalapril in mild-to-moderate essential hypertension. *Br J Clin Pharmacol* 1985;**19**:605–611.
26. Williams GH. Converting-enzyme inhibitors in the treatment of hypertension. *N Engl J Med* 1988;**319**:1517–1525.

27. Materson BJ, Reda DJ, Cushman WC *et al.* for the Department of Veterans Affairs Cooperative Study Group on Antihypertensive Agents. Single-drug therapy for hypertension in men: a comparison of six antihypertensive agents with placebo. *N Engl J Med* 1993;**328**:914–921.

28. Neaton JD, Grimm RH, Prineas RJ *et al.* for the Treatment of Mild Hypertension Study Research Group. Treatment of Mild Hypertension Study. Final results. *JAMA* 1993;**270**:713–724.

29. MacGregor GA, Markandu ND, Singer D *et al.* Moderate sodium restriction with angiotensin converting enzyme inhibition in essential hypertension: a double blind study. *Br Med J* 1987;**244**:531–534.

30. Singer DR, Markandu ND, Sugden AL *et al.* Sodium restriction in hypertensive patients treated with a converting enzyme inhibitor and a thiazide. *Hypertension* 1991;**17**:798–803.

31. Singer DRJ, Markandu ND, Cappuccio FP, Miller MA, Sagnella GA, McGregor GA. Reduction of salt intake during converting enzyme inhibitor treatment compared with addition of a thiazide. *Hypertension* 1995;**25**:1042–1044.

32. Epstein M, Bahris G. Newer approaches to antihypertensive therapy: use of fixed-dose combination therapy. *Arch Intern Med* 1996;**156**:1969–1978.

33. Textor SC. Renal failure related to angiotensin-converting enzyme inhibition. *Semin Nephrol* 1997;**17**:67–76.

References

6.5

Selective α_1-antagonists in the treatment of hypertension

HL Elliott

6

Introduction

It is generally accepted that the sympathetic nervous system plays a role in the initiation and maintenance of the increased peripheral vascular resistance which is characteristic of established essential hypertension [1,2]. Increases in arteriolar and venous tone, and hence blood pressure, are mediated by norepinephine released from sympathetic nerve terminals and acting at α_1-adrenoceptors located postjunctionally in the blood pressure wall [3,4]. Thus, in the treatment of hypertension, selective α_1-blockers interfere directly with sympathetically-mediated vasoconstrictor mechanisms and thereby promote a reduction in blood pressure.

Clinical pharmacology

Background

The first alpha-blockers were developed during the 1960s and were originally thought to be direct-acting vasodilators. Further developments through non-selective alpha-blocking drugs led to the identification of several agents, particularly the quinazoline derivatives, which were selective for the post-synaptic alpha-1 adrenoceptor (Figure 6.5.1). The particular advantage of selective α_1-antagonists, compared to non-selective agents, is that there is no interference with the negative feedback control mechanism mediated via the prejunctional α_2-adrenoceptor II [5,6]. Thus, catecholamine 'spill over' which occurs as a consequence of pre-synaptic α_2-adrenoceptor blockade is significantly reduced and, accordingly, the risk of reflex cardioacceleration during chronic treatment is reduced. Therefore, selective alpha-blockers appear to fulfil the required basic criteria for an effective antihypertensive agent since they reduce peripheral vascular resistance without interfering with myocardial contractility or exercise tolerance [7–9].

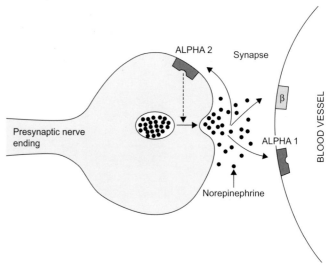

Fig. 6.5.1 Schematic representation of the pre- and postjunctional alpha adrenoceptors in the neuroeffector junction.

Alpha-blocker drugs (see Table 6.5.1)

Of the non-selective agents, only phentolamine and phenoxybenzamine retain an occasional clinical role in specialist circumstances. Of the selective α_1-blockers, the prototype drug prazosin has largely been superseded in the management of hypertension by the longer-acting quinazoline derivatives, particularly doxazosin.

Phentolamine and phenoxybenzamine

Both phentolamine (by parenteral administration) and the longer-acting agent, phenoxybenzamine (by oral administration) retain a role in the management of hypertension associated with pheochromocytoma, either as part of the perioperative management, or as a constituent of the long-term antihypertensive drug treatment when surgical correction is not possible. These drugs may also have a role in the treatment of hypertensive crises associated with, for example, overdosage of sympathomimetic drugs or the rebound hypertensive response which follows the abrupt withdrawal of chlonidine treatment.

Prazosin and quinazoline derivatives

Prazosin, the prototype quinazoline alpha-blocker, is a short-acting agent which requires multiple daily dosing (unless administered as a modified release formulation) whereas the newer quinazoline derivatives, including doxazosin and terazosin, are licensed for once-daily administration for the treatment of hypertension. In practical terms, and for the routine management of hypertensive patients, doxazosin is now the most important quinazoline derivative, and the most widely studied. Recently, to further improve the pharmacokinetic profile, a new modified release formulation (gastrointestinal therapeutic system, GITS) has been developed and is currently undergoing clinical studies [10]. For illustrative purposes the clinical pharmacokinetic parameters of doxazosin and prazosin are compared in Table 6.5.2.

Not only does doxazosin have a longer elimination half-life than prazosin but it attains its peak plasma concentrations more slowly, after

Table 6.5.1 Alpha-blocking drugs

Non-selective
Phenoxybenzamine
Phentolamine
Selective
Quinazoline derivatives
   Prazosin
   Doxazosin
   Terazosin
Non-quinazolines
   Indoramin
Multiple actions
   Carvedilol
   Labetalol

Table 6.5.2 Comparison of the clinical pharmacokinetics of doxazosin and prazosin

Parameters	Doxazosin	Prazosin
Bioavailability (%)	62–74	44–69
Clearance (ml/min/kg)	1–2	2–4
Elimination half-life (h)		
Single doses	9–16	2–4
Multiple doses	13–22	2–4
Volume of distribution (liters/kg)	62–74	44–69

about 2–4 hours, and this is associated with a more gradual onset of action. Specific pharmacokinetic studies have been undertaken in elderly patients and in patients with renal impairment. In summary, although there are some age-related differences in the disposition characteristics, neither the bioavailability nor clearance of doxazosin are significantly altered and the overall conclusion is that age is unlikely to influence the disposition of doxazosin to any clinically significant extent [11]. In patients with varying degrees of renal impairment there are no significant differences in half-life [12]. There is no evidence that the pharmacokinetics of doxazosin are either time- or dose-dependent and, for dosages between 1 mg and 16 mg, the steady-state pharmacokinetics show proportional increases in plasma concentration and in area under the concentration–time curve (AUC) [13].

The relationship between the response to doxazosin and either drug dose or plasma drug concentration has been investigated in several studies. For example, in a clinical study of antihypertensive efficacy a linear relationship was identified with a progressive increase in effect with oral doses of 2, 4 and 8 mg [13]. In a more detailed study, using integrated concentration–effect analysis (pharmacokinetic–pharmacodynamic modeling) linear relationships between dose, plasma drug concentration and blood pressure response were identified in individual hypertensive subjects [14]. The results of these studies confirm that doxazosin, despite its close structural similarities to prazosin, is qualitatively different with a gradual onset of action (even after intravenous administration) which is directly attributable to the parent drug and is not dependent upon an active metabolite. The consistency of the response to doxazosin has also been investigated in the same individual after oral and intravenous administration [15] and after single and multiple dosing [14]. The results of these studies confirm the consistency and reproducibility of the concentration–effect relationship such that the magnitude of the chronic blood pressure response to doxazosin is well correlated with that of the acute response.

Antihypertensive efficacy

First-line treatment

Comparative clinical studies of the antihypertensive efficacy of alpha-blockers have shown that the responses are similar to other antihypertensive drugs and usually considered to be equivalent. For

Table 6.5.3 Summary of the principal results in TOMHS (adapted from Neaton [16])

Drugs	Blood pressure reduction (mmHg)	Syncope (%)	Reported impotence (%)
Chlorthalidone	22/13	0	12
Acebutolol	20/14	1	8
Doxazosin	16/12	1	0
Enalapril	18/12	2	4
Amlodipine	18/13	1	3
Placebo	11/5	4	6

example, the Treatment of Mild Hypertension Study (TOMHS) was a randomized, placebo-controlled, parallel group study in 902 patients with mild (borderline) hypertension who were treated for four years with representative agents from the major antihypertensive drug classes, including the alpha-blocker, doxazosin [16]. There were modest blood pressure reductions with all active treatments and the principal blood pressure results are summarized in Table 6.5.3. Overall, the blood pressure reductions were similar with all active treatments and significantly greater than with placebo.

Some recent doubts have been cast on the effectiveness of doxazosin as a first-line antihypertensive agent not only in terms of blood pressure reduction but also in terms of risk reduction, particularly with respect to cardiac failure and stroke prevention. In the Antihypertensive and Lipid-Lowering Treatment to Prevent Heart Attack Trial (ALLHAT) [17], patients receiving doxazosin as their initial antihypertensive drug treatment were found to have poorer blood pressure control (by ~ 2–3 mmHg for systolic blood pressure) (Figure 6.5.2) and higher incidences of heart failure and stroke, relative to chlorthalidone-based treatment (Table 6.5.4). For this reason, doxazosin has been withdrawn as a first-line treatment in this trial.

ALLHAT is the first prospective clinical outcome trial to incorporate and evaluate first line treatment with an alpha-blocker and the result is of major importance. Whilst there were no differences in the primary outcome measures of fatal coronary heart disease (CHD) or non-fatal myocardial infarction there were significant outcome differences because of higher rates for stroke and congestive heart failure and for angina and coronary revascularization procedures. Whether or not this is a simple

Table 6.5.4 ALLHAT: outcomes per 100 patients per four years

End point	Chlorthalidone (n = 15 268)	Doxazosin (n = 9067)	
Primary end points Non-fatal myocardial infarction and fatal CHD	6.3	6.26	n.s.
Secondary endpoints Total mortality	9.08	9.62	n.s.
Coronary heart disease (CHD)	11.97	13.06	$P < 0.05$
Stroke	3.61	4.23	$P < 0.04$
Cardiovascular disease (CVD) (incl. congestive cardiac failure, CCF)	21.76	25.45	$P < 0.001$

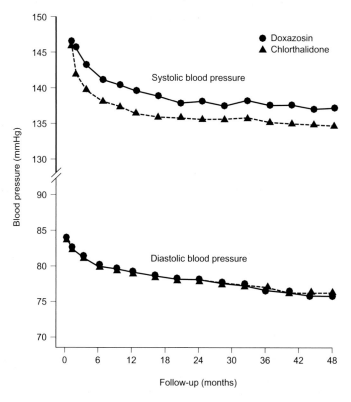

Fig. 6.5.2 Treatment blood pressure in ALLHAT: chlorthalidone vs. doxazosin.

and direct reflection of the small blood pressure difference in relatively high-risk patients remains unclear. With respect to tolerability there were some overall similarities between the two treatments. For example, the most common reasons offered by the patients for discontinuing medication during the four years of the trial were symptomatic adverse effects (20% in the chlorthalidone group and 19% in the doxazosin group), an unspecified refusal, 30% and 29% respectively, and because of abnormal laboratory values in 5% and 1% respectively. However, the target blood pressure of less than 140/90 mmHg was achieved in 64% of the chlorthalidone group, compared to 58% in the doxazosin group, and after four years of treatment the achieved blood pressures were respectively 135/76 and 137/76 mmHg.

Combination treatment regimens

As emphasized in several recent national and international guidelines, intensive treatment to provide 'tight' or optimal blood pressure control frequently requires combinations of antihypertensive drugs, particularly in high-risk patients. The preferred role of doxazosin now appears to be as a combination partner for a number of different antihypertensive drugs with the aim of improving blood pressure control. This combination role might be a particularly useful and important component of the regimens used in patients with renal impairment, for example, or with metabolic problems (particularly disorders of lipid and glucose metabolism) since other agents would be relatively contraindicated in such conditions.

Doxazosin and amlodipine

In clinical practice, usefully additive antihypertensive activity has been observed when doxazosin has been combined with representatives from other major antihypertensive drug classes. For example, a small-scale, three way double-blind crossover study in patients with moderate to severe hypertension investigated the effectiveness of amlodipine alone (10 mg daily), doxazosin alone (4 mg daily) and the combination of these two drugs [18]. There were significant additive effects with the combination, particularly on standing blood pressure, whereby an additional reduction of 10/8 mmHg was achieved with the combination, relative to amlodipine alone. There was no evidence of any significant reflex cardioacceleration nor any increased likelihood of postural hypotension.

Doxazosin and enalapril

Also of interest was a small but well-designed study investigating the combination of enalapril and doxazosin in nine hypertensive patients [19]. Standing blood pressure was reduced by 12/8 mmHg by doxazosin alone (4 mg daily) and by 9/6 mmHg with enalapril alone (20 mg daily). However, the combination of doxazosin and enalapril, with dosages constrained to respectively 1 mg and 5 mg daily, was associated with a significantly greater reduction of 23/20 mmHg ($P < 0.02$). These authors commented that the effectiveness of this combination might be particularly useful in the management of the diabetic hypertensive not only by virtue of the antihypertensive efficacy but also because of the combination of positive metabolic effects and the potential for nephroprotection. Thus, doxazosin now appears to be established as a combination partner for all antihypertensive drug treatments when blood pressure control requires to be improved.

Doxazosin as 'add-on' therapy

The usefulness and effectiveness of doxazosin as a general 'add-on' therapy was specifically studied in a double-blind, placebo-controlled study of 70 hypertensive patients who were inadequately controlled on existing treatment [20]. Sitting and standing blood pressures were significantly reduced by, on average, 12.4/4.9 and 10.5/3.8 mmHg respectively. Fatigue was the only symptomatic adverse effect which was reported significantly more often in the doxazosin group (24% vs 3%). There were small but significant reductions in LDL and total cholesterol during doxazosin treatment by approximately 4.8% and 9.1%, respectively (placebo adjusted).

6

Tolerability profile
Cardiovascular effects

The 'first-dose effect' with symptomatic orthostatic hypotension and possible syncope, accompanied by tachycardia and palpitations, is probably the most well-known adverse effect of alpha-blocking drugs. This well-recognized complication occurred on treatment initiation and was almost confined to short-acting and rapid-onset agents, particularly the prototype drug, prazosin. In retrospect, these dramatic (and worrying) hypotensive reactions were attributable to the use of unnecessarily high starting doses, particularly in patients who were salt/volume depleted or also receiving other antihypertensive treatment such as thiazide diuretics and beta-blockers. The newer agents, including doxazosin, with a more gradual onset of effect and longer duration of action, administered in initially low dosages, have minimized the risk of this dramatic early response. Unfortunately, whilst doxazosin continues to be associated to some extent with the 'bad publicity' which surrounded prazosin it is of particular interest that the incidence of syncope with doxazosin in the TOMHS study was identical to that of the other drug groups [16] (Table 6.5.3).

Effects on other systems

As with most antihypertensive drugs, non-specific upper gastrointestinal symptoms with nausea and abdominal discomfort have been reported. Similarly, drowsiness, fatigue, confusion and malaise have occasionally been reported. Because of the reputation for profound postural falls in blood pressure there have been concerns that alpha-blockers might impair cerebral perfusion particularly in elderly hypertensive. This concern has not been confirmed in clinical studies.

Alpha-blockers (particularly those with effects on the α_{1A}-receptor subtype) are well recognized to have effects on the genitourinary system. Accordingly, alpha-blockers are used for the relief of obstructive urinary symptoms in males with benign prostatic hypertrophy but, unfortunately, this predictable pharmacological effect may occasionally lead to urinary incontinence in females.

There is evidence also that male sexual dysfunction occurs less frequently with alpha-blockers than with other types of antihypertensive agent. This was seen in the TOMHS study where erectile dysfunction was reported in only 3% of patients receiving doxazosin compared to 17% of patients receiving chlorthalidone. There is no evidence that this effect can be used therapeutically although it may occasionally prove helpful to change to doxazosin treatment when a hypertensive male is having erectile problems during treatment with a thiazide diuretic.

Additional properties

With most antihypertensive drugs, claims have been made that non-hemodynamic pharmacological properties might lead to additional cardiovascular benefits. Beneficial or adverse effects on glucose and lipid metabolism have perhaps been most extensively studied but regression of left ventricular hypertrophy has often been assessed as an important surrogate index for improved cardiovascular outcome.

Metabolic effects

The small but potentially beneficial effects of alpha-blockers on glucose and lipid metabolism have been consistently identified. In fact, α_1-antagonist drugs are the only antihypertensive treatments which consistently have been shown to have beneficial effects on plasma lipid profiles with modest reductions in total and LDL-cholesterol and a small increase in HDL-cholesterol. For example, in the TOMHS study doxazosin was associated with a significant increase in the HDL/total cholesterol ratio by 2.6 compared to 1.2 with placebo ($P < 0.01$) and compared to 1.2 with acebutolol, 1.5 with amlodipine and 1.4 with chlorthalidone ($P < 0.01$). This metabolic benefit is linked to the beneficial effect which alpha-blockers have on insulin responsiveness leading to increased peripheral glucose uptake: thus, selective alpha-blockers may be particularly well suited for the treatment of the hypertensive patient with Type 2 diabetes mellitus [21,22]. Also linked to the effect on insulin responsiveness and of additional interest, was a more recent observation that doxazosin treatment in patients with CHD resulted in significant dose-dependent increases in tissue plasminogen activator (t-PA) concentration leading to a net increase in fibrinolytic potential [23]. However, whether such metabolic effects influence outcome remains uncertain.

Regression of left ventricular hypertrophy

Effective blood pressure reduction is the primary requirement for promoting the regression of left ventricular hypertrophy and whether or not different pharmacological properties lead to a greater effectiveness remains to be clearly established in clinical studies. The results of a meta-analysis indicate that treatment based upon alpha-blockers is correspondingly as effective as treatment based upon most types of antihypertensive drug [24] (Figure 6.5.3). This effect has also been demonstrated in a small study of 11 hypertensive patients over a six-month treatment period [25]. However, in this study, not only was there a significant reduction in left ventricular mass index, from 128.5 to 114 g/m² (a reduction of 12%), but left ventricular systolic and diastolic function were also shown to be improved.

Alpha-blockers in clinical practice

Alpha-blockers have the immediate attraction that there are no patient comorbidities which constitute absolute contraindications to their use. Thus, alpha-blockers can safely and appropriately be administered to hypertensive patients with concomitant disease states, such as diabetes mellitus or obstructive airway disease or renal impairment.

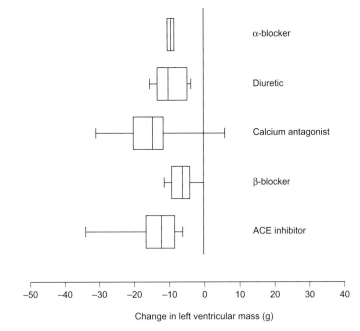

Fig. 6.5.3 Meta-analysis of the effectiveness of different types of antihypertensive drugs for promoting the regression of left ventricular hypertrophy.

Routine management of essential hypertension

Despite the improved pharmacodynamic profile with the more gradual onset and longer duration of action, alpha-blockers do not feature prominently in the list of the recommended automatic first choice agents. Additionally, whilst beneficial metabolic effects were thought to provide an added diversion for preventing CHD events there was no outcome evidence to confirm any such additional benefits. The results of ALLHAT are likely to reinforce this positioning. Thus, the current role for doxazosin (and other alpha-blockers) appears to be that of an additional treatment where improved blood pressure control is required, or as an alternative treatment where there are problems or relative contraindications to other types of antihypertensive drug, or as specific treatment in patients with metabolic derangements or in hypertensive males with prostatic problems.

Elderly hypertensives

The effectiveness of doxazosin in elderly patients, relative to young patients has been reviewed in a survey involving 1486 patients over 65 years of age. In brief, the blood pressure reduction of 23/15 mmHg in those patients aged more than 65 years was directly comparable to the reduction of 21/14 mmHg in the younger group. Importantly, this study also provided substantial support for the good overall tolerability profile of doxazosin even although the elderly group did report more frequent episodes of dizziness (10.9% vs. 5.1%). However, these authors concluded that this particular symptomatic complaint occurs more frequently in older patients in general and it did not constitute a particular problem in relation to the doxazosin treatment [26].

Diabetic hypertensives

The effectiveness of doxazosin has been compared with that of atenolol in a double-blind crossover comparative study involving 12 weeks of active treatment in hypertensive Type 1 diabetic patients. Overall, there were modest reductions in blood pressure at 12/9 mmHg with doxazosin and 12/8 mmHg with atenolol [27]. However, only during the doxazosin phase, was there any significant reduction in microalbuminuria. This potential benefit was not observed during the atenolol treatment phase. A number of other clinical studies have confirmed the effectiveness of doxazosin in the management of hypertensive Type 2 diabetic patients.

Conclusions

With particular reference to the quinazoline derivatives, no specific tissue or organ toxicity has been identified and there are no comorbid conditions which constitute contraindications to their use. The recent evidence favoring intensive blood pressure control has clearly identified the requirement for combination drug treatments if lower blood pressure targets are to be obtained. Furthermore, the evidence that patients with high levels of absolute cardiovascular risk – for example, those with diabetes mellitus or with concomitant hypercholesterolemia – benefit most from antihypertensive treatment indicates that an α_1-blocker should feature strongly in many antihypertensive treatment regimens by virtue of the favorable metabolic profile. However, it is difficult to ignore the results of ALLHAT whereby the principal antihypertensive alpha-blocker, doxazosin, should no longer be considered as a first-line agent but as an alternative or additional agent.

References

1. De Quattro V, Miura Y. Neurogenic factors in human hypertension: mechanism or myth? *Am J Med* 1973;**55**:362–378.
2. Philipp T. Sympathetic nervous systems in essential hypertension: activity and reactivity. In: *New Aspects in Hypertension: Adrenoceptors* (eds Meddeke M, Holzgreve H), pp. 91–102. Springer-Verlag: Berlin, 1986.
3. Van Zweiten PA, Timmermans PBMWM, Van Brummelen P. Role of alpha adrenoceptors in hypertension and in antihypertensive drug treatment. *Am J Med* 1984;**7**(Suppl. 4A):17–25.
4. Reid JL. Alpha-adrenoceptors in hypertension. In *Alpha and Beta Adrenoceptors and the Cardiovascular System* (eds Kobinger W, Ahlquist RP), pp. 161–171. Excerpta Medica: Amsterdam, 1984.
5. Langer SZ, Cavero I, Massingham R. Recent developments in non-adrenergic neurotransmission and its relevance to the mechanism of action of certain antihypertensive agents. *Hypertension* 1980;**2**:372–382.
6. Graham RM, Pettinger WA. Effects of prazosin and phentolamine on arterial pressure, heart rate, and renin activity. Evidence in the conscious rat for functional significance of the presynaptic alpha-blockade. *J Cardiovasc Pharamcol* 1982;**4**:44–52.

References

7. Lund-Johansen P. Haemodynamic changes at rest and during exercise in long term prazosin therapy for essential hypertension. *Postgrad Med J* 1975;**58**(Suppl.):45–52.

8. Lund-Johansen P, Omvik P, Haugland H. Acute and chronic haemodynamic effects of doxazosin in hypertension at rest and during exercise. *Br J Clin Pharmacol* 1986;**21**(Suppl. 1):45S–54S.

9. Hernandez RH, Armas de Hernandez MJ, Armas Padilla MC *et al.* Doxazosin in the treatment of arterial hypertension: its effects on exercise and spirometry. *Curr Ther Res* 1998;**43:610**(Suppl. 1):45S–54S.

10. Chung M, Vashi V, Puente J *et al.* Clinical pharmacokinetics of doxazosin in a controlled-release gastrointestinal therapeutic system (GITS) formulation. *Br J Clin Pharmacol* 1999;**48**:678–687.

11. Elliott HL, Meredith PA, Reid JL. Pharmacokinetic overview of doxazosin. *Am J Cardiol* 1987;**59**:786–818.

12. Bailey RR, Begg E, Carlson R, Sharman R. Single-dose pharmacokinetics of doxazosin in healthy volunteers and patients with renal insufficiency. *NZ Med J* 1985;**98**:248.

13. Cubeddu LX, Fuynmayor N, Caplan N, Ferry D. Clinical pharmacology of doxazosin in patients with essential hypertension. *Clin Pharmacol Ther* 1987;**41**:439–449.

14. Donnelly R, Elliott HL, Meredith PA, Reid JL. Concentration–effect relationships and individual responses to doxazosin in essential hypertension. *Br J Clin Pharmacol* 1989;**28**:517–526.

15. Meredith PA, Elliott HL, Kelman AW *et al.* Pharmacokinetic and pharmacodynamic modeling of the alpha adrenoceptor antagonist doxazosin. *Xenobiotica* 1988;**18**:123–129.

16. Neaton JD, Grimm JRH, Prineas RJ *et al.* Treatment of mild hypertension study. Final results. *J Am Med Ass* 1993;**270**:713–724.

17. The ALLHAT Collaborative Research Group. Major cardiovascular events in hypertensive patients randomised to doxazosin vs. chlorthalidone. *J Am Med Ass* 2000;**283**:1967–1975.

18. Brown MJ, Dickerson JEC. Alpha-blockade and calcium antagonism: an effective and well-tolerated combination for the treatment of resistant hypertension. *J Hypertension* 1995;**13**:701–707.

19. Brown MJ, Dickerson JEC. Synergism between α_1-blockade and angiotensin converting enzyme inhibition in essential hypertension. *J Hypertension* 1991;**6**(suppl):362–363.

20. Black HR, Sollins JS, Garofalo JL. The addition of doxazosin to the Therapeutic Regimen of Hypertensive Patients inadequately controlled with other antihypertensive medications: a randomised, placebo-controlled study. *Am J Hypertension* 2000;**13**:468–474.

21. Giorda C, Appendino M, Mason MG *et al.* Alpha-1 blocker doxazosin improves peripheral insulin sensitivity in diabetic hypertensive patients. *Metabolism* 1995;**44**:673–676.

22. Giordano M, Matsuda M, Sanders L *et al.* Effects of angiotensin-converting enzyme inhibitors, Ca^{2+} channel antagonists and alpha-adrenergic blockers on glucose and lipid metabolism in NIDDM patients with hypertension. *Diabetes* 1995;**44**:665–671.

23. Zehetgruber M, Christ G, Gabriel H *et al.* Effect of antihypertensive treatment with doxazosin on insulin sensitivity and fibrinolytic parameters. *Thromb Haemost* 1998;**79**:378–382.

24. Jennings GL, Wong J. Assessment of hypertensive organ damage. In: *Handbook of Hypertension*, Vol. 18 (eds Hansson L, Birkenhager WH). Amsterdam: Elsevier Science, 1997.

25. Agabati-Rosei E, Miuiesan ML, Eizzoni D *et al.* Reduction of left ventricular hypertrophy after long term antihypertensive treatment with doxazosin. *J Human Hypertension* 1992;**6**:9–15.

26. Langdon CG, Packard RS, Doxazosin in hypertension: results of a general practice study in 4809 patients. *Brit J Clin Prac* 1994;**48**:293–298.

27. Winocour PH. Contrasting renal and metabolic effects of alpha and beta-adrenergic blockade in mildly hypertensive Type 1 (insulin-dependent) diabetic subjects. *Nutr Metab Cardiovasc Dis* 1995;**5**:217–224.

6

Further reading

Fulton B, Wagstaff AJ, Sorkin EM. Doxazosin: an update of its clinical pharmacology and therapeutic applications in hypertension and benign hyperplasia. *Drugs* 1995;**49**:295–320.

Johnson S, Johnson FN. Doxazosin. *Rev Contemp Pharmacother* 1992; **3**(1).

6

6.6

Angiotensin II antagonists

JL Reid

6

Discovery and introduction
of angiotensin-receptor
antagonists

Discovery and introduction of angiotensin-receptor antagonists

The components of the renin–angiotensin–aldosterone system (RAAS) were first identified over a hundred years ago. The more recent elucidation of the role of the octapeptide angiotensin II in cardiovascular and renal function (see Chapter 2.3) has highlighted the contribution of angiotensin II to the pathophysiology of cardiovascular diseases including hypertension (Table 6.6.1). The potential for specific receptor blockers or antagonists to modify the action of angiotensin II was recognized in the 1970s when peptide analogs such as saralasin were synthesized and assessed both in experimental models of hypertension and in man. Such peptides were not orally absorbed, had a short duration of action and were unsuitable for use as therapeutic agents. In the late 1980s, Timmermans and colleagues [1] identified specific selective antagonists of angiotensin receptors which were orally active. Losartan (DuP 1753) which is a biphenyltetrazole was the first of these to be developed and introduced into clinical practice in 1995 as an antihypertensive agent. Subsequently, a large number of structures largely based on the same biphenyltetrazole lead compound have been identified [2,3]. Several are now available worldwide for clinical use (Table 6.6.2). During the development of these agents it was recognized that angiotensin II bound to at least two distinct subtypes of receptors [1]. This receptor heterogeneity is common for other classes of hormone and neurotransmitters (Table 6.6.3). All the previously known actions of angiotensin II including growth-promoting and trophic effects were found to be mediated by the AT_1 subtype [4]. The AT_2 subtype is now recognized to be expressed during early fetal development and in response to injury [5]. The AT_2 receptor may exert antigrowth, antiproliferation or pro-apoptotic actions. It should be emphasized that all the angiotensin-receptor antagonists currently available for clinical use have high AT_1 subtype selectivity.

The RAAS pathway is summarized in Figure 6.6.1. Angiotensin II can be generated in the circulation where it plays a circulating humoral role.

Table 6.6.1 Actions of angiotensin II

Tissue affected	Action
Artery	Stimulates contraction and growth
Adrenal zona glomerulosa	Stimulates secretion of aldosterone
Kidney	Inhibits release of renin
	Increases tubular reabsorption of sodium
	Stimulates vasoconstriction (angiotensin II more potent at efferent than afferent arteriole)
	Releases prostaglandins
Brain	Stimulates thirst and the release of vasopressin
Sympathetic nervous system	Increases central sympathetic outflow
	Facilitates peripheral sympathetic transmission
	Increases adrenal release of epinephrine
Heart	Increases contractility and heart rate
	Hypertrophy and remodeling
	Increase of collagen and matrix

Table 6.6.2 Angiotensin II receptor antagonists in clinical development

Generic	Compound	Company	Status
Losartan	Dup 753	Dupont Merck Pharmaceutical	Marketed 1994
Valsartan	CGP48933	Ciba-Geigy	Marketed 1996
Candesartan	TCV-116	Takeda/Astra	Marketed 1997
Irbesartan	SR-47436/BMS186295	Sanofi/BMS	Marketed 1997
Telmisartan	BIBR277	Boehringer Ingelheim	Marketed 1998
Eprosartan	SKF108566	Smith Kline Beecham	Phase III
Tasosartan	ANA-756	Wyeth Ayerst	Withdrawn
	E-4177	Elsa	Phase II
	SC-52458	Monsanto (Searle)	Phase II
	HN-65021	Halslund Nycomed	Phase II
	UP-2696	BMS (UPSA)	Phase II
	LR-B/081	Lusotarmaco (Menarini)	Phase II
	L-158,282/	Merck	Phase II
	GR-138950MK-996		Phase II

Table 6.6.3 Classification criteria of angiotensin-receptor subtypes

Property	AT_1	AT_2
Potency order	Angiotensin II > angiotensin III	Angiotensin II = angiotensin III
Selective agonists	L162017	CGP 42112
Selective antagonists	Losartan	PD 123177
	(Dup 753)	PD 123319
	SKF 108566	CGP 42112A
	EXP 3174	Partial agonist
Effector pathways	↑ Phospholipase C	↓ Guanylate
	↑ Phospholipase D	Cyclase
	↓ Adenylate cyclase	Regulation of ion currents
		Tyrosine
		Phosphorylation
Sensitivity to dithiothreitol (sulphydryl reducing agents)	↓ Binding	↑ Binding

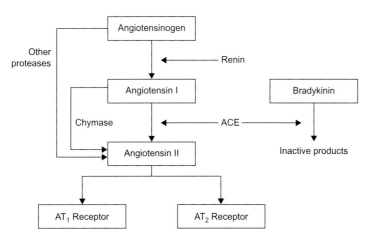

Fig. 6.6.1 Summary of renin–angiotensin–aldosterone system showing alternative pathways and the interaction with bradykinin.

6.6

Discovery and introduction
of angiotensin-receptor
antagonists

It can also be formed in many tissues where it appears to exert local autocrine or paracrine effects. Although the classical pathway of angiotensin II generation is via the decapeptide angiotensin I and subsequent cleavage by angiotensin-converting enzyme (ACE), there is increasing evidence for alternative non-ACE pathways including chymase [6]. These pathways appear to be of particular importance in man in tissues such as heart and blood vessels. The relevance of these non-ACE alternative pathways has still to be fully elucidated. One important therapeutic implication is that ACE inhibition may never be able to fully prevent the generation of angiotensin II and its actions. The alternative approach of angiotensin-receptor antagonism will block angiotensin II effects however it is generated. This is an important pharmacological difference between ACE inhibitors and angiotensin-receptor antagonists. Another difference is the recruitment of bradykinin effects with ACE inhibitors. ACE is identical to kininase II which breaks down bradykinin. An inevitable consequence of ACE inhibition is potentiation of the effects of endogenous and exogenous bradykinin. Angiotensin-receptor antagonists do not directly modify bradykinin metabolism. There is debate as to the therapeutic benefits or drawbacks of these bradykinin effects. In clinical studies it appears that bradykinin may be responsible for some adverse effects of ACE inhibitors including cough [7,8] and angio-oedema. Potential benefits of bradykinin including contributions to blood pressure lowering, and cardiac remodeling have been claimed in animal studies but not convincingly confirmed to date in clinical trials. However, bradykinin does contribute to the acute hypotensive effects of ACE inhibitors in man at least. The similarities and differences between ACE inhibition and angiotensin receptor blockade as practical therapeutic strategies are discussed further below.

At present several angiotensin-receptor blockers are licensed for use in hypertension (and less widely for heart failure). Recently angiotensin-receptor antagonists have been added to the list of possible first-line agents recommended for the treatment of hypertension by the WHO/ISH Working Party [9]. These drugs differ in a numbers of ways (see Table 6.6.4). However, all the clinically available agents (or their

Table 6.6.4 Pharmacological characteristics of clinically available angiotensin II (AT$_1$) receptor antagonists

Drug (active metabolite)	Relative AT$_1$ receptor affinity	Bioavailability	Food effect	Active metabolite	Plasma half-life (h)	Protein binding (%)	Dosage (mg)
Losartan (EXP 3174)	50 (10)	33%	Minimal	Yes	2 (6–9)	98.7 (99.8)	50–100 daily
Valsartan	10	25%	↓ 40–50%	No	6	95.0	80–320 daily
Candesartan (CV-11974)	280 (1)	42%	No	Yes	3.5–4 (3–11)	99.5	4–32 daily
Irbesartan	5	70%	No	No	11–15	> 90 (?)	150–300 daily
Telmisartan	10	n/a	n/a	No	~24	n/a	40–120 daily

n/a: not available.

metabolites) show insurmountable antagonism, a property which probably contributes to the long duration of action and successful once-daily dosing regimen of these agents. To date, there have been few pharmacological differences between these agents as far as angiotensin II blocking properties are concerned. However, losartan alone and not EXP.3174 or any of the others, has a well-documented uricosuric action which is independent of angiotensin II receptor mechanisms [10]. Uric acid levels in blood are lowered with long-term losartan. The therapeutic relevance is debatable but uric acid is re-emerging as an independent risk factor for cardiovascular disease [11].

Efficacy of angiotensin-receptor antagonists

Reduction of blood pressure is the essential feature of an effective antihypertensive drug. Blood pressure should be lowered throughout the dose interval and the onset and offset of effect should be gradual without dramatic swings in pressure. The antihypertensive effect must be maintained on long-term therapy. The clinically available angiotensin-receptor antagonists meet these criteria. Large-scale placebo-controlled trials have confirmed efficacy in the short and longer term [12,13]. Like other classes of antihypertensives, the fall observed depends on the magnitude of the starting blood pressure, and only 40–50% of mild–moderate hypertension (diastolic blood pressure 95–105 mmHg) will achieve targets of less than 90 mmHg with monotherapy. Large-scale, appropriately powered, comparative trials confirm that angiotensin-receptor antagonists are at least as effective in lowering blood pressure as beta-blockers, calcium antagonists, diuretics and ACE inhibitors when each is used in optimally titrated doses [12]. Three large trials comparing valsartan, candesartan and losartan to enalapril showed very similar efficacy in terms of the trough reduction in diastolic blood pressure [14–16] (Figure 6.6.2).

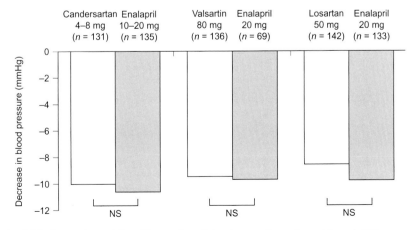

Fig. 6.6.2 Comparison of the efficacy of angiotensin-receptor antagonists and ACE inhibitors. (After [14]–[16].)

6

> **BOX 6.6.1 Within-class efficacy of angiotensin-receptor antagonists**
>
> Any review of efficacy (and safety) of angiotensin-receptor antagonists is dominated by the quantity of data from losartan compared to the others. This is inevitable as losartan was the first to be developed and was introduced several years before valsartan and even longer before the other agents. However, as far as efficacy is concerned, especially comparative efficacy overall, there is an homogeneity in the findings for the class [17]. Dose-ranging studies have identified for each agent the usual starting dose and in most cases a recommended dose increase to a higher dose. Angiotensin-receptor antagonists as a class do not show a steep dose–response at least within the limited range used to treat hypertension.

Once-daily dosing has been justified for these drugs based on ambulatory blood pressure (ABP) studies (Figure 6.6.3) [18]. In addition, using routine blood pressure measurements during controlled trials where the peak effect (usually 4–6 hours after dosing) and trough effect (at 22–24 hours after dosing and thus before the next dose) are recorded and the ratio (or per cent) of trough to peak effect is compared. A ratio of less than 0.5 or less than 50% suggests unacceptable fluctuation between doses and unsuitability of the selected (24-hour) dose interval. For losartan these ratios averaged over 0.7 (over 70%) for several controlled trials with 50 and 100 mg once daily (Table 6.6.5) [19].

Efficacy has been compared in men and women and in younger and older patients without evidence of any clinically relevant differences [12]. Angiotensin-receptor antagonists have been assessed in most ethnic groups and are effective in caucasian and orientals, but may be less effective as monotherapy in Afro-Americans, although there is only limited data available.

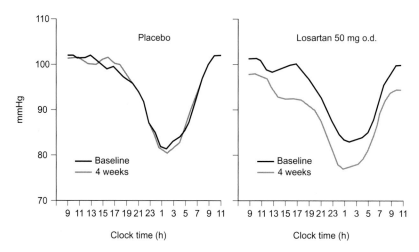

Fig. 6.6.3 Losartan – mean hourly diastolic blood pressure profiles. (Redrawn from Weber *et al.* [18].)

Table 6.6.5 Trough : peak ratio in double-blind studies of oral losartan once daily

Dose	Patients (*n*)	Trough : peak ratio (%)
50 mg	77	60
	93	87
	121	78
	122	73
50 mg and 100 mg	113	73
100 mg	86	72
Total	**612**	**74**

There is no evidence that angiotensin-receptor antagonists are relatively or absolutely contraindicated in any special patient population or group apart from pregnancy and patients with established or suspected unilateral renal artery stenosis. In these later conditions as with severe salt- and water-depletion angiotensin-receptor antagonists, like ACE inhibitors, should be avoided. In any clinical states where the RAAS is activated there may be an excessive fall in blood pressure associated with reversible impairment of renal function. However, angiotensin-receptor antagonists are safe and can be very useful in patients with chronic renal disease including diabetic nephropathy where they appear to exert similar renal protective effects to ACE inhibitors [20].

A corollary of the enhanced efficacy of angiotensin-receptor antagonists in the presence of an activated RAAS in that combination with low-dose thiazide diuretic (which activates the RAAS) enhances efficacy of angiotensin-receptor antagonists and may improve blood pressure control and achieve target pressure levels [21]. The increased antihypertensive effect achieved by adding low-dose thiazides to the starting dose of an angiotensin II antagonist, is significantly greater than the blood pressure lowering observed by increasing the dose of the receptor antagonist (Figure 6.6.4). If more stringent (lower) target

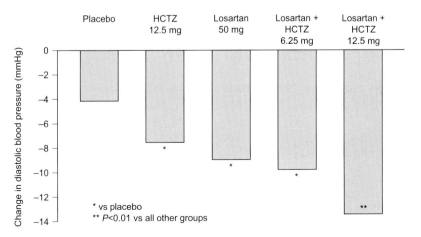

Fig. 6.6.4 Losartan and hydrochlorothiazide (HCTZ) alone and in combination. Change in diastolic blood pressure. (Redrawn from Mackay *et al.* [27].)

blood pressures are to result from the findings of the Hypertension Optimum Treatment (HOT) Study [22], then the combination of angiotensin-receptor antagonist with low-dose diuretic may be a very useful therapeutic option when monotherapy fails to achieve the goal (as may be the case in some ≥ 50% of patients).

Safety of angiotensin-receptor antagonists

Angiotensin-receptor antagonists have to date shown no 'class' side effects or any evidence of long-term toxicity. Early controlled trials undertaken for registration purposes showed a low level of complaints attributed to treatment [12]. In the case of losartan, the frequency of adverse effect was actually marginally lower than placebo-treated patients. This has been a consistent feature of the class. Good tolerability as indicated by low frequency of potentially drug-attributable side effects, has also been observed with longer term follow up in controlled trials. It appears that the low frequency of side effects translates into improved patient acceptability. Retrospective analysis of large data bases monitoring prescriptions for antihypertensive drugs for patients in US Health Maintenance Organizations indicates not only that patients on angiotensin-receptor antagonists are more likely to be compliant with medication but there is a significantly higher rate of persistence on the first drug prescribed at the end of one year compared to other drug classes [23]. The implication of higher persistency and compliance is more effective long-term blood pressure control and thus greater potential to improved long-term outcome.

One particular side effect of ACE inhibitors, the persistent dry cough which may afflict 10–20% of patients, does not occur with angiotensin-receptor antagonists. Several trials have unequivocally confirmed that the cough induced by ACE inhibitors does not recur with angiotensin-receptor antagonists any more frequently than it does with placebo or an active control of a thiazide diuretic (Table 6.6.6) [7,8]. These trials indicate that the ACE inhibitor cough is not related to angiotensin mechanisms and probably a consequence of bradykinin or other non-angiotensin vasoactive peptides.

Table 6.6.6 Angiotensin II receptor antagonists and cough in patients with ACE inhibitor-induced cough

Treatment	Patients (*n*)	Cough (%)
Lacourciere *et al.* [7]		
Losartan	48	29
Lisinopril	46	72*
Hydrochlorothiazide	41	34
Benz *et al.* [8]		
Valsartan	42	20
Lisinopril	45	69*
Hydrochlorothiazide	42	19

*$P < 0.01$ when lisinopril is compared to the other groups.

Angiotensin II antagonists

Effects on outcome of
long-term treatment with
angiotensin-receptor
antagonists

Effects on outcome of long-term treatment with angiotensin-receptor antagonists

Conclusions about long-term effects require long-term experience. This is a recently introduced class of drugs. While studies are underway to explore the effect of treatment on morbidity and mortality in hypertension [24], the results of these trials will not be available for some years. Meanwhile, there are promising results from studies of intermediate endpoints including reversal of left ventricular hypertrophy [25] as well as observations on outcome in heart failure. Intermediate endpoints in both cases, there are indications that angiotensin-receptor antagonists can favorably modify these 'targets' at least to a similar extent to ACE inhibitors and other drug classes (Figure 6.6.2). Preliminary observations are supported by experimental studies in animal models. Small studies confirm that angiotensin-receptor antagonists lower blood pressure and reduce proteinuria to a similar extent to ACE inhibitors in patients with renal disease (Figure 6.6.5) [20].

It is premature to conclude whether there are clinically meaningful differences between classes let alone within the class in effects on left ventricular hypertrophy or proteinuria. However, several large-scale comparative trials are currently underway which will assess outcome in patients with increased risk such as left ventricular hypertrophy or diabetes. These long-term trials in patients with target organ damage have the statistical power to assess cardiovascular outcome. They will be completed in the next few years. To date the only information on long-term outcome after angiotensin-receptor antagonists comes from trials in heart failure [26]. The Evaluation of Losartan in the Elderly (ELITE) trial reported a significantly better outcome which was largely due to a reduction in sudden death in older patients with heart failure treated with losartan compared to the ACE inhibitor captopril.

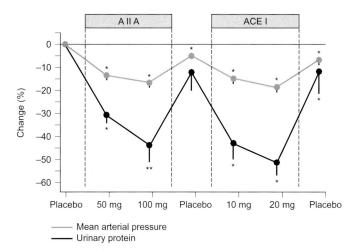

Fig. 6.6.5 The effects of angiotensin II antagonism (AIIA) (losartan) and ACE inhibition (ACEI) (enalapril) on blood pressure and proteinuria. (From Gansvoort *et al.* [20] with permission.)

Effects on outcome of
long-term treatment with
angiotensin-receptor
antagonists

Present role of
angiotensin-receptor
antagonists in
hypertension treatment

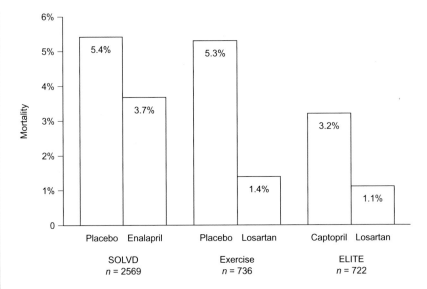

Fig. 6.6.6 Three-month mortality in heart failure studies (SOLVD, Exercise, ELITE) (From Pitt *et al.* [26] with permission.)

As outcome was only a secondary objective of the study which was not statistically powered to examine this endpoint, these conclusions await confirmation in a further larger *ELITE II* trial recently concluded. However, the mortality after three months in another losartan heart failure trial was also reduced compared to placebo (Figure 6.6.6). There is a strong internal consistency in the direction and magnitude of the results of these trials and a previously published trial of enalapril in heart failure (SOLVD). A conservative conclusion from present losartan experience is that the angiotensin-receptor antagonist is at least as effective in heart failure as the established ACE inhibitors captopril and enalapril.

Present role of angiotensin-receptor antagonists in hypertension treatment

Angiotensin-receptor antagonists are the newest class of drugs available to treat hypertension. As with any new development it takes time for practising doctors to identify their optimal role and use. Although losartan has been available for over six years in many countries and has subsequently been joined by at least four other agents, in some countries, notably Japan, the class has only been introduced recently. In the early years while clinical experience was being consolidated it was not unreasonable to reserve the new class for groups of patients who are poor responders or intolerant of other classes. Angiotensin-receptor antagonists are particularly indicated in patients who cannot tolerate ACE inhibitors because of cough. However, with further experience it is increasingly unjustified to reserve this very well tolerated and effective class to treatment failures and/or patients with side effects. In recent years, losartan and other angiotensin-receptor antagonists have been increasingly used as a first-line, first-choice, agents in their own right. The recent WHO/ISH Guidelines on Treatment of Hypertension recognize this by affording the new class the status of alternative first-step treatment (along with diuretics, beta-blockers, ACE inhibitors, calcium-channel blockers and alpha-blockers) [9].

As experience with the new class builds up, it is increasingly clear that good tolerability remains a key feature. Efficacy of monotherapy is similar to other first-line agents. In particular, efficacy of receptor antagonists is similar to those of ACE inhibitors – but without the side effect of cough. If there are any real clinical advantages or disadvantages in the long term of either bradykinin potentiation with ACE inhibitors or receptor blockade, these are not yet apparent but should emerge from the ongoing outcome trials.

Finally, at this stage is there any evidence of clinically important differences emerging between available agents within the angiotensin-receptor antagonist class? There are clearly differences in potency which require careful dose selection and adjustment to permit meaningful comparisons [1]. The introduction of a new class of drugs by several different companies not surprisingly has led to intense marketing activities. There is a tendency to highlight minor differences and exploit aberrant findings from small-scale trials. These strategies lead to claim and counter claim. They generate much 'heat' but little 'light'. An overview of the available published trials in over 6000 patients shows no statistical (or clinically meaningful) differences between the currently available angiotensin-receptor antagonists [17]. The fall in systolic and diastolic pressure is very similar at the usual starting doses. Very similar falls are observed with all agents when the higher doses are compared. In all cases, the addition of low-dose diuretic leads to a far greater response. Again, the blood pressure fall is similar with all the available antagonists from the class. Are there any groups or special populations where angiotensin-receptor antagonists are particularly useful? Are there any emerging contraindications? Angiotensin-receptor antagonists are effective in men and women, older and younger patients and are well tolerated, there is no reason to limit their use to specific populations. There are few relative or absolute contraindications or concomitant conditions apart from pregnancy or unilateral renal artery stenosis discussed above. The vast majority of patients are suitable for a treatment regimen based on an angiotensin-receptor antagonist with addition of low-dose diuretic where required for additional efficacy.

References

1. Timmermans P, Wong PC, Chin AT. Angiotensin II receptors and angiotensin II receptor antagonists. *Pharmacol Rev* 1993;**45**:205–251.
2. MacFadyen RJ, Reid JL. Angiotensin receptor antagonists as a treatment for hypertension. *J Hypertension* 1994;**12**:1333–1338.
3. Johnston CI. Angiotensin receptor antagonists: focus on losartan. *Lancet* 1995;**346**:1403–1407.

References

4. Goodfriend TL, Elliott ME, Catt KY. Angiotensin receptors and their antagonists. *N Engl J Med* 1996;**334**:1646–1654.
5. Dzau VJ, Mukoyama M, Pratt RE. Molecular biology of angiotensin II receptors: target for drug research? *J Hypertension* 1994;**12**:S1–S5.
6. Urata H, Nishimura, Ganten D. Chymase dependent angiotensin II forming system in humans. *Am J Hypertension* 1996;**9**:277–284.
7. Lacouciere Y, Brunner H, Irwin R *et al*. Effect of modulators on the renin angiotensin system on cough. *J Hypertension* 1994;**12**:1387–1393.
8. Benz J, Hofmann A. Valsartan, a new angiotensin II receptor antagonist: a double blind study comparing the incidence of cough with lisinopril and hydrochlorothiazide. *J Clin Pharmacol* 1997;**37**:101–107
9. 1999 Guidelines Committee World Health Organization – International Society of Hypertension Guidelines for the management of hypertension. *J Hypertension* 1999;**17**:151–183.
10. Burnier M, Rutschmann B, Nussberger J *et al*. Salt dependent renal effects of an angiotensin II antagonist in healthy subjects. *Hypertension* 1993;**22**:339–347.
11. Ward HJ. Uric acid as an independent risk factor in the treatment of hypertension. *Lancet* 1998;**352**:670–671.
12. McIntyre M, Caffe SE, Michalak RA, Reid JL. Losartan, an orally active angiotensin (AT$_1$) receptor antagonist. *Pharmacol Therapeut* 1997;**74**:181–194.
13. Oparil S, Dyke S, Harris F *et al*. The efficacy and safety of valsartan compared to placebo in the treatment of patients with essential hypertension. *Clin Therapeut* 1996;**18**:797–810.
14. Holwerda NJ, Fogari R, Angeli P *et al*. Valsartan, a new angiotensin II antagonist for treatment of essential hypertension: efficacy and safety compound with placebo and enalapril. *J Hypertension* 1996;**14**:1147–1151.
15. Zanchetti A, Ombon S, Di Biagio C. Candesartan, cilexetil and enalapril are of equivalent efficacy in patients with mild to moderate hypertension. *J Human Hypertension* **2**(Suppl. 2):S57–S60.
16. Tikkanen I, Omvik P, Jensen HA. Comparison of the angiotensin II antagonist losartan with the angiotensin converting enzyme inhibitor enalapril in patients with essential hypertension. *J Hypertension* 1995;**13**:1343–1351.
17. Conlin P, Spence JD, Williams B *et al*. Angiotensin II antagonists for hypertension: are there differences in efficacy? *Am J Hypertension* 1999;**13**:418–426.
18. Weber MA, Byyny RL, Pratt JH *et al*. Blood pressure effects of the angiotensin II receptor blocker losartan. *Arch Intern Med* 1995;**155**:405–411.
19. Elliott HL, Meredith PA. Clinical implications of the trough : peak ratio. *Blood Press Monitor* **1**(Suppl. 1):S47–S51.
20. Gansevoort RT, de Zeeuw D, de Jong PE. Is the antiproteinuric effect of ACE inhibition mediated by interference with the renin angiotensin system? *Kidney Int* 1994;**45**:861–867.
21. Soffer BA, Wright JT, Pratt JH *et al*. Effect of losartan on a background of hydrochlorothiazide in patients with hypertension. *Hypertension* 1993;**26**:112–117.
22. Hansson L, Zanchetti A, Carruthers SG *et al*. Effects of intensive blood pressure lowering and low dose aspirin in patients with hypertension: principal results of the Hypertension Optimal Treatment (HOT) randomized trial. *Lancet* 1993;**351**:1755–1762.
23. Bloom BS. Contribution of initial antihypertensive medication after 1 year of therapy. *Clin Therapeut* 1998;**20**:1–11.
24. Dahlof B, Devereux RB, Julius S *et al*. Characteristics of 9194 patients with left ventricular hypertrophy – The LIFE Study. *Hypertension* 1998; **32**:989–997.
25. Himmelmann A, Svensson A, Berglrant A, Hansson L. Long term effects of losartan on blood pressure and left ventricular function in essential hypertension. *J Human Hypertension* 1996;**10**:729–734.
26. Pitt B, Segal R, Martinez FA *et al*. Randomized trial of losartan versus captopril in patients over 65 with heart failure (Evaluation of Losartan in Elderly Study (ELITE)). *Lancet* 1997;**349**:747–752.
27. Mackay JH, Arcuri KE, Goldberg AI *et al*. Losartan and low dose hydrochlorothiazide in patients with essential hypertension. *Arch Intern Med* 1996;**156**:278–285.

6.7

Centrally acting antihypertensive drugs

PA van Zwieten

6

6.7

Introduction

Several receptors and neurotransmitters in the brain are involved in the regulation of peripheral blood pressure. However, only two of these receptor types are the targets of clinically used antihypertensive drugs.

Classic centrally acting antihypertensives, such as clonidine, guanfacine and α-methyldopa (via its active metabolite α-methylnorepinephrine) are agonists of α_2-adrenoceptors in the brainstem. Stimulation of these α_2-adrenoceptors causes peripheral sympathoinhibition and hence a fall of (elevated) blood pressure. These agents are effective antihypertensives with a favorable hemodynamic profile. However, their subjective side effects are unpleasant, thus influencing patient compliance in an unfavorable manner. For this reason they have lost much of their attraction and they can hardly or no longer compete with newer antihypertensives such as ACE inhibitors, the newer calcium antagonists and angiotensin II-receptor antagonists, which are also effective and much better tolerated than the classic α_2-adrenoceptor stimulants.

More recently a new type of centrally acting antihypertensives, the imidazoline (I_1)-receptor agonists has been introduced and developed clinically. Moxonidine and rilmenidine (Figure 6.7.1) are the prototypes of this newer category of centrally acting antihypertensives. They also cause peripheral sympathoinhibition, triggered by a central mechanism, but it may be hoped that their profile of side effects is more favorable than that of clonidine and α-methyldopa, owing to their weaker affinity for α_2-adrenoceptors. This latter receptor subtype is assumed to mediate the well-known side effects of the classic α_2-adrenoceptor stimulants, such as sedation, dry mouth and impotence.

BOX 6.7.1 Various types of centrally acting antihypertensives

- **Classic agents**
  α-methyldopa (α_2-agonist)
  Prodrug, acts via its active metabolite (α-methylnorepinephrine) effective antihypertensive, but not very well tolerated (sedation, dry mouth, impotence)
  Safe in pregnant women
  clonidine ($\alpha_2 + I_1$-agonist)
  Potent antihypertensive, but not very well tolerated (sedation, dry mouth, impotence)
  Risk of withdrawal phenomenon

- **Newer agents**: *imidazoline (I_1)-receptor agonists moxonidine and rilmenidine)*
  I_1-agonists, with lower affinity for α_2-adrenoceptors effective antihypertensives
  Better side-effect profile than the classic agents, no withdrawal phenomenon.

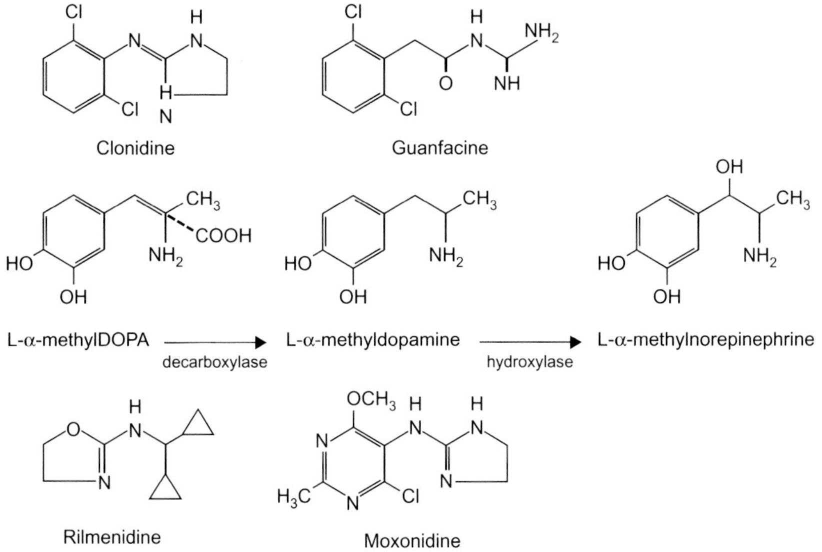

Fig. 6.7.1 Chemical structures of the various types of centrally acting antihypertensives.

Mode of action

The stimulation of central α_2-adrenoceptors in the region of the nucleus tractus solitarii (NTS) by clonidine or α-methylmorepinephrine (the active metabolite of α-methyldopa) causes sympathoinhibition in the periphery and hence a fall of (elevated) blood pressure. The plasma level of catecholamines is reduced. The stimulation of peripheral presynaptic α_2-adrenoceptors may contribute to the lowering of plasma norepinephrine levels and possibly also to the antihypertensive action.

Clonidine is a stimulant of both α_2-adrenoceptors and imidazoline (I_1)-receptors, and it therefore simultaneously triggers two mechanisms which both cause sympathoinhibition in the periphery. More selective imidazoline receptor agonists such as moxonidine and rilmenidine activate I_1-receptors in the region of the rostroventrolateral medulla (RVLM) and hence decrease the firing rate of the bulbospinal sympathoexcitatory neurons, thus causing peripheral sympathoinhibition, and a fall in blood pressure.

Accordingly, the stimulation of both α_2- and I_1-receptors in the central nervous system induces reduced activity of the peripheral sympathetic nervous system. It is very likely that the same final neuronal pathway of sympathoinhibition is involved, although the initial stimulation is triggered by two different populations of receptors in the central nervous system.

A schematic overview is shown in Figure 6.7.2. The receptor profiles of the most important drugs are listed in Table 6.7.1.

6

403

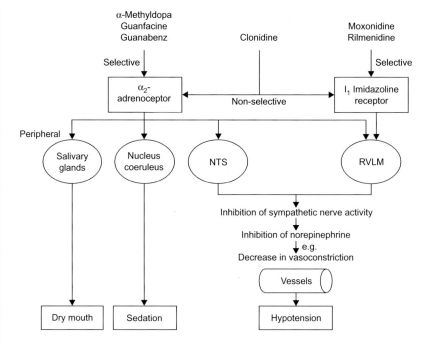

Fig. 6.7.2 Central antihypertensive mechanisms of various types of centrally acting antihypertensive drugs. Note the different targets of α_2-adrenoceptor agonists and I_1-imidazoline stimulants. The adverse reactions, dry mouth and sedation, are mediated by α_2-adrenoceptors but not by I_1-imidazoline receptors. NTS = nucleus tractus solitarii; RVLM = rostral ventrolateral medulla.

Table 6.7.1 Central nervous system receptors as targets of centrally acting antihypertensives

Compound	Receptors
α-Methyldopa*	α_2
Guanfacine	α_2
Guanabenz	α_2
Clonidine**	$\alpha_2 + I_1$
Moxonidine	$I_1 > \alpha_2$
Rilmenidine	$I_1 > \alpha_2$

* Through α-methylnorepinephrine.
** Mixed agonist.

Advantages and disadvantages of centrally acting antihypertensives

Pathophysiological considerations

Although complex, and not known in full detail, there exists a relationship between the centrally modulated, activated sympathetic nervous system and hypertensive disease. In more general terms sympathetic activation, as reflected by a high heart rate and elevated plasma catecholamine levels, is considered as a risk factor and therefore also as a potential target for drug treatment. This not only involves hypertensive disease, but also congestive heart failure and the recently recognized pathologic entity called 'the metabolic syndrome'. These arguments and assumptions would favor the use of centrally acting antihypertensives as a logical approach in drug treatment, based on the centrally triggered process of sympathoinhibition. Accordingly, centrally acting drugs causing peripheral sympathoinhibition are considered to approach to a certain degree a partly causative treatment of essential hypertension, congestive heart failure and the aforementioned metabolic syndrome.

Hemodynamic profiles

Another potential advantage of the centrally acting antihypertensives is offered by their hemodynamic profiles. The hemodynamic profiles of clonidine (and related drugs) and α-methyldopa may be briefly characterized as follows. The classic α_2-adrenoceptor agonists cause vasodilatation in the resistance vessels and hence reduce peripheral vascular resistance. For this reason (elevated) blood pressure is reduced. Heart rate remains unchanged or may be somewhat reduced. Cardiac output remains unchanged. Accordingly, in spite of the vasodilator action reflex tachycardia does not occur, probably as a result of the centrally induced sympathoinhibition in the periphery.

Single-dose studies with moxonidine and rilmenidine have shown that both centrally acting drugs are predominantly arterial vasodilators which reduce peripheral vascular resistance, in particular when this parameter is elevated, as in hypertensive patients (see Figure 6.7.3). A reduction in peripheral resistance is also found during long-term treatment of hypertension. Also during exercise both drugs cause vasodilatation and a reduction of peripheral vascular resistance.

The vasodilator and antihypertensive activities of both moxonidine and rilmenidine are clearly caused by sympathoinhibition, as reflected by a lowering of plasma norepinephrine levels. Moxonidine also caused

6

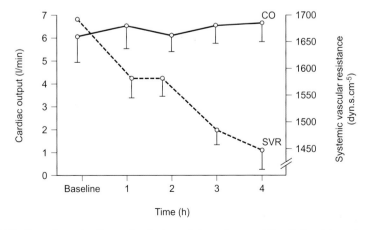

Fig. 6.7.3 Hemodynamic effects of a single oral dose of moxonidine (0.4 mg) in male patients (38–65 years; $n = 10$) with essential hypertension (WHO grade I or II). Systemic vascular resistance (SVR) is significantly reduced (* = $P < 0.01$), whereas cardiac output (CO) remains unchanged. From BNC Prichard, *The I_1-Imidazoline Receptor Agonist Moxonidine*, pp. 31–47. Royal Society of Medicine Press: London, 1996.

a reduction of plasma renin activity, whereas plasma concentrations of epinephrine, angiotensin II, aldosterone and atrial natriuretic peptide were not significantly diminished. Long-term treatment with both moxonidine and rilmenidine is associated with a partial regression of left ventricular hypertrophy (LVH). For moxonidine, a certain restoration of the impaired coronary vasodilator reserve (CVR) in hypertensives was found after 9–12 months of treatment.

These hemodynamic profiles of the two types of centrally acting antihypertensives are, at least on theoretical grounds, attractive in the treatment of hypertensive disease. In this connection it should be realized that elevated peripheral vascular resistance is the most consistent hemodynamic alteration observed in all types of established hypertensive disease. Accordingly, a reduction in peripheral resistance should be considered as a logical hemodynamic approach in the drug treatment of hypertension.

Antihypertensive efficacy

The antihypertensive efficacy of both the α_2-adrenoceptor agonists and the imidazoline (I_1)-receptor stimulants is beyond any doubt and has been confirmed in large numbers of patients with essential hypertension. Tachyphylaxis is not observed on long-term treatment. As stated previously, clonidine and α-methyldopa have lost much of their importance in the treatment of essential hypertension.

Clonidine may still be used in anesthesiology in order to suppress perioperative hypertension. α-Methyldopa is still sometimes used in the treatment of hypertension during pregnancy, because it is one of the few drugs for which safety in this condition has been documented by means of a clinical study.

Moxonidine and rilmenidine are effective antihypertensives in various types of patients of both genders, including those older than 65 years. Both moxonidine and rilmenidine can be administered once daily in order to achieve satisfactory 24-hour control of blood pressure. Both agents can be combined with several other types of antihypertensives. In comparative studies, moxonidine and rilmenidine proved as effective as low dose diuretics, beta-blockers, ACE inhibitors and calcium antagonists.

BOX 6.7.2 Potential advantages of centrally acting antihypertensives

- **Advantages**
  Hemodynamic profile
  Reduction of peripheral vascular resistance: no change in heart rate; circulatory reflexes remain intact; peripheral sympathoinhibition; regression of left ventricular hypertrophy.
  Metabolic aspects
  Lipid/glucose neutral; antagonism of the 'metabolic syndrome'.
  Drug combinations
  Effective antihypertensives, can be combined with virtually all other types of antihypertensive drugs.

BOX 6.7.2 *Continued*

- **Disadvantages**
  Side effects: sedation, dry mouth and withdrawal phenomenon (clonidine only).
  Moxonidine and rilmenidine (I_1 agonists) are better than clonidine with less sedation, less mouth dryness and no withdrawal phenomenon.

Adverse reactions

As mentioned before, the main disadvantages of the α_2-adrenoceptor stimulants are associated with their unpleasant adverse reactions. Sedation, dry mouth as a result of reduced salivary flow, and sexual impotence are well-known side effects of clonidine, guanfacine and α-methyldopa. These side effects, although not dangerous, are generally experienced as unpleasant and they therefore exert a negative influence on patient compliance. They are predominantly mediated by α_2-adrenoceptors located in regions other than those involved in the antihypertensive activity of these drugs.

Dry mouth, fatigue and drowsiness are also the most frequently reported side effects for the I_1-receptor stimulants moxonidine and rilmenidine. However, the incidence of these side effects of the I_1-stimulants appears to be significantly less than known to occur for clonidine. For treatment with rilmenidine, it has been claimed that dry mouth and drowsiness were the same as experienced by comparable patients on placebo. In more refined psychomotor tests, rilmenidine did not impair alertness.

Although it seems very likely that the incidence and severity of adverse reactions to moxonidine and rilmenidine are considerably less than those of clonidine or α-methyldopa, appropriately designed trials to quantitatively compare the side-effect profiles of both types of drugs remain to be performed. Both moxonidine and rilmenidine appear to be safe in patients with chronic obstructive pulmonary disease, diabetes mellitus or depression.

Clonidine rebound effect

The abrupt cessation of clonidine treatment, especially after prolonged use of high doses, may provoke a rebound phenomenon which is associated with sympathetic hyperactivation. Such a rebound phenomenon has never been reported for the cessation of moxonidine or rilmenidine treatment, and neither could it be evoked in animal models where the clonidine-rebound phenomenon could be demonstrated. Both moxonidine and rilmenidine are considered to be neutral with respect to plasma lipids. Blood glucose levels are unchanged by rilmenidine treatment, whereas under certain conditions moxonidine may even lower glucose levels via a combination of central and peripheral mechanisms.

6

Advantages and
disadvantages of centrally
acting antihypertensives

Adverse reactions

BOX 6.7.3 Interactions of centrally acting antihypertensive drugs with other drugs

- Interactions between centrally acting antihypertensives of both α_2-adrenoceptor agonists and I_1-receptor stimulants and other drugs are the following:
- The sedative effect is enhanced by a variety of drugs that depress the central nervous system, such as minor tranquillizers (benzodiazepines), hypnotics, barbiturates, antiepileptics, most H_1-antihistamines, neuroleptics, major tranquillizers, and also alcohol.
- Tricyclic antidepressants (imipramine, amitriptyline, etc.) reduce the antihypertensive action of clonidine and guanfacine, because they are antagonists of the central α_2-adrenoceptors which are stimulated by the antihypertensive drugs.
- The intestinal absorption of α-methyldopa and therefore its therapeutic effect is reduced by simultaneously ingested iron (Fe^{2+}) ions;
- The possibility that cessation of treatment with clonidine causes a rebound (withdrawal) phenomenon is enhanced by beta-blockers, in particular those which are not β_1-selective. For this reason beta-blockers should be stopped prior to clonidine when both drugs are used simultaneously.
- The combination of rilmenidine with monoamine oxidase (MAO) inhibitors should be avoided.

BOX 6.7.4 Practical use of centrally acting antihypertensives

Clonidine
Clonidine may be considered in patients where treatment with low-dose diuretics, beta-blockers, ACE inhibitors or calcium antagonists does not lead to satisfactory control of blood pressure.
Dosage
Initially 0.075 mg thrice daily, to be gradually increased to 0.15–0.6 mg daily in two or three doses.

In certain countries clonidine is also available as a patch preparation which releases 0.1–0.3 mg in 24 hours, to be used once daily.

Cessation of clonidine therapy should be carried out slowly over 2–5 days in order to avoid withdrawal (rebound) phenomena.

Clonidine can also be used in conditions of perioperative hypertension. Dosage is 0.15 mg in 10 ml saline, given in over 10 min, two to four times daily.

Guanfacine
Guanfacine is similar to clonidine.
Dosage
Initially 1 mg once daily, administered in the evening, to be gradually increased up to maximally 3 mg daily.

Withdrawal phenomena are probably significantly less pronounced than observed for clonidine.

α-methyldopa
The position of α-methyldopa in schedules of antihypertensive treatment is globally the same as that of clonidine.

Centrally acting antihypertensive drugs

Potentially new fields of
application of centrally
acting antihypertensives

BOX 6.7.4 *Continued*

Dosage
Initially two or three times daily 250 mg, orally; individual maintenance dose
0.5–2 g daily in two or three doses; α-methyldopa is considered to be safe in
pregnant women.

Moxonidine
Moxonidine is similar to clonidine, but *potentially* has side effects. Another
advantage of moxonidine is its pharmacokinetic profile, which allows once-
daily dosage in most patients.
Dosage
0.2 mg once daily (orally); if necessary the dosage can be slowly increased to
0.4 mg or 0.6 mg in two doses. The dose must be reduced to 0.2 mg or 0.4 mg
in patients with moderate renal insufficiency (glomerular filtration rate
60–30 ml/min).

Rilmenidine
Rilmendine is also similar to clonidine.
Dosage
1 mg per 24 hours, if necessary to be elevated to 2 mg in one oral dose. In
patients with renal insufficiency no dosage adjustment is necessary if the
creatinine clearance is higher than 15 ml/min.

Potentially new fields of application of centrally acting antihypertensives

- Clonidine may also be used in migraine prophylaxis, in order to
  suppress flushes during the climacterium, to suppress opioid-
  abstinence phenomena, and in the treatment of open-angle glaucoma.
- Clonidine and moxonidine have been investigated as experimental
  drugs in the treatment of congestive heart failure (CHF). CHF is
  known to be associated with activated sympathetic and/or
  renin–angiotensin–aldosterone systems. Sympathoinhibition by
  clonidine is assumed to be a beneficial approach to counteract the
  sympathetic hyperactivation in CHF patients.

BOX 6.7.5 The metabolic syndrome

This is characterized by the simultaneous occurrence of hypertension,
hyperglycemia, hyperinsulinemia, high plasma triglycerides and low plasma
levels of HDL-cholesterol. Both insulin resistance and a central nervous
activation of the sympathetic system have been proposed as important
pathophysiological mechanisms.

   Moxonidine has been proposed as a useful drug in the treatment of
hypertensive patients with an associated metabolic syndrome. This
presumption has been supported in animal models of the metabolic syndrome.
In a retrospective analysis, moxonidine was found to reduce plasma glucose
levels in patients with the metabolic syndrome. It so far remains unclear
whether central or peripheral mechanisms (or both) are involved.

Further reading

Further reading

Bousquet P, Esler M. I_1-agents in high blood pressure and cardioprotection management: the contribution of rilmenidine. *J Hypertension* 1998;**16**(Suppl. 3):S1–S62.

Prichard BNC. Clinical experience with moxonidine In: *The I_1-Imidazoline Receptor Agonist Moxonidine: A New Antihypertensive* (eds van Zwieten PA, Hamilton CA, Julius S, Prichard BNC), 2nd edn, pp. 49–77. Royal Society of Medicine Press: London, 1996.

Prichard BNC. Clinical pharmacology of moxonidine. In: *The I_1-Imidazoline Receptor Agonist Moxonidine: A New Antihypertensive* (eds van Zwieten PA, Hamilton CA, Julius S, Prichard BNC), 2nd edn, pp. 31–47. Royal Society of Medicine Press: London, 1996.

Rupp H, Maisch B, Brilla C. Drug withdrawal and rebound hypertension. Differential action of the central antihypertensive drugs moxonidine and clonidine. *Cardiovasc Drugs Ther* 1996;**10** (Suppl. 1):251–262.

United Kingdom Working Party on Rilmenidine. Rilmenidine in mild-to-moderate essential hypertension. *Curr Ther Res* 1990;**1**:194–211.

Van Zwieten PA, Thoolen MJMC, Timmermans PBMWM. The hypotensive activity and side-effects of methyldopa, clonidine and guanfacine. *Hypertension* 1984;**6**(Suppl. 11):28–33.

Van Zwieten PA, Thoolen MJMC, Timmermans PBMWM. The pharmacological base of the hypotensive activity and side-effects of α-methyl-DOPA, clonidine and guanfacine. *Hypertension* 1984;**6**:11–28.

Van Zwieten PA, Chalmers JP. Different types of centrally acting antihypertensives and their targets in the central nervous system. *Cardiovasc Drugs Ther* 1994;**8**:787–799.

Chapter

6.8

Other drugs

AC Pessina and E Casiglia

6

Introduction

This chapter includes two sessions: the first on the 'out-of-fashion' direct vasodilators and, the second on the new antihypertensive agents that are still under scrutiny (Table 6.8.1).

Direct vasodilators are no longer considered first-line drugs because of their side effects but may be employed in association with other more commonly used drugs in the so-called 'resistant hypertension'. Among the newer agents, special attention will be given to endopeptidase inhibitors and endothelin I antagonists because they act through mechanisms that are completely different from those of the presently available drugs. In the future they may become the first choice for the treatment of special forms of high blood pressure and of hypertension-related end organ damage.

Direct vasodilators

Direct vasodilators, such as hydralazine, dihydralazine, cadralazine and minoxidil, have been widely used in the past, mainly, in combination with a diuretic and a beta-blocker in the so-called 'triple drug therapy' for the treatment of severe hypertension [1]. The rationale for this association is outlined in Table 6.8.2. The use of direct vasodilators alone should be avoided because of their marked adrenergic hyperactivity, as well as sodium and water retention [2].

To date, hydralazine and dihydralazine (no longer available in many countries) are reserved for treatment of hypertension in pregnancy, while minoxidil is used only in association for patients with hypertension resistant to other treatments. They have also been employed in the past to treat hypertensive emergencies and pulmonary

Table 6.8.1 Direct vasodilators and new antihypertensive agents

Direct vasodilators	*Endothelin antagonists*
Hydralazine	Phosphoramidone
Dihydralazine	Bosentan
Cadralazine	BQ-123
Minoxidil	
Potassium-channel openers	*Neutral endopeptidase (NEP) inhibitors*
Nicorandil	Simple NEP inhibitors
Pinacidil	Sinorphan
Cromakalim	Candoxatrilat
Aprikalim	SCH-42495
Bimakalim	
KRN-4884	Vasopeptidase inhibitors*
Ki-1769	Omapatrilat
	MDL-100240
Renin inhibitors	Sampatmilat
Enalkiren	CGS-30440
Remikiren	SCH-34826
Terlakiren	Ecadotril
Zankiren	SCH-39370
CP-108 671	CCS-26303
	CGS-26393

*Formerly called 'dual inhibitors'.

6

Table 6.8.2 Rationale of combined use of direct vasodilators, diuretics and antiadrenergic drugs in so-called 'triple therapy'

Activity on:	Direct vasodilators	Diuretics	Antiadrenergic drugs	Net effect
Peripheral resistance	↓	↓ or =	↓ or =	↓↓
RAAS	↑	↑	↓↓	=
Circulating volume	↑	↓	=	=
Adrenergic drive	↑	↑	↓↓	=
Heart rate	↑	=	↓ or ↓↓	= or ↓
Cardiac output	↑	↓	= or ↓	=

=, no change.

hypertension. Pseudotolerance (see below) and side effects are the main reasons for their limited use.

Hydralazine and dihydralazine

Hydralazine as well as dihydralazine have in the short term an antihypertensive effect comparable to that of captopril and nifedipine. Unfortunately, the activation of the sympathetic drive and the increase of circulating volume rapidly lead to pseudotolerance. The use of hydralazine in monotherapy should therefore be avoided, particularly in subjects with coronary artery disease. Unwanted activation of sympathetic drive and of the renin–angiotensin–aldosterone system (RAAS) also leads to lack of regression of left ventricular and vascular hypertrophy. In several experimental studies, heart : bodyweight ratio and cardiac myocyte diameter even increased significantly after hydralazine therapy [2] which also increased or failed to reduce interstitial fibrosis. The lack of regression of left ventricular mass (LVM) appears to be associated with an increase in plasma norepinephrine.

Similarly, in the few studies that are available, hydralazine failed to normalize the media : lumen ratio probably because unable to abolish the upregulation of TR-mRNA expression. A further effect consists of an increase in abnormal high-velocity flow pattern associated with turbulence and vortex formation; for this reason, it is less effective than other drugs in preventing the occurrence of aortic atherosclerosis, even though it lowers blood pressure [3].

Hydralazine should not be used in subjects with intracranial hypertension because it increases cardiac output. In experimental studies it also appears to increase cerebral blood flow by 29%.

Finally, hydralazine may increase the risk of development of renal disease (relative risk 2.71 in men, 1.95 in women) as it stimulates fibronectin expression which contributes to the pathogenesis of renal glomerular sclerosis [4].

Incidence of side effects and frequency of withdrawal are as common with hydralazine as with other vasodilating drugs [5]. Apart from unwanted adrenergic activation and fluid retention, in chronic treatment the main side effect is systemic lupus erythematosus [6]. This is a dreadful but possibly reversible complication, whose incidence is dose dependent (5.4% of cases in patients taking 100 mg daily and

10.4% with 200 mg daily) and higher in women (11.6%, with peaks of 19.4% in those taking 200 mg/day) than in men (2.8%). Hydralazine elicits antinuclear antibodies and destabilizes duplex or triplex forms. It is, therefore, capable of stabilizing unusual high-order forms of DNA. Another rare and late complication is autoimmune constrictive pericarditis with antineutrophil cytoplasmic antibodies directed against myeloperoxidase.

Minoxidil

Minoxidil is a direct vasodilator which also shows important potassium-channel opening properties. Minoxidil is more potent than hydralazine and induces a more marked activation of adrenergic drive. A mean daily dose of minoxidil of 20 mg/day requires a beta-blocker and a diuretic in all patients to counteract tachycardia and fluid retention [7] (over 7 kg in many patients, more commonly in those with renal impairment). Even though minoxidil has been used in mild-to-moderate hypertension, the general opinion is that it should be used only in severe or intractable hypertension.

Side effects may be serious in patients receiving doses greater than 10 mg/day or in those with widespread atherosclerosis. When added to a diuretic and a beta-blocker (the only possible regimen), minoxidil is generally well tolerated. Hypertricosis due to vasodilatation of hair bulbs is very common. Some cases of pericarditis have also been described.

ST-segment depression or T-wave inversion may be observed during minoxidil therapy. They could simply be a consequence of sympathetic activation, but the possibility of an underlying coronary artery disease should always be kept in mind. In a study on 27 essential hypertensive patients with ST–T modifications during minoxidil, two had stenotic lesions by coronary angiography [8].

An increase in left ventricular mass (LVM) (V_3 type) by 15–22% despite normalization of blood pressure with minoxidil has been documented: this is due to cardiac overload as well as to adrenergic hyperactivity and is similar to that obtained in animals using isoproterenol. Minoxidil also increases the elastin content of the abdominal aorta, renal, and superior mesenteric arteries, secondary to a decrease in elastase activity. The effect on LVM is prevented by cotreatment with a beta-blocker, an ACE-inhibitor, or an AT_1-inhibitor. In combination with hydrochlorothiazide, minoxidil has sometimes caused concentric (rather than eccentric) left ventricular hypertrophy in animal models.

In humans, minoxidil generally improves renal function, or at least does not induce any significant worsening.

Nine deaths possibly related to treatment have been reported among subjects using topical formulations of minoxidil for baldness: five had cardiovascular abnormalities and two had acquired immunodeficiency syndrome-related pneumonia. The possibility that these deaths might be the result of the use of the drug cannot be excluded.

6

Potassium-channel openers

BOX 6.8.1 Potassium-channel openers

The opening of plasmalemma K^+-channels, with a resulting increase in K^+ conductance, shifts the membrane potential in a hyperpolarizing direction towards the K^+ equilibrium potential. Hyperpolarization reduces the opening probability of ion channels involved in membrane depolarization and excitation is reduced. Potassium-channel openers (KCO) are believed to hyperpolarize smooth muscle cells by a direct action on the cell membrane [9]. The clinical effect is relaxation of the blood vessels. KCO therefore act as potent precapillary vasodilators, and initial studies have emphasized their antihypertensive properties.

Nevertheless, as potassium channels are extremely diverse, not only with regards to their molecular structure but also to their function, KCO interfere with most of the physiological processes of the cardiac muscle, vascular smooth muscle and endothelial cells, leading to interesting accessory effects. For example, in the experimental setting, KCO afford cytoprotection during ischemia, an exciting property which opens a new field in clinical research [10]. Later studies have concentrated on selective coronary vasodilation and on the improvement of coronary blood flow produced by these substances, together with their protective effect on the ischemic myocardium.

The profound effects of the KCO *in vivo* has led to the suggestion that an endogenous KCO might exist and exert an important role in blood pressure homeostasis. The discovery of such a substance (endothelium-derived hyperpolarizing factor) has many implications, and its role in cardiovascular regulation is currently under investigation.

The best known members of the group called KCO are nicorandil, pinacidil, and cromakalim, but several new compounds are being evaluated. In addition, it has recently been shown that drugs belonging to other classes such as diazoxide and minoxidil exhibit KCO properties. To date, many potential clinical applications have been postulated for KCO. However, most available molecules do not seem to have a sufficient tissue selectivity to represent useful therapeutic alternatives to most of the commonly used drugs.

Pinacidil (P-1134, CAS-85371–64–8) has an overall potency two- to three times greater than that of hydralazine and induces a dose-dependent blood pressure fall which is preceded and superseded by a reduction of total peripheral resistance, as confirmed by a significant increase in calf blood flow. Pinacidil also increases brachial (+7%) and carotid diameters (+8%) and flows, and redistributes blood flow towards the muscular vascular bed, an effect that peaks at 4 hours and lasts 8 hours.

The pharmacodynamic profile of pinacidil is generally considered to be reminiscent of direct vasodilators [12], with stimulation of both sympathetic and RAAS, and an increase in heart rate, cardiac output and blood volume. However, during pinacidil treatment, plasma aldosterone has been observed to be occasionally reduced, while renin was not increased, and the heart rate remained unchanged.

In humans, vasodilatation and blood pressure reduction are accompanied by an increase in renal blood flow and a fall in fractional proximal tubular sodium excretion. A fall in pulmonary blood pressure has also been reported. Other accessory effects are a reduction in plasma cholesterol and triglycerides.

Pinacidil is indicated in the management of essential hypertension at a daily dose of 25–100 mg. Low (12.5–25 mg b.i.d.) doses are effective and safe as monotherapy and do not induce postural hypotension or rebound hypertension at withdrawal. Administered twice daily, pinacidil has been shown to achieve adequate blood pressure control both in previously untreated patients and in those with blood pressure inadequately controlled by beta-blockers or diuretics. In long-term comparative studies, it resulted at least as effective as hydralazine, prazosin, or nifedipine in maintaining blood pressure control [13]. A potential use in patients with secondary renal hypertension has also been postulated.

Adverse effects are quite frequent, but usually mild, transient and responding to reduction in dose. The main side effects are those due to peripheral vasodilation (headache, edema, palpitations, tachycardia) [7]. In monotherapy, the incidence of edema is 3% at a dosage of 12.5 mg/day and 26% at 25 mg/day, with significant attenuation when hydrochlorothiazide is added.

Nicorandil

Nicorandil lowers blood pressure by a dual mechanism (opening potassium channels and activation of guanidyl cyclase by its nitro group), and its antihypertensive effect is similar to that of pinacidil. At a dose of 2.5–10 mg orally, peak plasma concentration occurs in the first hour and a dose-related decrease in blood pressure is observed. Glomerular filtration rate and filtration fraction have been found to be unaltered, but fractional excretion of sodium tends to decrease with increasing doses. The cardioprotective effect of nicorandil has been particularly emphasized in patients with acute myocardial infarction undergoing reperfusion therapy [11].

Other KCO are cromakalim, aprikalim, bimakalim, KRN-4884 and KI-1769. Their effects do not substantially differ from those of pinacidil. However, the importance of these accessory effects in clinical practice has to be confirmed.

- Cromakalim has been shown to produce a shortening of atrial-to-His conduction time, atrial effective refractory period, ventricular effective refractory period, and PR-interval at a dose of 0.3 mg/kg [14].
- Aprikalim completely abates the coronary and cardiac depressant actions of free radicals, leading to further cardioprotection.
- Ki-1769 dose-dependently decreases coronary vascular resistance more than total peripheral resistance with a specificity greater than that of nifedipine.

Renin inhibitors

Inhibition of RAAS is one of the most interesting approaches for the treatment of arterial hypertension. Different levels of blockade of this system are possible today. Although renin catalyzes the first and rate-limiting step in the RAAS cascade (cleaving of angiotensinogen at Leu^{10}–Val^{11} bond, generating the decapeptide angiotensin), renin inhibitors have come last and clinical experience with them is limited. The major advantage of these drugs should be their high specificity for the RAAS.

Research has led to the synthesis of inhibitors with nano- or subnanomolar potency acting in blood or interstitium, rather than on cell surface (Table 6.8.3). When given parenterally, these drugs lowered blood pressure rapidly in a dose-related fashion both in animals and humans without causing tachycardia or tachyphylaxis. However, they do not seem to offer extra benefits when compared with other drugs acting on the RAAS. Table 6.8.3 compares the main characteristics of renin inhibitors, ACE inhibitors and angiotensin II antagonists.

Four classes of compounds have been shown to be renin inhibitors of high potency:

- specific antibodies;
- synthetic derivatives of the prosegment of renin precursor,
- pepstatin analogs; and
- angiotensinogen analogs.

The last are those that hold the greatest promise. Specific antibodies are currently no more than of experimental interest. The minimal substrate for renin has the sequence His-Pro-Phe-His-Leu-Val-Tyr; variants of this sequence have yielded competitive inhibitors. Remarkably active compounds have recently been synthesized by reducing the peptide bond that is cleaved by renin, or by incorporating the amino acid statine, found in pepstatin.

Dipeptide inhibitors of renin have been shown in the laboratory to be efficacious hypotensive agents when administered intravenously [15]. Recently smaller molecular weight and more stable structure components have been synthesized. *In vitro* potency has increased greatly, with several transition-state inhibitor designs yielding inhibitors

Table 6.8.3 Characteristics of different drugs acting on RAAS

Characteristic	Renin inhibitors	ACE inhibitors	Angiotensin II antagonists
Type of block	Angiotensinogen → angiotensin I	Angiotensin I → angiotensin II	AT_1 receptors
Effect on chymase	=	↓	=
Effect on plasma renin activity	↓	↑	↑
Effect on renal blood flow	↑↑	↑	↑
Receptor protein	In blood or interstitium	On cell surface	On cell surface
Effect on bradykinin	=	↑	=

=, no change.

6

417

with subnanomolar IC_{50} values. Most of the actual work is based on the design of peptide analogs of angiotensinogen, many of which contain statine or one of its variants. Substitutions at other sites in the molecule determine potency and species selectivity. Although some recently reported compounds demonstrate a certain degree of oral activity [15], oral bioavailability remains the main problem with these drugs. New compounds with improved pharmacokinetic profiles must be developed before renin inhibitors have a chance to compete with ACE inhibitors and AII antagonists.

Enalkiren (A-64662), the first orally-active compound studied in man, was found to be able to suppress plasma renin activity completely in essential hypertensive patients and to produce a dose-dependent hypotensive response without tachyphylaxis. High-renin sodium-depleted patients were reported to respond more vigorously than others. Unfortunately, the oral bioavailability in humans is ≤2%.

Remikiren (Ro-425892) is a very promising renin-inhibitor peptide whose activity could be localized in tissues rather than in plasma as for other compounds of this group. *In vivo*, despite its low oral bioavailability, it reduces blood pressure for more than 24 hours, and its antihypertensive efficacy is similar to that of ACE inhibitors (600 mg remikiren have the same effect as 20 mg enalapril). Co-administration of a diuretic or a restricted dietary sodium intake strongly increases its hypotensive effect [16]. After remikiren, glomerular filtration rate remains stable, whereas effective renal plasma flow rises; as a consequence, filtration fraction falls. These changes are more pronounced in individuals with a higher initial immunoreactive renin. Remikiren also induces a significant rise in the fractional excretion of sodium and lithium and a decrease in urinary albumin excretion.

Terlakiren (CP-80 794), specially studied in experimental animal models, shows an oral bioavailability that reaches 3% in suspension and 10% in solution [17].

Zankiren (A-72517), presently in clinical trials [15], has a dipeptide core with a very good oral bioavailability in different animal species (24% in the rat, 32% in the ferret, 53% in the dog) and acceptable (8%) in primates. Preliminary human data suggest that it is safe and active in hypertensive patients.

Modifications of chemical structure and physical properties of terlakiren has led to the synthesis of orally-active aminopiperidine. Further modifications to give enzymatic stability produced a benzylsuccinate, whose bioactive monomethylamine metabolite (called CP-108 671) has uniformly high oral bioavailability and activity [17].

Endothelin antagonists

The 1.8 to 3 kg of endothelium present in the human body produces a large amount of endothelin. Endothelin-1 (ET-1) is the most important isoform acting as a potent vasoconstrictor through ET_A receptors in vascular smooth muscle cells [18]. ET-1 also stimulates the generation of renin, angiotensin II, aldosterone and epinephrine. It is, therefore, not surprising that it could play a role in the pathogenesis of essential hypertension [18].

The possibility that ET-1 antagonists may be useful in the treatment of human hypertension has recently been demonstrated.

Phosphoramidone is an ET-1 converting enzyme inhibitor, able to decrease ET-1 formation from big endothelin. Clinical studies are limited to those conducted in patients undergoing cardioplegia: pretreatment with phosphoramidone significantly improves the postischemic recovery of coronary flow after 30 minutes of reperfusion. There are no studies on hypertension.

Bosentan (Ro-47–0203) is an orally-active, non-peptide, non-selective, competitive blocker of the ET_A and ET_B receptors obtained by structural optimization of the less potent Ro-46–2005. Preclinical studies demonstrated that the specific binding on ET_A receptors is 4.7 nM, versus 95 nM on ET_B. Its capability of reducing blood pressure has been repeatedly demonstrated in different animal models, and only sometimes denied. Its main hemodynamic effect is a reduction of systemic vascular resistance.

Experience in humans is, to date, very limited. In a study on healthy subjects [19], bosentan reversed the vasoconstrictor effect of ET-1 measured in the skin microcirculation and decreased blood pressure (–5 mmHg) in a dose-independent manner. In the only controlled study in essential hypertensive patients, 0.5–2 g/day bosentan reduced blood pressure similarly to 20 mg enalapril (–5.7 mmHg) without any increase in heart rate, norepinephrine, angiotensin II levels or plasma renin activity, testifying the absence of any reflex neurohormonal activation [20].

Bosentan has also been evaluated at a dose of 300 mg intravenously and 500 mg b.i.d. orally for two weeks in subjects with severe congestive heart failure taking standard triple therapy, where it improved hemodynamics due to systemic and venous vasodilation [21].

Special applications have been postulated for bosentan which appear to be partially independent from its antihypertensive effect. For example, in some hypertensive rat models, treatment with bosentan reduced the cross-sectional area of the media in small arteries from the coronary, renal, and mesenteric circulation, suggesting a possible favorable effect on human vascular hypertrophy complicating hypertension. It also reduced the vascular hypertrophy in kidneys and the extent of glomerular fibrinoid necrosis, suggesting that ET-1 inhibition could be useful in preventing hypertension-induced renal damage. In isolated human carotid arteries, bosentan showed a vasodilator effect entirely due to the ET_A blockade.

Preclinical studies with BQ-123 showed that it is an orally-active, non-peptide, selective, competitive blocker of the ET_A receptors. In the rat, it proved more effective than bosentan in reducing vasoconstriction induced by ET-1 intradermal injection.

Clinical experience is very limited. Cowburn *et al.* [22] used 100–200 mmol/min intravenous BQ-123 in human chronic heart failure and observed a systemic vasodilatation (peripheral resistance –12%) and cardiac index increase (+5%) without any change in heart rate.

6

Neutral endopeptidase inhibitors

Inhibitors of neutral endopeptidase (NEP), the major enzymatic pathway for degradation of natriuretic peptides, were developed with the aim of regulating endogenous levels of the atrial natriuretic peptide (ANP), which is also a vasodilatory hormone. The selective inhibitors (NEI) protect NEP from degradation and therefore enhance their plasma levels and biological activities. The most important action is on NEP in endothelial and smooth muscle cells, where the ANP-induced cGMP production is stimulated by NEI. These drugs also reduce bradykinin degradation and increase the bradykinin-stimulated release of arachidonic acid in fibroblasts and endothelial cells. These actions are the result of combined effects, as NEP metabolizes a variety of bioactive peptides.

In preclinical investigations, NEI lowered BP with an activity similar to that of exogenous ANP, i.e. quite low even in intravenous studies. In fact they cause marked natriuresis and diuresis and little reduction of blood pressure. Not only this, but it has also been shown that in some cases NEP inhibition may cause a progressive forearm vasoconstriction which may explain the failure to lower BP to any significant extent [23].

Since the demonstration that the combination NEI + ACE inhibitor produces cardiovascular effects greater than those elicited by selective inhibition of either enzyme alone, NEI have been especially employed in combination with ACE inhibitors. This has led to the production of dual metalloprotease inhibitors, i.e. single molecules that inhibit both NEP and ACE. Similarly, dual NEP/endothelin-converting enzyme inhibitors are becoming available.

Simple NEP inhibitors

Sinorphan is an orally-active inhibitor of NEP. When it was employed alone at a dose of 100 mg twice a day for four weeks, it failed to induce any appreciable result in patients with essential hypertension [24]. When sinorphan was combined with captopril (25 mg b.i.d.), a significant decrease both in systolic and diastolic blood pressure was observed, so as to suggest a synergistic effect [19].

Candoxatril is a prodrug, from which the active candoxatrilat (UK-79 300) is rapidly released. Systemic bioavailability is estimated to be 32% in man. Candoxatrilat has been shown to decrease blood pressure, enhance natriuresis and increase plasma ANP, plasma and urinary cGMP and plasma angiotensin II and aldosterone in humans. However, in other studies carried out in a double-blind placebo-controlled manner, candoxatrilat had little effect on blood pressure [3]. These conflicting results cast some doubts upon the usefulness of NEI in the treatment of unselected hypertensive patients. Most probably, the antihypertensive effect may be offset by the increase in RAAS and sympathetic nervous system activity. This is why the combination with ACE inhibitors potentiates its hypotensive effect.

SCH-42495 was investigated in a multicenter clinical trial in essential hypertensive patients aged 64 ± 1 years [25]. The administration of 50–200 mg twice daily for 8 days induced a significant blood pressure

6

reduction (from 171/100 to 146/84 mmHg) without any change in pulse rate. Efficacy rate was 44% with 50 mg b.i.d., 60% with 100 mg b.i.d., and 80% with 200 mg b.i.d. Adverse reactions such as headache and palpitation were observed in six patients (22.2%), with treatment discontinued in five. A significant correlation was observed between an increment in plasma ANP levels and blood pressure reductions, while an increase in plasma cGMP was positively correlated with increments in plasma ANP.

Vasopeptidase inhibitors (formerly dual inhibitors)

Omapatrilat (BMS-186716) is a peptidomimetic vasopeptidase inhibitor (the first of this group), blocking the cardiovascular effects of both NEP (with K_i 9 nmol/liter) and ACE (with K_i 6 nmol/liter). In rats, the intravenous injection of this drug inhibits the pressor response to angiotensin II with a potency and duration of action similar to those of fosinoprilat. The inhibition is 28% in sodium-depleted high-renin spontaneously hypertensive rats, 16% in deoxycorticosterone acetate-salt low-renin hypertensive rats and 15% in spontaneously normal-renin hypertensive rats.

To date, several clinical studies have been completed in man involving more than 2000 subjects [26,27]. In 108 normal volunteers, with oral doses ranging from 2.5 to 75 mg, blood pressure was reduced after the third hour, and ACE and NEP were inhibited for at least 24 hours. In patients with mild-to-moderate hypertension, 24-hour blood pressure was constantly reduced by 16.8/9.9 mmHg after 7 mg oral omapatrilat in comparison to placebo. Although side-effects (including angioedema) can always be observed with antihypertensive drugs [28], omapatrilat is generally well tolerated, with an incidence of adverse effects (32/125) similar to that of placebo but does cause cough.

MDL-100240, another vasopeptidase inhibitor, was administered intravenously to healthy volunteers in a four-period, dose-increasing (0, 1.56, 6.25 and 25 mg, and 0, 3.13, 12.5 and 50 mg, respectively) double-blind, placebo-controlled study. It induced a rapid, dose-related and sustained inhibition of ACE (–70% over 24 hours) and a transient decrease of mean supine blood pressure. The baroreceptor reflex, assessed by the response to exogenous angiotensin II challenge, remained unaltered.

Sampatrilat and CGS-30440 are other dual inhibitors of ACE and NEP, currently under development for the treatment of hypertension and congestive heart failure. SCH-34826 is a potent and selective NEI studied at the dose of 100 mg/kg in SHR rats. Interestingly, despite the lack of any antihypertensive activity, it reduced both the cardiac mass (–10%) and the amount of fibrotic tissue present in the left ventricle (–42%). As similar effects were observed after CGS-30440 and after ecadotril (another experimental NEI), this could indicate that chronic NEP inhibition *per se* interacts with the mechanisms causing myocardial hypertrophy and cardiac remodeling. SCH-39370 has been studied only in rats with heart failure. CGS-26303 and CGS-26393 could have an accessory inhibitory effect on the endothelin-converting enzyme.

Conclusions

Judging from the long list of the new antihypertensive drugs, it is clear that research in this field is still a top priority for many pharmaceutical companies. While waiting for a pharmacogenetic approach to the treatment of hypertension[29], the search for new drugs must be welcomed in view of the fact that there is still a number of patients who do not respond to any of the available agents and who complain of side effects with most of them. The persisting morbidity and mortality gap between well-treated hypertensive and normotensive patients is another reason that underlines the need for new drugs with a more potent effect on hypertension-related end organ damage and events.

References

1. Reams GP, Bauer JH. The effect of triple drug therapy on renal function in patients with essential hypertension. *J Clin Pharmacol* 1989;**29**:803–808.
2. Jablonskis LT, Howe PR. Plasma adrenaline responses to long-term modification of blood pressure in normotensive rats and hypertensive rats. *J Hypertension* 1995;**13**:319–325.
3. Spence JD. Hypertension and atherosclerosis: effects of antihypertensive drugs on arterial flow patterns. *J Cardiovasc Pharmacol* 1987;**10**(Suppl. 2):112–115.
4. Kai T, Kino H, Ishikawa K. Role of the renin–angiotensin system in cardiac hypertrophy and renal glomerular sclerosis in transgenic hypertensive mice carrying both human renin and angiotensinogen genes. *Hypertension Res* 1998;**21**:39–46.
5. Bevan EG, Connell JM, Doyle J *et al*. The effect of triple drug therapy on renal function in patients with essential hypertension. *J Hypertension* 1992;**10**:607–613.
6. Franks PJ, Hartley K, Bulpitt PF, Bulpitt CJ. Risk of serious morbidity associated with hydralazine versus methyldopa treatment in hypertensive patients. *Eur J Clin Pharmacol* 1991;**40**:327–331.
7. Mackay A, Isles C, Henderson I. Minoxidil in the management of intractable hypertension. *Q J Med* 1981;**50**:175–190.
8. Sanchez-Torres G, Panzzi ME, Kuri J *et al*. Acute electrocardiographic effects of minoxidil in hypertensive subjects. *Arch Inst Cardiol Mex* 1983;**53**:49–56.
9. Andersson KE. Clinical pharmacology of potassium channel openers. *Pharmacol Toxicol* 1992;**70**:244–254.
10. Escande D, Henry P. Potassium channels as pharmacological targets in cardiovascular medicine. *Eur Heart J* 1993;**14**(Suppl. B):2–9.
11. Kobayashi Y, Goto Y, Daikoku S *et al*. Cardioprotective effect of intravenous nicorandil in patients with successful reperfusion for acute myocardial infarction. *Jpn Circ J* 1988;**62**:183–189.
12. Nielsen CB, Pedersen EB. Effect of pinacidil on renal haemodynamics, tubular function and plasma levels of angiotensin II, aldosterone and atrial natriuretic peptide in healthy man. *Eur J Clin Pharmacol* 1998;**45**:29–35.
13. Friedel HA, Brogden RN. Pinacidil. A review of its pharmacodynamic and pharmacokinetic properties, and therapeutic potential in the treatment of hypertension. *Drugs* 1990;**39**:929–967.
14. D'Alonzo AJ, Darbenzio RB, Sewter JC *et al*. A comparison between the effects of BMS-180448, a novel K$^+$ channel opener, and cromakalim in rat and dog. *Eur J Pharmacol* 1995;**294**: 271–280.
15. Kleinert HD. Renin inhibitors: discovery and development. An overview and perspective. *Am J Hypertens* 1989;**2**:800–808.
16. Himmelmann A, Bergbrant A, Svensson A *et al*. Remikiren (Ro 42–5892) – an orally active renin inhibitor in essential hypertension. Effects on blood pressure and the renin–angiotensin–aldosterone system. *Am J Hypertension* 1996;**9**:517–522.

6

17. Hoover DJ, Lefker BA, Rosati RL *et al.* Discovery of inhibitors of human renin with high oral bioavailability. *Adv Exp Med Biol* 1995;**362**:167–180.

18. Schachter M. New ideas for treating hypertension. *J Hum Hypertension* 1995;**9**:663–667.

19. Weber C, Schmitt R, Birnboeck H *et al.* Pharmacokinetics and pharmacodynamics of the endothelin-receptor antagonist bosentan in healthy human subjects. *Clin Pharmacol Ther* 1996;**60**:124–137.

20. Krum H, Viskoper RJ, Lacourciere Y *et al.* The effect of an endothelin-receptor antagonist, bosentan, on blood pressure in patients with essential hypertension. Bosentan Hypertension Investigators. *N Engl J Med* 1998;**338**:784–790.

21. Sutsch G, Bertel O, Kiowski W. Acute and short-term effects of the nonapeptide endothelin-1 receptor antagonist bosentan in humans. *Cardiovasc Drugs Ther* 1997;**10**:717–725.

22. Cowburn PJ, Cleland JGF, McArthur JD *et al.* Short-term hemodynamic effects of BQ-123, a selective endothelin ET1-receptor antagonist, in chronic heart failure. *Lancet* 1998;**352**:201–202.

23. Ferro CJ, Spratt JC, Haynes WG, Webb DJ. Inhibition of neutral endopeptidase causes vasoconstriction of human resistance vessels *in vivo*. *Circulation* 1998;**16**:2323–2330.

24. Favrat B, Burnier M, Nussberger J *et al.* Neutral endopeptidase versus angiotensin converting enzyme inhibition in essential hypertension. *J Hypertension* 1995;**13**:797–804.

25. Ogihara T, Rakugi H, Masuo K *et al.* Antihypertensive effects of the neutral endopeptidase inhibitor SCH-42,495 in essential hypertension. *Am J Hypertension* 1994;**7**:943–947.

26. Data on File. Investigator brochure – Omapatrilat BMS-186,716. Bristol-Myers-Squibb Pharmaceutical Research Institute: Princeton, NJ, 1998.

27. McClean DR, Ikram H, Garlick AH *et al.* Effects of omapatrilat or systemic arterial function in patients with chronic heart failure. *Am J Cardiol* 2001;**87**:565–569.

28. Binder M, Kittler H. Angioedema and antihypertensive therapy. *Wien Klin Wochenschr* 2001;**113**:154–156.

29. Casiglia E, Tikhonoff V, Vinnicki M *et al.* Protocol and study design of the genetically oriented treatment optimisation (GOTO) study. *J Hypertension* 2001;**19**(Suppl 2):149.

6

Treatment strategies: selecting the proper therapeutic agent

7

Chapter

7.1

Goal blood pressure

A Zanchetti

7

Persistence of increased cardiovascular risk in treated hypertensives

A large number of randomized, controlled trials have documented the benefit of blood pressure lowering with antihypertensive drugs. Indeed, antihypertensive treatment is accompanied by a particularly striking reduction of fatal and non-fatal strokes, and a less marked, though significant, reduction in coronary events [1]. However, treated hypertensive patients are known to run a considerably higher risk of cardiovascular complications than matched normotensive subjects of the same age and sex. In the Dalby study, a significantly higher cardiovascular morbidity rate was found in most age groups when treated hypertensive patients in this southern Swedish community were compared with age- and sex-matched normotensive individuals from the same community in a three-year retrospective study [2]. In the Dalby study it was obvious that marked and highly statistically significant reductions in arterial pressure had been obtained in the treated individuals. However, despite this, blood pressure levels in the treated patients were still markedly and significantly higher than in the matched normotensive subjects. It is, therefore, likely that the failure to 'normalize' the risk in the treated patients may, to a certain extent, have been due to the failure of 'normalizing' blood pressure. A similar type of study investigated mortality in treated hypertensive patients in the Glasgow Blood Pressure Clinic [3]. The mortality in almost 4000 patients with non-malignant hypertension was compared to that of two control populations near Glasgow during a 6.5-year period. Somewhat disappointingly the mortality in the treated hypertensive patients was found to be two to five times higher than in the normal populations (Figure 7.1.1).

   Results of the kind shown in the Dalby and Glasgow studies, i.e. higher cardiovascular morbidity and mortality in treated hypertensive patients than in matched normotensive subjects, could be explained by several different circumstances. However, it is quite obvious from the two studies that the level of blood pressure in the treated patients was higher than in the normotensive subjects and that the benefits of treatment were greater in those patients in whom blood pressure had been reduced most. This suggests that insufficient lowering of the elevated blood pressure may have been an important explanation for the high morbidity and mortality found in the treated hypertensive patients. An additional obvious explanation is that treated hypertensives were likely to have differed from their normotensive counterparts for a higher prevalence of organ damage and additional risk factors.

The J-shaped curve hypothesis

Even if the results of a number of intervention trials in hypertension suggest that blood pressure had been lowered insufficiently in many instances and that this could be one explanation for the suboptimal results of antihypertensive treatment, the opposite opinion has been

7

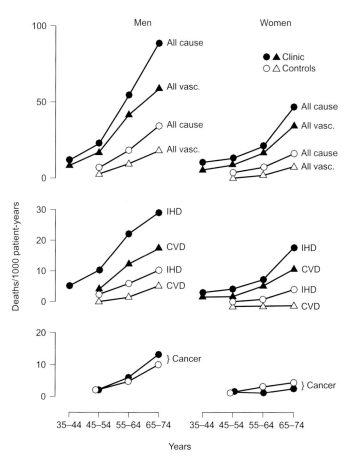

Fig. 7.1.1 Mortality rates in the Glasgow Clinic (closed symbols) and in Renfrew–Paisley control population (open symbols). IHD, ischemic heart disease; CVD, cerebrovascular disease; vasc, vascular disease. (From Isles *et al.* [3], reproduced with permission.)

expressed as well; in other words, it has been suggested that if blood pressure is lowered too vigorously, this could result in increased morbidity and mortality.

On theoretical grounds it must be assumed that the relationship between the level of blood pressure and the risk of any event, for instance of dying, must be J-shaped [4]. In 1979, Stewart [5] claimed in a retrospective analysis of 169 hypertensive patients that the risk of myocardial infarction was greater in patients in whom the diastolic blood pressure (fourth Korotkoff phase) was lowered to <90 mmHg as compared to 100–109 mmHg. In 1987, Cruickshank *et al.* [6] published a retrospective analysis of 939 treated hypertensive patients. From this analysis they claimed that, in patients with pre-existing ischemic heart disease, a lowering of the diastolic blood pressure to <85–90 mmHg was associated with an increase in fatal myocardial infarction (Figure 7.1.2). Support for this view appeared to be provided by the study by Alderman *et al.* [7], who followed 1765 previously untreated hypertensive patients during a 4.2-year observation period. They found

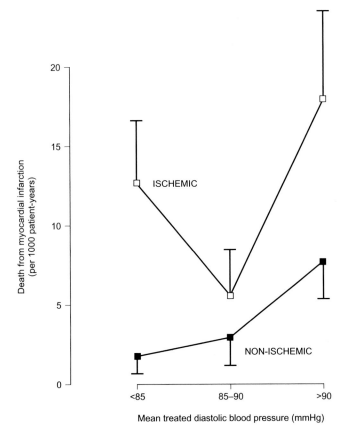

Fig. 7.1.2 Relationship between mortality rate (mean ±SE) from myocardial infarction in ischemic and non-ischemic patients, and treated diastolic blood pressure (age-adjusted). (From Cruickshank *et al.* [6], reproduced with permission.)

that the 39 fatal and non-fatal myocardial infarctions that occurred in this study were significantly more common in patients with a small (≤6 mmHg) or a large (≥18 mmHg) fall in diastolic blood pressure, whereas patients with a reduction of diastolic blood pressure between 7 and 17 mmHg had a significantly smaller risk. Some support for this view was also provided by the retrospective analysis by Samuelsson *et al.* [8]. Studies supportive of the J-shaped curve hypothesis have mostly been retrospective, often open, and commonly with too few events to reach significant conclusions. Furthermore, J-shaped relationships between cardiovascular events and blood pressure have also been described in untreated or placebo-treated patients, which suggests that increased event rates at lower blood pressure may be indicative of poor health conditions, particularly in the elderly. However, the real issue is not whether the relation between achieved blood pressure and cardiovascular risk is J-shaped (as mentioned above, it must be), but whether there are additional benefits, or risks, in lowering the blood pressure of patients with hypertension to fully normotensive levels, i.e. between 70 mmHg and 85 mmHg diastolic blood pressure.

Optimal blood pressure
Evidence from observational studies

The relationship between blood pressure and cardiovascular risk has
been investigated in a large number of prospective observational
studies. The overall information is provided by a meta-analysis of
these studies [9], as summarized in Figure 7.1.3: the relation between
stroke or coronary disease events and diastolic blood pressure is
continuous, without any lower threshold, at least within the range
76–105 mmHg. It will be noticed in Figure 7.1.3 that, although a larger
number of coronary events than of strokes occur at each given diastolic
blood pressure value, the relation of stroke incidence with diastolic
blood pressure is steeper, indicating a greater increase in the relative
risk of stroke for each increment of diastolic blood pressure. The
relation of cardiovascular risk with systolic blood pressure is also a
continuous one, without any evidence of a threshold, and it has
recently been stressed that this relation is even stronger than that with
diastolic blood pressure [10] (Figure 7.1.4). The increasing evidence of
the high risk of hypertension in the elderly, among whom isolated
systolic hypertension is frequent, indicates that isolated systolic
hypertension carries a greater risk of stroke than isolated diastolic
hypertension and combined systolic–diastolic hypertension [11]
(Figure 7.1.5).

These data have brought all current major guidelines on the
management of hypertension to define optimal blood pressure as values
<120 mmHg systolic and <80 mmHg diastolic [12,13].

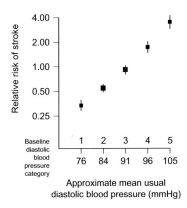
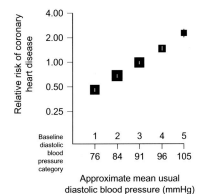

Fig. 7.1.3 Relative risk of stroke and of coronary events (CHD), estimated from combined
results of observational studies. Left: stroke and usual diastolic blood pressure (in five
categories defined by baseline diastolic blood pressure). Seven prospective observational
studies: 843 events. Right: coronary heart disease and usual diastolic blood pressure (in five
categories defined by baseline diastolic blood pressure). Nine prospective observational
studies: 4856 events. Solid squares represent risk of events relative to risk in the whole
population. Sizes of squares are proportional to number of events; 95% confidence
intervals are denoted by vertical lines. (From MacMahon *et al.* [9], reproduced with
permission.)

7

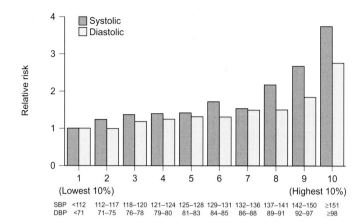

Fig. 7.1.4 Adjusted relative risk of coronary heart disease death according to deciles of baseline systolic and diastolic blood pressure in men from the MRFIT. (Drawn from data by Stamler *et al.* [10].)

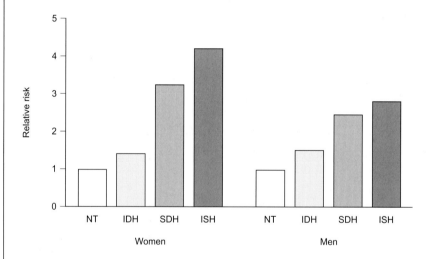

Fig. 7.1.5 Adjusted relative risk of stroke according to categories of baseline blood pressure in the subjects of the Copenhagen City Heart Study. NT, normotensive (systolic blood pressure <140 mmHg and diastolic blood pressure <90 mmHg); IDH, isolated diastolic hypertension (systolic blood pressure <160 mmHg and diastolic blood pressure ≥90 mmHg); SDH, combined systolic and diastolic hypertension (systolic blood pressure >160 mmHg and diastolic blood pressure ≥90 mmHg); ISH, isolated systolic hypertension (systolic blood pressure ≥160 mmHg and diastolic blood pressure <90 mmHg). (Drawn from data by Nielsen *et al.* [11].)

Evidence from interventional trials

The definition of the goal of antihypertensive treatment as that of achieving blood pressure levels defined as 'optimal' in a population requires the demonstration that lowering elevated blood pressure down or close to these optimal levels induces greater benefits than a more moderate blood pressure lowering, and that no J-shaped curve is

Table 7.1.1 Lack of blood pressure control in major trials of antihypertensive treatment.

Trial	Blood pressure goal*	Patients not at goal
HDFP	DBP < 90 mmHg	23–27%
Australian	DBP < 90 mmHg	36%
MRC-mild hypertension	DBP < 90 mmHg	23%
EWPHE	SDP/DBP < 160/90 mmHg	25–32%
IPPPSH	DBP < 90 mmHg	35%
HAPPHY	DBP < 95 mmHg	23%

*DBP = diastolic blood pressure: SBP = systolic blood pressure.

observed within the range of the blood pressure values achieved by more intensive blood pressure lowering.

Until recently, the information provided by trials was very scanty. Firstly, despite the fact that in most trials the blood pressure goal for active treatment was a diastolic blood pressure <90 mmHg, this goal was achieved in only 64–77% of patients, i.e. 23–36% of patients remained at definitely hypertensive levels [14] (Table 7.1.1). Secondly, the only trial that planned to compare a more with a less intensive lowering of blood pressure was the Hypertension Detection and Follow-up Program [15]. However, the trial design of randomizing patient to special care in specialized centers and to referred care by their practitioners resulted in a comparison of frequently treated versus infrequently treated hypertensive patients rather than in the comparison of blood pressure lowering to different goals.

The Hypertension Optimal Treatment (HOT) study

The HOT Study has been the first trial specifically designed to test the issue of how far blood pressure should be lowered to achieve the greatest reduction of cardiovascular morbidity and mortality, and in particular to answer the question whether there are additional benefits, or risks, in lowering blood pressure of hypertensive patients to fully normotensive levels (70–85 mmHg diastolic blood pressure) [16]. Altogether 18 790 hypertensive patients from 26 countries (mostly in Europe and North America), aged 50–80 years (mean 61.5 years), with baseline diastolic blood pressure 100–115 mmHg (mean 105 mmHg), were randomized to achieve three different diastolic blood pressure targets (≤90 mmHg, ≤85 mmHg, ≤80 mmHg). Treatment was carried out in five successive steps in order to achieve the randomized target:

Step 1. The calcium antagonist felodipine at the low dose of 5 mg once daily.
Step 2. Addition of a low dose of either an ACE inhibitor or a beta-blocker
Step 3. Increase of the felodipine dose to 10 mg once daily.
Step 4. Increase of the ACE inhibitor or of the beta-blocker dose.
Step 5. Addition of a diuretic or of another antihypertensive drug.

Randomized treatment was continued for an average of 3.8 years. The HOT study [14,17] has produced several clinically relevant findings. The first is that substantial reductions in both systolic and diastolic blood pressures were obtained, and diastolic blood pressure ≤90 mmHg was achieved in more than 90% of hypertensive patients with an intensive treatment regimen, based on a long-acting calcium antagonist, felodipine, and consisting in the combination of two or more drugs in about two-thirds of the patients. The medications administered were well tolerated, and a careful study of patients' well-being showed an overall improvement as compared with baseline; this improvement was greater in the ≤80 mmHg target group than in the other target groups. The feeling of well-being was also better the lower the achieved blood pressure was, and complaints of headache were fewer the lower the blood pressure was [18] (Figure 7.1.6).

Next, the between-group blood pressure differences were small (2 mmHg instead of the 5 mmHg expected), and consequently differences in event rates between target groups were also rather small. Table 7.1.2 shows that there was a trend for the rate of myocardial infarction to be lower at a lower target diastolic blood pressure (a 25% reduction in the target group ≤85 mmHg and 28% reduction in the target group ≤80 mmHg as compared with the target group ≤90 mmHg, for the trend $P = 0.05$). When the incidence of various types of events was related to the diastolic and systolic blood pressures achieved throughout the study (from end titration to event occurrence), confidence intervals were narrowest in the diastolic blood pressure range of 75–95 mmHg, and in the systolic blood pressure range of 130–140 mmHg, suggesting adequate precision of the estimated risk within these limits. As illustrated in Figure 7.1.7, the lowest risk for major cardiovascular events was at a mean achieved diastolic blood pressure of 82.6 mmHg and at a

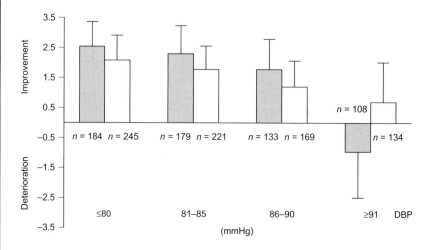

Fig. 7.1.6 The mean change (with standard error of the mean) in the Psychological General Well-Being Index total scores from baseline to six months correlated to actual diastolic blood pressure achieved. Per protocol (■) analysis included all patients that had evaluable data at baseline and at six months after entry; intention to treat (□) analysis also included patients who had isolated inclusion or follow-up dates. Pitman's non-parametric permutation test; correlation was significant ($P < 0.05$) for per-protocol analysis; $P = 0.11$ for intention-to-treat analysis. (From Wiklund *et al.* [18], reproduced with permission.)

7

Table 7.1.2 Events in relation to target blood pressure groups in the HOT study

Event	Number of events	Events/1000 patient-years	P for trend	Comparison	Relative risk (95% CI)
Major cardiovascular events					
≤90 mmHg	232	9.9		90 vs 85	0.99 (0.83–1.19)
≤85 mmHg	234	10.0		85 vs 80	1.08 (0.89–1.29)
≤80 mmHg	217	9.3	0.50	90 vs 80	1.07 (0.89–1.28)
All myocardial infarction					
≤90 mmHg	84	3.6		90 vs 85	1.32 (0.95–1.82)
≤85 mmHg	64	2.7		85 vs 80	1.05 (0.74–1.48)
≤80 mmHg	61	2.6	0.05	90 vs 80	1.37 (0.99–1.91)
All stroke					
≤90 mmHg	94	4.0		90 vs 85	0.85 (0.64–1.11)
≤85 mmHg	111	4.7		85 vs 80	1.24 (0.94–1.64)
≤80 mmHg	89	3.8	0.74	90 vs 80	1.05 (0.79–1.41)
Cardiovascular mortality					
≤90 mmHg	87	3.7		90 vs 85	0.97 (0.72–1.30)
≤85 mmHg	90	3.8		85 vs 80	0.93 (0.70–1.24)
≤80 mmHg	96	4.1	0.49	90 vs 80	0.90 (0.68–1.21)
Total mortality					
≤90 mmHg	188	7.9		90 vs 85	0.97 (0.79–1.19)
≤85 mmHg	194	8.2		85 vs 80	0.93 (0.77–1.14)
≤80 mmHg	207	8.8	0.32	90 vs 80	0.91 (0.74–1.10)

n = 6264, 6264 and 6262 in the target groups ≤90 mmHg, ≤85 mmHg and ≤80 mmHg, respectively. From Hansson *et al.* [17], courtesy of *The Lancet*.

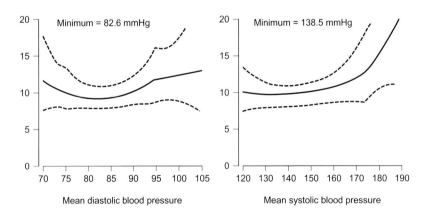

Fig. 7.1.7 Estimated incidence (continuous curves) and 95% confidence intervals (dashed curves) of major cardiovascular events in relation to achieved mean diastolic (left panel) and systolic blood pressure (right panel); averages of all blood pressure measurements from entry to event. Minimum indicates the blood pressure at the lowest point of the curve. (After Hansson *et al.* [17], reproduced with permission.)

mean systolic blood pressure of 138.5 mmHg, suggesting that the 'optimal' blood pressures for minimizing the risk of major cardiovascular events are between 80 and 85 mmHg for diastolic and between 135 and 140 mmHg for systolic blood pressure. However, there was no evidence of a significant increase of risk for any type of events at blood pressures lower than these 'optimal' levels (of course, within the ranges observed in the HOT study: down to 70 mmHg diastolic and 120 mmHg systolic blood pressure).

Thirdly, there were 1501 patients in the HOT study with diabetes mellitus at baseline, equally distributed in the three target diastolic blood pressure groups (diabetes was a factor used in randomization). A statistically significant decline in the rate of major cardiovascular events ($P = 0.005$) and in cardiovascular mortality rate ($P = 0.016$) was seen in relation to the target diastolic blood pressure groups. As illustrated in Figure 7.1.8, in the group randomized to ≤80 mmHg the risk of major cardiovascular events was halved in comparison with that of the target group ≤90 mmHg. The approximate halving of the risk was also observed for myocardial infarction, although the small number of events made it statistically insignificant; all stroke also showed a insignificant 30% decrease at the lowest target blood pressure. Cardiovascular mortality in the ≤80 mmHg target group was reduced to one-third of that occurring in the group randomized to ≤90 mmHg, and total mortality was reduced by 45%, a change close to statistical significance.

Finally, the event rate in the HOT study was very low. If event rates in the HOT study are compared with those in actively treated patients in the meta-analysis of all previous trials of antihypertensive treatment calculated by Collins and Peto [19], it is apparent that in HOT patients total mortality was 67%, cardiovascular mortality 58%, and myocardial infarction rate only 38% of the respective rates in actively treated patients of all previous studies, despite a higher mean age in the HOT study than in patients of the meta-analysis (61.5 years versus 56 years, respectively). Furthermore, a recent analysis of the baseline characteristics of the HOT patients [20] has shown that they were by no means low risk patients at baseline, 50% of them being classified as at high or very high risk according to World Health Organization/International Society of Hypertension guidelines [13]. It is, therefore, likely that the particularly low event rate found in the HOT study is due to the very effective blood pressure control achieved in this study, with only 8.5% of treated patients remaining at diastolic blood

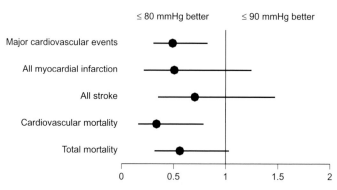

Fig. 7.1.8 Effects of intensive diastolic blood pressure lowering in the diabetic patients of the HOT study. Relative risk (filled circle) and 95% confidence limits (horizontal bars) of being randomized to ≤80 mmHg diastolic blood pressure rather than to ≤90 mmHg: (From Zanchetti [31], reproduced with permission.)

pressure >90 mmHg (versus 23% to 35% in the previous studies included in the meta-analysis).

The United Kingdom Prospective Diabetes Study (UKPDS)

In the UKPDS trial, 1148 patients with hypertension and diabetes were randomized to a less tight control of blood pressure, aiming at achieving values <180/105 mmHg, or to a tight control of blood pressure, with the aim of achieving blood pressure values <150/85 mmHg [21]. Tight control resulted in a 24% reduction ($P = 0.0046$) of all events, fatal or non-fatal, related to diabetes (Figure 7.1.9), in a 32% reduction ($P = 0.019$) of deaths related to diabetes, in a 44% reduction in stroke ($P = 0.013$) and in a 37% reduction in microvascular (mostly retinal) complications ($P = 0.0092$). There was no statistical difference in the benefits induced by tight treatment based either on an ACE inhibitor or a beta-blocker [22], but the study was underpowered to assess this issue.

Goals of treatment

Hypertension guidelines

The most recent international guidelines on the management of hypertension, such as those prepared by the Guidelines Subcommittee of the World Health Organization and International Society of Hypertension [13] make three important recommendations.

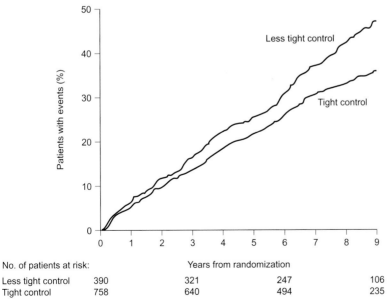

No. of patients at risk:				
Less tight control	390	321	247	106
Tight control	758	640	494	235

Fig. 7.1.9 Effects of less tight control or tight control of blood pressure in the diabetic patients of the UKPDS. Kaplan–Meier plots of proportions of patients with any clinical endpoint, fatal and non-fatal, related to diabetes. Reduction in risk with tight control 24% (95% CI is 8 to 38%) ($P = 0.0046$). (From UK Prospective Diabetes Study Group [21], reproduced with permission.)

The first is that the primary goal of treatment of the patient with high blood pressure should be to achieve the maximum reduction in the total risk of cardiovascular morbidity and mortality, and that this requires treatment of all reversible risk factors identified. The goal of controlling all modifiable factors for cardiovascular disease is also specified in the recent sixth report of the U.S. Joint National Committee [12].

The second recommendation concerns the values to which blood pressure should be brought by treatment. The sixth report of the Joint National Committee [12] recommends that one should achieve and maintain a systolic blood pressure below 140 mmHg and a diastolic blood pressure below 90 mmHg and lower if tolerated. The WHO/ISH guidelines [13] suggest it is desirable to achieve optimal or normal blood pressure in young, middle-aged or diabetic subjects (below 130/85 mmHg) and at least high normal blood pressure in elderly patients (below 140/90 mmHg). The recommendation of achieving values below 130/85 mmHg in young and middle-aged hypertensives is based on the observational epidemiological data summarized in Figure 7.1.3, showing a continuing relation between blood pressure and cardiovascular events without a lower threshold. The recommendation of achieving particularly low blood pressure levels in diabetics is founded on the data of the HOT study and of the UKPDS. Both studies have obtained the greatest benefits in randomized groups in which mean achieved diastolic blood pressure was 81 and 82 mmHg, respectively. It must be recognized that the benefit of reaching values below 130 mmHg systolic blood pressure has not yet been demonstrated by interventional trials, as even in the HOT study the mean systolic blood pressure of the diabetic patients randomized to the most intensive treatment was 142 mmHg (and 144 mmHg in the UKPDS). However, because of the indication that in diabetics the lower the blood pressure the greater the benefit, the recommendation to achieve systolic blood pressures lower than 130 mmHg appears a prudent one.

The third recommendation concerns the blood pressure values to be achieved when home or ambulatory blood pressure measurements are used to evaluate the efficacy of treatment. The WHO/ISH guidelines [13] highlight that daytime values provided by these methods (compared with office measurements) are on average around 10–15 mmHg lower for systolic blood pressure and 5–10 mmHg lower for diastolic blood pressure [23], and that treatment goals should be modified appropriately when these methods are used.

Medical practice

Unfortunately, experts' recommendations as summarized in guidelines have not produced the expected impact on medical practice, and insufficient lowering of blood pressure has been found in all countries of the world where suitable surveys have been carried out [24–29]. Indeed, these surveys report that the proportion of hypertensive patients with blood pressure values brought down by treatment to 140/90 mmHg or below is commonly between 20 and 25%, and sometimes much lower. It

7

Table 7.1.3 Possible reasons for the insufficient control of blood pressure in treated hypertensive patients

- Overestimation of hypertension prevalence in surveys
- The 'white coat' effect raises blood pressure in many patients during survey
- The observational nature of the evidence upon which intensive lowering of blood pressure is recommended
- Concern about the J-shaped curve effect
- Concern about cost-effectiveness of antihypertensive therapy
- Adverse effects of antihypertensive agents
- Infrequent use of combination therapy

is important to understand the reasons for this unfortunate gap, in order to devise a method to overcome it. Some of the possible reasons, as discussed by Zanchetti [30], are summarized in Table 7.1.3.

One possible reason is the definition of hypertension in surveys is not precise. In most, prevalence of hypertension is overestimated by a single measurement of blood pressure, with a consequent underestimation of the proportion of hypertensive subjects having a well-controlled blood pressure. On the other hand, our recent analysis of the PAMELA population [28], in which blood pressure was also measured by home and ambulatory monitoring techniques, makes it unlikely that a considerable proportion of treated but uncontrolled hypertensives is made of 'white coat' reactors. In the PAMELA population, a high proportion of uncontrolled treated hypertensives was also found with home or ambulatory blood pressure measurements, which are known to cause only minimal white coat reaction. The awareness that guideline recommendations are largely based, as far as goal blood pressure is concerned, on observational rather than interventional studies may be one reason weakening the strength of persuasion of this aspect of guidelines. A persistent belief in, or fear of, the J-shaped curve phenomenon, despite the strong evidence against it provided by the HOT study, may still play a role. An additional reason may be the debate on cost-effectiveness of antihypertensive therapy, and the discouragement of treating uncomplicated mild hypertension, which has unfortunately been fostered by national health services or health insurers in several countries, with the purpose of health-cost containment rather than that of health preservation. Undoubtedly, the adverse effects and even the annoying subjective disturbances often provided by most classes of antihypertensive agents play an important role in decreasing the compliance of patients toward antihypertensive treatment. Finally, combination therapy is seldom used in practice, while the excellent blood pressure control achieved in the HOT study was obtained thanks to the use of combination therapy (mostly two drugs, but sometimes three drugs) in about two-thirds of the patients.

Conclusion

The blood pressure goal of antihypertensive treatment has only been systematically researched recently. It is not surprising that more information is available on goal diastolic blood pressure. Most trials of antihypertensive therapy, with the exception of those on isolated systolic hypertension, have been based on diastolic blood pressure values both for recruitment and randomization, and for treatment titration.

There is no doubt that goal blood pressure should be lower than the levels commonly achieved in practice, where at best one out of four hypertensive patients achieve blood pressure levels lower than 140/90 mmHg.

Observational epidemiological studies support the recommendation that blood pressure values should be brought as close to optimal or normal blood pressure levels as tolerable.

Intervention studies indicate that the minimum goal should be blood pressure values lower than 140/90 mmHg. That this goal is indeed achievable, at least for diastolic blood pressure, has been shown by the large HOT study, in which 91.5% of the 18 790 patients achieved and maintained diastolic blood pressure ≤90 mmHg throughout the 3.8 years of the trial.

Blood pressure values lower than <130/85 mmHg should be maintained at least in special groups of patients, e.g. in diabetics, in whom the HOT study as well as the UKPDS have shown greater benefits for diastolic blood pressure values closer to 80 mmHg than to 85 mmHg. It is likely that incoming data will stress the benefit of further lowering the blood pressure goal in other groups of hypertensive patients.

References

1. Collins R, Peto R, MacMahon S *et al*. Blood pressure, stroke, and coronary heart disease. Part 2. Short-term reductions in blood pressure; overview of randomized drug trials in their epidemiological context. *Lancet* 1990;**335**:827–838.
2. Lindholm L, Ejlertsson G, Scherstén B. High risk of cerebrocardiovascular morbidity in well treated male hypertensives: a retrospective study of 40–59 year old hypertensives in a Swedish primary care district. *Acta Med Scand* 1984;**216**:251–259.
3. Isles CG, Walker LM, Beevers GD *et al*. Mortality in patients of the Glasgow Blood Pressure Clinic. *J Hypertension* 1986;**4**:141–156.
4. Zanchetti A. To what level should blood pressure be brought by antihypertensive treatment? *High Blood Press* 1992;**1**:197–200.
5. Stewart IM. Relation of reduction in pressure to first myocardial infarction in patients receiving treatment for severe hypertension. *Lancet* 1979;**i**:861–865.
6. Cruickshank JM, Thorp JM, Zacharias FJ. Benefits and potential harm of lowering blood pressure. *Lancet* 1987;**i**:581–584.
7. Alderman MH, Ooi WL, Madhavan S, Cohen H. Treatment-induced blood pressure reduction and the risk of myocardial infarction. *J Am Med Ass* 1989;**262**:920–924.
8. Samuelsson O, Wilhelmsen L, Andersson OK *et al*. Cardiovascular morbidity in relation to change in blood pressure and serum cholesterol levels in treated hypertension: results from the Primary Prevention Trial in Göteborg, Sweden. *J Am Med Ass* 1987;**258**:1768–1776.
9. MacMahon S, Peto R, Cutler J *et al*. Blood pressure, stroke and coronary heart disease. Part 1. Prolonged differences in blood pressure: prospective observational studies corrected for the regression dilution bias. *Lancet* 1990;**335**:765–767.
10. Stamler J, Stamler R, Neaton JD. Blood pressure, systolic and diastolic and cardiovascular risks. *Arch Intern Med* 1993;**153**:598–615.
11. Nielsen WB, Lindenstrom E, Vestbo J, Jensen GB. Is diastolic hypertension an independent risk factor for stroke in presence of normal systolic blood pressure in the middle-aged and the elderly? *Am J Hypertension* 1997;**10**:634–639.

7

12. Joint National Committee. The Sixth Report of the Joint National Committee on Prevention, Detection, Evaluation, and Treatment of High Blood Pressure. *Arch Intern Med* 1997;**157**:2413–2446.

13. WHO/ISH Guidelines Subcommittee. 1999 World Health Organization-International Society of Hypertension guidelines for the management of hypertension. *J Hypertension* 1999;**17**:151–183.

14. Zanchetti A, Hansson L. Hypertension Optimal Treatment (HOT) Study. In: *Clinical Trials in Hypertension* (ed. Black H), pp 357–394. Marcel Dekker: New York, 2001.

15. Hypertension Detection and Follow-up Program Cooperative Group. Five-year findings of the Hypertension Detection and Follow-up Program. I. Reduction in mortality of persons with high blood pressure, including mild hypertension. *J Am Med Ass* 1979;**242**:2562–2571.

16. Hansson L, Zanchetti A, for the HOT Study Group. The Hypertension Optimal Treatment Study (the HOT Study). *Blood Press* 1993;**2**:62–68.

17. Hansson L, Zanchetti A, Carruthers SG *et al.* for the HOT Study Group. Effects of intensive blood pressure lowering and low dose aspirin in patients with hypertension: principal results of the Hypertension Optimal Treatment (HOT) randomised trial. *Lancet* 1998;**351**:1755–1762.

18. Wiklund I, Halling K, Rydèn-Bergsten T, Fletcher A, on behalf of the HOT Study Group. Does lowering of blood pressure improve the mood? Quality-of-life results from the Hypertension Optimal Treatment (HOT) Study. *Blood Press.* 1997;**6**:357–364.

19. Collins R, Peto R. Antihypertensive drug therapy: effects on stroke and coronary heart disease. In: *Textbook of Hypertension* (ed. Swales JD), pp. 1156–1164. Blackwell Scientific Publications: Oxford, 1994.

20. Zanchetti A, Hansson L, Ménard J *et al.* for the HOT Study Group. Risk assessment and treatment benefit in intensively treated patients of the Hypertension Optimal Treatment (HOT) study. *J Hypertension* 2001;**19**:819–825.

21. UK Prospective Diabetes Study Group. Tight blood pressure control and risk of macrovascular and microvascular complications in Type 2 diabetes: UKPDS 38. *Br Med J* 1998;**317**:703–713.

22. UK Prospective Diabetes Study Group. Efficacy of atenolol and captopril in reducing risk of macrovascular and microvascular complications in Type 2 diabetes: UKPDS 39. *Br Med J* 1998;**317**:713–720.

23. Mancia G, Sega R, Bravi C *et al.* Ambulatory blood pressure normality: results from the PAMELA study. *J Hypertension* 1995;**13**:1377–1390.

24. Burt VL, Cutler JA, Higgins H *et al.* Trends in the prevalence, awareness, treatment, and control of hypertension in the adult US population. Data from the Health Examination Surveys, 1960 to 1991. *Hypertension* 1995;**26**:60–69.

25. Coca A. Actual blood pressure control. Are we doing the things right? *J Hypertension* 1998;**16**(Suppl. 1):S45–51.

26. Colhoun H, Dong W, Poulter NR. Blood pressure screening management and control in England: results from the Health Survey in England 1994. *J Hypertension* 1998;**16**:747–752.

27. Menotti A, Lanti M, Zanchetti A *et al.* on behalf of the Gubbio Study Research Group. Impact of the Gubbio population study on community control of blood pressure and hypertension. *J Hypertension* 2001;**19**:843–850.

28. Mancia G, Sega R, Milesi C *et al.* Blood pressure control in the hypertensive population. *Lancet* 1997;**349**:454–457.

29. Vaisse B, Renucci JF, Charmasson C *et al.* Efficacité du traitement antihypertenseur dans la population française. Enquête multicentrique. *Arch Maladies Coeur* 1992;**85**:1939–1942.

30. Zanchetti A. How far should blood pressure be lowered? *J Cardiovasc Pharmacol* 1999;**34**(Suppl. 3):S1–36.

31. Zanchetti A. The intensity of treatment of hypertension: the Hypertension Optimal Treatment (HOT) study. In: Harrison's online (ed. Braunwald E) McGraw-Hill; New York, 2000.

7

Lifestyle changes

LJ Beilin and V Burke

7

Why lifestyle changes?

Dietary and other lifestyle factors play a major role in the rise in blood pressure with age and hence the prevalence of so-called 'essential hypertension'. Up to 80% of the prevalence of hypertension in industrialized societies can be attributed to environmental factors. Although genetic influences are important in determining individual susceptibility to hypertension, the overall level of blood pressure in a community is largely dependent on dietary factors, physical activity levels, the prevalence of obesity and the amount of alcohol consumed[1]. Hypertension is a major risk factor for coronary heart disease and the most important factor predisposing to stroke. Therefore, there is clearly a major opportunity to reduce population morbidity and mortality by lifestyle modification, both in the population as a whole, and in individuals who have already developed elevated blood pressure. Many of the measures outlined below will have beneficial effects on cardiovascular risk over and above direct effects on blood pressure. This is especially likely to be the case with weight control, by dietary patterns characterized by reductions in saturated fat intake and increased fruit, vegetable and fish consumption, moderation of heavy alcohol intake and by increased physical activity. Smoking has a dominant effect in increasing cardiovascular risk in hypertensives and is probably the single most important factor to modify in terms of overall health.

Antihypertensive drug therapy does not usually fully normalize blood pressures even when multiple agents are used. Moreover, the risk of death from heart disease is only likely to be reduced by 13–24% by these drugs unless other risk factors are tackled simultaneously. Modification of lifestyle offers the possibility of avoiding drug therapy in many mild-to-moderate hypertensives and reducing drug requirements in those with more established hypertension. Consequent benefits include reduction in side effects and in costs of drugs and related investigations.

Indications for lifestyle changes in the management of hypertension

In contrast to drug therapy, there is no contraindication to lifestyle modification in the majority of hypertensives. Most hypertensives will exhibit one or more behaviors predisposing them to increased risk of cardiovascular disease. Risk behavior tend to cluster, such that smokers are more likely to drink heavily, be physically inactive, and eat less healthily than non-smokers[2]. The metabolic syndrome, of which hypertension is a part, along with dyslipidemia and glucose intolerance, is largely determined by obesity and physical inactivity. Most hypertensives carry excess body fat and are relatively inactive. The majority of people in Western societies do not meet current dietary recommendations as regards to dietary salt, total and saturated fat consumption, fruit, vegetables and fibre intake; hypertensives are no exception.

Lower socioeconomic groups and disadvantaged indigenous groups are at particular risk of hypertensive cardiovascular disease due to dietary and risk behaviors. Hypertensives are more likely to drink alcohol above so-called 'safe levels'. Smoking rates range from 30 to 70%, and are at the upper end of this range in countries with the largest populations such as China and in the former Eastern Bloc, where stroke and coronary death rates are still increasing.

Lifestyle measures appropriate to the individual are indicated in all degrees of hypertension, in both primary and secondary hypertension, and at all ages. Hypertensives who have multiple risk factors and/or have already experienced cardiovascular events such as angina, myocardial infarction and stroke should be targeted for lifestyle changes to prevent progression and recurrence of disease. The objectives are to lower blood pressure, to minimize antihypertensive drug needs, to reduce the overall risk of cardiovascular disease and to improve quality of life.

BOX 7.2.1 Objectives of lifestyle changes in hypertension

- Lower blood pressure
- Minimize drug use
- Reduce overall cardiovascular risk
- Improve outcome
- Maintain or improve quality of life

The evidence

Role of weight control

In population studies, weight or body mass index (BMI) predict blood pressure[3], and the prevalence and incidence of hypertension. Based on data from the Framingham study, 78% of hypertension in men and 65% in women is attributable to obesity.

In clinical trials, blood pressure falls with weight loss[4]. Although the initial level of weight loss is usually not maintained, the Trials of Hypertension Prevention[4] found benefits associated with a weight-loss program, even if weight returned to preintervention levels, relative to the control group who gained weight over the same period. In that study lower blood pressure, a 20% lower incidence of hypertension and lower requirements for antihypertensive drugs were seen up to two years after beginning the weight-loss program. Additive effects on blood pressure are seen when weight loss is combined with restriction of alcohol intake[5], increased fish consumption[6] or moderate sodium restriction (TONE study) and with exercise[7].

In the Framingham Study, both weight and weight gain increased the risk of hypertension. In the Nurses Health Study, a longitudinal study involving more than 120 000 women in the United States[8], the risk for hypertension was related to current BMI, BMI at the age of 18 years and change in weight up to fifty years later. The risk of hypertension decreased by 26% for a 10-kg weight loss from the age of 18 years and increased by 74% for a weight gain of 5–10 kg.

Although cut-off points are widely used to define overweight and obesity, there is, in fact, a continuum of risk[9]; weight gain is associated with increased risk even if the resulting BMI is within the 'normal' range. In the Nurses Health Study[8], risk of hypertension increased by an estimated 12% for each unit increase in current BMI, by 8% for each unit increase in BMI at the age of 18 years and by 5% for each 1 kg of weight gain in the long term.

Distribution of body fat

Hypertension, insulin resistance and dyslipidemia, along with increased risk for coronary heart disease, are associated with central obesity[10]. Visceral obesity is most accurately shown by methods such as magnetic resonance imaging, however, waist : hip ratios (WHR) give a reasonable estimate of visceral fat. Central obesity may be present with body weight or BMI within the normal range, particularly in smokers. Measurement of the waist midway between the rib margin and the iliac crest and of the hip at the level of the greater trochanters is widely used and is readily applied to monitoring patients

Weight loss and weight cycling

Findings from large epidemiological studies suggested that weight loss and large fluctuations in body weight i.e. 'weight cycling', may be associated with greater mortality in the longer term, particularly for cardiovascular disease. However, these studies were not specifically designed to address this question, nor did they allow recognition of involuntary weight loss caused by coincident disease. In contrast, Williamson *et al.*[11] found decreased mortality among obese women who lost weight intentionally. Weight loss clearly benefits several cardiovascular risk factors and has a major role in the non-pharmacological management of hypertension. However, the associations between weight gain and risk for hypertension and the difficulty of achieving and maintaining weight loss point to prevention of weight gain as the ideal.

Achieving weight control

Although reduction of energy intake can achieve weight loss in the short term, compliance is difficult to maintain and it is common for weight lost to be gradually regained[4]. Diet, behavioral modification and exercise all have a role in maintaining long-term weight loss. Overall, integration of physical activity programs with energy restriction appears to have the greatest longer-term success, while conferring other benefits associated with exercise. Even modest weight loss of the order of 3–5 kg has substantial benefits and patients should not be set unrealistic goals.

BOX 7.2.2 Benefits of weight control for hypertension

- Lower blood pressure
- Lower drug requirements
- Improved glucose tolerance
- Improved lipid profile
- Lower left ventricular load and strain
- Lower risk of arterial thrombosis

Exercise and physical activity

Exercise, regular physical activity and measures of fitness have all been associated, in population studies, with lower blood pressure as well as with lower risk for cardiovascular disease[12]. However, cross-sectional studies may be confounded by other lifestyle factors such as healthier diets, lower rates of smoking and lower alcohol intake among individuals who exercise regularly. In randomized controlled trials in the short term, meta-analysis indicates that exercise training can lead to a fall in clinic systolic blood pressure of 10 mmHg in hypertensives and 3 mmHg in normotensives[13]. Meta-analyses, however, have emphasized deficiencies in the design of many of these studies[14] and findings have been inconsistent, particularly in normotensives. Studies employing ambulatory blood pressure have also yielded inconsistent results[15].

Exercise programs may lead to additional benefits when combined with other lifestyle interventions. The combination of weight loss with exercise training led to additive falls in blood pressure in hypertensives while, in obese subjects, weight loss and exercise resulted in more prolonged reduction in 24-hour ambulatory blood pressure. In longer-term studies, the systolic blood pressure fell by 10 mmHg in hypertensives and 7 mmHg in normotensives with a combination of weight control, quitting smoking, salt restriction and physical activity. Salt restriction, weight loss, reduced alcohol intake and exercise resulted in falls of 11 mmHg systolic in mild hypertensives. In Type 2 diabetics, an exercise program attenuated mild impairment of glycemic control associated with dietary marine oils.

Although regular exercise may decrease blood pressure, effects on other cardiovascular risk factors, including decreased insulin resistance, decreased coagulation and increased HDL-cholesterol, also play a role in modifying cardiovascular risk. Regular physical activity is promoted as an important part of adopting a healthy lifestyle. High-intensity exercise is not needed to produce health benefits and vigorous exercise may, in fact, attenuate blood pressure lowering. Lower intensity exercise and the incorporation of physical activity into regular daily activities, such as walking to work and climbing stairs, are usually recommended. Although there have been variations in suggested intensity, duration and frequency of exercise needed to achieve lowering of blood pressure[15], the health benefits of moderate exercise for at least 30 minutes at least three times a week are now widely endorsed.

7

BOX 7.2.3 Exercise

- Physical activity is associated with lower cardiovascular morbidity and mortality
- Blood pressure-lowering effects of exercise are greater in hypertensives
- Regular exercise also benefits other cardiovascular risk factors by:
  decreasing insulin resistance;
  decreasing coagulation; and
  increasing HDL-cholesterol
- Moderate-intensity exercise for at least 30 minutes at least three times a week is recommended to achieve health benefits

---

Dietary sodium and potassium

The relationship between dietary salt and blood pressure levels in populations is now well established[16]. Much of the earlier controversy relates to poor methods for assessing individual sodium consumption and confounding issues such as the fact that overall nutrient consumption is largely determined by energy expenditure or physical activity and the latter is inversely related to blood pressure levels. There is also some evidence that a high dietary salt intake may predispose to left ventricular hypertrophy over and above its effects on blood pressure.

Randomized, controlled trials in treated and untreated hypertensives (with initial systolic blood pressures of 140–160 mmHg) have shown blood pressure falls of 6 mmHg systolic when sodium intake is reduced from 170 to 70–90 mmols/day[17]. A dose–response effect has been demonstrated in older hypertensives with reductions of sodium of 50 and 100 mmols/day[18]. These effects are likely to be greater in those with higher pressures and appear independent of age. The effects have been shown to be sustained over many months. Sodium restriction has been shown to potentiate the effects of diuretics, beta-blockers and angiotensin-converting enzyme inhibitors.

Concerns about the safety of moderate sodium restriction are most likely misplaced and based on results of short term studies of extremes of salt depletion and poorly designed cohort studies. The recent TONE study from the USA showed that overweight elderly hypertensives could substantially reduce their antihypertensive drug requirements without adverse effects by either sodium restriction averaging 40 mmols/day or weight control, with the greatest effect if both lifestyle changes were combined[19] (Figure 7.2.1).

Potassium intake, which is largely related to fruit and vegetable consumption, tends to be inversely associated with salt intake. Population studies suggest that dietary potassium consumption is independently related to blood pressure levels and that the effects are amplified by a dietary salt. A high intake of salt and low consumption of food containing potassium is a particular feature of poorer communities such as American Blacks. It has been claimed that dietary potassium may help protect against stroke independent of effects on blood

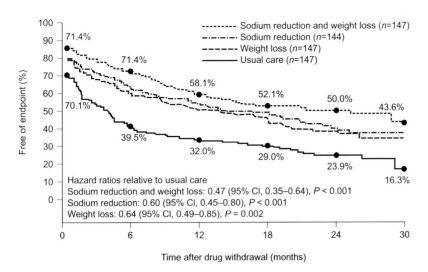

Fig. 7.2.1 Percentages of the 144 participants assigned to reduced sodium intake, the 147 assigned to weight loss, the 147 assigned to reduced sodium intake and weight loss combined, and the 147 assigned to usual care (no lifestyle intervention) who remained free of cardiovascular events and high blood pressure and did not have an antihypertensive agent prescribed during follow-up. CI indicates confidence interval. (Reproduced with permission from Whelton PK *et al.*[19].)

pressure; however, there is a strong possibility of confounding in population studies due to the high covariance of potassium and other dietary constituents. Nonetheless, there are animal data to back up this hypothesis.

Randomized, controlled trials of potassium supplements show useful blood pressure lowering effects in hypertensives[20]. However, it is generally recommended that potassium intake be increased by increasing fruit and vegetable consumption from which additional cardiovascular and other health benefits may accrue.

Dietary *n*3 fatty acids

Dietary *n*3 fatty acids are found principally in marine animals and to a lesser extent in some plants, such as rapeseed. Eicosapentanoic (EPA) and docosahexanoic (DHA) acids are the two compounds best studied and between them have a range of biological properties potentially protective against atherosclerosis, thrombosis and hypertension. These effects include inhibition of platelet aggregation, reduction in VLDL-cholesterol synthesis and triglyceride levels, elevation in HDL_2-cholesterol, improved endothelial vasomotor function, diminished vascular reactivity to pressor stimuli, and antiarrhythmic and anti-inflammatory effects. Although earlier studies suggested that only very large doses of *n*3 fatty acids were antihypertensive, recent large randomized placebo-controlled trials with mixtures of EPA and DHA in oil have been shown to be effective in doses of 3.5–5 g day in untreated mild hypertensives and in non-insulin-dependent diabetics resulting in blood pressure falls of 4–5 mmHg systolic[21].

> **BOX 7.2.4 Some effects of *n*3 fatty acids**
>
> - Reduce platelet aggregation
> - Lower triglycerides
> - Increased HDL_2
> - Improved endothelial function
> - Lower blood pressure
> - Antiarrhythmic effect (in animals)
> - Anti-inflammatory effect

Palatable amounts of daily servings of fish rich in *n*3 fatty acids can provide equivalent quantities of *n*3 fatty acids. A recent controlled trial in overweight treated hypertensives compared effects of a daily fish meal either alone or in combination with a reducing diet[6]. There were independent effects of fish and 5–6 kg weight loss on 24-hour ambulatory systolic blood pressure of the order of 5 mmHg. When a daily fish meal was incorporated into a weight-losing regime, there was an additive effect on daytime blood pressure which fell by 13/9 mmHg compared with control subjects. The two modalities also produced the greatest reduction in cardiovascular risk overall with a 38% fall in serum triglycerides, a 20% increase in HDL_2-cholesterol and the improvement in glucose tolerance. Taking these results together with the known effects of *n*3 fatty acids on platelet function it would appear that measures to increase consumption of oily fish could lead to significant reductions in blood pressure and substantial reduction in cardiovascular risk, particularly in overweight or diabetic hypertensives. Substituting fish for meat several times a week is also likely to lead to a reduction in total and saturated fat intake with consequent benefit to cardiovascular health.

Complex dietary changes

Links between blood pressure and diet have been recognized in population studies, most of which initially explored associations with nutrients and micronutrients. In general, lower blood pressure is related to higher dietary fiber, potassium, magnesium and calcium[22] while, in some studies, total or saturated fat intake correlates positively with blood pressure. Inverse associations between protein intake and blood pressure have also been reported.

Studies in vegetarians who, in both population studies and clinical trials, have lower blood pressure[23], are consistent with these reports. Vegetarian diets differ, not only in their source of protein, but in containing more cereal, fruit and vegetables and provide more fiber, complex carbohydrates, potassium, magnesium, folic acid and antioxidants and have a higher polyunsaturated to saturated fatty acid ratio. Several clinical trials have explored these differences in nutrients and micronutrients, but no single dietary component responsible for lower blood pressure in vegetarians has been identified. Lowering of blood pressure must either depend on a combination of dietary components, or involve some component not yet identified. In either case, dietary recommendations based on foods rather than nutrients are appropriate, as well as being more readily applied to health promotion.

Interpreting the effects of dietary components is complicated by the coexistence of multiple nutrients and micronutrients in foods. For example, fruit and vegetables contain fiber, potassium and magnesium and antioxidant vitamins, all of which have been linked, individually, to lower blood pressure. When data from population studies are examined in terms of foods, intake of fruit and vegetables is associated with lower blood pressure. Consumption of fish and fish oils is also related to lower blood pressure but associations with other foods have been less consistent. Epidemiological studies also support the cardiovascular benefits of a 'Mediterranean' diet[24]. This type of diet is high in fruit, vegetables and whole-grain cereals and low in animal products with saturated fat replaced to a large extent by monounsaturated fat as olive oil and is associated with a moderate intake of alcohol.

In addition to studies of vegetarian diets, clinical trials support the benefits of a diet low in fat and high in fruit and vegetables. A low-fat, high-fiber diet achieved by changing to low-fat dairy products, decreasing intake of meat, increasing fish consumption and increasing intake of fruit and vegetables led to a fall of 6 mmHg in systolic blood pressure in young men after six months. Among hypertensives, comparison of diets low in fat, low in sodium, high in fiber or combining all three modifications showed the greatest fall in blood pressure with the combination diet along with the greatest fall in requirements for antihypertensive drugs.

The Dietary Approaches to Stop Hypertension (DASH) study was a multicenter trial, carried out in the United States, designed to examine the effects on blood pressure of dietary patterns reported to be associated with lower blood pressure[25]. This study focused on foods, rather than individual nutrients or micronutrients. A diet relatively low in potassium, magnesium, calcium and fiber with no modification of fat content was compared to a diet high in fruit and vegetables with no modification of fat and to a diet high in fruit and vegetables and low-fat dairy foods with fat content reduced to 25% energy[25]. An eight-week increase in fruit and vegetables lowered blood pressure by ~ 3/1 mmHg (systolic/diastolic), while the low-fat, high-fruit and vegetable diet lowered blood pressure by ~ 6/3 mmHg. Effects were even more obvious in hypertensives with a fall of 7/3 mmHg in the group with increased fruits and vegetables and 11/6 mmHg with both increased fruit and vegetables and lower fat intake.

A diet rich in fruit and vegetables and fish, and low in total and saturated fat and salt confers benefits extending beyond the effects on blood pressure. Improvements in blood lipids, lowering of plasma homocysteine and increased antioxidant activity are all associated with a diet of this type and more favorable outcomes, in terms of both cardiovascular disease and cancer, are seen in prospective studies.

The evidence
Dietary *n*3 fatty acids

7

451

BOX 7.2.5 Changing diet

- Blood pressure is lower in vegetarians
- No single blood pressure-lowering dietary component is recognized
- Diets high in fruit and vegetables and low in fat are associated with lower blood pressure
- Such diets lower cardiovascular risk with additional benefits on glycemic control and lipids

---

Alcohol and hypertension

Population studies from around the world show a consistent relation between the amount of alcohol consumed, blood pressure levels and the prevalence of hypertension. The relationship is seen in all ethnic groups studied, in men and women, and with all types of alcohol beverage. Although some earlier studies suggested a J-shaped association with blood pressure, subsequent work indicates that the relationship is linear throughout the entire range of consumption[26]. The effect of alcohol on blood pressure increases with age and with cigarette smoking and is additive to effects of obesity. Heavier drinkers may show some withdrawal hypertension in the 48 hours after a binge.

Randomized controlled trials of effects of reducing alcohol consumption from the equivalent of five or six standard drinks (10 g ethanol/drink) to one or two drinks a day show blood pressure falls of ~ 5 mmHg systolic within one or two weeks in treated or untreated hypertensives or normotensive subjects[26,27]. Combining alcohol moderation with 7-kg weight loss in obese subjects with borderline hypertension resulted in falls of 10–14 mmHg systolic and 9 mmHg diastolic sustained over four months[5] compared with controls (Figure 7.2.2)[5]. Resistant hypertension in heavier drinkers may be due to direct pressor effects of alcohol as well as problems with compliance with therapy.

The effects of alcoholic beverages on cardiovascular disease processes are complex. Regular drinking of the equivalent of up to three to five standard drinks a day is associated with some reduction in the risk of coronary events[20] despite a three-fold increase in the risk of hypertension. Most of any benefit on coronary risk is probably due to effects of alcohol *per se*; the much popularized but unproven role of antioxidants in wine requires more critical research. Light-drinking patterns are associated with decreased risk of ischemic stroke in some, but not, all studies. On the other hand, there is a linear increase in the risk of hemorrhagic stroke with alcohol, while binge drinking increases the risk of both cerebral infarction and hemorrhage[29]. Heavier drinking patterns can also lead to cardiomyopathy and arrhythmias.

In summary, regular alcohol drinking is a major contributor to hypertension and stroke. Light-drinking patterns may afford some protection against coronary heart disease and ischemic stroke. These observations need to be seen in the overall context of effects of alcohol on other medical and psychosocial issues.

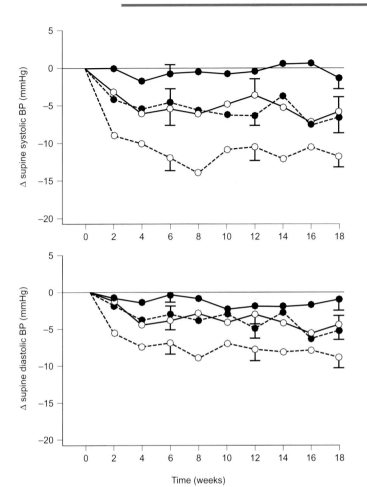

Fig. 7.2.2 Line graphs show change in mean ± SEM systolic (top) and diastolic (bottom) blood pressure (BP) in four study groups. ●——●, normal alcohol intake/normal caloric intake (*n* = 20); ●----● normal alcohol intake/low caloric intake (*n* = 22); ○——○ low alcohol intake/normal caloric intake (*n* = 21); ○-----○ low alcohol intake/low caloric intake (*n* = 23). (Reproduced with permission from Puddey *et al.*[5].)

BOX 7.2.6 Alcohol

- Alcohol is an important and reversible cause of hypertension
- Regular alcohol consumption can increase antihypertensive drug requirements
- Lower levels of alcohol consumption may protect against coronary heart events
- Alcohol increases the risk of hemorrhagic stroke
- Binge-drinking patterns increase the risk of all stroke types
- Hypertensive drinkers should be advised to restrict intake to one or two standard drinks a day

Caffeine-containing beverages

Reported effects of caffeine-containing beverages on blood pressure have been inconsistent. Caffeine, tea and coffee have each been examined, but may not be equivalent, as both tea and coffee are rich in pharmacologically active compounds.

There is general agreement that caffeine-containing drinks will increase blood pressure acutely in individuals who are 'caffeine-naïve', with exaggerated responses in hypertensives[30]. Within a few days of resuming caffeine consumption, this pressor effect is reported to disappear as tolerance develops. However, caffeine has a half-life of about 5 hours, and overnight abstinence may be enough to reach a 'caffeine-naïve' state.

Clinical trials of longer-term effects have mostly examined coffee or caffeine. Myers[31], in reviewing studies based on measurement of clinic blood pressure, concluded that the evidence, overall, indicates no long-term effects of caffeine on blood pressure. However, most of these reports do not relate to the elderly nor to hypertensives.

Several trials using ambulatory blood pressure monitoring (ABPM) have reported a pressor effect of caffeine (see James[32] for summary), exacerbated by smoking and stress. However, other studies using ABPM have been negative[32] with inconsistent findings in both normotensives and hypertensives.

Although impairment of baroreceptor function and greater responses to caffeine are more likely in the elderly, effects of age have received little attention. In a controlled trial, we found that blood pressure in elderly treated or untreated hypertensives increased over a period of two weeks with continued coffee intake but fell with abstinence; no pressor effects were observed in elderly normotensives. It is possible that some of the inconsistencies in previous studies are explained by interactions between hypertension and age.

BOX 7.2.7 Caffeine

- Caffeine increases blood pressure acutely in the 'caffeine naïve' state
- Long-term pressor effects of caffeine are more obvious in elderly hypertensives
- Hypertensives should be advised to limit their intake of caffeine.
- The combination of smoking and caffeine intake should be avoided.

Smoking and blood pressure

Smoking substantially influences the risk of cardiovascular disease directly[33] and through adverse health behaviors that tend to cluster in smokers such as physical inactivity, diets high in fat and low in fiber and greater alcohol consumption[34]. Smoking cessation has been estimated to lead to a reduction of 43% in prevalence of coronary heart disease[33].

7

Hypertension is more difficult to control in smokers, and non-selective beta-blockers, in particular, are less effective. Hypertensive smokers also have a worse prognosis and a greater risk of developing both renovascular and accelerated hypertension. However, in population studies, smokers are usually reported to have lower blood pressure and to have a lower prevalence of hypertension. Lower body mass index (BMI) in smokers may, in part, explain this association. Smoking cessation followed by weight gain can lead to an increase in blood pressure, but blood pressure may be unchanged. In contrast, smoking causes an acute rise in blood pressure with a reported increase in mild hypertensives of 10/7 mmHg (systolic/diastolic) lasting 15 minutes after smoking two cigarettes. This increase is greater and more sustained if smoking is combined with drinking coffee. Acute effects of smoking are linked mainly to nicotine which brings about an increase in cardiac output and in peripheral resistance.

Ambulatory blood pressure monitoring suggests a possible explanation for the apparent difference in acute and longer-term associations between smoking and blood pressure. In mild hypertensives, daytime blood pressure is higher among smokers than non-smokers, whilst clinic blood pressure is, in fact, lower in smokers[35]. Greater daytime ambulatory blood pressure, with no significant difference in night-time ambulatory blood pressure has been found in hypertensives, borderline hypertensives and normotensives.

Cessation of smoking reduces morbidity and mortality for cardiovascular disease within two years[36] and should be a high priority, especially in hypertensive smokers. Smokers should also receive advice about other health behaviors, given the tendency for clustering of adverse health choices in smokers. Interactions between coffee drinking and smoking suggest that this combination should be avoided, particularly in hypertensive smokers.

BOX 7.2.8 Smoking

- Quitting smoking should be a high priority in lowering risk for cardiovascular disease
- Prognosis is worse and blood pressure more difficult to control in hypertensive smokers
- Risk is reduced within two years of quitting smoking
- Advice about alcohol, weight control, diet and exercise should be combined with efforts to stop smoking

---

Stress modification and coping mechanisms

The role of stress and personality in long-term blood pressure regulation and the genesis of hypertension remains unclear despite widespread public perceptions that they are closely related[37]. Acute blood pressure elevation with acute mental stress is undoubted. Chronic depressive personalities if anything have lower blood pressures than average. Those who suppress hostile emotions seem more prone to higher blood pressure. Part of the problem in this area is defining stress; one man's potion is another's poison in emotional terms. Using the Karacek model of job stress and strain, Pickering's group[38] have found that job strain and blood pressure are related in male drinkers but not women or non-drinkers. Ambulatory blood pressure studies suggest that women with both home, family and work commitments are more likely to have sustained blood pressure elevation. However, it is still not clear whether these are direct effects of stress on blood pressure regulation or indirect effects mediated by unhealthy dietary and lifestyle habits. That the latter may be the case was suggested by a study from Western Australia of 800 income tax workers in whom no relation was found between job stress and blood pressure[39]. However, job stress was related to coping mechanisms which in turn related to blood pressure. These coping mechanisms included those determining dietary, drinking, exercise and smoking habits which are known to directly influence blood pressure and risk of heart disease.

Various approaches have been used to reduce blood pressure by stress reduction techniques. These approaches have often involved a mixture of physical and psychological maneuvers such as muscle relaxation, breathing techniques, yoga, transcendental meditation and biofeedback. Very few of these studies have been adequately controlled or used ambulatory blood pressure measurements. With the occasional exception, the better designed trials have been negative, but perhaps the targets are wrong. The Australian studies suggest that it may be more rewarding to tackle maladaptive and adaptive mechanisms for coping with stress.

Strategies for behavioral change in clinical practice

Who should do it, how, and who pays? These are the critical questions. Who should do it? Clearly the patient. This is one area of the doctor–patient relationship where responsibility for their actions and health has to be accepted by the patient. The incentives of reduced drug requirements, improved health, an enhanced feeling of wellbeing and a greater control of one's own destiny are not insubstantial.

Who should help them is perhaps an equally important question. Doctors clearly have a vital role but are often hampered by a lack of conviction, lack of education of behavioral modification techniques and in many countries lack of financial incentives to spend the time required. In the field of smoking addiction, the benefit of even the briefest exhortation to stop smoking by a doctor has been clearly demonstrated, especially when combined with ancillary measures such as nicotine patches or gum, to help overcome withdrawal symptoms. However, in many instances allied health professionals may be a more cost-effective alternative, particularly, but not exclusively, in developing countries.

How should behavioral change be achieved? Models derived from the addiction field are now being applied to diet, weight control and exercise in people with hypertension and related cardiovascular

Lifestyle changes

Strategies for behavioral
change in clinical practice
References

problems. These models include concepts such as Prochaska's Stages of (or readiness to) Change and Self Efficacy or confidence in one's ability to achieve changes in behavior. Setting achievable goals and promoting self-esteem appear to be important elements of more successful programs. These techniques can be applied by suitably trained nurses or other allied health professionals as well as doctors[40]. Imparting a sense of guilt has been the traditional medical approach and is clearly counterproductive. Sustained lifestyle changes can be achieved in hypertensives and have been shown in earlier studies to reduce antihypertensive drug requirements over periods of four years or more. However, these approaches are still relatively labour-intensive and new techniques need to be developed and assessed for cost effectiveness.

In many instances, healthy lifestyle changes will only be more readily achieved by social and structural changes in society. This has already been illustrated in relation to laws relating to tobacco smoking in North America and Australia. Changes in dietary salt will require the cooperation of the food industry and governments. The growing fast food industry can play a more critical role in promoting healthier foods than at present. Facilities for safer walking, cycling and other recreational sports may help stem the tide of physical inactivity that accompanies advances in technology and car transport.

References

1. Beilin LJ (Editorial) The Fifth Sir George Pickering Memorial Lecture. Epitaph to essential hypertension – a preventable disorder of known aetiology? *J Hypertension* 1988;**6**:85–94.
2. Burke V, Milligan RAK, Beilin LJ *et al*. Clustering of health-related behaviours in 18-year-old Australians. *Prevent Med* 1997;**26**:724–733.
3. Stamler R, Stamler J, Riedlinger WF *et al*. Weight and blood pressure. Findings in hypertension screening of 1 million Americans. *J Am Med Ass* 1978;**240**:1607–1610.
4. The Trials of Hypertension Prevention Collaborative Research Group. Effects of weight loss and sodium reduction intervention on blood pressure and hypertension incidence in overweight people with high-normal blood pressure. *Arch Intern Med* 1997;**157**:657–667.
5. Puddey IB, Parker M, Beilin LJ *et al*. Effects of alcohol and caloric restrictions on blood pressure and serum lipids in overweight men. *Hypertension* 1992;**20**:533–541.
6. Bao DQ, Mori TA, Burke V *et al*. Effects of dietary fish and weight reduction on ambulatory blood pressure in overweight hypertensives. *Hypertension* 1998;**32**:710–717.
7. Cox KL, Puddey IB, Morton AR *et al*. Exercise and weight control in sedentary overweight men: effects on clinic and ambulatory blood pressure. *J Hypertension* 1996;**14**:779–790.
8. Huang Z, Willett WC, Manson JE *et al*. Body weight, weight change and risk for hypertension in women. *Ann Intern Med* 1998;**128**:81–88.
9. Willett WC, Manson JE, Stampfer MJ *et al*. Weight, weight change and coronary heart disease in women. *J Am Med Ass* 1995;**273**:461–465.
10. Kaplan NM. Obesity, insulin and hypertension. *Cardiovasc Risk Factors* 1994;**4**:133–139.
11. Williamson DE, Pamuk E, Thun M *et al*. Prospective study of intentional weight loss and mortality in never-smoking overweight US white women aged 40–64 years. *Am J Epidemiol* 1995;**141**:1128–1141.
12. Paffenbarger RS Jr, Hyde RT, Wing AI *et al*. The association of changes in physical activity level and other lifestyle characteristics with mortality in men. *N Engl J Med* 1993;**328**:538–545.

7

References

13. Fagard RH. The role of exercise in blood pressure control: supportive evidence. *J Hypertension* 1995;**13**:1223–1227.

14. Arroll B, Beaglehole R. Does physical activity lower blood pressure?: a critical review of the clinical trials. *J Clin Epidem* 1992;**45**:439–447.

15. Puddey IB, Cox K. Exercise lowers blood pressure – sometimes? Or did Pheidippides have hypertension? *J Hypertension* 1995;**13**:1229–1233.

16. Law MR. Epidemiological evidence on salt and blood pressure. *Am J Hypertension* 1997;**10**:42S–45S.

17. Cutler JA, Follman D, Alexander PS. Randomised controlled trials of sodium reduction: an overview. *Am J Clin Nutr* 1997;**65**(Suppl):643S–651S.

18. Cappuccio FP, Markandu ND, Carney C *et al*. Double-blind randomised trial of modest salt restriction in older people. *Lancet* 1997;**350**(9081):850–854.

19. Whelton PK, Appel LJ, Espeland MA *et al*. Tone Collaborative Research Group: sodium reduction and weight loss in the treatment of hypertension in older persons. A randomized controlled Trial of Nonpharmacologic Interventions in the Elderly (TONE). *J Am Med Ass* 1998;**279**(11):839–846.

20. Geleijnse JM, Witteman JC, Bak AA *et al*. Reduction in blood pressure with a low sodium high potassium, high magnesium salt in older subjects with mild to moderate hypertension. *Br Med J* 1994;**309**:436–440.

21. Bønaa KH, Kjerve KS, Straume B *et al*. Effect of eicosapentanoic acid and docosahexanoic acid on blood pressure in hypertension. A population based intervention trial from the Tromsø study. *N Engl J Med* 1990;**322**:795–801.

22. Ascherio A, Hennekens C, Willett WC *et al*. Prospective study of nutritional factors, blood pressure, and hypertension among US women. *Hypertension* 1996;**27**:1065–1072.

23. Burke V, Beilin LJ. Vegetarian diets and high blood pressure – an update. *Nutrition Metab Cardiovasc Dis* 1994;**4**(2):103–112.

24. Kushi LH, Lenart EB, Willett WC. Health implications of Mediterranean diets in the light of contemporary knowledge. 1. Plants and dairy products. *Am J Clin Nutr* 1995;**61**(Suppl. 6):1407S–1415S.

25. Appel LJ, Moore TJ, Obarzanek E *et al*. A clinical trial of the effects of dietary patterns on blood pressure. *N Engl J Med* 1997;**336**:1117–1124.

26. Puddey IB, Beilin LJ, Rakic V. Alcohol, hypertension and the cardiovascular system: A critical appraisal. *Addiction Biol* 1997;**2**:159–170.

27. Puddey IB, Beilin LJ, Vandongen R. Regular alcohol use raises blood pressure in treated hypertensive subjects – a randomized controlled trial. *Lancet* 1987;**i**:647–651.

28. Thun MJ, Peto R, Lopez AD *et al*. Alcohol consumption and mortality among middle-aged and elderly US adults. *N Engl J Med* 1997;**337**:1705–1714.

29. Donahue RP, Abbott RD, Reed DM, Yano K. Alcohol and haemorrhagic stroke: The Honolulu Heart Program. *J Am Med Ass* 1986;**255**:2311–2314.

30. Pincomb GA, Lovallo WR, McKey BS *et al*. Acute blood pressure elevations with caffeine in men with borderline systemic hypertension. *Am J Cardiol* 1996;**77**:2704.

31. Myers MG. Effects of caffeine on blood pressure *Arch Intern Med* 1988;**148**:1189–1193.

32. James JE. Is habitual caffeine use a preventable cardiovascular risk factor? *Lancet* 1997;**349**:279–281.

33. Hopkins PN, Williams RR. Identification and relative weight of cardiovascular risk factors. *Cardiol Clin* 1986;**4**:3–31.

34. Prattala R, Karisto A, Berg MA. Consistency and variation in unhealthy behaviour among Finnish men. *Social Sci Med* 1994;**39**:115–122.

35. Narkiewicz K, Maraglino G, Biasion T *et al*. Interactive effect of cigarettes and coffee on daytime systolic blood pressure in patients with mild essential hypertension HARVEST Study Group. *J Hypertension* 1995;**13**:965–970.

36. Kawachi I, Colditz GA, Stampfer MJ *et al*. Smoking cessation and time course of decreased risks of coronary heart disease in middle-aged women. *Arch Intern Med* 1994;**154**:169–175.

37. Nyklicek I, Vingerhoets JJM, Van Heck GL. Hypertension and objective and self-reported stressor exposure: a review. *J Psychosom Res* 1996;**40**:585–601.

38. Pickering TG, Devereux RB, James GD *et al*. Environmental influences on blood pressure and the role of job strain. *J Hypertension* 1996;**14**(Suppl. 5):S179–S185.

7

39. Lindquist TL, Beilin LJ, Knuiman MW. Influence of lifestyle, coping and job stress on blood pressure in men and women. *Hypertension* 1997;**29**:1–7.
40. Woollard J, Beilin L, Lord T *et al*. A controlled trial of nurse counselling on lifestyle change for hypertensives treated in general practice: Preliminary results. *Clin Exp Pharmacol Physiol* 1995;**22**:466–468.

References

7

7.3

The stepped-care approach: pros and cons

BJ Materson

7

Introduction

The stepped-care approach to the therapy of hypertension was an outgrowth of highly successful clinical trials that demonstrated the efficacy of drug treatment. Simplicity and relatively low cost were attractive features, but the inflexibility of the algorithm was problematic. In this chapter, we review the history of the development of the stepped-care algorithm, its advantages and disadvantages in the treatment of hypertension, and some of the modern alternatives for tailoring antihypertensive therapy to the characteristics of the individual patient.

History

Shift from single-drug therapy to polypharmacy

In the days before science became a full partner in the practice of the art of medicine, polypharmacy was the accepted standard of drug therapy. It was common for complex prescriptions to be compounded by pharmacists in an attempt to cure or alleviate disease by means of an interaction of the component chemicals. As science advanced, this approach became intellectually unsatisfactory and therapeutic 'magic bullets' were sought that were specific to the problem at hand. Until thiazide diuretics became available in 1958, there were no safe magic bullets for the treatment of hypertension. Thiocyanate, severe sodium restriction, surgical sympathectomy, veratrum alkaloids, and ganglionic blocking agents were available for severe complicated or malignant hypertension but at a considerable cost to the patient's quality of life. Hydralazine and rauwolfia alkaloids became available in 1953, but high doses were required for effect and were accompanied by a high incidence of adverse drug reactions.

Diuretics changed the entire approach to the treatment of hypertension and, because of the ability of diuretics to enhance the efficacy of other antihypertensive drugs, ushered in an era of polypharmacy specific to the treatment of hypertension[1].

BOX 7.3.1 Shift of the therapeutic paradigm

In the late 1950s ganglionic blocking agents, veratrum alkaloids, reserpine, and hydralazine were used for the treatment of severe hypertension. Serious disabilities, such as orthostatic hypotension, bowel and bladder dysfunction, visual changes, and sexual dysfunction, had made it extremely unlikely that a previously asymptomatic patient would accept such treatment even on the promise of prolongation of his or her life. In fact, about the only hypertension worth treating was that of the severe, accelerated, malignant, or already complicated variety. These patients tended to be highly symptomatic and frequently had irreversible target organ disease. By the early 1960s, veratrum alkaloids and ganglionic blocking agents would be outdated. The advent of diuretic drugs and newer antihypertensive agents had made it possible to treat hypertension without disabling the patient[1].

Impact of Freis and the VA Cooperative Study

Edward D. Freis chaired the seminal VA Cooperative Study[2], which proved, in 1967, that treatment of severe hypertension was associated with a striking reduction of target organ damage when compared to a comparable group of patients who were randomly assigned to blinded treatment with placebo. Even though many experts in the early 1960s believed that Freis' study was unethical and that there was no benefit to treating hypertension, the study was stopped prematurely for ethical reasons when the dramatic beneficial results became apparent. Subsequent publications in 1970[3] and 1972[4] confirmed the benefit of treatment, although less dramatic, for moderate and mild hypertension. The Freis study had used hydrochlorothiazide, reserpine, and hydralazine in combination. This provided a firm basis for the stepped-care concept.

National High Blood Pressure Education Program (1973) and stepped care

Freis had the opportunity to interact with Secretary of State Elliott Richardson and philanthropist Mary Lasker. He helped to convince them of the importance of taking the results of the VA hypertension studies to the entire population. This was at least part of the impetus for the National High Blood Pressure Education Program of the National Heart, Lung, and Blood Institute. Task Force I of that group, chaired by H. Mitchell Perry, Jr., arrived at a consensus document that was the foundation of the stepped-care algorithm[5]. The VA research data were thereby translated into an action plan that was promulgated to physicians nationwide.

The Joint National Committee and stepped care

The Joint National Committee on the Detection, Evaluation, and Treatment of High Blood Pressure (JNC) is composed of representatives from numerous scientific and governmental bodies. Its recommendations, like those of Task Force I, are consensus statements and may not represent the opinion of each individual committee member. Nevertheless, that consensus is derived from considerable expert input and, to the extent possible, is evidence-based.

The first JNC report[6] in 1977 confirmed the stepped-care algorithm and included Figure 7.3.1 as the visual version of the algorithm. A thiazide diuretic was the foundation of the steps. In 1980 the second JNC report[7] greatly expanded the committee information about hypertension and its treatment, but maintained the basic stepped-care philosophy. The third report[8], published in 1984, took advantage of new data regarding the use of beta-adrenergic blocking agents as single-drug therapy for hypertension. They changed the first step to a choice of either a diuretic or a beta-blocker. By 1988, newer drugs such as angiotensin-converting enzyme (ACE) inhibitors, calcium antagonists, and α_1-peripheral adrenergic blockers had become available. JNC IV[9]

7

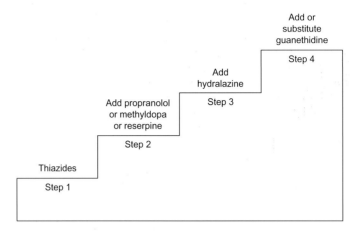

Fig. 7.3.1 Concept of stepped care from the 1977 Joint National Committee on Detection, Evaluation, and Treatment of High Blood Pressure. (Redrawn from[6].)

modified the stepped-care algorithm so that the first step included a choice of a diuretic, beta-blocker, ACE inhibitor, or calcium antagonist. Some experts argued that the α_1-peripheral adrenergic blockers should have been included as well. By the time of the JNC V[10] in 1993, the philosophy had changed to one of strongly evidence-based recommendations. There was inadequate scientific support for the first step use of drugs other than diuretics and beta-blockers because only the latter two drugs had been demonstrated to reduce cardiovascular events, especially stroke. This report created considerable controversy, but the 1997 JNC VI report[11] essentially verified the basis for recommending either a diuretic or beta-blocker as the first step unless there were some compelling reasons to do otherwise.

BOX 7.3.2 Major studies on hypertension used a stepped-care protocol

The legitimacy of the stepped-care algorithm was supported by major prospective randomized clinical trials of treatment of hypertension that used one or another type of stepped care in their protocol. Unlike the clinical practice of medicine, research trials demand rigorous regimens that can be followed identically by different investigators in multiple sites. It is not unusual for these sites to be in more than one country or even on more than one continent. The Hypertension Detection and Follow-up Program (HDFP)[12] compared a stepped-care algorithm using low-dose chlorthalidone as the first step with usual care in the community. The stepped-care protocol effected a greater reduction in diastolic blood pressure (−12.9 vs −8.6 mmHg) and that decrease was associated with 26% fewer deaths from all cardiovascular diseases. Furthermore, the HDFP stepped-care protocol reduced all-cause mortality by 19% for Black hypertensive men and 28% for women[13]. The favorable impact of HDFP was greatest in the group at highest risk, Blacks of lowest socioeconomic status.

BOX 7.3.2 *Continued*

Other major trials such as the Medical Research Council Trial[14] and the European Working Party on High Blood Pressure in the Elderly (EWPHE)[15] contributed additional favorable information on reduction of stroke and cardiovascular mortality by diuretics and beta-blockers.

The Systolic Hypertension in the Elderly Program (SHEP)[16] used chlorthalidone 12.5 mg as a step-one drug and atenolol 25 mg as the starting step-two drug. This effected a 36% reduction (absolute five-year benefit 30 events per 1000 participants) in total stroke compared to placebo. Major cardiovascular events were reduced with a five-year absolute benefit of 55 events per 1000 participants. There was a dramatic reduction in fatal and non-fatal congestive heart failure (relative risk 0.51) that was even more impressive (relative risk 0.19) in patients who had a prior myocardial infarction[17].

On the other hand, the Multiple Risk Factor Intervention Trial (MRFIT)[18] offered some controversial data that diuretics (at least hydrochlorothiazide) might actually be harmful. At the same time, the promotional efforts for newer antihypertensive medications tended to emphasize the negative aspects of diuretics and beta-blockers and to denigrate the concept of a stepped-care algorithm.

Advantages of stepped care

The stepped-care algorithm for treatment of hypertensive patients has been one of the great successes of pharmacologic management of a disease. There is no question that the stepped-care philosophy is effective in lowering blood pressure. One can reasonably expect a 40–60% success rate with a diuretic alone, approximately an 80% success rate when a second drug is added, and better than 90% success rate using three drugs[19].

Table 7.3.1 displays the results of the addition of drugs stepwise in three different VA cooperative studies. Better results may be obtained by careful selection of the patient population matched to the drug or drugs as discussed below, but these excellent results are in populations

Table 7.3.1 Demonstration of the effect of hydrochlorothiazide in combination with other drugs in early VA cooperative studies.

Drug or drug combination	Controlled*
Reserpine + hydrochlorothiazide	88%
Propranolol	52%
Propranolol + hydrochlorothiazide	81%
Propranolol + hydralazine	72%
Propranolol + hydrochlorothiazide + hydralazine	92%
Bendroflumethiazide	46%
Nadolol	49%
Bendroflumethiazide + nadolol	85%
Nadolol + hydralazine	75%
Nadolol + hydralazine + bendroflumethiazide	93%

* 'Controlled' is defined as achieving a diastolic blood pressure of less than 90 mmHg. Data derived from[19] and[20].

selected only by being male ambulatory veterans with mild-to-moderate hypertension and no study exclusions.

An appropriately constructed stepped-care algorithm has very clear rules for initiation of drug therapy, for titration of the first drug, for the addition of a second drug and its titration, and for the addition of subsequent drugs. The algorithm may include 'decision nodes' at which point a physician must become involved. This allows the algorithm to be operated by military corpsmen, pharmacists, nurses, and other non-physician personnel with the appropriate training and qualifications. Its beauty lies in both its efficacy and simplicity.

As healthcare costs rise, the low cost of the drugs included in most stepped-care algorithms becomes very attractive to payers (especially governmental payers) for healthcare. The difference in cost is by no means trivial. A standard stepped-care approach to treatment may cost less than $100 per patient year for medication in contrast to hundreds or even thousands of dollars per patient per year for combinations of newer, very expensive antihypertensive medications.

BOX 7.3.3 Advantages of stepped-care

- The algorithm is highly effective in reducing blood pressure
- The algorithm is simple and well suited for use by non-physician personnel with appropriate physician supervision at 'decision nodes'
- The rules for initiation of therapy, titration of the first drug, initiation and titration of the second and subsequent drugs are very clear
- In general, stepped-care algorithms have used less expensive drugs and may result in substantial monetary savings

---

Disadvantages of stepped care

The hypertensive population is not homogeneous. It is unrealistic to expect that a 'one-drug-fits-all' approach would be the best approach. We now know that patients of different races, older or younger age, degrees of obesity, differing volume status, specific indications or contraindications for various drugs, concomitant disease and other special conditions (see Section 8) should be treated more specifically than stepped-care permits.

Therefore, there are a number of disadvantages to using the strict stepped-care algorithm. These negatives have become more problematic with the continuing introduction of more and more new drug classes that permit greater 'fine tuning' of antihypertensive therapy:

- Stepped care generally requires that the first drug be pushed to its maximum dose (or to toxicity) if the blood pressure is not controlled before the next step drug is added. Starting with a thiazide diuretic in a young White patient, the chances are that potentially toxic doses will be reached and that efficacy might not be achieved. On the other hand, a beta-blocker or angiotensin-converting enzyme inhibitor might be effective at a low dose in such a patient.

BOX 7.3.4 Disadvantages of stepped-care

The hypertensive population is not homogeneous. There are:
different races;
older versus younger age;
thin versus obese;
volume-constricted versus volume-replete;
presence of concomitant diseases;
indications or contraindications for specific drugs;
individual quality of life issues;
cost considerations

Therefore stepped-care:

- may titrate each drug to toxicity before adding the next drug
- does not consider the underlying mechanisms of hypertension
- is not intellectually satisfying in that it does not challenge the practitioner to make the best drug match for that particular patient
- is relatively inflexible
- does not permit the use of patient characteristics to tailor therapy to that individual patient

---

- Stepped care does not consider the underlying mechanism of the hypertension. A diuretic should not be the drug of first choice in a patient likely to have high renin hypertension nor should an ACE inhibitor be the drug of first choice in a patient likely to have low-renin hypertension.
- Stepped care, while highly effective and free from the necessity for a great deal of thoughtful reflection, is not intellectually satisfying because it does not challenge the practitioner to make the best drug match for that particular patient.
- Stepped care is relatively inflexible. Its basic design is to bring the patient and non-physician therapist to 'decision nodes' that require the interaction of a physician. There is little room for maneuvering.
- Finally, stepped care does not allow for the modern ability of the practitioner to use multiple patient characteristics in order to tailor therapy to the needs of that individual patient. This requires much greater knowledge of the drugs and the underlying mechanisms of hypertension for that particular patient, but the opportunity for success in controlling the blood pressure without adverse effects is greater.

BOX 7.3.5 Plasma renin profiling

In the early 1970s. John Laragh and his colleagues[21] promulgated the hypothesis that hypertensive patients could be placed somewhere on a continuum of vasoconstriction or volume expansion and that this could be determined by doing plasma renin profiling. That procedure required collection of a 24-hour urine specimen plus a blood sample. When performed and interpreted correctly, plasma renin profiling was useful in helping to select the appropriate antihypertensive drug for the patient. However, its inconvenience and expense prevented it from being very widely used by practicing physicians.

Joint National Committee VI algorithm

The Sixth Joint National Committee on Prevention, Detection, Evaluation and Treatment of High Blood Pressure (JNC VI)[11] used evidence-based medicine concepts and a large panel of experts to arrive at a consensus document that includes an algorithm for the treatment of hypertension (Figure 7.3.2). Like any product of a large committee, the consensus statements may not be the actual opinion of all of the participating experts. Nevertheless, this document makes clear, evidence-based recommendations for a logical approach to the treatment of hypertensive patients.

JNC VI makes a strong argument for population-based methods to prevent hypertension in the first place and for a base of non-pharmacologic healthy lifestyle changes for all patients with hypertension. They recommended initial treatment with a diuretic or beta-blocker for the majority of patients who did not respond to lifestyle changes and who had no other special or compelling indications for other drugs(Table 7.3.2). Their algorithm is clear, reasonably easy to use, and provides considerable discretion to the treating physician (Table 7.3.3).

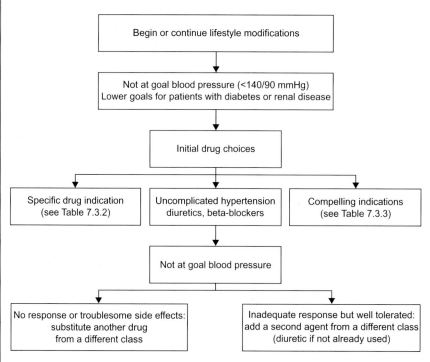

Fig. 7.3.2 Basic hypertension treatment algorithm from the 1997 Joint National Committee on Prevention, Detection, Evaluation, and Treatment of High Blood Pressure. (Redrawn from[11].)

VA age by race interaction
for the selection of initial
drug therapy

Table 7.3.2 Specific indications for selection of an initial medication other than a diuretic or beta-blocker. (After[11].)

- Angina, atrial tachycardia and fibrillation: beta-blockers, calcium antagonists (non-dihydropyridine for arrhythmia)
- Essential tremor, hyperthyroidism, migraine, preoperative hypertension: beta-blockers (usually non-selective)
- Prostatism: α-blockers
- Osteoporosis: thiazides
- Renal insufficiency: ACE inhibitors

Table 7.3.3 Compelling indications for selection of an initial medication other than a diuretic or beta-blocker. (After[11].)

- Diabetes mellitus (Type 1) with proteinuria: ACE inhibitors
- Heart failure: ACE inhibitors, diuretics
- Isolated systolic hypertension: diuretics (preferred), long-acting dihydropyridine calcium antagonists
- Myocardial infarction: beta-blockers (non ISA (intrinsic sympathomimetic activity)), ACE inhibitors (with systolic dysfunction)

VA age by race interaction for the selection of initial drug therapy

In 1993, the Department of Veterans Affairs Cooperative Study Group on Antihypertensive Agents published the results of their study of representatives of six classes of antihypertensive drugs and placebo in 1292 ambulatory men[22]. The key finding was that consideration of all 1292 men together gave a misleading picture of response to the various drugs. In contrast, separating the patients into four age by race subgroups provided far more information as to the drug most likely to be effective for that given subgroup. The two races were Caucasian (White) and African-American (Black). No Blacks from countries other than the United States were included and there were too few Asians for separate analysis. Younger was defined as less than 60 years of age and older as 60 years or greater.

The seminal results were that younger Blacks responded best to the calcium antagonist (diltiazem-SR), while younger Whites responded best to the beta-blocker (atenolol) or ACE inhibitor (captopril) and slightly less well to the calcium antagonist or α_1-blocker (prazosin). Older Blacks had an excellent response to the calcium antagonist and also did well with the diuretic (hydrochlorothiazide); they responded poorly to the beta-blocker and not at all to the ACE inhibitor. Older Whites seemed to respond similarly to all of the drug classes, including the beta-blocker and ACE inhibitor (Figure 7.3.3). Although Whites responded particularly well to the central α_1-agonist (clonidine), they had a very high level of adverse effects and removals from the study because of drug intolerance.

The robust database generated by the VA study has permitted additional analyses that pertain directly to patient care. The study contained an arm that required treatment of patients who failed to

7

VA age by race interaction for the selection of initial drug therapy

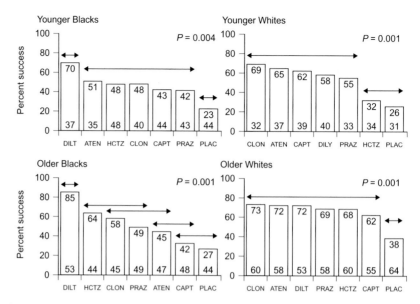

Fig. 7.3.3 Younger Black patients, younger White patients, older Black patients, and older White patients classified as treatment success (diastolic blood pressure less than 90 mmHg at end-titration and less than 95 mmHg at one year) in each of the study groups. The arrows group the medications whose effects do not differ from each other by more than 15%. ATEN = atenolol, CAPT = captopril, CLON = clonidine, DILT = diltiazem-SR, HCTZ = hydrochlorothiazide, PLAC = placebo, and PRAZ = prazosin. (Reproduced with permission from Elsevier Science from Materson *et al.*[6]. Copyright 1995 American Journal of Hypertension Ltd.)

respond to the first randomly allocated drug with a second randomly assigned drug (but not placebo)[24]. The results validated the initial findings and strongly suggested a role for a strategy of substitution or sequential treatment of hypertension (see Chapter 7.4). There was a final arm that included patients who had failed treatment with both the first and the second drug[25]. The two drugs were carefully combined in this group of 102 patients. Despite the fact that they had failed two separate single drug treatments, 58% responded to a combination of two drugs (Figure 7.3.4). When a diuretic was one of the two drugs, the systolic blood pressure response rate was significantly higher than in patients who received two non-diuretic drugs. The diastolic blood pressure response rate was also better in the diuretic than non-diuretic group, although not statistically significant (Figure 7.3.4).

Analysis of 24-hour urine protein excretion strongly suggested that the ACE inhibitor used (captopril) did not cause proteinuria[26]. In fact, the combination of proteinuria and hypertension, especially in patients with concomitant diabetes mellitus, is a strong indication for the use of an ACE inhibitor.

Analysis of sophisticated serum lipid and lipoprotein data demonstrated that, over a one- to two-year period, diuretic drugs did not significantly perturb these substances toward a more cardiotoxic profile[27].

Serial echocardiograms were performed in the majority of the patients (Figure 7.3.5). These demonstrated that hydrochlorothiazide

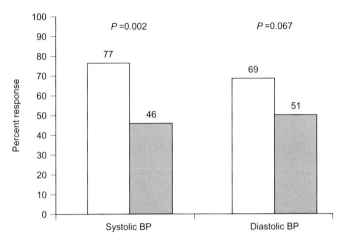

VA age by race interaction for the selection of initial drug therapy

Fig. 7.3.4 Number and percentage of patients who responded with a systolic blood pressure less than 140 mmHg and diastolic blood pressure less than 90 mmHg while taking two medications. The open bars depict combinations in which one of the two medications was hydrochlorothiazide. The shaded bars depict combinations of two non-diuretic medications. (Reconstructed from data in Materson *et al.*[25].)

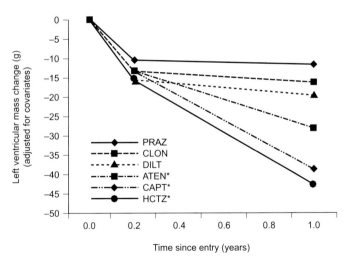

Fig. 7.3.5 Left ventricular mass changes in patients with the highest tertile of left ventricular mass, adjusted for patient covariates. The asterisk indicates medications that were associated with significant reductions in left ventricular mass. (Reproduced with permission from Gottdiener *et al.* and *Circulation*[28].)

caused substantial reduction of left ventricular mass for patients in the highest tertile of left ventricular mass at baseline; captopril and atenolol had a significant, but somewhat lesser effect[28]. For those patients with left atrial enlargement, the same three drugs effected significant regression in left atrial size[29].

All of the above data lend support to the position taken by JNC VI regarding diuretics as a first line agent, absent other factors.

Finally, the study protocol included plasma renin profiling of all of the patients[30]. We compared the ability of plasma renin profiling versus the age by race model to predict response to a single antihypertensive drug in patients with stage 1 hypertension. The age by race model proved to be at least as good as plasma renin profiling and, in one analysis, was marginally better. Determining a patient's age and race is simple, cheap, rapid, and non-invasive.

Conclusions

The stepped-care algorithm is highly effective and inexpensive when used by non-physicians in large populations without easy access to sophisticated medical care. There are better algorithms for the treatment of hypertension. The JNC VI model can be strongly recommended but it should be modified by use of the age by race paradigm for purposes of improving the likelihood of success with the first drug.

References

1. Materson BJ. Perspectives on contemporary management of hypertension. In: *Management of Hypertension: A Multifactorial Approach* (ed. Hollenberg NK), p. 21. Scientific Therapeutics Information: Springfield, NJ, 1987.
2. Veterans Administration Cooperative Study Group on Antihypertensive Agents. Effects of treatment on morbidity in hypertension. I. Results in patients with diastolic blood pressure averaging 115 through 129 mmHg. *J Am Med Ass* 1967;**202**:1028–1034.
3. Veterans Administration Cooperative Study Group on Antihypertensive Agents. Effects of treatment on morbidity in hypertension. II. Results in patients with diastolic blood pressure averaging 90 through 114 mmHg. *J Am Med Ass* 1970;**213**:1143–1152.
4. Veterans Administration Cooperative Study Group on Antihypertensive Agents. III. Influence of age, diastolic pressure, and prior cardiovascular disease: further analysis of side effects. *Circulation* 1972;**45**:991–1004.
5. Perry HM. Recommendations for a National High Blood Pressure Program Data Base for Effective Antihypertensive Therapy. Report of Task Force I. DHEW publication No. (NIH) 75–593. US Department of Health, Education, and Welfare: Bethesda, MD, 1973.
6. Joint National Committee on Detection, Evaluation, and Treatment of High Blood Pressure. Report of the Joint National Committee on Detection, Evaluation, and Treatment of High Blood Pressure: A cooperative study. *J Am Med Ass* 1977;**237**(3):255–261.
7. Joint National Committee on Detection, Evaluation, and Treatment of High Blood Pressure. The 1980 Report of the Joint National Committee on Detection, Evaluation, and Treatment of High Blood Pressure. *Arch Intern Med* 1980;**140**(10):1280–1285.
8. Joint National Committee on Detection, Evaluation, and Treatment of High Blood Pressure. The 1984 Report of the Joint National Committee on Detection, Evaluation, and Treatment of High Blood Pressure. *Arch Intern Med* 1984;**144**(5):1045–1057.
9. Joint National Committee on Detection, Evaluation, and Treatment of High Blood Pressure. The 1988 Report of the Joint National Committee on Detection, Evaluation, and Treatment of High Blood Pressure. *Arch Intern Med* 1988;**148**(5):1023–1038.
10. Joint National Committee on Detection, Evaluation, and Treatment of High Blood Pressure. The Fifth Report of the Joint National Committee on Detection, Evaluation, and Treatment of High Blood Pressure (JNC V). *Arch Intern Med* 1993;**153**(2):154–183.
11. Joint National Committee on Prevention, Detection, Evaluation, and Treatment of High Blood Pressure. The Sixth Report of the Joint National Committee on Prevention,

7

Detection, Evaluation, and Treatment of High Blood Pressure. *Arch Intern Med* 1997;**157**:2413–2446.

12. Hypertension Detection and Follow-up Program Cooperative Group. Five-year findings of the hypertension detection and follow-up program. I. Reduction in mortality of persons with high blood pressure, including mild hypertension. *J Am Med Ass* 1979;**242**(23):2562–2571.

13. Moorman PG, Hames CG, Tyroler HA. Socioeconomic status and morbidity and mortality in hypertensive blacks. *Cardiovasc Clin* 1991;**21**(3):179–194.

14. Medical Research Council Working Party. MRC trial of treatment of mild hypertension: principal results. *Br Med J* 1985;**291**:97–104.

15. Amery A, Birkenhäger W, Brixko P *et al*. Mortality and morbidity results from the European Working Party on High Blood Pressure in the Elderly trial. *Lancet* 1985;**i**(8442):1349–1354.

16. SHEP Cooperative Research Group. Prevention of stroke by antihypertensive drug treatment in older persons with isolated systolic hypertension. Final results of the Systolic Hypertension in the Elderly Program (SHEP). *J Am Med Ass* 1991;**265**(24):3255–3264.

17. Kostis JB, Davis BR, Cutler J *et al*. Prevention of heart failure by antihypertensive drug treatment in older persons with isolated systolic hypertension. SHEP Cooperative Research Group. *J Am Med Ass* 1997;**278**(3):212–216.

18. Multiple Risk Factor Intervention Trial Research Group. Mortality after 10 1/2 years for hypertensive participants in the Multiple Risk Factor Intervention Trial. *Circulation* 1990;**82**(5):1616–1628.

19. VA Cooperative Study Group on Antihypertensive Agents. Propranolol in the treatment of essential hypertension. *J Am Med Ass* 1977;**237**(21):2303–2310.

20. VA Cooperative Study Group on Antihypertensive Agents. Efficacy of nadolol alone and combined with bendroflumethiazide and hydralazine for systemic hypertension. *Am J Cardiol* 1983;**52**(10):1230–1237.

21. Laragh JH. Modification of stepped care approach to antihypertensive therapy. *Am J Med* 1984;**77**(2A):78–86.

22. Materson BJ, Reda DJ, Cushman WC *et al*. Single-drug therapy for hypertension in men. A comparison of six antihypertensive agents with placebo. *N Engl J Med* 1993;**328**:914–921.

23. Materson BJ, Reda DJ, Cushman WC for the Department of Veterans Affairs Cooperative Study Group on Antihypertensive Agents. Department of Veterans Affairs Single-Drug Therapy of Hypertension study: revised figures and new data. *Am J Hypertension* 1995;**8**:189–192.

24. Materson BJ, Reda DJ, Preston RA *et al*. for the Department of Veterans Affairs Cooperative Study Group on Antihypertensive Agents. Response to a second single antihypertensive agent used as monotherapy for hypertension after failure of the initial drug. *Arch Intern Med* 1995;**155**:1757–1762.

25. Materson BJ, Reda DJ, Cushman WC, Henderson WG for the Department of Veterans Affairs Cooperative Study Group on Antihypertensive Agents. Results of combination antihypertensive therapy after failure of each of the components. *J Human Hypertension* 1995;**9**:791–796.

26. Preston RA, Materson BJ, Reda DJ, Hamburger RJ, Smith MH for the Department of Veterans Affairs Cooperative Study Group on Antihypertensive Agents. Proteinuria in mild to moderate hypertension: results of the VA cooperative study of six antihypertensive agents and placebo. *Clin Nephrol* 1997;**47**:310–315.

27. Lakshman MR, Reda D, Materson BJ *et al*. for the Department of Veterans Affairs Cooperative Study Group on Antihypertensive Agents. Comparison of plasma lipid and lipoprotein profiles in hypertensive Black versus White men. *Am J Cardiol* 1996;**78**:1236–1241.

28. Gottdiener JS, Reda DJ, Massie BM *et al*. Effect of single-drug therapy on reduction of left ventricular mass in mild to moderate hypertension: comparison of six antihypertensive agents. The Department of Veterans Affairs Cooperative Study Group on Antihypertensive Agents. *Circulation* 1997;**95**:2007–2014.

29. Gottdiener JS, Reda DJ, Williams DW *et al*. for the VA Cooperative Study Group on Antihypertensive Agents. Effect of single-drug therapy on reduction of left atrial size

References

7

References

in mild to moderate hypertension: comparison of six antihypertensive agents. The Department of Veterans Affairs Cooperative Study Group on Antihypertensive Agents. *Circulation* 1998;**98**:140–148.

30. Preston RA, Materson BJ, Reda DJ *et al.* Age–race subgroup compared to renin profile as predictors of blood pressure response to antihypertensive therapy in 1031 patients: results of a VA cooperative study. *J Am Med Ass* 1998;**280**:1168–1172.

7

Chapter

7.4

Substitution of therapy and other approaches

PW de Leeuw and AA Kroon

7

Introduction

Although a large amount of information is available about the type of drugs that can be used to treat hypertensive patients, far less is known about optimal management strategies. In particular, there is little data concering the therapeutic options once initial treatment has failed. While monotherapy is to be preferred in the 'average' hypertensive patient, it should be realized that the response rate with any antihypertensive agent (in terms of blood pressure reduction without unacceptable side effects) is usually not much greater than 50–60%, and often lower. For instance, in the Treatment of Mild Hypertension Study (TOMHS), five antihypertensive agents were evaluated against placebo[1]. The results showed that 72% of patients given active drug treatment continued on their initial medication as monotherapy over a period of four years (range 66–82% for the various forms of treatment). This may seem substantial, but in the placebo group this figure was 59%. Thus, when corrected for the placebo response, active drugs given as single agents were effective in only a modest proportion of patients. Likewise, in the SYST-EUR trial only 31% of patients who were followed for four years were still taking the initial (active) drug as monotherapy as compared to 14% of those taking placebo[2]. Similar conclusions can be drawn when analyzing other trials. Translated into daily practice, this means that it may frequently be necessary to adjust medication in hypertensive patients in whom existing treatment is not effective enough or causes too many side effects. This calls for some reflection on how this could or should be done and on the preferred types of treatment.

Initial treatment of hypertension

For the treatment of hypertension, several classes of drugs are now available (Table 7.4.1). Currently, the most important of these are diuretics, beta-blockers, calcium-channel blockers and ACE inhibitors because of their favorable effect on long-term prognosis. However, it is not an easy task to choose among the various categories. In coming to a sound decision, the physician may take several courses, approaching the problem from a drug-related or a patient-related perspective.

Table 7.4.1 Classes of antihypertensive drugs (in alphabetical order) and prognosis (as demonstrated in large trials)

Class	Beneficial effect on prognosis
ACE inhibitors	Yes
Alpha-blockers	No
AT_1-receptor antagonists	No
Beta-blockers	Yes
Calcium-entry blockers	Yes
Centrally acting agents	No
Direct vasodilators	No
Diuretics	Yes

7

Drug-oriented approach

Efficacy of available drugs

In essence, only double-blind randomized trials can provide the evidence upon which it is possible to base rational treatment decisions. Numerous such trials have been performed comparing different classes of drugs or different agents within classes. Although there are some gradual differences in efficacy between individual drugs, by and large they produce comparable falls in blood pressure (Figure 7.4.1). In terms of hypotensive potential, therefore, there is little if any evidence that one agent is much better than the other[1]. In the end, however, it is the reduction in cardiovascular morbidity and mortality that counts. For certain categories, e.g. alpha-blockers, the effect on long-term prognosis is uncertain and in some aspects perhaps even unfavorable[3]. On the other hand, large trials conducted in the last 25 years have shown that treatment with diuretics and/or beta-blockers confers prognostic benefit[4]. Recently, the results from other trials have provided evidence that newer agents such as calcium-channel blockers and ACE inhibitors also improve cardiovascular

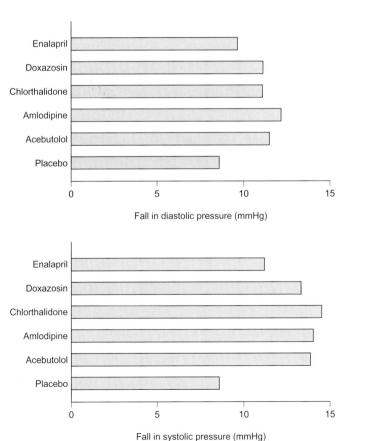

Fig. 7.4.1 Decrease in systolic and diastolic blood pressure produced by placebo and five different antihypertensives. (Data taken from the TOMHS trial[1].)

Table 7.4.2 Relative risk (and 95% confidence intervals) of cardiovascular mortality and morbidity: comparison of conventional* and newer drugs

Mortality/Morbidity	All newer drugs	ACE inhibitors	Calcium-entry blockers
Total mortality	1.01 (0.89–1.14)	1.02 (0.89–1.18)	0.99 (0.86–1.15)
Cardiovascular mortality	0.99 (0.84–1.16)	1.01 (0.84–1.22)	0.97 (0.80–1.17)
All stroke	0.89 (0.76–1.04)	0.90 (0.74–1.08)	0.88 (0.73–1.06)
All myocardial infarction	1.04 (0.86–1.26)	0.90 (0.72–1.13)	1.18 (0.95–1.47)
All major cardiovascular events	0.96 (0.86–1.08)	0.94 (0.82–1.07)	0.99 (0.87–1.12)

* 'Conventional' drugs include beta-blockers and diuretics.
Data taken from the STOP-2 study[5]. Adjusted for age, sex, diabetes, diastolic blood pressure, and smoking.

prognosis[2,5] to the same degree as 'conventional' drugs (Table 7.4.2). However, whether this holds true for the still newer AT_1-receptor antagonists is yet to be established.

Taking the position that only drugs that have proven to reduce cardiovascular mortality and morbidity should be prescribed initially, then at present the choice is between diuretics, beta-blockers, ACE inhibitors and calcium-channel blockers. Any fine-tuning of the choice will have to be based on additional arguments.

Pharmacological considerations

One of the factors that may favour the choice of a particular hypotensive drug relates to its pharmacological profile. Presently, full 24-hour coverage of the blood pressure-lowering effect with single doses is seen as a great advantage. Once-daily dosing has the additional benefit of improving patients' compliance. However, many of the available antihypertensives still have to be dosed at least twice a day and, although this does not necessarily reduce compliance[6,7], it may put them somewhat lower on the list.

A related matter may be the duration of action in case of 'missed' doses. In one study, for instance, the ACE inhibitor trandolapril appeared to provide a longer effect than enalapril on the day of a missed dose[8]. Unfortunately, such information is still lacking for the majority of available medications.

Finally, another factor that needs to be taken into account is whether the drug lowers blood pressure smoothly and, preferably, without causing orthostatic hypotension. In this respect, centrally acting agents and alpha-adrenergic blockers are less desirable.

Ancillary properties

Another argument that may be weighed is the alleged ancillary properties of a particular drug. However, of the various properties that have occasionally been linked to certain drugs such as inhibition of platelet aggregation, stimulation of fibrinolysis or improvement of insulin sensitivity, none has been substantiated to the extent that it can play an overriding role in treatment decisions.

Costs

Today, diuretics are still the cheapest antihypertensive medication and this has led several authoritative bodies to recommend this class of drugs as first-line therapy. One should bear in mind, though, that this aspect has only relative merit since there is more to costs than only the price per tablet per day. The need for patient monitoring and the possible occurrence of metabolic derangements such as hypokalemia may increase total costs relative to medications which need less surveillance.

Patient-oriented approach

Age and race

Several studies have suggested that age and race may influence the antihypertensive response to a number of drugs[9]. For instance, diuretics and calcium-channel blockers may do better in elderly patients and beta-blockers and ACE inhibitors in younger subjects. For reasons that are incompletely understood, Black patients tend to respond better to diuretics and to be more resistant to ACE inhibitors. However, there is great interindividual variability in patients' responses, and claims about demographic features being predictive of the responsiveness of individual patients to antihypertensive agents have never been convincingly substantiated in cross-over trials.

On the other hand, age may argue against the use of certain drugs. Especially in the elderly, for instance, one should avoid medications that may induce profound falls in standing blood pressure (e.g. alpha-blockers or centrally acting agents).

Pathophysiological profile

The most logical approach to treatment would be to adjust medication according to the pathophysiological profile of the patient. This means that, for example, in younger patients with a relatively high cardiac output a beta-blocker should be tried first, while in older subjects with a high peripheral vascular resistance a vasodilator would be more appropriate. Also, plasma renin activity has often been put forward as a powerful predictor of responsiveness in the sense that low levels would call for diuretic therapy and high levels for beta-blocker treatment or a drug that interferes with the renin–angiotensin–aldosterone system. From another angle, patients with signs of volume expansion or salt-sensitive hypertension would likely respond better to a diuretic. Despite several claims that such rational choices can be made, these are not corroborated by scientific evidence. In other words, individual hypertensive patients cannot be fully classified on the basis of a few mechanistic findings and attempts to match treatment with such findings are bound to yield disappointing results[10].

Some investigators believe that the presence of target organ damage should have a major impact on the choice of antihypertensive medication. For instance, regression of left ventricular hypertrophy may

7

be better achieved with an ACE inhibitor than with other drugs[11], although, again, this is not without dispute. It seems reasonable to state that all four major drug classes are still appropriate choices in patients with target organ damage.

Comorbidity

Concomitant diseases may have an overriding role in the decision with which drug to treat the patient. For instance, insulin resistance or frank diabetes often occur together with hypertension. In such cases ACE inhibitors, AT_1-receptor antagonists and some calcium-entry blockers are attractive choices. ACE inhibitors have sometimes even been found to prevent the development of new diabetes[12]. Similarly, disturbances in lipid metabolism may argue against the use of diuretics and beta-blockers and favor the prescription of ACE inhibitors, AT_1-receptor antagonists and calcium entry blockers. Although there is a general feeling that drugs which are metabolically neutral are to be preferred in the treatment of hypertension, there is no scientific evidence that they are absolutely better as far as long-term prognosis is concerned. On the contrary, in this respect the four major drug classes (diuretics, beta-blockers, ACE inhibitors and calcium entry blockers) seem to be comparable[5].

Other conditions that may influence therapeutic decisions are ischemic heart disease, congestive heart failure, renal disease, obstructive lung disease and prostatic hypertrophy. Potential first-line treatments in such cases are listed in Table 7.4.3.

Contraindications, side effects and quality of life

Potential contraindications may lead one not to use certain drugs. Some of these are obvious: beta-blockers, for instance, should be avoided in obstructive lung disease and ACE inhibitors in patients with significant

Table 7.4.3 Hypertension and concomitant diseases: preferred choice of treatment

Coexisting disease	Preferred treatment	Less advisable
Diabetes mellitus	ACE inhibitor AT_1-receptor blocker Calcium-entry blocker	Diuretic
Ischemic heart disease	Beta-blocker ACE inhibitor Calcium-entry blocker (verapamil, diltiazem)	Diuretic
Congestive heart failure	ACE inhibitor AT_1-receptor blocker Beta-blocker (some) Diuretic	Alpha-blocker Calcium-entry blocker
Renal disease	ACE inhibitor (*caution!*) Calcium-entry blocker Diuretic	Beta-blocker
Obstructive lung disease	ACE inhibitor Calcium-entry blocker	Beta-blocker
Prostatic hypertrophy	Alpha-blocker	Diuretic

renal artery stenosis. Others are less obvious or even theoretical such as diuretics being less advisable in patients with lipid abnormalities.

Besides contraindications, side effects may limit the usefulness of a particular drug. Although these may differ in frequency and severity between various agents, available data indicate that no single drug stands out as being more acceptable than others[1,9]. A possible exception may be the class of AT_1-receptor blockers which presently seems to be the one with the least side effects[13]; together with ACE inhibitors, the AT_1-receptor blockers are better tolerated than the older drugs. Therefore, AT_1-receptor blockers have the potential to become first-line treatment, once they have proven to reduce definite cardiovascular endpoints.

With long-term treatment, quality of life becomes an increasingly important issue when it comes to the choice of medication. Surely, there is no treatment without adverse effects on well-being, but in a meta-analysis by Beto and Bansal concerning five measures of quality of life, the overall effect size was reassuringly positive with the exception of sexual function[14]. There was also very little difference between the six types of agents, included in this analysis.

Genetic aspects

An interesting new development is the matching of treatment with certain genetic characteristics of a patient. It has been thought, for instance, that certain polymorphisms in the *ACE* gene would predict responsiveness to ACE inhibition or polymorphisms in sodium channel genes to diuretics. So far, however, no unequivocal relationships between such polymorphic markers and responsiveness to antihypertensive drugs have been established and it is too early to build a therapeutic regimen upon the genetic make-up of the patient.

Treatment approach based on prognostic indices

Is is increasingly recognized that decisions about *whether* to start treatment should take estimates of absolute (cardiovascular) risk into account[15]. To a certain extent, this may also apply to the question of *how* to start treatment. In other words, one should always weigh the potential prognostic benefit incurred by active treatment against the long-term complications of such treatment. When it is anticipated that drug therapy will be necessary for many years, it would be unwise to choose a class which has been linked to such life-threatening complications as carcinoma, gastrointestinal bleeding or even the occurrence of cardiovascular events. Whilst discussions about these aspects continue in the literature, at this point there is no compelling evidence that any of the available antihypertensives truly has an adverse effect on overall prognosis.

Taking all of the above together, there is, as yet, no justification to promote any one class of antihypertensive drugs as the absolute first-line priority. Moreover, no one variable can predict with enough certainty a patient's response to a given antihypertensive drug. Thus,

7

Table 7.4.4 Choice of first drug in hypertension (without other specific indications) as propagated in the guidelines from different countries

Country	Authoritative body	Initial treatment recommendation
Australia	High Blood Pressure Research Council of Australia[21]	Diuretics, beta-blockers, ACE inhibitors, calcium-entry blockers
Canada	Canadian Hypertension Society[22]	Diuretics, beta-blockers
Great Britain	British Hypertension Society[23]	Diuretics, beta-blockers
Netherlands	Kwaliteitsinstituut voor de Gezondheidszorg CBO[27]	Diuretics, beta-blockers
New Zealand	National Advisory Committee on Core Health and Disability Support Services[24]	Diuretics, beta-blockers
USA	Joint National Committee VI[25]	Diuretics, beta-blockers
–	World Health Organization/ International Society of Hypertension[15]	ACE inhibitors. AT_1-receptor blockers, alpha-blockers, beta-blockers, calcium-entry blockers and diuretics (no preference for any)

the practice of treating hypertension remains empirical[16]. In this respect, an individualized approach, taking into account contraindications and side effects, should prevail above rigid recommendations based on alleged rather than documented evidence. Nevertheless, the guidelines from different countries are remarkably consistent in their recommendation to use diuretics or beta-blockers as first-choice agents (Table 7.4.4). An alternative view comes from the World Health Organization/International Society of Hypertension and states that all classes of drugs are acceptable as first-line agents with no preference for any of these. Since all guidelines were produced well before the results of newer studies on the effects of ACE inhibitors and calcium-entry blockers on long-term prognosis had been published, national recommendations may become a bit more liberal in the near future, if drug prices do not become prohibitive.

When low-dose monotherapy fails

Whatever the drug of first choice, it is usual to start with a low dose. Even though this may bring blood pressure down, the effect may not be large enough to reach the preset target. When low-dose monotherapy fails to control blood pressure adequately, there are at least three options to proceed:

- increasing the dosage (dose titration),
- switching to another drug (sequential monotherapy) or
- adding another drug (combination therapy).

These options will be described in more detail below.

Dose titration

Assuming that treatment has started with a low dose of a particular drug, failure to control blood pressure may be remedied simply by increasing drug dose. Of course, this may be effective but there is also the risk of introducing (more) side effects. Moreover, better efficacy can only be expected when the initial dose was really low, i.e. well below the point where the dose–response relationship begins to plateau[17]. However, it should be noted that for most drugs, the clinically recommended doses are already at (or close to) the flat portion of the dose–response curve so that it would seem in the office as if there was no such dose–effect relation.

Sequential monotherapy

In 1990, Brunner and colleagues made a firm plea for sequential monotherapy[17], a form of treatment in which several drugs are prescribed sequentially until an optimal regimen is found[18]. The rationale for such an approach is that, since no antihypertensive drug is entirely free of side effects, it seems preferable to evaluate the efficacy of the components individually instead of formulating a combination regimen. Especially in patients with only mild blood pressure elevation, some form of monotherapy is likely to be adequate and it would be unwise, therefore, to proceed to combination therapy or to increase the dose (with perhaps induction of side effects), once the first drug remains without success. Moreover, the proportion of the hypertensive population that can be treated with only one drug may increase to 70 or 80% when various drugs are tested one after the other[17]. Although sequential monotherapy looks very attractive, there is still no direct evidence to prove its superiority over other methods. However, the practical advantages of this approach are clear and substitution rather than addition has become a rather popular method of treatment. Its major drawback, of course, is that it may take many weeks or even months before the 'right' drug is found. Nevertheless, this is time well spent, considering that this medication will be continued for a very long time.

This substitution strategy does not necessarily have to involve drugs that belong to different classes of antihypertensive agents. A representative from one class could be replaced by another from the same class.

Substitution within classes

Replacement of one drug by another from the same class is justifiable only when there are reasonable *a priori* expectations of differences in efficacy. These could be based, for instance, upon differences in pharmacokinetic profiles, dosing, routes of elimination, or certain pharmacodynamic properties. In this respect, experiences with beta-blockers are perhaps the most telling[19]. In the past, many trials have been performed in which different beta-blockers and ACE inhibitors have been compared with each other. Most of these, however, show about equal efficacy of the drugs under scrutiny and usually similar response rates. Unfortunately, it is not always possible to determine whether the same patients would respond similarly to the two drugs. In

7

other words, even though response rates may be the same for two drugs, a direct comparison may reveal that responsive patients differ during the two types of treatment. Since such comparisons are not made routinely, there is insufficient data to absolutely 'forbid' a within-class substitution. Only when certain patient characteristics make it highly unlikely that this particular class will exert little, if any, effect should another class be considered. However, as explained above, inefficacy on the basis of class alone is very difficult to ascertain.

Substitution between classes

The same reasoning as above applies for the substitution of one drug by another from a different class. Again, individual patients may have varying responses to different drugs even though overall responsiveness of groups of patients to these drugs is similar. In this respect one could follow the '*n* of 1 trial' approach as advocated by Jaeschke and Guyatt[20]. With this approach the physician treats the patient during successive periods with an active drug and matching placebo. Both the patient and the doctor are blind to the active treatment, the choice being made by the pharmacist. Provided that the effect of the various treatment periods is assessed properly, it should be possible to determine the agent that is most effective and well tolerated. Using this approach one could either test a considerable number of drugs to look for the one which gives the best results or stop the trial when an effective agent has been found. The latter, of course, seems preferable.

Combination treatment

Data from several large-scale trials have shown that a considerable number of patients cannot be controlled with only one drug (Figure 7.4.2). In those cases, a second antihypertensive should be added and, if necessary, more. The options are to combine low doses of each drug or

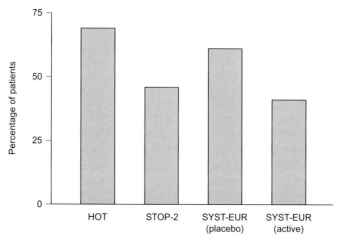

Fig. 7.4.2 Percentage of patients who needed combination treatment in some recent trials. Data taken from the HOT[26], STOP-2[5] and SYST-EUR[2] studies.

7

	ACE inhibitor	AT₁ receptor blocker	Alpha-blocker	Beta-blocker	Calcium-entry blocker	Diuretic
ACE inhibitor		?	+	+	++	++
AT₁ receptor blocker	?		+	+	++	++
Alpha-blocker	+	+		++	+	±
Beta-blocker	+	+	++		+ (V,D) ++ (DHP)	++
Calcium-entry blocker	++	++	+	+ (V,D) ++ (DHP)		+
Diuretic	++	++	±	++	+	

Possible combinations of antihypertensive drugs

? = Effect of combination not well known
± = Combination acceptable, but caution needed
+ = Fair combination
++ = Very effective combination
V = Verapamil
D = Diltiazem
DHP = Dihydropyridines

Fig. 7.4.3 Possible combinations of antihypertensive drugs.

When low-dose monotherapy fails

Combination treatment

to use maximal tolerable doses of every agent. Whereas the former approach is usually recommended to minimize dose-related side effects, there is no compelling evidence against the latter. Figure 7.4.3 illustrates some of the possible combinations.

When combining several types of drugs, two approaches are possible: the stepped-care approach or a 'liberal' combination scheme. Since the stepped-care approach is discussed at length elsewhere in this book (Chapter 7.3), we will restrict ourselves here to only a few remarks. The basic assumption with this approach is that it is the reduction in blood pressure which counts and that the means or mechanisms by which this is achieved are less important. In this view, the best way to treat hypertension is by systematically prescribing drugs according to a prespecified scheme. Traditionally, this includes the addition of other drugs if the first one does not work, rather than replacing one drug by another. The justification for such a scheme is not so much driven by the evidence that this is a better way to manage hypertension (in fact, there is no such evidence) but by the notion that an individualized approach may lead to chaotic ways of treatment. The major and most obvious criticism against the stepped-care approach, however, is the fact that simply adding one drug to the other increases the potential for side

7

effects. There is also the potential for adding three or four antihypertensive agents while none of these is really effective. For these reasons, many clinicians will prefer to try such agents sequentially as described above.

Another way of combining several medications is to utilize drug classes that work through different, and preferably supplemental, mechanisms, e.g. an ACE inhibitor with a diuretic. It is wise to avoid combinations in which the drugs may produce similar types of side effects.

Conclusions

The treatment of hypertension remains enigmatic. Although for many agents it is known how far they lower the average blood pressure in a selected group of patients, it is impossible to predict responsiveness to a certain drug in the individual. The doctor who is faced with such an therapeutic dilemma may either follow a rigid stepwise protocol which is applicable to nearly everybody or individualize treatment. In the latter case, the choice of medication can only be based upon subjective arguments. A few characteristics of the patient or of the drug which is going to be prescribed may help in coming to a final decision, but overall it remains a matter of trial and error. Substitution of drugs rather than addition offers the opportunity to evaluate the efficacy of an array of drugs in a particular patient. With this approach, the physician must be able to select that type of medication that is most beneficial for the patient.

References

1. Neaton JD, Grimm RHJ, Prineas RJ *et al*. Treatment of Mild Hypertension Study. Final results. *J Am Med Ass* 1993;**270**:713–724.
2. Staessen JA, Fagard R, Thijs L *et al*. for the Systolic Hypertension in Europe (SYST-EUR) Trial Investigators. Randomised double-blind comparison of placebo and active treatment for older patients with isolated systolic hypertension. *Lancet* 1997;**350**:757–764.
3. Messerli FH. Implications of discontinuation of doxazosin arm of ALLHAT. *Lancet* 2000;**355**:863.
4. Psaty BM, Smith NL, Siscovick DS *et al*. Health outcomes associated with antihypertensive therapies used as first-line agents. A systematic review and meta-analysis. *J Am Med Ass* 1997;**277**:739–745.
5. Hansson L, Lindholm LH, Ekbom T *et al*. for the STOP-Hypertension-2 study group. Randomised trial of old and new antihypertensive drugs in elderly patients: cardiovascular mortality and morbidity the Swedish Trial in Old Patients with Hypertension-2 study. *Lancet* 1999;**354**:1751–1756.
6. Cramer JA, Mattson RH, Prevey ML *et al*. How often is medication taken as prescribed? A novel assessment technique. *J Am Med Ass* 1989;**261**:3273–3277.
7. Eisen SA, Miller DK, Woodward RS *et al*. The effect of prescribed daily dose frequency on patient medication compliance. *Arch Intern Med* 1990;**150**:1881–1884.
8. Meredith P. Implications of the links between hypertension and myocardial infarction for choice of drug therapy in patients with hypertension. *Am Heart J* 1996;**132**:222–228.
9. Materson BJ, Reda DJ, Cushman WC *et al*. for the Department of Veterans Affairs Cooperative Study Group on Antihypertensive Agents. Single-drug therapy for hypertension in men. A comparison of six antihypertensive agents with placebo. *N Engl J Med* 1993;**328**:914–921.

7

References

10. Kaplan NM. *Clinical hypertension*, 7th edn. Williams & Wilkins: Baltimore, MD, 1998.
11. Schmieder RE, Martus P, Klingbeil A. Reversal of left ventricular hypertrophy in essential hypertension. A meta-analysis of randomized double-blind studies. *J Am Med Ass* 1996;**275**:1507–1513.
12. Hansson L, Lindholm LH, Niskanen L *et al.* for the Captopril Prevention Project (CAPPP) study group. Effect of angiotensin-converting-enzyme inhibition compared with conventional therapy on cardiovascular morbidity and mortality in hypertension: the Captopril Prevention Project (CAPPP) randomised trial. *Lancet* 1999;**353**:611–616.
13. Birkenhäger WH, De Leeuw PW. Non-peptide angiotensin type 1 receptor antagonists in the treatment of hypertension. *J Hypertension* 1999;**17**:873–881.
14. Beto JA, Bansal VK. Quality of life in treatment of hypertension. A metaanalysis of clinical trials. *Am J Hypertension* 1992;**5**:124–133.
15. Guidelines Subcommittee. 1999 World Health Organization-International Society of Hypertension Guidelines for the Management of Hypertension. *J Hypertension* 1999;**17**:151–183.
16. Guyatt G, Sackett D, Taylor DW *et al.* Determining optimal therapy: randomized trials in individual patients. *N Engl J Med* 1986;314:889–892.
17. Brunner HR, Ménard J, Waeber B *et al.* Treating the individual hypertensive patient: considerations on dose, sequential monotherapy and drug combinations. *J Hypertension* 1990;**8**:3–11.
18. Krakoff L. Changing strategies in the management of hypertension. *Cardiovasc Rev Rep* 1983;**4**:319–324.
19. Man in't Veld AJ, Van den Meiracker AH, Schalekamp MADH. Do beta-blockers really increase peripheral vascular resistance? Review of the literature and new observations under basal conditions. *Am J Hypertension* 1988;**1**:91–96.
20. Jaeschke R, Guyatt GH. Randomized trials in the study of antihypertensive drugs. *Am J Hypertension* 1990;**3**:811–814.
21. Hypertension Guidelines Committee. Hypertension, diagnosis, treatment and maintenance. Guidelines endorsed by the High Blood Pressure Research Council of Australia. Royal Australian College of General Practitioners: Adelaide, 1991.
22. Ogilvie RI, Burgess ED, Cusson JR *et al.* Report of the Canadian Hypertension Society Consensus Conference: 3. Pharmacologic treatment of essential hypertension. *Can Med Ass J* 1993;**149**:575–584.
23. Ramsay LE, Williams B, Johnston GD *et al.* for the British Hypertension Society. Guidelines for management of hypertension: report of the third working party of the British Hypertension Society. *J Human Hypertension* 1999;**13**:569–592.
24. National Advisory Committee on Core Health and Disability Support Services. Guidelines for the management of mildly raised blood pressure in New Zealand. Ministry of Health: Wellington, 1995.
25. Joint National Committee. The Sixth Report of the Joint National Committee on Prevention, Detection, Evaluation, and Treatment of High Blood Pressure. *Arch Intern Med* 1997;**157**:2413–2446.
26. Hansson L, Zanchetti A, Carruthers SG *et al.* Effects of intensive blood-pressure lowering and low-dose aspirin in patients with hypertension: principal results of the Hypertension Optimal Treatment (HOT) randomised trial. HOT Study Group[see comments]. *Lancet* 1998;**351**:1755–1762.
27. Herziening Richtlijn Hoge Bloeddruk; Alphen aan den Rijn: Van Zuiden Communications, BV, 2000.

7

Combination treatment in hypertension

G Mancia and G Grassi

7

Introduction

A large number of controlled studies have conclusively shown that treatment of hypertension is beneficial. In virtually all hypertensive conditions, drugs that lower diastolic and/or systolic blood pressure reduce cardiovascular morbidity and mortality[1,2]. However, this is counterbalanced by the evidence that current management of hypertension is unable to bring the cardiovascular risk of the treated hypertensive patient back to the level of the nomotensives[3]. Although several factors are believed to be responsible for this finding, a likely candidate is poor blood pressure control, i.e. by the fact that blood pressure levels of treated hypertensives remain, almost invariably, higher than those of normotensive controls. However, this limitation can be overcome by a therapeutic strategy based on combination of two or more antihypertensive drugs, which allows achieving a better blood pressure control (and thus a greater cardiovascular protection) in a much larger fraction of hypertensive patients than would be achievable with monotherapy[4].

This chapter will discuss the theoretical background and the main requirements for an effective antihypertensive drug combination treatment. It will then examine the advantages and disadvantages of fixed versus extemporaneous combinations of two antihypertensive drugs. Finally, it will focus on the drug combinations as first-line treatment and outline the two-drug combinations that are regarded as being of priority use by the recent guidelines on the treatment of hypertension[5].

Features of combination treatment

Rationale

Combination therapy plays a fundamental role in the overall treatment of hypertension because, although initial monotherapy effectively lowers blood pressure only in a limited fraction of the hypertensive population, combined administration of two or three drugs achieves a successful antihypertensive response in about 80% and 90% of cases, respectively. This is not limited to clinical practice (and thus to the possible incorrect use of single-drug regimens) because combination treatment with two and three drugs has also been commonly employed to achieve optimal blood pressure in controlled studies. This is exemplified in Figure 7.5.1, which shows the high percentage of hypertensive patients under treatment with more than one drug in various trials[6].

The importance of administering more than one drug to achieve the goal of 'normalizing' blood pressure in a large number of hypertensive patients is acknowledged by guidelines on the treatment of hypertension. The latest World Health Organization/International Society of Hypertension Guidelines[5] give priority to combination therapy over other approaches that might be considered once conventional monotherapy fails, i.e. a progressive increase in the dose of the single drug being employed or a switch to other monotherapies until an

7

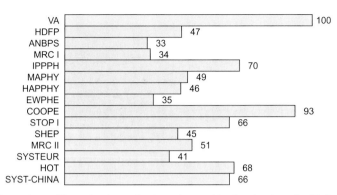

Fig. 7.5.1 Percentage of hypertensive patients under combination treatment with two or more drugs in various clinical trials. (Modified from Mancia and Grassi[6].)

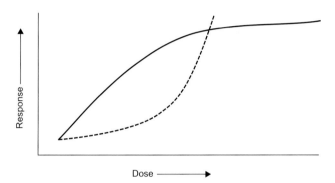

Fig. 7.5.2 Dose-response curves for the blood pressure lowering (continuous line) and the side effects (hatched line) of an antihypertensive drug. (Modified from Mancia *et al.*[9].)

antihypertensive response is obtained. The latter two approaches are associated with problems that detract from the practicality and advisability of their use. For example, if the dose of some antihypertensive drugs (e.g. calcium antagonists) is progressively increased, the blood pressure-lowering effect may increase but at the risk of an increased rate of side effects. Moreover, if the dose of other agents (e.g. diuretics) is increased, an increase only in the medicine of side effects may be seen because a dose–response curve will achieve an early plateau only for the antihypertensive effect (Figure 7.5.2). Finally, if an approach based on sequential monotherapy is employed, the success rate may increase because some patients who are unresponsive to one class of drug may respond to another (Figure 7.5.3)[7], but at the price of wasted time and decreased adherence of the patient to the treatment itself[2].

Requirements

Optimal two-drug combinations are characterized by five main requirements.

- First, the drugs to be combined should have mechanisms of action that are different but complementary.

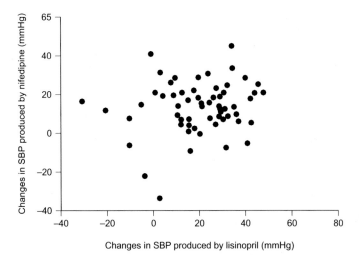

Fig. 7.5.3 Relationship between the systolic blood pressure (SBP) reductions induced by lisinopril and by nifedipine in essential hypertensives in whom these drugs were administered in monotherapy on a sequential basis. (Modified from Sever[7].)

- Second, they should, when given together, produce an antihypertensive effect that is greater than, or equal to, the sum of the antihypertensive effect of the individual combination components, although an effect that is just greater than that of either drug alone may also be acceptable.
- Third, there should also be total or partial summation of their ability to protect aganist the organs that are damaged by hypertension, e.g. they should produce a regression of left ventricular hypertrophy or a reduction in proteinuria greater than can be achieved by the individual combination components.
- Fourth, they should reciprocally reduce (or at least not increase) their side effects.
- Fifth, they should have untoward hemodynamic and humoral effects.

Fixed combinations

Fixed combinations have advantages, but also disadvantages, over the separate administration of the same drugs (Table 7.5.1). It is obvious that extemporaneous combinations allow flexible dosing of the components, e.g. the dose of one drug may be increased while keeping the other

Table 7.5.1 Advantages of fixed versus extemporaneous combinations of two antihypertensive drugs

Fixed	Extemporaneous
Simplicity of treatment	Flexibility of dosing of combination components
Reduced price	Better awareness of combination constituents
Acceptance by doctors	Reduced risk of administering contraindicated drugs
	Better identification of drug responsible for side effects

constant, if this is felt to be useful. They also facilitate a greater awareness, by the physician, of the constituents of the combination treatment[8], thus reducing the risk of administering contraindicated drugs and allowing better identification of which drug is responsible for the side effects that may appear during treatment[9]. Except for the flexibility of dosing, these advantages, however, are not in principle incompatible with fixed-dose combinations, provided that doctors receive proper information.

However, fixed combinations have specific advantages. It should be remembered that fixed combinations allow blood pressure control to be achieved with a reduced number of daily tablets compared with extemporaneous combinations, thus simplifying the therapeutic approach. This is of great potential advantage because in the hypertensive population blood pressure control is unsatisfactory, i.e. in only a minority of the hypertensive population diastolic blood pressure is reduced by antihypertensive treatment to 90 mmHg or less[10–14] (Figure 7.5.4). This is even more evident for systolic blood pressure which is only controlled in a minute number of hypertensive individuals, with no trend towards any improvement in the last few years (Figure 7.5.5)[15]. This is due largely to poor compliance with long-term treatment due to a number of factors, among which the complexity of the treatment scheduled. An example is given in Figure 7.5.6, which shows treatment compliance to decrease progressively with the increase of the daily dosing frequency[16].

Other favorable features of fixed combination are represented by a reduced treatment cost as compared to the cost of using the same drugs on a separate basis, with further advantages for compliance. This has been acknowledged by the World Health Organization/International Society of Hypertension Guidelines[5] which mention fixed combinations as an asset for antihypertensive treatment and a further means to improve the remarkably poor blood pressure control in the hypertensive population.

7

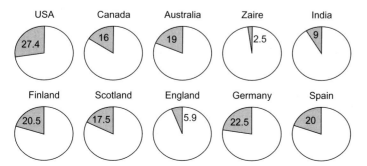

Fig. 7.5.4 Percentage of hypertensive patients (expressed by numbers in each panel) with controlled blood pressure values 140/90 mmHg) in different countries[21]. *Over 65 years.

Combination therapy in
clinical practice

Combinations of priority
use

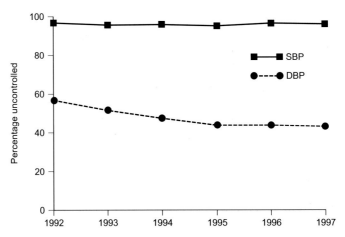

Fig. 7.5.5 Percentage of treated hypertensive patients with uncontrolled systolic blood pressure (SBP) > 140 mmHg or diastolic blood pressure (DBP) > 90 mmHg over time. (Modified from Swales[15].)

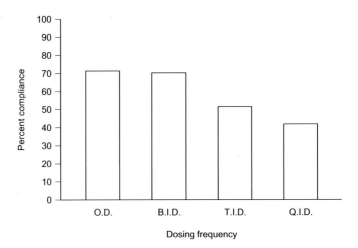

Fig. 7.5.6 Compliance to antihypertensive drugs with different treatment regimens (o.d. = 1 tablet per day; b.i.d. = 2 tablets per day; t.i.d. = three tablets per day; q.i.d = 4 tablets per day). (Modified from Rudd[16].)

Combination therapy in clinical practice
Combinations of priority use

According to the World Health Organization/International Society of Hypertension Guidelines[5], the priority combinations are the following:

1. A thiazide diuretic and an ACE inhibitor (or an angiotensin II-receptor antagonist).
2. A thiazide diuretic and a beta-blocker.

3. A beta-blocker and an α_1-blocker.
4. A calcium antagonist of the dihydropyridine type and a beta-blocker.
5. A thiazide diuretic and an α_1-blocker.
6. A calcium antagonist and an ACE inhibitor.

All these combinations meet most of the requirements for an optimal two-drug combination therapy previously mentioned, although they do not cover all possible useful combinations that can be used in the clinical practice, pending scientific evidence on their superior effectiveness and tolerability over monotherapy.

Combination as the first-line treatment

The World Health Organization/International Society of Hypertension Guidelines[5] do not yet recommend that antihypertensive treatment starts with two drugs because this may result in some patients who are responsive to monotherapy taking more pharmacological agents than they need. It should be emphasized, however, that combination treatment is likely to be used even more frequently in the future because of the evidence that in a number of conditions a more drastic reduction in systolic and diastolic blood pressure below 140/90 mmHg may be more protective to the patient.

One of these conditions is hypertension associated with diabetes mellitus, in which a diastolic blood pressure reduction for values close to 80 mmHg (and the systolic blood pressure reduction close to 140 mmHg) may markedly reduce diabetic-related macro- and microvascular complications as compared to more traditional blood pressure goals[17]. Another condition is nephropathy in which a diastolic blood pressure reduction (to 120/75 mmHg) may guarantee renal survival more than a less drastic one, particularly in the presence of proteinuria[18–20]. Finally, there are reasons to believe that a blood pressure reduction well below 140/90 mmHg (to less than 130/85 mmHg) may provide a greater protection also in the more general hypertensive population, also because a more ambitious blood pressure goal is accompanied by achievement of the less ambitious one (<140/90 mmHg) in a greater number of individuals[17]. This has led the World Health Organization/International Society of Hypertension guidelines[5] to suggest blood pressure goals <130/80 mmHg in hypertension and diabetes or nephropathy and to define target values < 130/85 mmHg as desirable at least in middle-aged and young hypertensive patients. Clearly, these lower blood pressure targets require greater use of combination treatment[21]. In nephropathic and diabetic patients this goal is virtually always achieved by use of multiple drug therapy. This was also the case in the Hypertension Optimal Treatment (HOT) study in which achievement of optimal blood pressure control for the initially elevated values was made possible by combination treatment in two-thirds of the cases. Combination treatment was necessary in three-quarters of the cases when the goal was to reduce blood pressure to particularly low values (diastolic <80 mmHg) (Figure 7.5.7)[17].

7

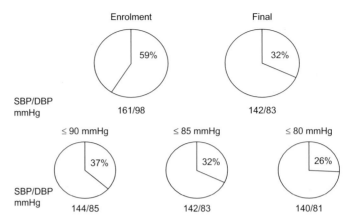

Fig. 7.5.7 Percentage of hypertensive patients in monotherapy (open symbols) or in combination treatment (closed symbols) in the Hypertension Optimal Treatment (HOT) Study, according to different goal blood pressure values. SBPs systolic blood pressure; DBP = diastolic blood pressure. (Modified from Hansson *et al.*[17].)

High- versus low-dose combination

It is a common experience, in both large-scale intervention trials and in clinical daily practice, that high doses of almost all antihypertensive drugs neither necessarily enhance the effectiveness of antihypertensive treatment nor increase the incidence and severity of adverse effects. This also applies to combination therapy, which in its low-dose formulations has been shown to achieve an antihypertensive efficacy greater than high-dose monotherapy or high-dose combination. This has been recently shown in the HOT study in which target diastolic blood pressure was achieved in a large fraction of patients with low dose combination of two antihypertensive drugs[17]. Finally, it should be underlined that low-dose combination is associated with a much better tolerance which is, as mentioned above, of key importance for patient's compliance to treatment and thus for the success of antihypertensive therapy.

References

1. MacMahon S, Rodgers A. The effects of antihypertensive treatment on vascular disease: reappraisal of evidence in 1994. *J Vasc Med Biol* 1993;4:265–271.
2. Mancia G, Stella ML, Pozzi M, Grassi G. Treatment of hypertension: general aspects. *J Cardiovasc Pharmacol* 1996;**28**(Suppl. 4):S23–S28.
3. Isles CG, Walker LM, Beevers GD *et al.* Mortality in patients of the Glasgow Blood Pressure Clinic. *J Hypertension* 1986;4:141–156.
4. Mancia G. Improving the management of hypertension in clinical practice. *J Human Hypertension* **9**(Suppl. 2):S29–S31.
5. Guidelines Sub-Committee of the WHO/ISH mild hypertension Liaison Committee. WHO/ISH guidelines for the management of hypertension. *J Hypertension* 1999;**17**:151–183.
6. Mancia G, Grassi G. Combination treatment in antihypertensive drug trials. *Cardiovasc Drug Therapy* 1997;**11**:517–518.

7. Sever P. The heterogeneity of hypertension: why doesn't every patient respond to every antihypertensive drug? *J Human Hypertension* 1995;**9**:S33–S36.

8. Materson BJ, Reda DJ, Cushman VC *et al.* Single-drug therapy for hypertension in men. *N Engl J Med* 1993;**328**:914–921.

9. Mancia G, Failla M, Grappiolo A, Giannattasio C. Present and future role of combination treatment in hypertension. *J Cardiovasc Pharmacol* **3**(Suppl. 2):S41–S44.

10. Smith WCS, Cutler JA, Higgins M *et al.* Trends in the prevalence, awareness treatment and control in hypertension in the adult US population. Data from the Health Examination Surveys, 1960 to 1991. *Hypertension* 1995;**26**:60–69.

11. Joint National Committee on Prevention, Detection, Evaluation and Treatment of High Blood Pressure. The Sixth Report of the Joint National Committee on Prevention, Detection, Evaluation and Treatment of High Blood Pressure (JNC VI) *Arch Intern Med* 1997;**157**:2413–2466.

12. Mancia G, Sega R, Milesi C *et al.* Blood pressure control in hypertensive population. *Lancet* 1997;**349**:454–457.

13. Chockalingham A, Fodor JG. Treatment of raised blood pressure in the population. The Canadian experience. *Am J Hypertension* 1998;**11**:747–749.

14. Colhoun HM, Dong W, Poulter NR. Blood pressure screening, management and control in England: results from the healthy survey for England 1994. *J Hypertension* 1998;**16**:747–752.

15. Swales JD. Current clinical practice in hypertension: the EISBERG (Evaluation and Intervention for Systolic Blood Pressure Elevation–Regional and Global) project. *Am Heart J* 1999;**138**:S231–S237.

16. Rudd P. Clinicians and patients with hypertension: unsettled issues about compliance. *Am Heart J* 1995;**130**:572–579.

17. Hansson L, Zanchetti A, Carruthers SG *et al.* Effects of intensive blood pressure lowering and low-dose aspirin in patients with hypertension: principal results of the Hypertension Optimal Treatment (HOT) randomised trial. *Lancet* 1998;**351**:1755–1762.

18. Lewis EJ, Hunsiker LG, Bain RP. Rohde RD for the Collaborative Study Group. The effects of angiotensin converting enzyme inhibition on diabetic nephropathy: the Collaborative Study Group. *N Eng J Med* 1993;**329**:1456–1462.

19. Giatras I, Lau J, Levey AS for the Angiotensin Converting Enzyme Inhibition and Progressive Renal Disease Study Group. Effect of angiotensin-converting-enzyme inhibitors on the progression of nondiabetic renal disease: a meta-analysis of randomized trials. *Ann Intern Med* 1997;**127**:337–345.

20. UK Prospective Diabetes Study Group. Tight blood pressure control and risk of macrovascular and microvascular complications in Type 2 diabetes: UKPDS 38. *Br Med J* 1998;**317**:703–713.

21. Mancia G, Omboni S, Grassi G. Combination treatment in hypertension. *Am J Hypertension* 1997;**10**:153S–158S.

Further reading

Mann SJ, Blumenfeld JD, Laragh JH. Issues, goals and guidelines for choosing first-line and combination antihypertensive drug therapy. In: *Hypertension: Pathophysiology, Diagnosis and Management* (eds Laragh JH, Brenner BM). Raven Press: New York, 1995.

References

Further reading

7

7.6

The problem of compliance with antihypertensive therapy

B Waeber, M Burnier and HR Brunner

7

Introduction

A number of drugs are now available to lower blood pressure by a variety of different mechanisms[1]. Given alone, or in combination, these medications allow control of blood pressure in most hypertensive patients. This is true at least in drug trials, which are generally performed by physicians who have a special interest in the field of hypertension and who, most likely, include motivated patients in the study. For example, in the Hypertension Optimal Treatment (HOT) study, more than 90% of patients had their diastolic blood pressure below 90 mmHg after a mean follow-up of 3.6 years[2]. There is, however, still a major gap between the rate of blood pressure normalization achieved in close to 'ideal' clinical settings, and that observed in the community[3]. Thus, even in industrialized countries, only a fraction of hypertensive patients have their blood pressure normalized by the treatment. In the USA, 27% of hypertensive patients have their systolic and diastolic blood pressure below 140 and 90 mmHg, respectively[1]. The situation is worse in the UK, the corresponding figure being only 6%[4].

Several reasons account for the poor blood pressure control seen in everyday practice. Doctors may not adhere strictly enough to the official recommendations and set the target blood pressure too high[5]. Also, the guidelines of a given country, for instance those prevailing in the UK, may propose upper limits for normal blood pressure, higher than those currently accepted[6]. Another potential explanation is poor efficacy of available antihypertensive drugs. However, this should not be a problem if physicians are prepared or permitted to use the available drugs[2].

Another confounding factor coud be related to the 'white-coat' effect on blood pressure[7]. It is true that some treated patients might be seemingly hypertensive when facing their doctor, but show normal blood pressures when undergoing their usual daily activities away from the medical setting. An additional explanation for an unsatisfactory blood pressure control could be a poor compliance with antihypertensive therapy[8]. Compliance can be defined as 'the extent to which a person's behavior coincides with medical or health advice'[9]. Interestingly, failure of bringing blood pressure under control is attributed by 70% of doctors to a problem of adherence to therapy[3]. This differs drastically from the view of the patients, of whom 81% claim to 'always take their medication'. Clearly, the patient's and the doctor's perception of compliance with antihypertensive therapy is not identical. Compliance remains in everyday practice very difficult to assess: it remains frequently a 'black box' for the doctor and represents often an unrecognized source of misunderstanding between the doctor and his or her patient.

How to assess compliance?

There is no ideal way to assess compliance[9,10]. Several methods have been used, mainly in clinical trials (Table 7.6.1).

Table 7.6.1 Methods of measuring compliance

Parameter	Usefulness in:	
	clinical trials	everyday practice
Follow up	+	+
Outcome of therapy	−	−
Direct questioning	+	++
Pill count	+	+
Drug assays, chemical markers	+	−
Prescription refills	+	++
Electronic medication monitoring	+++	+++*

* If available.

Follow up

The way the patient keeps an appointment given by a doctor can be taken as an indicator of the patient's compliance. Patients included in clinical trials may be particularly well motivated. Thus, in the Medical Research Council trial, no more than 5% of patients allocated to placebo withdrew during the five-year follow up[11]. Based on the experience of a large hypertension clinic, it might be expected there would be a loss of follow up of one out of four patients over a three-year period[12]. It is, however, difficult to extrapolate from these observations the drop-out rate of hypertensive patients treated by a practicing physician according to usual local habits. In the USA, approximatively 15% of hypertensives are aware of having an abnormally high blood pressure, but are not on antihypertensive therapy[1]. The majority of these patients are most likely poor compliers who have decided, for whatever reason, to interrupt treatment.

Outcome of therapy

The fact that a patient does not have his or her blood pressure controlled during antihypertensive therapy cannot be taken as an evidence of poor compliance. Any medication, even if taken regularly, is ineffective in approximately half of the patients. Even a perfect complier may be unresponsive to a multiple drug therapy. The occurrence of drug-specific effects such as slowing of heart rate with beta-blockers may indicate that the given drug has been taken. However, it does not give any information on the dynamic of compliance. Futhermore, it does not confirm good compliance to concomitant treatments.

Direct questioning

The easiest way to evaluate compliance is to interview the patient about his or her habits in taking the prescribed treatment. This approach is unsuitable as long as a patient claims a good adherence to treatment. However, it becomes meaningful if a patient voluntarily admits a non-compliance behavior. Unfortunately, doctors are reluctant to start a discussion about compliance with their patients since such a discussion is often felt to be a potential source of conflict. Direct questioning appears especially effective when a patient is followed regularly for months or years by the same physician, which helps to develop a valuable patient–doctor relationship. In clinical trials there is only a weak link between the rate of blood pressure normalization and the reported degree of compliance[13].

Pill count

Pill count has, traditionally, been used to monitor compliance in drug trials. It tends to overestimate compliance, mainly because a patient may deliberately discard tablets before returning the container to his or her doctor[10]. There is some evidence that compliance assessed by pill count must be 80% or more in order to obtain significant blood pressure reductions[14]. Pill count is no longer advocated to assess compliance: it reflects only poorly compliance monitored more precisely using electronic devices (see below).

Drug assays and chemical markers

The measurement of plasma or urine concentrations of antihypertensive drugs or their metabolites as a marker of compliance is attractive. This is also true for the determination of chemical markers[10]. The major drawback of this approach is the possible existence of a 'toothbrush effect', which relates to the fact that a non-complier may resume a perfect compliance a few days before the next visit[15].

Prescription refills

Monitoring prescriptions of antihypertensive drugs may be useful to evaluate compliance. This can hardly be done with the individual patient if the doctor is not at the same time prescriber and dispenser of the medications. This technique is especially appropriate to assess compliance in a community of hypertensive patients, for example those belonging to a given medical care system[16–19].

Electronic medication monitoring

It is now possible to monitor compliance using electronic medication dispensers that record each time at which the container is opened. Most of the experience accumulated so far with 'realtime' compliance has been gained using the Medication Event Monitoring System (MEMS)[20]. It is assumed that the patient ingests the tablet(s) as prescribed each time he or she is removing the cap with microcircuity incorporated.

Figure 7.6.1 illustrates two different patterns of compliance observed using the MEMS in hypertensive patients asked to take one tablet each day for three months. In the upper panel is depicted a perfect complier. This patient opened the box at almost the same time every day. In the lower panel the pattern is very erratic, with large variations in timing. This patient also omitted doses for several days to several weeks. Of

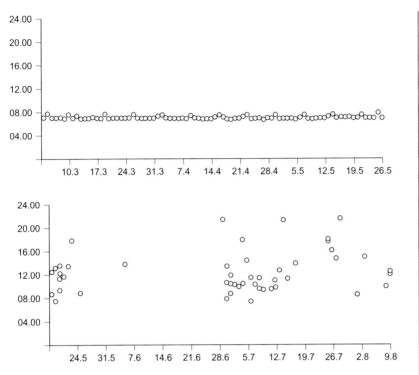

Fig. 7.6.1 Examples of patterns of compliance monitored for three months using an electronic device. The ordinate shows the time of the day at which the drug dispenser was opened and the abcissa the date (month and day). On the upper panel is illustrated a perfect complier and on the lower panel a poor complier.

note is that the patient took occasionally one to three extra doses per day. These two examples have been gathered from a trial carried out by practicing physicians[21]. The patients were informed about the proper use of the electronic device and knew that their compliance with the prescribed drug would be monitored. It is, therefore, impressive to see how the compliance behavior can differ from patient to patient, even during a short-term follow up.

This new method of monitoring compliance with antihypertensive therapy is more reliable than conventional pill count, as exemplified by the result of a study in which 81 African American hypertensive patients were treated for at least three months with either a once-a-day or a twice-a-day drug regimen[22]. Adherence to the once-a-day and twice-a-day dosing was considered acceptable if 80% of the time intervals between MEMS openings were within 24 ± 6 hours or 12 ± 3 hours, respectively. Pill count adherence level was defined as acceptable if comprised between 80% and 100%. Figure 7.6.2 shows that the percentage of patients found adherent by pill count is more than double that determined by the MEMS.

Another advantage of electronic monitoring of compliance is that it also collects information on dosing intervals and, by knowing the duration of action of a given antihypertensive drug, it is possible to

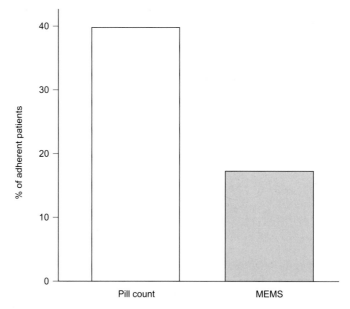

Fig. 7.6.2 Percentage of patients found to be adherent by pill count and electronic monitoring using the MEMS (adapted from[22]).

calculate the therapeutic coverage[20,23,24]. This is an important issue since a smooth and sustained blood pressure reduction during 24 hours is highly desirable to provide an optimal cardiovascular protection.

Non-compliance and cardiovascular risk

Low compliance with antihypertensive drug regimens is a common cause of inadequate blood pressure control and may explain the suboptimal benefit of even strict intervention efforts. Data from the Systolic Hypertension in the Elderly Program (SHEP) pilot study indicate that a pill count compliance above 80% is associated with a greater probability of achieving the target systolic blood pressure reductions[25].

BOX 7.6.1 Non-compliance and cardiovascular complications

Two recent studies point to an immediate relationship between therapeutic non-compliance and the occurrence of cardiovascular complications. In the first, the impact of underutilization of antihypertensive drugs and acute-care readmissions was evaluated in 113 patients[26]. All patients had been hospitalized with a primary or secondary diagnosis of hypertension. They were then observed for readmission for the next 18 months. During this period, the non-compliance rate of each patient was calculated as the ratio of the number of days when the patient had no antihypertensive drugs (based on pharmacy records) divided by the number of days of observation. The non-compliance rate averaged 39% in the 28 patients who had to be readmitted, which was significantly higher than the corresponding rate (11%) seen in patients (*n* = 85) who were not rehospitalized.

Parameter	Readmission	No readmission	P value
Number of cases	28	85	
Number of days in study (SE)	185 (23)	293 (14)	0.0001
Number of lack-of-drug days (SE)	49 (8)	26 (4)	0.003
Noncompliance rate (SE)	39 (7)%	11 (2)%	0.001

SE = standard error of the mean.

The second study deals with the influence of noncompliance with antihypertensive therapy on healthcare costs[16]. This is a key issue since the economic consequences of compliance errors in the field of hypertension are largely unknown[27]. Paid claims data from the California Medicaid program were used for the analysis. The primary outcome variable was the total cost of healthcare during the first year after initiation of antihypertensive therapy in patients aged 40 and over (*n* = 6419). Approximately 86% of the patients (*n* = 5504) interrupted or discontinued purchasing any blood pressure lowering drug during this period. Each of these patients consumed on the average $873 more than patients who filled the prescriptions regularly during the study period (*n* = 915). The increased costs were essentially related to hospital expenditures ($637), indicating that withdrawal of therapy led to serious complications. These observations reflecting a real-life experience are of great interest: they clearly show that non-compliance represents for hypertensive patients a high-risk situation and that hospitalization is frequently required if antihypertensive treatment is discontinued.

The different processes of compliance with antihypertensive therapy

In considering preventive lifestyle measures and long-term pharmacological treatment of hypertension, three different steps can be identified[28]:

1. The adoption.
2. The execution.
3. The discontinuation process.

This is illustrated in Figure 7.6.3.

The adoption process

A difficult step for the patient is to accept the diagnosis of hypertension and its therapeutic implication, that is to initiate a lifelong non-pharmalogical or pharmalogical treatment. At that time the patient has generally no symptoms and no cardiovascular complications. The doctor plays a key role in the adoption process, having to make the patient understand the hypertension-related risk, the benefits expected from lowering blood pressure and the need for a continual blood pressure control even if there is no obvious immediate advantage of therapy. With

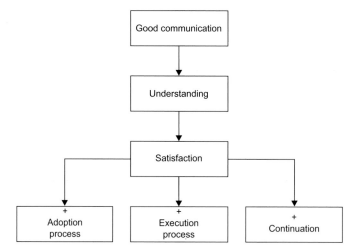

Fig. 7.6.3 Good communication between doctor and patient reinforces the adoption and the execution processes. It also helps the patient to continue the treatment.

regard to the risk attributable to hypertension, the doctor has to evaluate not only the likelihood of developing an overt cardiovascular disease, but also the potential severity of the cardiovascular complication.

BOX 7.6.2 The three steps in cardiovascular risk evaluation[29]

Hedner and Falk have identified three steps in evaluating cardiovascular risk.

1. The traditional risk assessment which is aimed to determine the relative and the absolute risk of the patient.
2. The appraisal of the global burden from the risk by identifying all factors potentially beneficial or detrimental for the acceptance of a long-term intervention.
3. The prescription of therapeutic measures.

Going through these three steps implies a close and time-consuming interaction between doctor and patient. An excellent patient–doctor relationship is a priority at this stage to promote adoption of the prescribed treatment[30].

The execution process

The execution process is by far the most difficult for patients since it deals with their daily life for years. Each day the patient has to take the prescribed treatment as recommended by the doctor. During this phase the doctor has still to motivate the patient, but multiple interventions may be useful to improve compliance, for example by other healthcare professionals, in particular nurses and pharmacists[30]. The multidisciplinary approach helps to recognize the patient's barriers, and therefore to direct efforts to facilitate compliance in taking into account social, cultural psychological and economic factors. During this phase, a

Table 7.6.2 Hypertensive patients recalling and adhering to selected medical recommendations (adapted from[36])

Area of recommendation	Recalled recommendations*	Adherence to recommendation	
		If recalled recommendation	If did not recall recommendation
Drug therapy: take prescribed medication?	94.6%	90.0%	51.6%
Diet therapy			
Follow a low-salt diet?	74.2%	72.8%	51.4%
Follow a low-fat or weight-loss diet?	62.0%	47.6%	26.1%
Exercise regularly?	62.7%	20.6%	20.0%
Avoidance of tobacco and alcohol			
Stop/cut down on smoking?	79.8%	5.2%	17.9%
Cut down on alcohol?	39.9%	18.4%	16.5%

* Expressed as a percentage of the total

number of strategies may improve compliance, including educational tools, self-monitoring of blood pressure, telephone follow up and electronic monitoring of compliance[30–35]. The main sequential factors that oppose long-term adherence to antihypertensive therapy are a poor communication between the patient and doctor, low motivation (from either the patient, doctor or both), logistical barriers (e.g. excessive costs), the occurrence of side effects, complex and/or ineffective drug regimens, an insufficient periodical reinforcement of compliance and a poor continuity of the healthcare system (e.g. a different doctor on each visit or too large an interval between appointments[8]). Patients also frequently forget what they were being told during the consultation. This is illustrated in Table 7.6.2[36].

BOX 7.6.3 The execution process: patient forgetfullness[36]

Data have been gathered on a total of 1751 patients with chronic medical conditions, half of them hypertensive. The physicians monitoring the patients had to give disease-specific recommendations to each of the patients included in the study. A telephone interview was performed thereafter to assess whether the patients recalled the recommendations. Within the following three to four months the patients were then asked to complete a questionnaire to evaluate the extent to which they had performed the recommended behaviors during the past four weeks. It is rather alarming that a large number of patients did not recall the recommendations. Moreover, those patients who did not recall recommendations were also more likely not to adhere to the medical advice. This was especially true for the advice that the medication(s) should be taken as prescribed.

An important task for the doctor is therefore to make their patients understand and remember what having a high blood pressure means. This is an effective way to improve compliance[29].

The discontinuation process

A substantial fraction of patients treated for hypertension decide, for various reasons, to discontinue therapy. Most of these patients are lost to follow up. The responsibility of such treatment failure has to be shared by patients and health providers, especially doctors. Possibly not enough time is reserved for educating and counselling activities[30].

Patient–physician communication

Doctors often do not feel comfortable talking about compliance with their patients. They are concerned with the possibility that some patients might consider questions related to compliance as an intrusion of privacy and, even worse, as a lack of confidence in the way the patient responds to medical recommendations. However, there is clearly something wrong in this perception. Doctors should recognize that defective compliance is the norm. There is, therefore, no reason for doctors to be disappointed if patients do not take medication(s) as prescribed and no systematic reason to doubt the willingness of patients to be treated. With this in mind, doctors should discuss compliance in a constructive way, with the primary goal being to help patients better adhere to medical advice.

The influence of antihypertensive drug regimen on compliance

Tolerability

Any antihypertensive drug may occasionally cause adverse effects and, therefore, have a negative impact on compliance. This can be illustrated by the results of a study in which 632 patients on antihypertensive therapy were surveyed for one year[37]. The aim was to assess using a questionnaire the prevalence of patient-initiated modifications of drug instructions (use of lower dosage and/or fewer drugs than prescribed) in relation to the occurrence of problems (symptoms of high blood pressure, adverse drug effects, perceived memory problems with drug taking, perceived negative patient role and/or barriers to drug taking in everyday life). Figure 7.6.4 shows that the prevalence of modifications increased linearly as a function of the number of problems experienced.

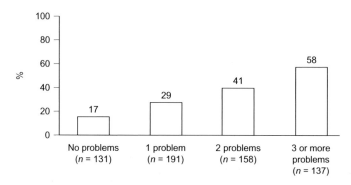

Fig. 7.6.4 Percentage of patients modifying drug instructions according to the number of reported problems (adapted from[37]).

7

In another study, the reasons for stopping or altering antihypertensive therapy were investigated in the UK by surveying a total of 178 family doctors and 948 hypertensive patients[38]. The doctors felt that 18% of their hypertensive patients did not comply with the antihypertensive therapy and that, of these non-compliant patients, 22% were not adhering to treatment because of side effects. Among the patients, 34% reported that they had experienced unacceptable side effects. The majority of these patients (78%) advised their doctor of the side effects while a few patients (9%) spontaneously stopped taking their medication.

These observations highlight the necessity of tailoring the drug regimen to the individual patient, the goal being to normalize blood pressure of each patient without interfering adversely with quality of life.

Type of antihypertensive agent

The class of agents used to initiate antihypertensive therapy might influence long-term compliance, possibly because of more or less favorable side-effect profiles. Several studies have addressed this question by analyzing the repeat prescription (refill) failure in managed-care organizations. Figure 7.6.5 shows the odds ratio for good compliance (adjusted for age, race and gender) in patients described in Box 7.6.4[17]. The compliance observed during diuretic therapy was taken as reference value. All medications given as monotherapy were associated with a significantly better compliance as compared with diuretics, ACE inhibitors being the best in this respect. Interesting findings were also that good compliance was inversely related to comorbid cardiac disease as well as to the need of multiple drug therapy.

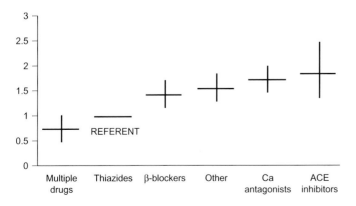

Fig. 7.6.5 Initial drug choice as a factor related to antihypertensive therapy compliance. The ordinate shows the odds ratio for good compliance (⩾80% of days covered) for patients beginning antihypertensive therapy. For each class of antihypertensive medication, the odds ratio is indicated by the horizontal line and the 95% confidence interval by the vertical line (adapted from[17]).

The influence of
antihypertensive drug
regimen on compliance

Type of antihypertensive
agent

BOX 7.6.4 Refill failure

In a cohort of hypertensive patients who were enrollees of Tennessee's Medicaid managed-care program, refill failure (i.e. if a refill was not obtained within 36 days of the last prescription for that medication) occurred in 33% of 7413 refill opportunities[18]. The frequency of refill failure was 30% for beta-blockers, 29% for calcium-channel blockers, 35% for ACE inhibitors and 34% for thiazide diuretics. The refill opportunities for these four major classes of antihypertensive agents were 199, 2806, 602 and 3272, respectively. Manifestly, this large disparity in refill opportunities between the different treatments renders the interpretation of the results difficult.

More meaningful are the observations made in 27 364 hypertensive patients aged 40 and over and living in Saskatchewan[19]. All these patients received, for the first time, an antihypertensive treatment which consisted mainly of diuretics (40%), beta-blockers (10%), ACE inhibitors (30%) or calcium antagonists (13%). Overall, 78% of patients were still on the same treatment after one year. Patients who had an ACE inhibitor as initial drug were, however, significantly more likely to remain on the same medication after one year in comparison with patients receiving treatment with the other types of antihypertensive agents.

A retrospective analysis of prescriptions was also performed in 8643 elderly hypertensives (aged 65 to 99 years) belonging to the New Jersy Medicaid and Medicare programs[17]. Compliance was defined as the number of days in which antihypertensive therapy was available to the patient during the 12 months following the initiation of treatment. Patients were considered good compliers when compliance was 80% or higher. Diuretics were the most frequently prescribed drugs (50%), followed by beta-blockers (12%), calcium antagonists (12%) and ACE inhibitors (5%). Other medications accounted for 17% and 4% of patients had multiple drugs as initial therapy.

Simplification of treatment might be expected to facilitate long-term compliance, and in this respect once-daily dosing would appear desirable. There are now numerous antihypertensive drugs available with a prolonged duration of action allowing control of blood pressure throughout the day when given once a day. Whether difference exists in compliance between a once-a-day and a twice-a-day drug regimen has been tested recently using the MEMS device. In a prospective crossover study performed in a general practice environment compliance with two calcium antagonists, one given twice a day (slow-release nifedipine) and the other one once a day (amlodipine) was assessed[23]. A total of 113 patients with hypertension or stable angina pectoris were treated for two consecutive four-week periods (initially with nifedipine and thereafter with amlodipine). Figure 7.6.6 depicts the percentage of patients having taken the drugs as prescribed in more than 90% of the days. There was a clear-cut advantage in favor of the once-a-day medication. Most likely the difference would have been even greater if the treatment periods were longer. Actually a better compliance for a once-a-day as compared with a twice-a-day regimen as also been found using the MEMS in African American hypertensive patients followed for an average of 4.6 months[22].

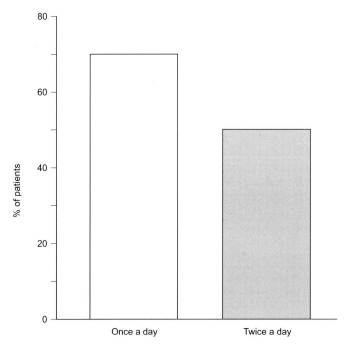

Fig. 7.6.6 Percentage of patients having taken the drugs as prescribed (either once a day or twice a day) in more than 90% of the days (adapted from[23]).

Electronic monitoring of compliance

As already pointed out, 'realtime' monitoring of compliance makes it possible not only to evaluate precisely the percentage of prescribed doses taken, but also to measure the intervals between doses as well as to assess the extent to which some intervals may be longer than the drug's duration of action, in which case drug action is interrupted. It also enables errors in dosings such as skipping one or more sequential doses (drug holidays), to be detected[20,24,28]. Electronic monitoring of compliance is particularly useful in clinical trials[10]. Non-compliers generally go undetected and are often misjudged as 'non-responders'. The identification of such patients can therefore be very helpful to interpret the observations.

Electronic monitoring of compliance should not be regarded as an intrusion into the privacy of the patient's life, but rather as a privilege, an occasion for discussion between the patient and physician. The objective record of drug intake can reinforce the patient's motivation and improve compliance with medication regimens. In this regard the results of a recent trial carried out by practicing physicians are noteworthy[21]: 35 patients remaining hypertensive for at least eight weeks despite the once-a-day administration of an antihypertensive drug (either as monotherapy or as fixed-dose combination therapy) were asked to continue the same treatment for three additional months. The patients were explained how to take the medication using a MEMS, which obliged the doctors in charge of the patients to raise the potential

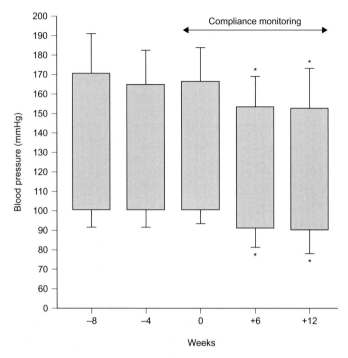

Fig. 7.6.7 Blood pressure effect of a three-month electronic monitoring in patients taking one medication per day. *$P < 0.001$ versus week 0. Means ± SD. (adapted from[21]).

problem of non-compliance. A significant fall in blood pressure was seen during the three-month observation period, even though the patients appeared previously resistant to the used medication (Figure 7.6.7). At the end of the study, 20 patients had their diastolic blood pressure <90 mmHg (against 3 before compliance monitoring) and 13 had their systolic blood pressure <140 mmHg (against 1 before compliance monitoring). Compliance was expressed as the percentage of days with one opening/day over the three-month follow up. All patients taken together, compliance averaged 81%.

Figure 7.6.8 depicts the percentage of patients who exhibited during the study a compliance ≥50%, ≥60%, ≥70%, ≥80% or ≥90%. These data provide important information. They show that it is really not easy for the patients to adhere perfectly to the treatment, even if it consists of one tablet per day only, and even if the patients know that their compliance with the prescribed medication is being monitored. They also point to the potential usefulness of compliance monitoring in routine everyday practice to discuss with the patient medication-taking behavior and, thereby, to improve the patient's adherence to treatment

Conclusions

The treatment of hypertension remains a difficult task. There are still too many patients who have their blood pressure unsatisfactorily controlled. A frequent reason is poor adherence to the drug regimen. The doctor

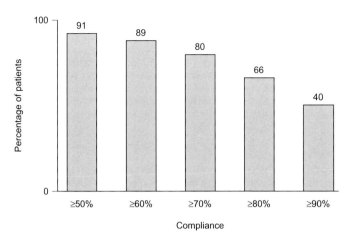

Fig. 7.6.8 Percentage of patients with a compliance ≥50%, ≥60%, ≥70%, ≥80% or ≥90% during a three-month observation period. Compliance was defined as the percentage of days with one opening of the electronic monitoring device (adapted from[21]).

should always keep in mind the problem of poor compliance when prescribing antihypertensive agents. This will urge the doctor to inquire regularly about barriers to optimal compliance and help the patient to seek solutions for improving adherence to the prescribed medication(s).

References

1. Joint National Committee on Prevention, Detection, Evaluation, and Treatment of High Blood Pressure. The Sixth Report of the Joint National Committee on Prevention, Detection, Evaluation, and Treatment of High Blood Pressure. *Arch Intern Med* 1997;**157**:2413–2446.
2. Hansson L, Zanchetti A, Carruthers SG *et al*. Effects of intensive blood-pressure lowering and low-dose aspirin in patients with hypertension: principal results of the Hypertension Optimal Treatment (HOT) randomised trial. HOT Study Group. *Lancet* 1998;**351**:1755–1762.
3. Ménard J, Chatellier G. Limiting factors in the control of blood pressure: why is there a gap between theory and practice? *J Human Hypertension* 1995;**9**(Suppl. 2):19–23.
4. Colhoun HM, Dong W, Poulter NR. Blood pressure screening, management and control in England: results from the health survey for England 1994. *J Hypertension* 1998;**16**:747–752.
5. Dickerson REC, Brown MJ. Influence of age on general practitioners definition and treatment of hypertension. *Br Med J* 1995;**30**:574.
6. Sever P, Beevers G, Bulpitt C *et al*. Management guidelines in essential hypertension: report of the second working party of the British Hypertension Society. *Br Med J* 1993;**306**:983–987.
7. Waeber B, Rutschmann B, Nussberger J, Brunner HR. Evaluation of antihypertensive therapy: discrepancies between office and ambulatory recorded blood pressure. *J Hypertension* 1991;**9**(Suppl. 3):53–56.
8. Rudd P. Clinicians and patients with hypertension: unsettled issues about compliance. *Am Heart J* 1995;**130**:572–589.
9. Urquhart J. Patient non-compliance with drug regimens: measurement, clinical correlates, economic impact. *Eur Heart J* 1996;**17**(Suppl. A):8–15.
10. Van der Stichele. Measurement of patient compliance and the interpretation of randomized trials. *Eur J Clin Pharmacol* 1991;**41**:27–35.

7

References

11. Medical Research Council. Adverse reactions to bendrofluazide and propranolol for the treatment of mild hypertension. Report of Medical Research Council Working Party on Mild to Moderate Hypertension. *Lancet* 1981;**ii**:539–543.

12. Degoulet P, Menard J, Vu HA *et al*. Factors predictive of attendance at clinic and blood pressure control in hypertensive patients. *Br J Med* 1983;**287**:88–93.

13. Hershey JC, Morton BG, Davis JB, Reichgott MJ. Patient compliance with antihypertensive medication. *Am J Public Health* 1980;**70**:1081–1089.

14. Sackett DL, Haynes RB, Gibson ES *et al*. Randomised clinical trial of strategies for improving medication compliance in primary hypertension. *Lancet* 1975;**i**:1205–1207.

15. Feinstein AR. On white-coat effects and the electronic monitoring of compliance. *Arch Intern Med* 1990;**150**:1377–1378.

16. McCombs JS, Nichol MB, Newman CM, Sclar DA. The costs of interrupting antihypertensive drug therapy in a Medicaid population. *Med Care* 1994;**32**:214–226.

17. Monane M, Bohn RL, Gurwitz JH *et al*. The effects of initial drug choice and comorbidity on antihypertensive therapy compliance: results from a population-based study in the elderly. *Am J Hypertension* 1997;**10**:697–704.

18. Bailey JE, Lee MD, Somes GW, Graham RL. Risk factors for antihypertensive medication refill failure by patients under Medicaid managed care. *Clin Ther* 1996;**18**:1252–1262.

19. Caro JJ. Stepped care for hypertension: are the assumptions valid? *J Hypertension* 1997;**15**(Suppl. 7):35–39.

20. Urquhart J. The electronic medication event monitor. Lessons for pharmacotherapy. *Clin Pharmacokinet* 1997;**32**:245–256.

21. Waeber B, Vetter W, Darioli R *et al*. Improved blood pressure control by monitoring compliance with antihypertensive therapy. *J Clin Pract* 1999;**53**:37–38.

22. Lee JY, Kusek JW, Greene PG *et al*. for the AASK Pilot Study Investigators. Assessing medication adherence by pill count and electronic monitoring in the African American Study of Kidney Disease and Hypertension (AASK) Pilot Study. *Am J Hypertension* 1996;**9**:719–725.

23. Waeber B, Erne P, Saxenhofer H, Heynen G. Use of drugs with more than a twenty-four-hour duration of action. *J Hypertension* 1994;**12**(Suppl. 8):67–71.

24. Meredith PA. Therapeutic implications of drug 'holidays'. *Eur Heart J* 1996;**17**(Suppl. A):21–24.

25. Black DM, Brand RJ, Greenlick M *et al*. Compliance to treatment for hypertension in elderly patients: the SHEP pilot study. *J Gerontol* 1987;**42**:552–557.

26. Maronde RF, Chan LS, Larsen FJ *et al*. Underutilization of antihypertensive drugs and associated hospitalization. *Med Care* 1989;**27**:1159–1166.

27. Mancia G, Giannattasio C. Benefit and costs of anti-hypertensive treatment. *Eur Heart J* 1996;**17**(Suppl. A):25–28.

28. Waeber B, Brunner HR, Metry JM. Compliance with antihypertensive treatment: implications for practice. *Blood Press* 1997;**6**:326–331.

29. Hedner T, Falk M. Physician and patient evaluation of hypertension-related risks and benefits from treatment. *Blood Press* 1997;**6**(Suppl. 1):26–34.

30. Miller NH, Hill M, Kottke T, Ockene IS. The multilevel compliance challenge: recommendations for a call to action. A statement for healthcare professionals. *Circulation* 1997;**95**:1085–1090.

31. Edmonds D, Foerster E, Groth H *et al*. Does self-measurement of blood pressure improve patient compliance in hypertension? *J Hypertension* 1985;**3**(Suppl. 1):31–34.

32. Binstock ML, Franklin KL, Formica EK. Therapeutic adherence program improves compliance and lowers blood pressure. *J Hypertension* 1986;**4**(Suppl. 5):375–377.

33. McKenney JM, Munroe WP, Wright JT, Jr. Impact of an electronic medication compliance aid on long-term blood pressure control. *J Clin Pharmacol* 1992;**32**:277–283.

34. Cramer JA. Microelectronic systems for monitoring and enhancing patient compliance with medication regimens. *Drugs* 1995;**49**:321–327.

35. Friedman RH, Kazis LE, Jette A *et al*. A telecommunications system for monitoring and counseling patients with hypertension. Impact on medication adherence and blood pressure control. *Am J Hypertension* 1996;**9**:285–292.

36. Kravitz RL, Hays RD, Sherbourne CD *et al*. Recall of recommendations and adherence to advice among patients with chronic medical conditions. *Arch Intern Med* 1993;**153**:1869–1878.

7

37. Wallenius SH, Vainio KK, Korhonen MJ *et al*. Self-initiated modification of hypertension treatment in response to perceived problems. *Ann Pharmacother* 1995;**29**:1213–1217.
38. Lip GY, Beevers GD. Doctors, nurses, pharmacists and patients. The Rational Evaluation and Choice in Hypertension (REACH) survey of hypertension care delivery. *Blood Press* 1997;**6**(Suppl. 1):6–10.

References

Treatment in special conditions

8

8.1

Hypertension in children and adolescents

B Falkner

8

Introduction

Hypertension may occur at any time during childhood, from infancy through adolescence. Significant elevation of blood pressure, relative to age and body size, during childhood is a clinical sign which may indicate an underlying cardiovascular, endocrine, or renal disorder. High blood pressure in these situations is considered as 'secondary hypertension'. Blood pressure levels which exceed the normal blood pressure range in childhood may also be an expression of a disorder, termed 'essential' or 'primary hypertension'. Essential hypertension had generally been considered to be a problem of adults. With the development of more clinical and epidemiologic knowledge, the perspective on the origin and expression of primary hypertension has shifted, with more attention directed toward the young. Whether hypertension is detected in childhood or later adulthood, the consequences of sustained blood pressure elevation render hypertension a significant health problem both for individual patients from a clinical perspective and for populations from a public health perspective.

Definition and epidemiology

Historically, measurement of blood pressure has not been part of routine healthcare in children. In the absence of reference data on blood pressure which defined the normal range of blood pressure in childhood in the past, the adult criteria of >140/90 mmHg applied to children to define hypertension. Children will this degree of blood pressure elevation were usually symptomatic and had, by current standards, severe hypertension. Clinical evaluation of children with severe hypertension frequently detected an underlying abnormality which was determined to be the cause of the hypertension. Hypertension in childhood which is due to an underlying renal, cardiac, endocrine, or neurologic disorder is termed 'secondary hypertension'. Secondary hypertension can be detected more frequently in children compared to adults and is characterized by a more severe degree of hypertension. For these children, rigorous evaluation and management is indicated to treat the underlying cause and control the blood pressure. 'Primary' or 'essential' hypertension had been thought to be rare in childhood. However, with better understanding of the normal range of blood pressure, along with routine measurement of blood pressure throughout childhood, this view has changed.

Several epidemiologic studies have been conducted which have measured blood pressure in healthy children and adolescents[1–5]. Blood pressure distribution curves in populations of healthy children demonstrate a progressive rise in the blood pressure level with increasing age throughout childhood. The increase in blood pressure with increasing age in childhood is very similar to the normal age-related increase height and weight throughout childhood. These data made it clear that the normal range of blood pressure in children was well below the standard adult cut-off point of 140/90 mmHg. It was also apparent that normal blood pressure level in childhood was determined by body size and growth. By using the 95th percentile for age and sex as the level to define higher than normal blood pressure, a more appropriate definition of hypertension during childhood began to emerge. With expansion of the epidemiologic data and further analysis of the correlates of blood pressure in healthy children, it became apparent that the strongest correlate of blood pressure in children and adolescents was height. Children of a given age have a broad variation in height, so that accurate assessment of blood pressure in a child requires adjustment for height as well as age and sex[3].

BOX 8.1.1 When to measure blood pressure

It is currently recommended that all children have their blood pressure measured as part of regular health assessments beginning at three years of age. In addition, any child who is sick or symptomatic should have their blood pressure measured regardless of age. In childhood and adolescence, hypertension is defined as systolic and/or diastolic blood pressure equal to or above the 95th percentile for age, sex, and height. Due to the known blood pressure variability in the young, the blood pressure should be at or above the 95th percentile on at least three separate measurements. Normotension is defined as systolic and diastolic blood pressure below the 90th percentile for age, sex, and height. Blood pressure levels (systolic or diastolic) between the 90th and 95th percentile are considered to be high normal and warrant further monitoring.

Newborn blood pressure

There are limited data on blood pressure in newborn infants. Early reports, which examined the level of blood pressure in infants, were based on single measurements of blood pressure[4–6]. A few reports described the relationship of blood pressure with birth weight in large numbers of infants[7,8] which indicated a direct relationship between blood pressure and birth weight. These reports, however, showed wide variability in the data. Hulman *et al.*[9] examined blood pressure in healthy newborns on the day of birth and repeatedly on consecutive days in the nursery. There was a rapid and consistent increase in blood pressure during the first five days of life which reflect a hemodynamic transition from intrauterine to extrauterine life. These observations were replicated in a larger study on newborn infants comprising a broad range of birth weight and gestational age[10]. There is a direct relationship of blood pressure with both birth weight and gestational age at birth. In all infants, regardless of birth weight or gestational age at birth, there is a transition, reflected by an increase in blood pressure, which occurs over the first five days of post-natal life. Subsequently, there is a direct relationship of blood pressure with weight or gestational age (Figure 8.1.1).

8

Methodology of blood
pressure measurement in
the young

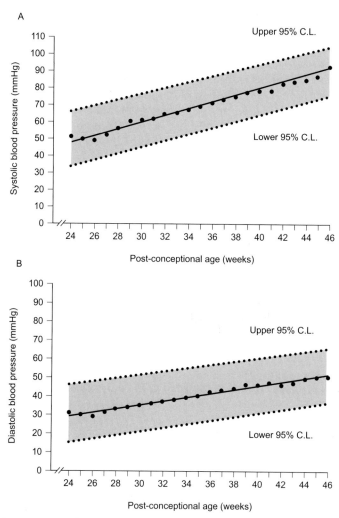

Fig. 8.1.1 Postconceptional age (gestational age in weeks + weeks after delivery) is computed daily for each infant (8568 daily records) and regressed against mean systolic blood pressure (SBP) (A) and diastolic blood pressure (DBP) (B) for that day. Regression lines and equations are presented in terms of postconceptional weeks, which is more useful clinically. Regression equations are SBP = (0.255 × postconceptional age in weeks × 7) + 6.34, $r = 0.61$, $P < 0.0001$ and DBP = (0.151 × postconceptional age in weeks × 7) + 3.32, $r = 0.46$, $P < 0.0001$. Observed means of SBP and DBP for each postconceptional week are also plotted. C.l., Confidence limits. (After Zubrow et al.[10].)

Methodology of blood pressure measurement in the young

Table 8.1.1 provides reference blood pressure levels for boys and Table 8.1.2 provides the reference blood pressure levels for girls on which determination is made of normotension, high normal blood pressure, and hypertension in children and adolescent[3]. Use of these tables depends on measurement of blood pressure using a standardized

8

Table 8.1.1 Blood pressure levels for the 90th and 95th percentiles of blood pressure for boys age 1 to 17 years by percentiles of height† (see also text)

Age (years)	Height percentiles*	systolic blood pressure (mmHg)							Diastolic blood pressure (mmHg)						
		5%	10%	25%	50%	75%	90%	95%	5%	10%	25%	50%	75%	90%	95%
1	90th	94	95	97	98	100	102	102	50	51	52	53	54	54	55
	95th	98	99	101	102	104	106	106	55	55	56	57	58	59	59
2	90th	98	99	100	102	104	105	106	55	55	56	57	58	59	59
	95th	101	102	104	106	108	109	110	59	59	60	61	62	63	63
3	90th	100	101	103	105	107	108	109	59	59	60	61	62	63	63
	95th	104	105	107	109	111	112	113	63	63	64	65	66	67	67
4	90th	102	103	105	107	109	110	111	62	62	63	64	65	66	66
	95th	106	107	109	111	113	114	115	66	67	67	68	69	70	71
5	90th	104	105	106	108	110	112	112	65	65	66	67	68	69	69
	95th	108	109	110	112	114	115	116	69	70	70	71	72	73	74
6	90th	105	106	108	110	111	113	114	67	68	69	70	70	71	72
	95th	109	110	112	114	115	117	117	72	72	73	74	75	76	76
7	90th	106	107	109	111	113	114	115	69	70	71	72	72	73	74
	95th	110	111	113	115	116	118	119	74	74	75	76	77	78	78
8	90th	107	108	110	112	114	115	116	71	71	72	73	74	75	75
	95th	111	112	114	116	118	119	120	75	76	76	77	78	79	80
9	90th	109	110	112	113	115	117	117	72	73	73	74	75	76	77
	95th	113	114	116	117	119	121	121	76	77	78	79	80	80	81
10	90th	110	112	113	115	117	118	119	73	74	74	75	76	77	78
	95th	114	115	117	119	121	122	123	77	78	79	80	80	81	82
11	90th	112	113	115	117	119	120	121	74	74	75	76	77	78	78
	95th	116	117	119	121	123	124	125	78	79	79	80	81	82	83
12	90th	115	116	117	119	121	123	123	75	75	76	77	78	78	79
	95th	119	120	121	123	125	126	127	79	79	80	81	82	83	83
13	90th	117	118	120	122	124	125	126	75	76	76	77	78	79	80
	95th	121	122	124	126	128	129	130	79	80	81	82	83	83	84
14	90th	120	121	123	125	126	128	128	76	76	77	78	79	80	80
	95th	124	125	127	128	130	132	132	80	81	81	82	83	84	85
15	90th	123	124	125	127	129	131	131	77	77	78	79	80	81	81
	95th	127	128	129	131	133	134	135	81	82	83	83	84	85	86
16	90th	125	126	128	130	132	133	134	79	79	80	81	82	82	83
	95th	129	130	132	134	136	137	138	83	83	84	85	86	87	87
17	90th	128	129	131	133	134	136	136	81	81	82	83	84	85	85
	95th	132	133	135	136	138	140	140	85	85	86	87	88	89	89

* Height percentile determined by standard growth curves.
† Blood pressure percentile determined by a single measurement.
From National High Blood Pressure Education Program Working Group[3].

method. The tables are based on blood pressure measurements obtained by auscultation with an inflatable blood pressure cuff. This method is recommended for screening and standard office measurement of blood pressure in children. Similar tables for children based on oscillometric or other instrumentation for blood pressure measurement are unavailable due to insufficient data. The auscultatory method for measuring blood pressure is also recommended because the instruments for measurement are inexpensive and easily available. The automated instruments have appropriate clinical use in hospital settings, critical care units, and in situations where the measurement of blood pressure by auscultation is particularly difficult.

Methodology of blood pressure measurement in the young

8

Table 8.1.2 Blood pressure levels for the 90th and 95th percentiles of blood pressure for girls age 1 to 17, years by percentiles of height† (see also text)

Age (years)	Height percentiles*	systolic blood pressure (mmHg)							Diastolic blood pressure (mmHg)						
		5%	10%	25%	50%	75%	90%	95%	5%	10%	25%	50%	75%	90%	95%
1	90th	97	98	99	100	102	103	104	53	53	53	54	55	56	56
	95th	101	102	103	104	105	107	107	57	57	57	58	59	60	60
2	90th	99	99	100	102	103	104	105	57	57	58	58	59	60	61
	95th	102	103	104	105	107	108	109	61	61	62	62	63	64	65
3	90th	100	100	102	103	104	105	106	61	61	61	62	63	63	64
	95th	104	104	105	107	108	109	110	65	65	65	66	67	67	68
4	90th	101	102	103	104	106	107	108	63	63	64	65	65	66	67
	95th	105	106	107	108	109	111	111	67	67	68	69	69	70	71
5	90th	103	103	104	106	107	108	109	65	66	66	67	68	68	69
	95th	107	107	108	110	111	112	113	69	70	70	71	72	72	73
6	90th	104	105	106	107	109	110	111	67	67	68	69	69	70	71
	95th	108	109	110	111	112	114	114	71	71	72	73	73	74	75
7	90th	106	107	108	109	110	112	112	69	69	69	70	71	72	72
	95th	110	110	112	113	114	115	116	73	73	73	74	75	76	76
8	90th	108	109	110	111	112	113	114	70	70	71	71	72	73	74
	95th	112	112	113	115	116	117	118	74	74	75	75	76	77	78
9	90th	110	110	112	113	114	115	116	71	72	72	73	74	74	75
	95th	114	114	115	117	118	119	120	75	76	76	77	78	78	79
10	90th	112	112	114	115	116	117	118	73	73	73	74	75	76	76
	95th	116	116	117	119	120	121	122	77	77	77	78	79	80	80
11	90th	114	114	116	117	118	119	120	74	74	75	75	76	77	77
	95th	118	118	119	121	122	123	124	78	78	79	79	80	81	81
12	90th	116	116	118	119	120	121	122	75	75	76	76	77	78	78
	95th	120	120	121	123	124	125	126	79	79	80	80	81	82	82
13	90th	118	118	119	121	122	123	124	76	76	77	78	78	79	80
	95th	121	122	123	125	126	127	128	80	80	81	82	82	83	84
14	90th	119	120	121	122	124	125	126	77	77	78	79	79	80	81
	95th	123	124	125	126	128	129	130	81	81	82	83	83	84	85
15	90th	121	121	122	124	125	126	127	78	78	79	79	80	81	82
	95th	124	125	126	128	129	130	131	82	82	83	83	84	85	86
16	90th	122	122	123	125	126	127	128	79	79	79	80	81	82	82
	95th	125	126	127	128	130	131	132	83	83	83	84	85	86	86
17	90th	122	123	124	125	126	128	128	79	79	79	80	81	82	82
	95th	126	126	127	129	130	131	132	83	83	83	84	85	86	86

* Height percentile determined by standard growth curves.
† Blood pressure percentile determined by a single measurement.
From National High Blood Pressure Education Program Working Group[3].

Methodology of blood pressure measurement in the young

The tables are used in the following way: first, the child's height is measured and plotted on standard growth curves. The appropriate height percentile for age and sex is determined. The child's blood pressure is measured using methods appropriate for children (see above). The child's systolic blood pressure and diastolic blood pressure are compared to the blood pressure levels in the tables according to the child's sex, age, and height percentile. The child is normotensive if both systolic and diastolic blood pressures are less than the 90th percentile. If either systolic or diastolic blood pressure is above the 95th percentile, the child may be hypertensive. If either systolic or diastolic blood pressure are between the 90th and 95th percentile, the child has high normal blood pressure.

8

Hypertension in children and adolescents

Methodology of blood
pressure measurement in
the young

BOX 8.1.2 Measurement of blood pressure

Blood pressure should be measured in a calm and controlled environment
after the patient has been seated for 3–5 minutes. Ideally the blood pressure
should be measured twice and the average of the values used to estimate the
blood pressure level[3]. The cuff used for a patient must be appropriately-
sized. The cuff label (e.g. 'infant', 'child') may not correctly designate the
appropriate cuff for a child of the designated age range. The bladder, not the
cloth covering, is the key determinant of correct size. For each child the
bladder width of the cuff should be approximately 40% of the arm
circumference midway between the olecranon and the acromion. This size of
cuff bladder will cover 80–100% of the circumference of the arm. This ensures
that the brachial artery is completely compressed during inflation, and avoids
premature blood flow through the artery during deflation of the bladder[3]. A
cuff which is too small for a patient will result in falsely elevated readings;
however, a cuff which appears somewhat large for a patient will not obscure
elevated values[2]. Oversized adult cuffs may be necessary in obese or large
muscular adolescents. Careful attention to correct cuff size is key to accurate
assessment of blood pressure in children and adolescents.

Measurement of diastolic blood pressure in children is sometimes
difficult. The determination of diastolic blood pressure depends on which
Korotkoff sound is considered the most accurate estimate of diastolic
blood pressure. The fourth Korotkoff sound (K4) is defined as the
muffling of the auscultated pulsation; the fifth Korotkoff sound (K5) is
defined as the disappearance of the auscultated pulsation. In adults K5 is
used to determine the diastolic blood pressure. However, in younger
children there may be a wide gap between K4, the muffling of the
Korotkoff sounds, and K5, the disappearance of the Korotkoff sounds. In
some children, K5 may be heard to near 0 mmHg. Because of the large
difference between K4 and K5 in some children, K4 had been the
recommended measure of diastolic blood pressure in children under the
age of 13 years and K5 had been the recommended measure of diastolic
blood pressure in adolescents aged 13 years and over. In the recent Task
Force Report, however, K5 was recommended as the measure of diastolic

---

BOX 8.1.3 Measuring blood pressure at the 90th and 95th percentile

An 8-year-old girl whose height is 50 in (127 cm) is at the 50th percentile for
height on the standard pediatric growth chart. For her age and height, the
90th percentile for systolic blood pressure is 111 mmHg and the 95th
percentile 115 mmHg (see Table 8.1.2); the 90th percentile for diastolic blood
pressure is 71 mmHg and the 95th percentile 75 mmHg. If her measured
blood pressure is 118/68 mmHg, she could be hypertensive. However, a
single measurement of blood pressure in the elevated range is not sufficient
to diagnose hypertension in childhood. Unless the blood pressure is
extremely elevated or the child is symptomatic, multiple measurements of
blood pressure on several occasions are necessary to verify a diagnosis of
hypertension.

8

blood pressure. The available data were considered sufficient to derive accurate blood pressure distribution based on K5 for diastolic blood pressure. In measurement of blood pressure, K5 is more easily distinguishable than K4. In children who do have a large difference between K4 and K5, elevated diastolic blood pressure is rarely an issue. Therefore, to detect elevated diastolic blood pressure, K5 is regarded as an accurate measure of diastolic blood pressure in children as well as adolescents and adults. More clinical observation and prospective data will be necessary to decide whether K4 or K5 is a more reliable predictor of risk for future hypertension.

Secondary hypertension in childhood

The prevalence of secondary forms of hypertension is greater during childhood than any other period of life. In one report on hypertensive children less than 10 years of age, 90% had identifiable or secondary causes and only 10% were attributed to essential hypertension[11]. In contrast, another series, which included both children and adolescents, reported the prevalence of secondary hypertension in the adolescents as 65%, and that of essential hypertension 35%[12]. Thus, secondary etiologies of hypertension predominate during childhood and the expression of essential hypertension increases with age.

Although detection of high blood pressure at a younger age should raise the suspicion of a secondary cause of hypertension, the degree of elevation of the blood pressure is also important.

A blood pressure level that is 8–10 mmHg beyond the 95th percentile indicates significant hypertension; and a blood pressure level that is more than 15 mmHg above the 95th percentile indicates severe hypertension in children and adolescents. When significant or severe hypertension is documented in childhood, a secondary cause should be strongly considered. For example, a four-year-old boy at the 50th height percentile with a blood pressure of 126/84 mmHg has severe hypertension and requires a careful evaluation to uncover a probable secondary etiology. A general rule to guide the evaluation of high blood pressure in the pediatric population is that the higher the blood pressure and the younger the child, the more likely a secondary cause is responsible[2].

The most frequent cause of secondary hypertension in children is renal disease. Although renovascular, cardiovascular, endocrine, neurogenic, and pharmacologic abnormalities do cause hypertension in children, these categories account for far fewer subjects. Some of the more common causes of secondary hypertension in the pediatric population are shown in Table 8.1.3. Although many pathologic conditions have been associated with hypertension in childhood, the majority of these disorders can be attributed to renal disease. Moreover, within the pediatric age range, certain causes of hypertension are typically seen at particular ages.

Neonates

Although hypertension is uncommon in the neonatal period, certain infants are at increased risk of hypertension. Newborn infants who

Table 8.1.3 Secondary causes of hypertension

Chronic hypertension	Acute hypertension
Renal	*Renal*
Chronic glomerulonephritis	Post infectious glomerulonephritis
Focal segmental glomerulosclerosis	Schönlein–Henoch purpura
IgA nephropathy	Hemolytic uremic syndrome
Interstitial nephritis	Acute tubular necrosis
Collagen vascular diseases	
Alport syndrome	*Vascular*
Reflux nephropathy	Renal or renal vascular trauma
Polycystic kidney disease	
Medullary cystic disease	*Neurogenic*
Hydronephrosis	Increased intracranial pressure
Hypoplastic/dysplastic kidney	Guillain–Barré syndrome
Endocrine	*Drugs*
Hyperthyroidism	Cocaine
Pheochromcytoma	Phencyclidine
Primary aldosteronism	Amphetamines
	Jimson weed
Cardiac and Vascular	
Coarctation of aorta	*Miscellaneous*
Patent ductus arteriosa	Burns
Renal artery stenosis	Orthopedic surgery
Takayasu arteritis	Urologic surgery
Neurogenic	
Dysautonomia	
Drugs	
Non-steroidal anti-inflammatory drugs	
Corticosteroids	
Alcohol	
Appetite suppressants	
Anabolic steroids	
Oral contraceptive	
Nicotine	
Syndromes	
Williams (renovascular lesions)	
Turner (coarctation or renovascular)	
Tuberous sclerosis (cystic renal)	
Neurofibromatosis (renovascular)	
Adrenogenital syndromes	
Little syndrome	
Miscellaneous	
Heavy-metal poisoning	

require umbilical artery catheterization in the neonatal period are at risk from thromboembolic events, leading to abnormalities in renal blood flow, sometimes acute renal failure, and resultant hypertension[13,14]. Low birth-weight infants who have developed bronchopulmonary dysplasia may also develop hypertension, sometimes related to sodium retention from steroid therapy[15]. In general, the most frequent detectable causes of neonatal hypertension include renal artery stenosis, renal artery thrombosis, congenital renal malformations, coarctation of the aorta, and bronchopulmonary dysplasia[2]. Although diagnostic

8

evaluation in some neonates with hypertension, fails to identify an etiology, these infants require blood pressure control and monitoring.

Infancy to ten years

Renal parenchymal diseases, coarctation of the aorta, and renal artery stenosis, are the most frequent diagnoses. From 6 to 10 years of age, renal artery stenosis and renal parenchymal diseases are the most common causes of elevated diastolic pressure. Essential hypertension, causing milder elevations in blood pressure, also begins to occur in this age range. During childhood an acute elevation in blood pressure can also be seen with renal diseases such as hemolytic uremic syndrome or acute postinfectious glomerulonephritis. These acute elevations may require prompt intervention and in-hospital management. Some conditions, such as hemolytic uremic syndrome, can also cause permanent renal dysfunction, resulting in chronic hypertension.

Adolescence

Renal parenchymal diseases are the leading cause of secondary hypertension. The other major cause of hypertension during the teenage years is essential hypertension. The renal diseases during adolescence are quite varied. More chronic diseases, such as chronic pyelonephritis, reflux nephropathy, or focal segmental glomerulosclerosis (FSGS), may manifest during adolescence. Renal disease associated with systemic illnesses, such as systemic lupus erythematosus, may also occur during these years.

There are other important aggravating, if not causative, factors related to hypertension in adolescents. Any form of nicotine, whether cigarette smoking or smokeless tobacco[16,17], may contribute to elevated blood pressure. Illicit substance use, especially cocaine and amphetamine-related compounds, may also cause hypertension. To achieve rapid increases in muscle strength and bulk, some teenage athletes use anabolic steroids, which commonly result in blood pressure elevation[18]. Other substances associated with hypertension in adolescents include appetite suppressants (both over-the-counter and prescription), oral contraceptive pills, and ethanol, when used excessively.

BOX 8.1.4 Coarctation of the aorta

A frequently missed diagnosis in children and adolescents is coarctation of the aorta. In a review of 50 consecutive cases of coarctation, Ing *et al.*[19] found that most children had systolic blood pressures in an upper extremity which was greater than the 95th percentile. The most consistent sign of coarctation on physical examination is a systolic blood pressure gradient of more than 10 mmHg between the arms and legs. Detection and correction of coarctation is important because early childhood repair of coarctation is associated with an improved long-term outcome[20,21].

Essential hypertension in children and adolescents

Essential hypertension of adulthood has its roots in childhood. This concept has been inferred from blood pressure tracking studies[22–28] which suggest that children with elevated blood pressure will continue to have elevated blood pressure as adults. Therefore, an important aspect of blood pressure surveillance in the young is to distinguish between elevated blood pressure signalling an underlying disease i.e. secondary hypertension, and when it is an early expression of primary (essential) hypertension.

Children and adolescents with essential hypertension generally demonstrate several clinical characteristics or associated risk factors. The degree of blood pressure elevation is generally mild, approximating the 95th percentile and there is often considerable variability in blood pressure over time. Laboratory and observational studies have also demonstrated a marked cardiovascular response to stress, including increased heart rate and blood pressure responses to stimuli[29–32]. A consistent clinical observation in children exhibiting mild essential hypertension is a positive history of hypertension in parents and/or grandparents[23,33,34].

In both children and adults, body weight and increases in body weight correlate with blood pressure[35,36]. Essential hypertension in children is frequently associated with obesity, which appears to be a contributory factor since even a modest reduction in excess adiposity in such children is accompanied by a reduction in blood pressure[37,38]. The cluster of mild blood pressure elevation, a positive family history of hypertension, and obesity is a typical pattern in children and adolescents with essential hypertension. However, obesity is not always present, particularly in adolescent males expressing mild blood pressure elevation and a positive family history of hypertension. These children and adolescents should be considered at risk of developing chronic hypertension and may benefit from lifestyle changes to reduce their cardiovascular risk[39].

At present the prevalence of childhood obesity is increasing[40]. Obesity does have an adverse effect on risk for cardiovascular disease and warrants attention for prevention and health promotion. This is supported by a study by Daniels *et al.*[41] who examined cardiac structure by echocardiography in young adolescents with essential hypertension. These investigators found a significant incidence of left ventricular hypertrophy (14%). The adolescents with cardiac hypertrophy, despite mild blood pressure elevation were all obese males.

Over the past two decades the literature on hypertension and cardiovascular disease in adults has focused on the overlap of hypertension, non-insulin-dependent diabetes mellitus, atherosclerosis, and obesity. This constellation within individuals and within populations has been described as the insulin-resistance syndrome[42–44]. Children as well as adults may exhibit characteristics of the insulin-resistance syndrome[38,45,46]. Some investigators have detected the insulin-resistance syndrome in non-obese offspring of

8

hypertensive parents[47,48], indicating an hereditary component to the syndrome. The characteristics of the insulin-resistance syndrome are also congruent with the overweight child having a strong family history of hypertension or early heart disease. These children often have higher than normal plasma lipids levels. Although these children are not at risk for immediate adverse effects of the higher than normal blood pressure, they should be considered at risk for future cardiovascular disease[49]. There is likely benefit to these children from efforts to control excess adiposity, modify diet, and increase physical activity. These health behaviors improve insulin action.

The cause of essential hypertension is believed to be multifactorial and the outcome of an interplay of genetic and environmental factors. However, there is an association of hypertension and ischemic heart disease in adults with a low recorded birth weight. It has been proposed that lower birth weight, within the normal range of birth weights and gestational ages, reflects alteration in the intrauterine nutritional environment. The impairment in optimal fetal growth affects an alteration in organ structure and an impairment in organ function in later life[50,51]. Higher blood pressure is considered to be the link between compromised intrauterine growth and the long term risk for cardiovascular disease[50]. Despite the reports, based on retrospective data, which support the low birth weight–high blood pressure hypothesis[50–53], this concept is in conflict with the body of data in childhood as well as adulthood, which consistently demonstrate a direct relationship between body weight and blood pressure[22,54,55]. Furthermore, the observation of blood pressure tracking in childhood[22,24,27,28] is in conflict with the low birth weight–high blood pressure hypothesis. Reports from studies on small cohorts, which have examined birth weight as a determinant of blood pressure in childhood, adolescence, or young adulthood have not detected a significant correlation[56,57]. Despite the appeal of this novel concept, investigations will be necessary to obtain prospective data and rigorously examine the relationship of intrauterine nutritional environment and fetal growth effect on blood pressure and the risk for cardiovascular disease in later life.

Evaluation of hypertension in children and adolescents

Once sustained hypertension in a child is established a decision must be made regarding the extent of further evaluation. The degree of investigation is usually determined by the type of hypertension one suspects. When a secondary cause is considered, an extensive, comprehensive array of studies may be necessary. On the other hand, when the patient's elevated blood pressure is more likely to be an early expression of essential hypertension, a few screening studies may be sufficient. The key, then, is to determine whether the characteristics of a patient's presentation indicate essential hypertension or reflect a secondary, potentially correctable cause.

Children, in whom a secondary cause for hypertension is possible, may have certain characteristics. Young children with significant or severe hypertension generally have an identifiable underlying cause. As noted above, the higher the blood pressure and the younger the child, the more likely a secondary cause is present. A two-month-old infant with a blood pressure of 120/82 mmHg, for example, has severe hypertension, and requires a thorough evaluation to identify the etiology of the hypertension. On the other hand, a 12-year-old with the same blood pressure of 120/82 mmHg has, depending upon his or her height percentile, mild elevation in blood pressure and is less likely to have a secondary cause.

A particular symptom complex revealed in the history or findings on physical examination, may also prompt a thorough investigation. In these patients, the direction of the evaluation is dictated by the particular symptom complex or physical examination findings. For instance, a 16-year-old female with declining school performance, weight loss, tachycardia, emotional lability, and a 'fullness' of her thyroid requires a focused evaluation for hyperthyroidism. Any pediatric patient who is hypertensive and is not growing normally should also undergo an evaluation for secondary causes. Although it is often difficult to determine the precise onset of hypertension from the history, a sudden onset of elevated blood pressure in a previously normotensive child should always prompt a search for secondary causes. Further, evidence of target organ injury implies a level of severity and/or chronicity of hypertension that mandates a survey for secondary etiologies. When no family history of hypertension exists, the likelihood that the child has essential hypertension is less. Absence of a positive family history of hypertension should increase the level of suspicion for an underlying disorder and widen the extent of the evaluation.

In contrast, another set of findings tends to characterize children and adolescents with essential hypertension. These characteristics include: slight to mild elevations in blood pressure; a strong family history of essential hypertension; elevated resting heart rate; variable blood pressure readings upon repeated measurement; and obesity. Clusters of these characteristics often help to identify children with essential hypertension. If no other abnormalities are found on history or physical examination, these children and adolescents require less extensive evaluations than those in whom secondary causes are suspected. For example, an obese 15-year-old female with a blood pressure of 140/92 mmHg, two parents with primary hypertension, and no additional findings on history or physical examination will not usually require invasive studies or an extensive evaluation. On the other hand, a slender eight-year-old female with a blood pressure of 140/92 mmHg and no family history of hypertension requires a thorough evaluation for secondary causes. Although the evaluation plan may be different, both children require monitoring and management to control blood pressure. The 15-year old requires few diagnostic studies. On the other hand, the eight-year old requires careful examination and diagnostic studies to determine an etiology.

Medical history

The medical history and physical examination are used to detect clues to determine if the blood pressure elevation is secondary or essential. It is also helpful to determine whether the hypertension is long-standing or of acute onset. The information obtained from the medical history and physical examination assists in determining the extent and direction of the evaluation.

The family history is particularly important. In both first- and second-degree relatives, the family history of essential hypertension, myocardial infarction, stroke, renal disease, diabetes, and obesity should be obtained. It can be relevant to the diagnosis in a hypertensive child if relatives had an onset at an early age of any of the above conditions. Children of parents who have early-onset coronary artery disease, may be at high risk for lipid abnormalities. Parents should also be asked about conditions in family members which are inheritable and have hypertension as a component (e.g. polycystic kidney disease, neurofibromatosis, pheochromocytoma). Another recently-recognized familial type of hypertension is glucocorticoid-remediable aldosteronism, an autosomal dominant condition, which should be considered when multiple family members have early-onset hypertension associated with hypokalemia or stroke[58,59].

Details regarding the child's hospitalizations and operations should be obtained. In younger children with hypertension, the neonatal history is especially important. A history of prolonged mechanical ventilation or umbilical artery catheterization may suggest bronchopulmonary dysplasia or a thromboembolic complication, respectively. A history of urinary tract infections is important as there may be associated reflux nephropathy, renal scarring, and resultant hypertension.

A history of medications used can be helpful. Patients may not consider over-the-counter preparations as medications and therefore need to be specifically asked. The most common misused products are cold preparations containing pseudoephedrine or phenylpropanolamine[60,61]. Adolescents need to be discreetly questioned about the use of 'street' drugs, smokeless tobacco, oral contraceptive pills, cigarette smoking, diet aids, ethanol, and anabolic steroids. It is also useful to gather information about the patient's usual diet, level of activity, and lifestyle.

The review of systems should be directed at uncovering chronic symptoms and establishing whether any symptoms associated with hypertension-causing diseases are present. For example, the complex of headaches, palpitations, weight loss and excessive sweating suggests pheochromocytoma.

Physical examination

The physical examination for a hypertensive child should be comprehensive. An assessment of the child's general growth rate and growth pattern should be made. To determine whether a child is

Hypertension in children and adolescents

Evaluation of hypertension
in children and adolescents
Physical examination
Diagnostic testing

underweight or overweight, the child's weight and accompanying percentile ranking for age should be compared to his or her height percentile. A decrease in the weight or height percentile may indicate a more chronic or insidious disease process associated with hypertension. Abnormalities in growth which are associated with hypertension can be seen with chronic renal disease, hyperthyroidism (causing primarily systolic hypertension), pheochromocytoma, adrenal disorders, or certain genetic abnormalities such as Turner syndrome.

To rule out coarctation of the aorta, the evaluation of every child for hypertension should include upper- and lower-extremity blood pressure measurements taken with appropriately-sized cuffs. The cuffs appropriate for thigh measurements in adolescents or overweight children often need to be very large and oversized. Normally the leg blood pressure levels are slightly higher than the arm blood pressure levels. A child with coarctation will have systolic hypertension in an upper extremity, sometimes absent or decreased femoral or other lower extremity pulses, and, more reliably, a blood pressure differential greater than 10 mmHg between the upper and lower extremities[19]. In older infants and children, extensive collateral circulation may have developed so that femoral pulses are still easily palpated. During simultaneous palpation of the radial and femoral pulses, however, a delay in the femoral pulse timing can sometimes be detected[21].

Other clues that can suggest a particular secondary etiology can be found on physical examination[62]. Abnormal facies or dysmorphic features may suggest a syndrome, some of which are linked with specific lesions causing hypertension. For example, both Turner and Williams syndromes are associated with renovascular or cardiac lesions which cause hypertension. A retinal examination should be performed to determine the presence of hypertensive vessel injury. Renal vascular lesions may sometimes have an audible abdominal bruit detectable by auscultation of the abdomen. Skin lesions are sometimes the first manifestations of disorders such as tuberous sclerosis and systemic lupus erythematosus.

Diagnostic testing

If the history and physical examination provide clues for a specific underlying cause for the hypertension, such as an endocrine or cardiac disorder, the testing should be directed to the area of clinical suspicion. Other important historical information such as a history of urinary tract infections might dictate studies to evaluate vesicoureteral reflux and renal scarring. In the absence of clues, however, renal parenchymal disease should be considered a likely etiology as this diagnosis is the most frequent cause of secondary hypertension in the pediatric population. The initial evaluation of children with possible secondary hypertension should therefore include a screen for renal abnormalities. This screen should include a full urinalysis, electrolytes, creatinine, complete blood count, urine culture, and renal ultrasound. In addition, the other important component of the initial evaluation includes an

8

Diagnostic testing

Management of hypertension in children and adolescents

assessment of target-organ injury. The presence of target-organ injury provides a measure of chronicity and severity (characteristics sometimes difficult to ascertain from the history) and will later aid in deciding whether pharmacologic therapy should be instituted. This is best accomplished with echocardiography and/or an ophthalmologic evaluation. Echocardiography is a sensitive means to detect interventricular septal and posterior ventricular wall thickening[63–66]. Chest X-ray and ECG are much less sensitive measures of left ventricular hypertrophy. Not as well appreciated is the usefulness of a thorough ophthalmologic examination. In a study of 97 children and adolescents with essential hypertension, Daniels and associates found that 51% displayed retinal abnormalities[67]. The usefulness of microalbuminuria, sometimes used as a marker for renal injury in adults[68], has not been determined for children. The remainder of the evaluation should be directed by specific findings on history and physical examination as well as results of initial screening studies. The use of 24-hour ambulatory blood pressure monitoring has become increasingly used in the evaluation of adults with hypertension[69]. Standards for ambulatory blood pressure values in children and adolescents have not been fully developed and for this reason ambulatory blood pressure monitoring is not recommended for screening or routine assessment in healthy children[3]. However, with the available data there are some situations in which this method may be useful[70]. For example, in children or adolescents with intermittent significant elevations in blood pressure, ambulatory blood pressure monitoring may prove useful in determining how consistently blood pressure readings are elevated over a 24-hour period and aid in assessing the urgency for implementing pharmacologic therapy.

Management of hypertension in children and adolescents

Children and adolescents with a mild elevation of blood pressure and without end-organ damage, or with cases of probable early essential hypertension, should begin treatment with non-pharmacologic interventions which include weight reduction, exercise, and diet modification. Obesity is often associated with mild hypertension in childhood and adolescence, and the benefits of weight reduction have been demonstrated in obese children. Using a program of both behavior modification and parental involvement, Brownell *et al.* showed that weight loss in obese adolescents was associated with a significant decrease in blood pressure[71]. Exercise training alone in both school-aged children and in adolescents also lower both systolic and diastolic blood pressures[72–74]. Compared with a regimen of caloric restriction alone, Rocchini and colleagues showed that a program integrating both caloric restriction and exercise produced the greatest decrease in blood pressure as well as a reversal of structural changes in forearm resistance vessels[37]. Weight reduction can be extremely difficult and is usually best accomplished in conjunction with comprehensive programs which combine the input of a nutritionist with dietary education, emotional support, information about exercise, and family involvement. Power weightlifting should be discouraged in hypertensive adolescents because of its potential to induce marked blood pressure elevation. Participation in other sports should be encouraged as long as blood pressure is under reasonable control, regular monitoring of blood pressure occurs, and a thorough examination has been conducted to exclude cardiac conditions[18].

The guidelines for dietary modifications in the pediatric population are less clear than in adults. There may be, as in adults, a subset of hypertensive children who are 'salt sensitive'[38]. Yet, data, with regard to children, on the effects of salt on blood pressure are not as definitive as in adults. In general, significant correlations have not been demonstrated between sodium intake and blood pressure in children and adolescents. There does seem to be, however, a subset of adolescents, particularly those who are obese, who demonstrate blood pressure sensitivity to salt as well as other risk factors for hypertension[38]. Most likely sodium does not act as an isolated factor but rather in conjunction with other factors to influence blood pressure. As the usual dietary intake of sodium for most children and adolescents in the USA far exceeds nutrient requirements, it is reasonable to restrict sodium intake to less than 4 g/day by decreasing fast-food consumption and refraining from adding salt to cooked foods[75].

Our current understanding with regard to the effects of potassium and calcium intake on blood pressure are even less definitive. Some evidence exists to suggest that a diet high in potassium and calcium may help to lower blood pressure[76], yet no study has definitively shown this effect in children or adolescents. The dietary intervention clinical trial, Dietary Approach to Stop Hypertension (DASH) reported results that could be relevant to diet benefits in children. This study, which was conducted on adults with mild hypertension, demonstrated a significant reduction in both systolic and diastolic blood pressure in subjects consuming a diet high in fruits, vegetables, and low-fat dairy products compared to the subjects consuming their usual diet. There was no difference in sodium intake and no weight loss occurred in either group. These results indicate that a benefit on blood pressure occurs from diets that are high in potassium, calcium, magnesium, and other vitamins[77]. A similar approach may be of benefit for children and investigations to examine this issue would be appropriate.

Pharmacologic therapy

If non-pharmacologic approaches are unsuccessful, or when a child is symptomatic, has severe hypertension, or end-organ damage, pharmacologic therapy is indicated. In addition, a child with diabetes mellitus or chronic renal disease may benefit from the 'renal protective' effects of antihypertensive treatment to maintain the blood pressure below the 90th percentile for age, sex, and height.

8

8.1

Most of the medications used for adults can be used for children. However, efficacy data, as well as long-term safety data, are limited for the pediatric population. The choice of antihypertensive medication must be individualized and depends upon the child's age, the etiology of the hypertension, the degree of blood pressure elevation, adverse effects, and concomitant medical conditions. In most patients therapy is begun with a single agent. The dose is titrated upward until control of the blood pressure is attained. Blood pressure control, in most instances, is defined as maintaining systolic and diastolic pressure below the 90th percentile. If control cannot be achieved using the maximum dose of a single agent, a second medication can be added or, alternatively, another agent from a different class selected. The more commonly used medications for chronic antihypertensive therapy in children are listed in Table 8.1.4 and those for use in acute, hypertensive emergencies in Table 8.1.5. The dosing recommendations for children have been largely based upon practitioner experience, not on large, multicenter trials.

Table 8.1.4 Antihypertensive drug therapy for chronic hypertension in children*

Drug	Dose (mg/kg/day)		Dosing interval
	Initial	**Maximum**	
Adrenergic-blocking agents			
Alpha-/beta-blocker			
Labetalol	1	3	6–12 h
Alpha-blocker			
Prazosin	0.05–0.1	0.5	6–8 h
Beta-adrenergic blockers			
Atenolol	1	8	12–24 h
Propranolol	1	8	6–12 h
Alpha-agonist			
Clonidine	0.05–0.1**	0.5–0.6†	6 h
Calcium antagonists			
Nifedipine	0.25	3	4–6 h
Nifedipine XL	0.25	3	12–24 h
Converting enzyme inhibitors			
Captopril			
Children	1.5	6	8 h
Neonates	0.03–0.15	2	8–24 h
Enalapril	0.15	not established	12–24 h
Diuretics			
Bumetanide	0.02–0.05	0.3	4–12 h
Furosemide	1	12	4–12 h
Hydrochlorothiazide	1	2–3	12 h
Metolazone	0.1	3	12–24 h
Spironolactone	1	3	6–12 h
Triamterene	2	3	6–12 h
Vasodilators			
Hydralazine	0.75	7.5	6 h
Minoxidil	0.1–0.2	1	12 h

* Listed in alphabetical order by drug class. Other drugs are available in some classes, but data on dosage in children have not been published.
** Total initial dose in mg.
† Total daily dose in mg.
From National High Blood Pressure Education Program Working Group[3].

Table 8.1.5 Antihypertensive drug therapy for hypertensive emergencies in children

Drug	Dose
Nifedipine	0.25–0.5 mg/kg oral when required. May be repeated two times, if no response.
Sodium nitroprusside	0.5–1 µg/kg/min i.v. initially. May be increased stepwise to 8 µg/kg/min maximum.
Labetalol	0.2–1 mg/kg/dose i.v. may be increased incrementally to 1 mg/kg/dose until response achieved. 0.25–2 mg/kg/h maintenance, either bolus or i.v. infusion.
Esmolol	500–600 µg/kg i.v. load dose over 1–2 min then 200 µg/kg/min. May be increased by 50–100 µg/kg each 5–10 min to maximum of 1000 µg/kg.
Diazoxide	1–5 mg/kg/dose i.v. bolus up to maximum of 150 mg/dose.
Hydralazine	0.2–0.4 mg/kg i.v. when required. May be repeated two times if no response.
Minoxidil	0.1–0.2 mg/kg oral.

From National High Blood Pressure Education Program Working Group[3].

Beta-adrenergic blockers, such as propranolol and atenolol, are good choices in some non-asthmatic children, yet are not well tolerated by athletes in whom exercise tolerance may be decreased. More frequently, first line medications are either angiotensin-converting enzyme (ACE) inhibitors or calcium-channel blockers. ACE inhibitors rarely cause side effects (e.g. cough, rash, neutropenia) in children, are usually well tolerated, and some formulations have the advantage of once-a-day dosing. Not only are they effective at controlling blood pressure, but may have beneficial effects on renal function, peripheral vasculature, and cardiac function[78]. Importantly, children with diabetes and those with chronic renal disease may be at special risk for progressive renal deterioration and may benefit from low doses of ACE inhibitors[79,80]. Because of their vasodilator effects on the efferent arteriole, ACE inhibitors can severely reduce glomerular filtration and should therefore be used with caution in patients with renal artery stenosis, a solitary kidney, or a transplanted kidney[81]. ACE inhibitors are contraindicated during pregnancy because of teratogenic effects upon the lungs, kidneys, and brain of the fetus[82]. Therefore, these agents should be used with special caution in adolescent females.

Of the calcium-channel blockers, nifedipine, is most commonly used in pediatrics. The appropriate dose for small children is often lower than the strength of available capsules, so that nifedipine is more practical to use in older children and adolescents. Both short-acting and longer-acting forms are available. Although the use of short-acting forms have adverse effects in some adults[83,84], the same data are unavailable in children. Until more information becomes available, use of short-acting calcium-channel blockers should be limited to children with acute hypertension, such as occurs with acute glomerulonephritis. When calcium-channel blockers are needed for blood pressure control in chronic hypertension, long-acting preparations are preferred, provided that the correct dosage preparation can be used.

8

Conclusion

Children and adolescents with suspected secondary hypertension may require a more extensive evaluation compared to children and adolescents expressing characteristics of essential hypertension. Whether the hypertension is determined to be secondary or essential these children require careful monitoring, interventions to control the blood pressure, and long-term follow up. Considering the long-term morbidity and mortality associated with essential hypertension, major efforts which focus on blood pressure control beginning in the young are needed[85]. Essential hypertension may be found to encompass several distinct pathophysiological entities, each with its own genetic basis and management approach. With continuing research, the knowledge on hypertension in the young as well as adults will continue to expand.

References

1. National Heart, Lung, and Blood Institute. Report of the Task Force on Blood Pressure Control in Children. *Pediatrics* 1977;**59**:797–820.
2. Task Force on Blood Pressure Control in Children: Report of the Second Task Force on Blood Pressure Control in Children, 1988. *Pediatrics* 1987;**79**:1–25.
3. National High Blood Pressure Education Program Working Group Report on Hypertension Control in Children and Adolescents. The Update on the 1987 Task Force Report on High Blood Pressure in Children and Adolescents: A Working Group Report from the National High Blood Pressure Education Program. *Pediatrics* 1996;**98**:649–658.
4. deSwiet M, Fayers P, Shinebourne. Blood pressure survey in a population of newborn infants. *Br Med J* 1976;**ii**:9–11.
5. Schachter J, Kuller LH, Perfetti C. Blood pressure during the first five years of life: relation to ethnic group (black or white) and to parental hypertension. *Am J Epidemiol* 1984;**119**:541–553.
6. Zinner SH, Rosner B, Oh WO. Significance of blood pressure in infancy. *Hypertension* 1985;**7**:411–416.
7. Versmold HT, Kitterman JA, Phibbs RH *et al*. Aortic blood pressure during the first 12 hours of life in infants with birth weight 610 to 4220 grams. *Pediatrics* 1981;**67**:607–613.
8. Tan KL. Blood pressure in full-term healthy neonates. *Clin Pediatr* 1987;**26**:21–24.
9. Hulman S, Edwards R, Chen Y *et al*. Blood pressure patterns in the first three days of life. *J Perinatol* 1991;**11**:231–234.
10. Zubrow AB, Hulman S, Kushner H, Falkner B. Determinants of blood pressure in infants admitted to neonatal intensive care units: A prospective multicenter study. *J Perinatol* 1995;**15**:470–479.
11. Hanna JD, Chan JCM, Gill JR, Jr. Hypertension and the kidney. *J Pediatr* 1991;**118**:327–340.
12. Arar MY, Hogg RJ, Arant BS, Jr, Seikaly MG. Etiology of sustained hypertension in children in the southwestern United States. *Pediatr Nephrol* 1994;**8**:186–189.
13. Plumer LB, Kaplan GW, Mendoza SA. Hypertension in infants – a complication of umbilical arterial catheterization. *J Pediatr* 1976;**89**:802–805.
14. Vailas GN, Brouillette RT, Scott JP *et al*. Neonatal aortic thrombosis: recent experience. *J Pediatr* 1986;**109**:101–108.
15. Abman SH, Warady BA, Lum GM, Koops BL. Systemic hypertension in infants with bronchopulmonary dysplasia. *J Pediatr* 1984;**104**:928–931.
16. Adelman RD. Smokeless tobacco and hypertension in an adolescent. *Pediatrics* 1987;**79**:837–838.
17. Blachley JD, Knochel JP. Tobacco chewer's hypokalemia: Licorice revisited. *N Engl J Med* 1980;**302**:784–785.

8

References

18. Committee on Sports Medicine and Fitness: Athletic participation by children and adolescents who have systemic hypertension. *Pediatrics* 1997;**99**:637–638.
19. Ing FF, Starc TJ, Griffiths SP, Gersony WM. Early diagnosis of coarctation of the aorta in children: a continuing dilemma. *Pediatrics* 1996;**98**:378–382.
20. Strafford MA, Griffiths SP, Gersony WM. Coarctation of the aorta: a study in delayed detection. *Pediatrics* 1982;**69**:159–163.
21. Thoele DG, Muster AJ, Paul MH. Recognition of coarctation of the aorta. *Am J Dis Child* 1987;**141**:1201–1204.
22. Lauer RM, Clarke WR, Beaglehole R. Level, trend, and variability of blood pressure during childhood. The Muscatine Study. *Circulation* 1984;**69**:242–249.
23. Shear CL, Burke GL, Freedman DS, Berenson GS. Value of childhood blood pressure measurements and family history in predicting future blood pressure status: results from 8 years of follow-up in the Bogalusa Heart Study. *Pediatrics* 1986;**77**:862–869.
24. Michels V, Bergstralh E, Hoverman V *et al*. Tracking and prediction of blood pressure in children. *Mayo Clin Proc* 1987;**62**:875–881.
25. Julius S, Jamerson K, Mejia A *et al*. The association of borderline hypertersion with target organ changes and higher coronary risk. Tecumseh Blood Pressure Study. *J Am Med Ass* 1990;**264**:354–358.
26. Mahoney LT, Clarke WR, Burns TL, Lauer RM. Childhood predictors of high blood pressure. *Am J Hypertension* 1991;**4**:6085.
27. Nelson M, Ragland D, Syme S. Longitudinal prediction of adult blood pressure from juvenile blood pressure levels. *Am J Epidemiol* 1992;**136**:633–645.
28. Lauer RM, Clarke WR, Maloney LT, Witt J. Childhood predictors for high adult blood pressure: the Muscatine Study. *Pediatr Clin N Am* 1993;**40**:23–40.
29. Falkner B, Onesti G, Angelakos ET *et al*. Cardiovascular response to mental stress in normal adolescents with hypertensive parents. *Hypertension* 1979;**1**:23–30.
30. Warren P, Fischbein C. Identification of labile hypertension in children and hypertensive parents. *Conn Med* 1980;**44**:77–79.
31. Matthews KA, Manuck SB, Saab PG. Cardiovascular responses of adolescents during a naturally occurring stressor and their behavioral and psychophysiological predictors. *Psychophysiology* 1984;**23**:198.
32. Falkner B, Kushner H. Racial differences in stress induced reactivity in young adults. *Health Psychol* 1989;**8**:613–617.
33. Falkner B, Lowenthal DT. Dynamic exercise response in hypertensive adolescents. *Int J Ped Nephrol* 1980;**1**:161–165.
34. Munger R, Prineas R, Gomez-Marin O. Persistent elevation of blood pressure among children with a family history of hypertension: The Minneapolis children's blood pressure study. *J Hypertension* 1988;**6**:647–653.
35. Himes JH, Dietz WH. Guidelines for overweight in adolescent preventive services: recommendations from an expert committee. *Am J Clin Nutr* 1994;**59**:307–316.
36. Havlik R, Hubert H, Fabsity R, Feinleib M. Weight and hypertension. *Ann Intern Med* 1983;**98**:855–859.
37. Rocchini AP, Katch V, Anderson J *et al*. Blood pressure in obese adolescents: effect of weight loss. *Pediatrics* 1988;**82**:16–23.
38. Rocchini AP, Key J, Bondie D *et al*. The effect of weight loss on the sensitivity of blood pressure to sodium in obese adolescents. *N Eng J Med* 1989;**321**:580–585.
39. Sinaiko AR. Hypertension in children. *N Engl J Med* 1996;**335**:1968–1973.
40. Troiano RP, Flegal KM, Kuczmarski RJ *et al*. Overweight prevalence and trends for children and adolescents. *Arch Pediatr Adolesc Med* 1995;**149**:1085–1091.
41. Daniels SR, Loggie JMH, Khoury P, Kimball TR. Left ventricular geometry and severe left ventricular hypertrophy in children and adolescents with essential hypertension. *Circulation* 1998;**97**:1907–1911.
42. DeFronzo R, Tobin J, Andres R. Glucose clamp technique: A method for quantifying insulin secretion and resistance. *Am J Physiol* 1979;**237**:E214–E223.
43. Ferrannini E, Buzzigoli G, Bonadonna R *et al*. Insulin resistance in essential hypertension. *N Eng J Med* 1987;**317**:350–357.
44. Reaven GM. Role of insulin resistance in human disease. *Diabetes* 1988;**37**:1595–1607.

8

References

45. Berenson GS, Wattigney WA, Bao W *et al.* Epidemiology of early primary hypertension and implications for prevention: The Bogalusa Heart Study. *J Human Hypertension* 1994;**8**(5):303–311.

46. Falkner B, Hulman S, Tannenbaum J, Kushner H. Insulin resistance and blood pressure in young Black men. *Hypertension* 1990;**16**:706–711.

47. Ferrari P, Weidmann P, Shaw S *et al.* Altered insulin sensitivity, hyperinsulinemia, and dyslipidemia in individuals with a hypertensive parent. *Am J Med* 1991;**91**:589–596.

48. Grunfeld B, Balzareti M, Romo M *et al.* Hyperinsulinemia in normotensive offspring of hypertensive parents. *Hypertension* 1994;**23**(Suppl. I):12–15

49. Bao W, Srinivasan SR, Wattigney WA, Berenson GS. Persistence of multiple cardiovascular risk clustering related to syndrome X from childhood to young adulthood. *Arch Intern Med* 1994;**154**:1842–1847.

50. Barker DJP, Osmond C, Golding J *et al.* Growth *in utero*, blood pressure in childhood and adult life, and mortality from cardiovascular disease. *Br Med J* 1989;**298**:564–567.

51. Law CM, Shiell AW. Is blood pressure inversely related to birth weight? The strength of evidence from a systematic review of the literature. *J Hypertension* 1996;**14**:935–941.

52. Barker DJP, Gluckman PD, Godfrey KM *et al.* Fetal nutrition and cardiovascular disease in adult life. *Lancet* 1993;**341**:938–941.

53. Osmond C, Barker DJP, Winter PD *et al.* Early growth and death from cardiovascular disease in women. *Br Med J* 1993;**307**:1519–1524.

54. Harlan WR, Cornoni Huntley J, Leaverton PE. Blood pressure in childhood. National Health Examination Survey. *Hypertension* 1979;**1**:566–571.

55. Katz SH, Hediger MC, Schall HI *et al.* Blood pressure, growth and maturation from childhood to adolescence. *Hypertension* 1980;**2**(Suppl):55–69.

56. Falkner B, Hulman S, Kushner H. Birth weight vs childhood growth as determinants of adult blood pressure. *Hypertension* 1998;**31**(1):145–150.

57. Hulman S, Kushner H, Katz S, Falkner B. Can cardiovascular risk be predicted by newborn, childhood, and adolescent body size? An examination of longitudinal data in urban African Americans. *J Pediatr* 1998;**132**:90–97.

58. Rich GM, Ulick S, Cook S *et al.* Glucocorticoid-remediable aldosteronism in a large kindred: clinical spectrum and diagnosis using a characteristic biochemical phenotype. *Ann Intern Med* 1992;**116**:813–820.

59. Lifton RP, Dluhy RG, Powers M *et al.* Hereditary hypertension caused by chimeric gene duplications and ectopic expression of aldosterone synthase. *Nature Genet* 1992;**2**:66–74.

60. Kroenke K, Omori DM, Simmons JO *et al.* The safety of phenylpropanolamine in patients with stable hypertension. *Ann Intern Med* 1989;**111**:1043–1044.

61. Lake CR, Gallant S, Masson E, Miller P. Adverse drug effects attributed to phenylpropanolamine: A review of 142 case reports. *Am J Med* 1990;**89**:195–208.

62. Hurley JK. A pediatrician's approach to the evaluation of hypertension. *Pediatr Ann* 1989;**18**:542, 544–546, 548–549.

63. Laird WP, Fixler DE. Left ventricular hypertrophy in adolescents with elevated blood pressure: assessment by chest roentgenography, electrocardiography and echocardiography. *Pediatrics* 1981;**67**:255–259.

64. Shieken RM, Clark WR, Lauer RM. Left ventricular hypertrophy in children with blood pressures in the upper quintile of the distribution: the Muscatine Study. *Hypertension* 1981;**3**:669–675.

65. Zahka KG, Neill CA, Kidd L *et al.* Cardiac involvement in adolescent hypertension. *Hypertension* 1981;**3**:664–668.

66. Culpepper WS, Sodt PC, Messerli FH *et al.* Cardiac status in juvenile borderline hypertension. *Ann Intern Med* 1983;**98**:1–7.

67. Daniels SR, Lipman MJ, Burke MJ, Loggie JM. The prevalence of retinal vascular abnormalities in children and adolescents with essential hypertension. *Am J Ophthalmol* 1991;**111**:205–208.

68. Yudkin JS, Forrest RD, Jackson CA. Microalbuminuria as predictor of vascular disease in non-diabetic subjects. *Lancet* 1988;**ii**:530–533.

69. Townsend RR, Ford V. Ambulatory blood pressure monitoring: coming of age in nephrology. *J Am Soc Nephrol* 1996;**7**:2279–2287.

8

References

70. Harshfield GA, Alpert BS, Pulliam DA *et al*. Ambulatory blood pressure recordings in children and adolescents. *Pediatrics* 1994;**94**:180–184.

71. Brownell KD, Kelman JH, Stunkard AJ. Treatment of obese children with and without their mothers: changes in weight and blood pressure. *Pediatrics* 1983;**71**:515–523.

72. Hagberg JM, Goldring D, Ehsani AA *et al*. Effect of exercise training on the blood pressure and hemodynamic features of hypertensive adolescents. *Am J Cardiol* 1983;**52**:763–768.

73. Hansen HS, Froberg K, Hyldebrandt N, Nielson JR. A controlled study of eight months of physical training and reduction of blood pressure in children: the Odense Schoolchild Study. *Br Med J* 1991;**303**:682–685.

74. Shea S, Basch CE, Gutin B *et al*. The rate of increase in blood pressure in children 5 years of age is related to changes in aerobic fitness and body mass index. *Pediatrics* 1994;**94**:465–470.

75. Falkner B, Michel S. Blood pressure response to sodium in children and adolescents. *Am J Clin Nutr* 1997;**65**(Suppl):618S–621S.

76. Sinaiko AR, Gomez-Marin O, Prineas RJ. Effect of low sodium diet or potassium supplementation on adolescent blood pressure. *Hypertension* 1993;**21**:989–994.

77. Appel LJ, Moore TJ, Obarzanek E *et al*. For the DASH Collaborative Research Group. A clinical trial of the effects of dietary patterns on blood pressure. *N Engl J Med* 1997;**336**(16):1117–1124.

78. Doyle AE. Angiotensin-converting enzyme (ACE) inhibition: benefits beyond blood pressure control. *Am J Med* 1992;**92**(4B):1S–107S.

79. Krolewski AS, Canessa M, Warram JH *et al*. Predisposition to hypertension and susceptibility to renal disease in insulin-dependent diabetes mellitus. *N Engl J Med* 1988;**318**:140–145.

80. National High Blood Pressure Education Program. Working group report on hypertension and diabetes. *Hypertension* 1994;**23**:145–158.

81. Hricik DE, Dunn MJ. Angiotensin-converting enzyme inhibitor-induced renal failure: causes, consequences, and diagnostic uses. *J Am Soc Nephrol* 1990;**1**:845–858.

82. Pryde PG, Sedman AB, Nugent CE, Barr M. Angiotensin-converting enzyme inhibitor fetopathy. *J Am Soc Nephrol* 1993;**3**:1575–1582.

83. Furberg CD, Psaty BM, Meyer JV. Nifedipine: dose-related increase in mortality in patients with coronary heart disease. *Circulation* 1995;**92**:1326–1331.

84. National Heart, Lung, and Blood Institute. New Analyses Regarding the Safety of Calcium-Channel Blockers: A Statement for Health Professionals From the National Heart, Lung, and Blood Institute. National Institutes of Health: Bethesda, MD, 1995.

85. Arbeit ML, Johnson CC, Mott DS *et al*. The heart smart cardiovascular school health promotion; behavior correlates of risk factor change. *Prevent Med* 1992;**21**:18–32.

8

Chapter

8.2

Hypertension in the elderly

T Grodzicki and FH Messerli

8

Introduction

Increasing life expectancy has resulted in more elderly and fragile people who are seeking help in clinics and hospitals everyday around the world. The appropriate assessment of their needs as well as differentiation between ontogenetic changes associated unequivocally with aging from pathologic processes can mean the difference between health and disease, or frequently, even between life and death.

Although for years treated as a 'natural' feature of aging, increased blood pressure is a major risk factor for cardiovascular and renal complications, and blood pressure values exceeding 140 mmHg for systolic pressure and 90 mmHg for diastolic pressure are now widely accepted as pathological even in the elderly. The decision-making process concerning diagnosis and proper treatment of hypertension in the elderly is more complicated than in young or middle-aged patients because of higher variability of blood pressure, the increased prevalence at secondary hypertension, frequent comorbidity and concomitant drug therapy in the elderly.

In the USA the prevalence of hypertension exceeds 50% in the elderly population[1], indicating that the majority of this population should receive some form of antihypertensive therapy. However, the results of the recently published observation from a Veterans Administration study in New England are not encouraging: a meager 40% of elderly men had blood pressure equal to or below 160/90 mmHg despite more than six hypertension-related office visits per year[2]. In spite of this, intensification of antihypertensive therapy occurred in only 7% of all visits. Thus, physician and patient inertia alike seem to contribute to the inappropriate blood pressure control and the subsequent excessive cardiovascular morbidity and mortality in the elderly.

Pathophysiology of hypertension in the elderly

A variety of pathophysiologic changes are associated with aging *per se* and longstanding hypertension. Consequently, it is often difficult to disassociate the effects of aging from those of hypertension itself in a given patient (Table 8.2.1). However, antihypertensive therapy may have a beneficial effect on some of these pathophysiologic findings, regardless of whether they are the result of an increased hemodynamic burden from arterial hypertension or aging. Thus, from a somewhat simplistic point of view, it could be stated that arterial hypertension accelerates the cardiovascular effects of aging, thereby setting the biological clock at a faster pace, whereas antihypertensive therapy prevents or reduces cardiovascular effects of aging, thereby (hopefully) slowing down the biological clock.

Hypertension in the elderly is characterized by low cardiac output, low heart rate and increased peripheral resistance[3]. The heart often shows left ventricular hypertrophy of the concentric type with impaired filling, impaired systolic function, ventricular arrhythmias and diminished coronary reserve. In the kidney, renal blood flow, and to a

Table 8.2.1 The effects of aging compared with the effects of hypertension

Parameter	Aging	Hypertension
Hemodynamics	+	++
↓ heart rate		
↓ cardiac output		
Left ventricular hypertrophy	+	++
↓ left ventricular filling	+	++
↓ systolic function	+	++
ventricular arrhythmias	+	++
↓ coronary reserve	+	++
Nephrosclerosis	+	++
↓ renal blood flow	+	++
↑ glomerular filtration rate	+	+
↓ plasma volume	+	+
↓ arterial compliance	+	↓

Pathophysiology of
hypertension in the elderly

The results of the major
placebo-based trials –
implications and
limitations

lesser extent glomerular filtration rate, are reduced and microproteinuria is increasingly common[3,4]. The vascular tree is characterized by increased stiffness, loss of Windkessel function in the aorta, macrovascular and microvascular changes, and endothelial dysfunction. Total body fluid volume and intravascular volumes are reduced. The activity of the plasma renin angiotensin system is decreased, whereas plasma norepinephrine levels increase with age. Beta-receptor responsiveness is diminished. Most of these features occur with aging *per se* and are accelerated by the presence of hypertension[5].

Baroreceptor dysfunction also occurs in the elderly, and although much neglected means that they are often unable to maintain blood pressure within safe limits and, therefore, are prone to episodes of orthostatic and postprandial hypotensive episodes[6]. However, orthostatic hypotension clearly cannot be neglected and has been shown to be a powerful predictor of cardiovascular morbidity and mortality in elderly men.

The main age-related pathophysiologic changes that accelerate the clinical course of hypertension in the elderly are:

● Increased left ventricular mass;
● Diminished arterial compliance;
● Loss of renal function;
● Decreased baroreceptor and beta-receptor function; and
● Impaired endothelial function.

The results of the major placebo-based trials – implications and limitations

During the last two decades multiple trials involving elderly subjects with hypertension have been conducted to validate the thesis that treatment of high blood pressure in older patients will prevent cardiovascular events[7–14]. The subjects included in these studies represent a diverse population of older citizens from Europe (West and East), the United States, Australia, and East Asia (Japan and China), aged between 60 and 84 years, with diastolic, systolodiastolic and

The results of the major
placebo-based trials –
implications and
limitations

Table 8.2.2 Benefits of antihypertensive therapy in STONE, SYST-EUR, SYST-CHINA

Morbid events	Reduction in risk
Cardiovascular events	16–40%
Stroke	25–59%
Coronary events	13–26%
Congestive heart failure	51–55%
Dementia	0–50%

isolated systolic hypertension. The antihypertensive agents that proved to be efficacious in reducing cardiovascular risk were diuretics (both in large and smaller doses) but not beta-blockers, and in three recent trials (STONE, SYST-EUR, SYST-CHINA) long-acting dihydropyridine calcium antagonists. A summary of documented benefits of these trials is presented in Table 8.2.2.

The result of these trials documented that antihypertensive therapy in the elderly is characterized by a high benefit : risk ratio. This ratio is higher in the elderly than in the younger or middle-aged patient, which means that considerably fewer older than younger patients will have to be exposed to antihypertensive therapy to prevent cardiovascular events. Thus, antihypertensive therapy is more cost efficient in the elderly than in the young.

Unfortunately, careful analysis of exclusion criteria to these trials as well as comparison of an average included patient with the general elderly population shows that the results presented in Table 8.2.2 pertain to the highly selected group of patients only. A patient who qualified for being enrolled in the trials should be remarkably healthy. Exclusion criteria included the presence of secondary hypertension, congestive heart failure, myocardial infarction or stroke within last 12 months, neoplasm, dementia, renal failure, any condition prohibiting a sitting or standing position, or other cardiovascular or non-cardiovascular disease.

Table 8.2.3 compares the incidence of comorbid conditions observed in the general elderly population[15], in subjects enrolled in the trials[7–13], in hypertensive aged patients[16] and in residents of nursing homes with hypertension[17]. Even taking into account that

Table 8.2.3 Incidence of comorbid conditions

Disease	General population* 65–74 years	Trials 60–84 years	Hypertensive elderly subjects 65–89 years	Residents of nursing homes 65–74 years of age
Angina	14.7% (m), 8.6% (w)	12.3%	12.2 (m), 16% (w)	20%
Post-myocardial infarction	11.1% (m), 4.4% (w)	1.2–5%	11.9% (m), 4.6% (w)	
Congestive heart failure	2.0% (m), 1.3% (w)	0%	3% (m), 4.9% (w)	16%
Post-stroke	3.5% (m), 1.3% (w)	1.4–3.5%	9.5% (m), 4.9% (w)	40%
Diabetes	22.9% (m), 20.1% (w)	10.5%	20.1% (m), 15.2% (w)	36%
Dementia	7%	0–1.6%	10%	29%
Depression	15%	4.4%	10%	23.9%
Limitation in ADL**	4.5% (m), 7.3% (w)	5%	15%	83%

* m = men; w = women.
** ADL = activities of daily living.

presented data originating from different papers and diagnostic criteria differed significantly, the health status of a typical hypertensive patient enrolled in the prospective double-blind trials was much better than that of an average old person without hypertension. This difference is even more striking when residents of elderly nursing homes are considered[17]. Thus, the results of major trials conducted in the elderly allow us to conclude that high blood pressure should be treated and lowered to below 140/90 mmHg in the aged but otherwise healthy hypertensive patients. In many other elderly patients with comorbid conditions, the decision about treatment must be highly individual (and *horribile dictu* not evidence-based). Some subgroup analysis of the above-mentioned trials as well as smaller studies may be helpful to arrive at a therapeutic decision. The longitudinal epidemiological observations documented increased risk of non-fatal and fatal cardiovascular events in subjects with high blood pressure and concomitant diseases[16,18].

Diagnosis of hypertension in the elderly

In addition to routine diagnostic procedures performed in all hypertensive patients, the elderly should be carefully screened in order to exclude presence of pseudohypertension, white coat hypertension, hypotensive episodes, and secondary hypertension.

Especially in the elderly, hypertension is associated with increased arterial stiffness. In some cases the excessive increase in stiffness may lead to falsely elevated blood pressure readings. In one of our studies, cuff blood pressure measurements were shown to exceed intra-arterial blood pressure by 10–54 mmHg[19]. Such pseudohypertensive patients can be diagnosed by a simple Osler's maneuver: assessment of the palpability of the pulseless radial (or brachial) artery distal to the point of occlusion by cuff pressure. Patients found to be Osler-positive remain at risk of vital organ hypoperfusion when treatment is based on traditionally measured cuff blood pressure values.

High variability of blood pressure remains another consequence of increased stiffness of large arteries. Deterioration in baroreceptor function in elderly hypertensive subjects as well as diminished blood volume and dysfunction of beta-receptors may contribute to an increased blood pressure variability in those patients. The clinical consequences are often serious and include:

- orthostatic fall in blood pressure;
- postprandial fall in blood pressure;
- exaggerated hypotensive response to antihypertensive treatment;
- exaggerated hypertensive reactions to isometric and other stress; and
- white coat hypertension.

As a consequence, in patients with a history of falls, dizziness, vertigo or syncope, or high blood pressure values without target organ involvement, 24-hour blood pressure monitoring or home blood pressure measurements (four or five times during a day) should be considered[5,20,21].

8

Secondary hypertension in the elderly

The Sixth Report of the Joint National Committee recommended that age should be considered as one of the factors suggesting the presence of secondary causes of hypertension[22]. In fact, the results of Anderson *et al.*, who assessed prevalence of secondary hypertension in 4429 patients aged 18 to more than 70 years, demonstrated a significant increase in the prevalence of secondary hypertension with age. In subjects 70 years and older this rate was more than 3.5-fold than for age 18–29 years[23]. One-day evaluation consisted of history and physical examination and measurement of serum sodium, potassium, creatinine, thyroxine, thyroid-simulating hormone, stimulated plasma renin activity, plasma catecholamines (recumbent and upright), blood pressure response after saralasin, and plasma cortisol and aldosterone (after 3–4 hours' infusion of saline). Among the secondary forms of hypertension, renal insufficiency, renovascular hypertension and hypothyroidism were the most frequent in the elderly. Hypothyroidism, a possible cause of high blood pressure, was found in 6.5% of hypertensive subjects 60–69 years old and in less than 2% of patients aged 18–39 years.

Practical considerations concerning treatment

Education

Education of a patient and his or her family or caregivers remains the first important step in antihypertensive therapy. The implementation of a teaching program results in a substantial improvement of the compliance to both non-pharmacological and pharmacological treatment and results in a significant improvement in blood pressure control. In a study by Gruesser *et al.*, who implemented a program developed at the University of Düsseldorf at 43 primary healthcare practices and trained 466 patients (mean age 59 years), a significant reduction in body weight and in systolic and diastolic blood pressure and increase in self blood pressure measurements were observed after 22 weeks[24]. Taking into account the cost-effectiveness of a comprehensive antihypertensive therapy, it seems, therefore, reasonable to spend some time with a patient, or with the family, to discuss the risks associated with hypertension and benefits from therapy.

Non-pharmacologic therapy

In every elderly patient in whom blood pressure values exceed 140/90 mmHg, non-pharmacological treatment should be attempted as the first step. Lifestyle modifications including weight reduction, increased physical activity, moderation of dietary sodium, decreased alcohol intake, and limitation in consumption of non-steroidal anti-inflammatory drugs may in some elderly patients help to effectively reduce blood pressure. However, such an approach is prone to face many limitations due to age-related changes such as lack of sensitivity of taste buds and concomitant diseases like heart failure, osteoarthrosis, neurologic diseases (Parkinson's disease), dementia or post-stroke physical disability that limit participation in exercise programs. Last, but not least, depression and anxiety, and the reluctance to consider any changes in a very established and rigid daily schedule, as well as the fear of being injured or assaulted cannot be neglected. Despite these potential pitfalls, it seems worthwhile to motivate elderly subjects to change their lifestyle and to encourage them to participate in a regular physical fitness program. The improvement in physical strength and better social interactions may improve quality of life even if the influence on blood pressure level remains minimal.

Drug treatment

If non-pharmacological procedures fail, drug therapy should be considered in otherwise healthy patients with systolic blood pressures over 140 mmHg, and/or diastolic blood pressure above 90 mmHg since their risk of complications is markedly higher. Pharmacological treatment should start earlier in patients with systolic blood pressure over 140 mmHg with coexistence of diabetes, angina pectoris, left ventricular hypertrophy or failure, and renal failure.

The drug regimen should be simple, starting with a low dose (about half of that used in younger patients) of a single long-acting drug that is up titrated slowly, if necessary, until a systolic blood pressure below 140 mmHg is attained and diastolic blood pressure is below 90 mmHg. Such an approach will minimize the incidence of orthostatic and postprandial hypotension. Any exaggerated reduction in blood pressure may compromise cerebral and coronary perfusion in elderly hypertensive patients, in whom the brain and coronary arteries are frequently narrowed by obstructive atherosclerotic lesions, and in whom a hypertrophied ventricle may pose higher demands on the supply of oxygen[25].

Optimal antihypertensive therapy in the elderly should:

- be hemodynamically compatible, i.e. preserve or improve systemic flow while reducing total peripheral resistance;
- reduce arterial stiffness and improve endothelial dysfunction;
- preserve or improve target organ blood flow and prevent or reduce target organ damage;
- reduce sympathetic activity and be metabolically neutral;
- cover at least a full 24-hour period with a smooth onset of action;
- be well tolerated – preserve or improve quality of life;
- have no interaction with other commonly used drugs in the elderly; and
- be affordable.

Treatment of uncomplicated hypertension

The guidelines for antihypertensive therapy of elderly patients are based on the results of previously described major trials. Agents such as diuretics or long-acting dihydropyridines are efficacious in preventing

Practical considerations concerning treatment

Non-pharmacologic therapy

Drug treatment

stroke and major cardiovascular events. However, beta-blockers considered for a long time as efficacious seem less appropriate. In a recently published meta-analysis, we showed that beta-blockers were ineffective in preventing coronary heart disease, cardiovascular and all-cause mortality and much less effective than diuretics in preventing cerebrovascular events and fatal stroke[26]. Therefore, in contrast to diuretics and dihydropyridine calcium antagonists, beta-blockers should no longer be considered appropriate first line therapy of uncomplicated hypertension in the elderly.

The systolic pressure in the elderly patients with isolated systolic hypertension (ISH) can be specifically lowered by actively decreasing arterial stiffness, by reducing pulsewave velocity and delaying the return of the reflected pressure waves to the ascending aorta. Vasoactive drugs that reduce smooth muscle tone in the large arteries actively increase arterial compliance. This effect has been demonstrated for calcium antagonists, angiotensin-converting enzyme (ACE) inhibitors, nitrates and beta-blockers with intrinsic sympathomimetic activity. Systolic pressure can also be lowered in patients with ISH by decreasing the blood volume ejected from the left ventricle during each heart cycle. Diuretics decrease both plasma and stroke volume, which may explain their efficacy in reducing systolic blood pressure in patients with ISH. Apart from these pathophysiologic considerations, diuretics and calcium antagonists (long-acting dihydropyridines) have been shown to be effective as first choice therapy in double-blind trials in older subjects. ACE inhibitors were used in two trials (SYST-EUR, SYST-CHINA) and beta-blocker (in the SHEP study) as add-on therapy.

Complicated hypertension

The selection of the first-line antihypertensive agent in subjects with coexistent diseases should also be based on a careful assessment of the drug's potential influence on the clinical course of coexistent diseases. Table 8.2.4 briefly outlines the indications for various antihypertensive agents depending on some comorbid conditions seen frequently in the elderly.

Combination therapy

The significant reduction in cardiovascular complications observed in previously cited trials was achieved through rigid control of blood

Table 8.2.4 Indications for various antihypertensive agents

Disorder	First choice	Second choice
Angina post-myocardial infarction	beta-blockers	Non-dihydropyridine calcium antagonists, ACE inhibitors
Heart failure	ACE inhibitors, diuretics	Carvedilol, long-acting dihydropyridine calcium antagonists
Diabetes	ACE inhibitors	Calcium antagonists
Renal failure	ACE inhibitors	Calcium antagonists, diuretics

Table 8.2.5 Initial blood pressure values, changes in blood pressure and the number of subjects who required combination therapy in recently published trials

Trial	Initial blood pressure (mmHg)	Change in blood pressure (mmHg)	Subjects on combination therapy
STOP-Hypertension[6]	195/102	27/10	66%
SHEP[9]	170/77	27/9	64%
SYST-EUR[10]	174/86	23/7	45%
HOT[27]	170/105	26/20	60%

STOP = Swedish Trial in Old Patients with Hypertension;
SHEP = Systolic Hypertension in the Elderly Program;
SYST-EUR = Systolic Hypertension in Europe;
HOT = Hypertension Optimal Treatment (group with target diastolic blood pressure ≤90 mmHg)

pressure (Table 8.2.5). Therefore, it seems reasonable to assume that one-half to two-thirds of elderly subjects with hypertension will need combination therapy to keep their blood pressure level below 140/90 mmHg. Based on the data from presented trials as well as pathophysiologic features of hypertension in elderly patients, a combination of low dose of thiazide diuretics with either ACE inhibitor or long-acting dihydropyridine calcium antagonists should be preferred. However, the combination of a calcium antagonist with an ACE inhibitor has been particularly useful in our experience. The ACE inhibitor has been shown to antagonize the vasodilatory edema, which is not an uncommon feature of calcium antagonists. Thus, in combination with an ACE inhibitor, a much higher dose of a calcium antagonist is often tolerated. In some cases such as in post-myocardial infarct patients, a beta-blocker or non-dihydropyridine calcium antagonist might be combined with an ACE inhibitor.

BOX 8.2.1 Hazards of combination therapy in the elderly

Combinations that might be hazardous and should be avoided are:

- A beta-blocker and non-dihydropyridine calcium antagonist (e.g. verapamil) because of possible left ventricular dysfunction and bradyarrhythmia.
- ACE inhibitor and potassium-sparing diuretic because of possible renal failure and hyperkalemia.
- Alpha-blocker and dihydropyridine calcium antagonist because of possible orthostatic hypotension.

8

A simple algorithm might be useful in the decision-making process in the elderly hypertensive subjects (Table 8.2.6). We conclude that in elderly hypertensive patients, both the proper choice of the antihypertensive agent and the modalities of therapy should be highly individualized (and often therefore cannot be evidence-based). The evolution of knowledge concerning the processes associated with human aging showed that we have to change our approach to high blood pressure in the elderly and to treat it very early and vigorously, but be aware at some pitfalls associated with too low blood pressure.

Table 8.2.6 An algorithm for the decision-making process in elderly hypertensive patients

Step	Aim	Especially important in the elderly
1	Proper diagnosis	Exclusion of secondary hypertension, white coat hypertension, pseudohypertension
2	Assessment of risk	Coexistent diseases, especially dementia, depression, history of falls, concomitant drug therapy
3	Education	Directed not only to a patient but also to the caregivers
4	Non-pharmacological therapy	Multiple additional benefits
5	Drug treatment	Uncomplicated: diuretics, calcium antagonists
		Complicated: choice dependent on coexistent diseases
		Combination: calcium antagonist + ACE inhibitor or angiotensin-receptor blocker diuretics + ACE inhibitor or angiotensin-receptor blocker

References

1. Burt VL, Cutler JA, Higgins M *et al*. Trends in the prevalence, awareness, treatment and control of hypertension in the adult US population. Data from the Health Examinations Surveys, 1960 to 1991. *Hypertension* 1995;**26**(1):60–69.
2. Berlowitz DR, Ash AS, Hickey EC *et al*. Inadequate management of blood pressure in a hypertensive population. *N Engl J Med* 1998;**339**(27):1957–1963.
3. Messerli FH, Sundgaard-Riise K, Ventura HO *et al*. Essential hypertension in the elderly: haemodynamics, intravascular volume, plasma renin activity, and circulating catecholamine levels. *Lancet* 1988;**ii**(8357):983–986.
4. Schmieder RE, Schachinger H, Messerli FH. Accelerated decline in renal perfusion with aging in essential hypertension. *Hypertension* 1994;**23**:351–357.
5. Grodzicki T, Michalewicz L, Messerli FH. Ageing and essential hypertension: effect of left ventricular hypertrophy on cardiac function. *Am J Hypertens* 1998;**11**(4 Pt 1):425–429.
6. Masaki KH, Schatz IJ, Burchfiel CM *et al*. Orthostatic hypotension predicts mortality in elderly men: the Honolulu Heart Program. *Circulation* 1998;**98**(21):2290–2295.
7. Dahlof B, Lindholm LH, Hansson L *et al*. Morbidity and mortality in the Swedish Trial in Old Patients with Hypertension (STOP-Hypertension). *Lancet* 1991;**338**(8778):1281–1285.
8. Fletcher A, Amery A, Birkenhager W *et al*. Risks and benefits in the trial of the European Working Party on High Blood Pressure in the Elderly. *J Hypertens* 1991;**9**(3):225–230.
9. Gong L, Zhang W, Zhu Y *et al*. Shanghai trial of nifedipine in the elderly (STONE). *J Hypertens* 1996;**14**(10):1237–1245.
10. SHEP Cooperative Research Group. Prevention of stroke by antihypertensive drug treatment in older persons with isolated systolic hypertension. Final results of the Systolic Hypertension in the Elderly Program (SHEP). *JAMA* 1991;**265**(24):3255–3264.
11. Staessen JA, Fagard R, Thijs L *et al*. Subgroup and per-protocol analysis of randomized European Trial on Isolated Systolic Hypertension in the Elderly. *Arch Intern Med* 1998;**158**(15):1681–1691.
12. MRC Working Party. Medical Research Council trial of treatment of hypertension in older adults: principal results. *Br Med J* 1992;**304**(6824):405–412.
13. Liu L, Wang JG, Gong L *et al*. Comparison of active treatment and placebo in older Chinese patients with isolated systolic hypertension. Systolic Hypertension in China (SYST-CHINA) Collaborative Group. *J Hypertens* 1998;**16**(12 Pt 1):1823–1829.
14. Forette F, Seux ML, Staessen JA *et al*. Prevention of dementia in randomised double-blind placebo-controlled Systolic Hypertension in Europe (SYST-EUR) trial. *Lancet* 1998;**352**(9137):1347–1351.
15. Bild DE, Fitzpatrick A, Fried LP *et al*. Age-related trends in cardiovascular morbidity and physical functioning in the elderly: the Cardiovascular Health Study. *J Am Geriatr Soc* 1993;**41**(10):1047–1056.

8

16. Kannel WB. Hypertension in the elderly: epidemiologic appraisal from the Framingham Study. *Cardiol Elderly* 1993;**1**:359–363.
17. Gambassi G, Lapane K, Sgadari A *et al*. Prevalence, clinical correlates, and treatment of hypertension in elderly nursing home residents. SAGE (Systematic Assessment of Geriatric Drug Use via Epidemiology) Study Group. *Arch Intern Med* 1998;**158**(21):2377–2385.
18. Skoog I, Lernfelt B, Landahl S *et al*. 15-year longitudinal study of blood pressure and dementia. *Lancet* 1996;**347**(9009):1141–1145.
19. Messerli FH, Ventura HO, Amodeo C. Osler's maneuver and pseudohypertension. *N Engl J Med* 1985;**312**(24):1548–1551.
20. Ferrara LA, Cicerano U, Marotta T *et al*. Postprandial and postural hypotension in the elderly. *Cardiol Elderly* 1993;**1**:33–37.
21. Grodzicki T, Rajzer M, Fagard R *et al*. Ambulatory blood pressure monitoring and postprandial hypotension in elderly patients with isolated systolic hypertension. Systolic Hypertension in Europe (SYST-EUR) Trial Investigators. *J Hum Hypertens* 1998;**12**(3):161–165.
22. The Sixth Report of the Joint National Committee on Prevention, Detection, Evaluation, and Treatment of High Blood Pressure. *Arch Intern Med* 1997;**157**(21):2413–2446.
23. Anderson GH Jr, Blakeman N, Streeten DH. The effect of age on prevalance of secondary forms of hypertension in 4429 consecutively referred patients. *J Hypertens* 1994;**12**(5):609–615.
24. Gruesser M, Hartmann P, Schlottmann N *et al*. Structured patient education for out-patients with hypertension in general practice: a model project in Germany. *J Hum Hypertens* 1997;**11**(8):501–506.
25. Grossman E, Messerli FH, Grodzicki T, Kowey P. Should a moratorium be placed on sublingual nifedipine capsules given for hypertensive emergencies and pseudoemergencies? *JAMA* 1996;**276**(16):1328–1331.
26. Messerli FH, Grossman E, Goldbourt U. Are β-blockers efficacious as first-line therapy for hypertension in the elderly? A systematic review. *JAMA* 1998;**279**(23):1903–1907.
27. Hansson L, Zanchetti A, Carruthers SG *et al*. Effects of intensive blood-pressure lowering and low-dose aspirin in patients with hypertension: principal results of the Hypertension Optimal Treatment (HOT) randomised trial. HOT Study Group. *Lancet* 1998;**351**(9118):1755–1762.

Further reading

1. Black HR. Antihypertensive therapy and cardiovascular disease. Impact of effective therapy on disease progression. *Am J Hypertens* 1998;**11**(1 Pt 2):3S–8S.
2. Bulpitt CJ. A risk-benefit analysis for the treatment of hypertension. *Postgrad Med J* 1993;**69**(816):764–774.
3. Grodzicki T, Messerli FH. The elderly hypertensive. In: *Individualized Therapy of Hypertension* (eds Kaplan N, Ram CVS), pp. 47–63. Marcel Dekker: New York, 1995.
4. Kay DWK. The epidemiology of age-related neurological disease and dementia. *Rev Clin Gerontol* 1995;**5**:39–56.
5. Lakatta EG. Cardiovascular regulatory mechanisms in advanced age. *Physiol Rev* 1993;**73**(2):413–467.
6. Messerli FH. Osler's maneuver, pseudohypertension, and true hypertension in the elderly. *Am J Med* 1986;**80**(5):906–910.
7. Mulrow CD, Cornell JA, Herrera CR *et al*. Hypertension in the elderly. Implications and generalizability of randomized trials. *JAMA* 1994;**272**(24):1932–1938.
8. O'Connell JE, Gray CS. Treatment of post-stroke hypertension. A practical guide. *Drugs Aging* 1996;**8**(6):408–415.
9. Safar ME, London GM, Asmar R, Frohlich ED. Recent advances on large arteries in hypertension. *Hypertension* 1998;**32**(1):156–161.
10. Turnheim K. Drug dosage in the elderly. Is it rational? *Drugs Aging* 1998;**13**(5):357–379.
11. Vidt DG. Renal disease and renal artery stenosis in the elderly. *Am J Hypertens* 1998;**11**(3 Pt 2):46S–51S.
12. Wei JY. Age and the cardiovascular system. *N Engl J Med* 1992;**327**(24):1735–1739.

References

Further reading

Chapter

8.3

The patient with multiple risk factors

GLR Jennings

8

Introduction

Hypertension is a major risk factor for coronary heart disease, stroke, aneurysm, and other atherosclerotic vascular diseases. In turn, there are specific risk factors for hypertension. Some of these predispose to hypertension, but have no separate propensity to cause atherosclerosis. An example of this is excessive alcohol intake which is associated with high blood pressure and increased risk of stroke but not with increase in coronary heart disease rates above those seen in those who drink no alcohol, or have a modest intake. High sodium intake may be a similar example[1,2]. On the other hand, some factors predispose to atherosclerosis over and above their effects on blood pressure. Examples are obesity and sedentary lifestyle. Both are associated with increase in blood pressure, but are also risk factors for coronary heart disease independent of their pressor effects as a result of metabolic and other effect.

Other important cardiovascular risk factors are not associated with blood pressure but are common in the hypertensive population. These include dyslipidemias and diabetes (Figure 8.3.2). The importance of coexisting hypertension in these patients lies in the interaction between major risk factors (Figure 8.3.1). Combinations have greater effects on the probability of disease than would be predicted by the risk associated with a given risk factor acting alone[3].

Multiple risk factors

The interaction between multiple risk factors in patients with hypertension is of great importance in management, not only because of the consequences for risk stratification of the individual patient, but also because aggregations of risk factors are common. Hypertension is

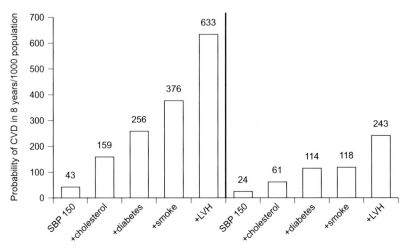

Fig. 8.3.1 Framingham Study 18-year follow up – risk of cardiovascular disease (CVD) in eight years in 45-year-old males and females at a systolic blood pressure (SBP) of 150 mmHg but varying other major risk factors: cholesterol 4.8 mmol/liter elevated to 8.5 mmol/liter; left ventricular hypertrophy (LVH) assessed by electrocardiogram[4].

The patient with multiple risk factors

Multiple risk factors
The metabolic syndrome
Smoking

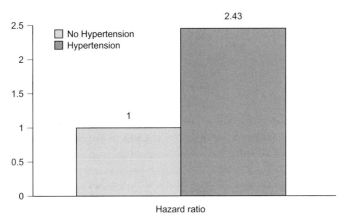

Fig. 8.3.2 Diabetes is more common in hypertensive than normotensive subjects. Data from subjects with hypertension aged 45–64 years followed for six years[9].

common in most communities. Hyperlipidemias and other risk factors are also common, so their coexistence in many patients is inevitable. In addition, there are predisposing lifestyle factors common to hypertension, hyperlipidemia, and diabetes, increasing the frequency with which the clinician will encounter patients with multiple risk factors still further. Furthermore there are specific clusters of risk factors that often occur together due to both genetic and environmental influences.

The metabolic syndrome

The most important risk factor cluster is the metabolic syndrome[5]. which is characterized by insulin resistance, high blood triglyceride and low high-density lipoprotein (HDL) levels and high blood pressure. Abdominal obesity is also a common feature of the phenotype. The metabolic syndrome occurs in all populations but in some areas of the world, e.g. parts of Asia, the Pacific and indigenous populations such as Australian aborigines it is the predominant predisposing risk factor profile for atheroschlerosis and coronary heart disease[6]. The metabolic syndrome (Table 8.3.1) is a major public health problem and may be increasing in frequency due to nutritional changes and reduction in physical activity.

Smoking

Of the major cardiovascular risk factors, smoking has a unique relationship to blood pressure. Smoking greatly exaggerates the *risks* of

Table 8.3.1 Features of the metabolic syndrome

- Increased triglyceride
- Decreased high-density lipoprotein
- Increased blood pressure
- Abdominal obesity
- Insulin resistance

8

hypertension, but in general tobacco smokers have slightly[7] lower blood pressure than non-smokers. Cessation of smoking is a major priority in the management of hypertension even though success in an individual patient will not generally improve blood pressure control and indeed many patients will gain weight.

Other risk factors

Hypertension can also be associated with risk markers such as left ventricular hypertrophy[8] or increased carotid artery wall thickness. These indicate a degree of risk of complications of hypertension over and above that of the blood pressure level as they provide objective evidence that a given individual has begun the transformation from being risk prone but healthy, to developing hypertension with target-organ damage.

Blood pressure variables

Both systolic and diastolic blood pressure are continuously related to the risk of stroke, coronary heart disease, death and non-fatal myocardial infarction. Blood pressure is also related to the risk of heart failure and of renal disease. There is some debate over the best blood pressure variable to predict risk. Systolic blood pressure may be more predictive than diastolic or mean pressures. Progressive increase in systolic blood pressure and fall in diastolic blood pressure with age may be particularly adverse. Pulse pressure, the difference between systolic and diastolic blood pressure is also positively associated with coronary heart disease. This is an indirect measure of arterial stiffness. The latter may be predictive of cardiovascular disease independently of blood pressure. However, blood pressure variables are strongly interrelated and statistical considerations imply that it may be the measurement with the lowest variance that bears the strongest correlation to cardiovascular disease, rather than the most biologically important.

Although high blood pressure has traditionally been regarded as a single risk factor, there are reasons for considering a patient with, say, systolic hypertension and diastolic hypertension, or systolic hypertension and wide pulse pressures as having 'multiple' risk factors.

Pre-existing cardiovascular disease

This is the most important predictor of future risk of major cardiovascular events in patients with hypertension[10]. Patients with advanced congestive heart failure face the highest risks and those with left ventricular hypertrophy, post-myocardial infarction, stroke, transient ischemic attack or peripheral vascular disease have higher risks than other patients with hypertension. Other non-cardiovascular diseases that increase the risks of future events in hypertensives are renal disease, as indicated by elevated serum creatinine, microalbuminuria and proteinuria and diabetes.

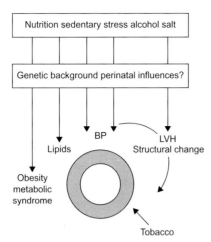

Fig. 8.3.3 Risk factor profiling in hypertension. The major risk factors interacting with hypertension.

The management of these diverse conditions is beyond the scope of this chapter. However, many have implications in the choice of antihypertensive drugs (Figure 8.3.3) and without exception control of blood pressure assists to reduce adverse outcomes[10].

Non-modifiable risk factors

The risks of cardiovascular disease in hypertensive patients increase with age. Men are more at risk than women from both stroke and coronary heart disease at least up until the mid 70s. Beyond that age the risk of death from stroke and coronary heart disease are similar.

In older patients with hypertension the best outcome data at the present time pertain to diuretic drugs and with dihydropyridine calcium-channel blockers. Salt moderation[13] may be particularly effective in older hypertensives.

Modifiable risk factors
Cigarette smoking

Cigarette smoking increases cardiovascular risk in both hypertensive and non-hypertensive subjects. The effect on cardiovascular mortality is an increase of about 50% over non-smokers, and cardiovascular events are doubled. Cigarette smokers have on average a blood pressure that is similar or even lower than non-smokers, perhaps because of lower body weight. However, smoking impairs endothelial function[14], which may adversely affect risk and is associated with increase in fibrinogen levels in the blood and lower HDL-cholesterol. Cigarette smoking is a particular risk factor for peripheral artery disease and the odds ratio in smokers over non-smokers is over five for arterial occlusion adjusted for age and sex. In smokers with reversible airways obstruction beta-adrenergic antagonists should be avoided[10].

8

Exercise

Sedentary lifestyle is an independent risk factor for coronary heart disease and fatal myocardial infarction and a secondary risk factor due to its effects on other risk factors such as blood pressure itself, obesity, lipids and type 2 diabetes. All of the above can be prevented with regular physical exercise[15]. Paradoxically, some young athletes may have higher systolic blood pressure. The reason for this is not known nor whether it is associated with increased risk of cardiovascular events later in life in this particular subgroup. The increase in systolic blood pressure may be related to higher stroke volume as a result of exercise training. In strength-trained competitive athletes, it may also be a consequence of concentric left ventricular hypertrophy and even steroid use. Experience with rehabilitation programs suggests that regular exercise is also beneficial in patients who have previously suffered cardiovascular events. Blood pressure may be unchanged or fall after myocardial infarction. The latter is adverse in its consequences for prognosis as it may reflect loss of cardiac muscle sufficient to cause left ventricular dysfunction. Meta-analysis of the combined trials of cardiac rehabilitation involving exercise has suggested that some reduction in overall death rates with exercise after myocardial infarction although this may be at the cost of a slight excess in non-fatal myocardial infarction.

Recommendations for physical activity in the general population have largely been based on epidemiological studies. In a report of the US Surgeon General on Physical Activity and Health Services in 1996[16] the level of exercise recommended for optimal benefit was that required to expend their energy by an additional 150 kcal/day or 1050 kcal/week. This was associated with reduction in coronary heart disease mortality by about one-third in epidemiological studies. A similar level of exercise training has been associated with a reduction in onset of new cases of non-insulin-dependent diabetes mellitus (NIDDM) by about 20%.

In studies in hypertensive subjects regular exercise at the level of 30–40 minutes, three times a week at 50–60% of maximum work capacity is associated with fall in blood pressure, improvement in insulin sensitivity and reduction in sympathetic activity[13]. There is no indication in the studies performed to date that regular aerobic exercise is particularly hazardous in patients with hypertension. However, it is prudent to recommend moderate levels that are within the capacities of the patients and avoidance of highly intense and unaccustomed or severe isometric stress in patients with hypertension.

Patients on antihypertensive therapy can perform moderate aerobic exercise safely and derive benefit. Dehydration must be avoided, especially in diuretic-treated patients. Those on beta-blockers may have reduced exercise tolerance and higher muscle fatigability.

Obesity

Throughout the world many populations are progressively increasing their body fat. Obesity is a contributor towards rates of hypertension in the general community. However, it is also, independently a risk factor for cardiovascular disease. The most adverse form of obesity may be that which is largely localized to the abdomen. As outlined above this can be related to hyperinsulinemia, low HDL, insulin resistance and the metabolic syndrome. In some populations, microalbuminuria is another marker of this metabolic syndrome.

Some obese subjects take diuretics regularly or intermittently in the hope of losing weight. It is not clear that any particular antihypertensive drug group is of special value in the obese hypertensive.

Lipid-associated risks

Increased levels of total and low-density lipoprotein (LDL)-cholesterol are associated with increasing risks of coronary heart disease at all ages as are low levels of HDL lipoprotein. There is overrepresentation of lipid abnormalities in the hypertensive population. What may in part, reflect common lifestyle factors such as high fat intake and obesity, lack of physical activity and the associations of the metabolic syndrome occurring in some population.

It has been regarded as important to avoid thiazides and beta-antagonists in hypertensives[17] with hyperlipidemia because they may increase triglyceride levels and/or lower HDL-cholesterol in the short term. Outcome studies, including studies of older patients and of diabetics have, however, provided strong reassurances of overall benefit.

Alcohol

There is a paradox in that the risk of coronary heart disease appears to be reduced among regular light consumers of alcohol, for example 5–30 g/day in men. However, there is probably a linear relationship between alcohol consumption and blood pressure and higher levels of alcohol consumption are associated with increased risk of stroke. This is particularly likely after binge drinking.

Other risk factors

There are many other risk factors for coronary heart disease and because of common environmental factors they tend to be found in a high proportion of hypertensives. These include elevated plasma fibrinogen which is positively associated with the risk of coronary heart disease and ischemic stroke. In many patients, this is associated with cigarette smoking. Other risk factors include passive smoking, specific lipoprotein defects such as elevated Lp(a) and elevated homocysteine. These may be genetic indicators of risk. An important risk factor for hypertension in the mind of the lay population is emotional stress. Although there is no doubt that this is associated with acute increases in blood pressure, the evidence that sustained blood pressure is a consequence of psychological stress has been more controversial. There is strong interrelationship between other lifestyle factors influencing blood pressure including adverse diet, lack of exercise and obesity in response to emotional stress in some patients.

Modifiable risk factors
Obesity
Lipid-associated risks
Alcohol
Other risk factors

8

Multiple risk factor models

It is most important in managing hypertensive patients with multiple risk factors to keep in the mind the overall risk. This is the arithmetic sum of the positive and negative influences affecting the likelihood of future events. For example, patients with very mild elevations of multiple risk factors may be at higher risk than those with major elevations of a single risk factor. Assessment of multivariate risk may be useful in counselling patients with hypertension who can be shown the likely benefits of various interventions. A number of models have been proposed as useful screening tools to identify individuals at risk and quantitate the benefits of therapy. They always rely on assumptions and are derived from prospective studies of risk factors for coronary heart disease that estimate the risk in the absence and presence of a set of factors or treatment. The usual analysis is a linear logistic model that estimates the odds ratio and permits adjustment to relevant covariates. Causal relationships are largely inferred from experimental data and analysis of longitudinal population studies and clinical trials with therapeutic agents. Application of the statistical associations does involve the assumption of causality. This assumption is on stronger grounds when it is supported by a high level of association and appropriate temporal sequence, evidence of a dose–response effect, consistency, biological plausibility and specificity. However, reversing the risk factor has not been shown to lower the risk in all cases. Typically data from the Framingham, MRFIT or PROCAM Studies[18] have been used to derive the coefficients of the logistic regression analysis. Although care needs to be used in applying computer programs or risk algorithms derived in this way, it may be a very useful tool for practitioners to determine the priorities and agree on targets with individual patients.

Management of patients with multiple risk factors

Patients with hypertension and coexisting risk factors may require medications for multiple conditions (Figure 8.3.4). Blood pressure targets are also commonly lower in these patients and combination antihypertensive drug therapy is frequently required. There are formidable barriers to implementation of lifestyle measures and maintenance of healthy lifestyle long term in patients with hypertension. The considerable literature on compliance suggests that these barriers may not be as great as we make them and an important component is to re-evaluate the medical consultation process. The interaction needs to be successful from the point of view of the patient and requires the provision of simple and intelligible prescription, clear instruction, follow-up monitoring including reminders and rewards, and maximizing social support. The practitioner need not act alone in this process but should enlist wherever possible the full resources of the health system and local community support.

Effective management of multiple risk factors requires a strategic approach. If the practitioner attempts to control all of the adverse

8

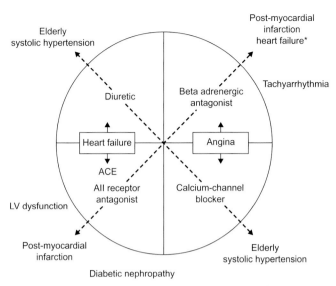

Fig. 8.3.4 Preferred antihypertensive drug choices in patients with hypertension and coexisting cardiovascular disease or other risk factors (modified from WHO-ISH guidelines[10] and adapted from Sudhir and Jennings[11] and Whitworth *et al.*[12]).

lifestyle and other risk factors at once, there is a risk of overwhelming the patient. It is often preferable to address risk factors in order of priority, accepting that it may take some months to achieve every goal of therapy. A specific example is cessation of cigarette smoking, which is often followed by weight gain and therefore it is important to warn the patient this may happen and to reassure them that there is an overall benefit in risk profile.

References

1. Wannamethee SG, Shaper AG. Patterns of alcohol intake and risk of stroke in middle-aged British men. *Stroke* 1996;**27**:1033–1039.
2. Law MR. Epidemiological evidence on salt and blood pressure. *Am J Hypertens* 1997;**10**(Suppl.):42S–45S.
3. Stamler J, Vaccaro O, Neaton JD, Wentworth D for the Multiple Risk Factor Intervention Research Group. Diabetes, other risk factors, and 12-year cardiovascular mortality for men screened in the Multiple Risk Factor Intervention Trial. *Diabetes Care* 1993;**16**:434–444.
4. Levy D, Garrison R, Savage D *et al.* Prognostic implications of echocardiographically determined left ventricular mass in the Framingham Heart Study. *N Engl J Med* 1990;**322**:1561–1566.
5. Stern MP, Haffner SM. Body fat distribution and hyperinsulinemia as risk factors for diabetes and cardiovascular disease. *Arteriosclerosis* 1986;**6**:123–130.
6. Wahi S, Gatzka CD, Sherrard B *et al.* Risk factors for coronary heart disease in a population with a high prevalence of obesity and diabetes: a case-control study of the Polynesian population of Western Samoa. *J Cardiovasc Risk* 1997;**14**:173–178.
7. Doll R, Peto R, Wheatley K *et al.* Mortality in rleation to smoking: 40 years observation on male British doctors. *BMJ* 1994;**309**:901–911.
8. Jennings G, Wong J. Reversibility of left ventricular hypertrophy and malfunction by antihypertensive treatment. In: *Handbook of Hypertension*, Vol 18. *Assessment of hypertensive organ damage* (eds Hansson L, Birkenhager W), pp. 184–223. Elsevier Science BV, 1997.

8

References

9. Gress TW, Nieto FJ, Shahar E *et al.* Hypertension and antihypertensive therapy as risk factors for type 2 diabetes mellitus. Atherosclerosis Risk in Communities Study. *N Engl J Med* 2000;**342**:905–912.
10. Alderman M, Arakawa K, Beilin L *et al.* for the Guidelines Subcommittee. World Health Organisation–International Society Hyeprtension Guidelines for the Management of Hypertension. *J Hypertension* 1999;**17**:151–183.
11. Sudhir K, Jennings GL, Bruce A. Cardiovascular risk reduction: initial diuretic therapy compared with calcium-antagonist (felodipine) therapy for primary hypertension. *Med J Aust* 1989;**151**:277–279.
12. Whitworth JA, Clarkson D, Dwyer T *et al.* for the Australian Consensus Panel. The management of hypertension: a consensus statement. *Med J Aust* 1994;**160**(S21):S1–S16.
13. Whelton PK, Appel LJ, Espeland MA *et al.* for the TONE Collaborative Research Group. Sodium reduction and weight loss in the treatment of hypertension in older persons: a randomised controlled trial of non pharmacologic interventions in the elderly (TONE). *JAMA* 1998;**279**:839–846.
14. Raitakari OT, Adams MR, McCredie RJ *et al.* Oral vitamin C and endothelial function in smokers: short-term improvement, but no sustained beneficial effect. *J Am Coll Cardiol* 2000;**35**:1616–1621.
15. Jennings G, Nelson L, Nestel P *et al.* The effects of changes in physical activity on major cardiovascular risk factors, haemodynamics, sympathetic function, and glucose utilisation in man: a controlled study of four levels of activity. *Circulation* 1986;**73**:30–40.
16. Centers for Disease Control Surgeon General's Workshop on Health Promotion and Aging: summary recommendations of Physical Fitness and Exercise Working Group. *JAMA* 1989;**262**:2507–2510.
17. Lithell HO. Hyperinsulinemia, insulin resistance, and the treatment of hypertension. *Am J Hypertens* 1996;**9**(Suppl.):150S–154S.
18. Anderson KM, Wilson PWF, Odell PM, Kannel WB. An updated coronary risk profile: A statement for health professionals. *Circulation* 1991;**83**:356–362.

8

Hypertension and diabetes mellitus

ME Cooper and P Chattington

8

Introduction

The hypertensive diabetic patients must be considered at high risk for vascular disease. The combination of hypertension and diabetes is associated with at least a two-fold increase in a range of vascular complications including coronary artery disease, stroke and peripheral vascular disease. This increased risk of atherosclerotic-related disorders has led to diabetes being considered a factor for more aggressive blood pressure reduction. This issue has been addressed specifically in a range of new guidelines recently distributed by both the World Health Organization–International Society of Hypertension [1] and the Joint National Committee on Prevention, Detection, Evaluation, and Treatment of High Blood Pressure [2]. Although prevention of macrovascular complications is an important aim of treating hypertension in the diabetic patient, it is now evident that systemic hypertension is also a major factor in the progression of microvascular complications, including nephropathy and retinopathy.

Definition of hypertension in the presence of diabetes

The diagnostic criteria for hypertension in diabetes have changed over the last twenty years from 160/95 (1983 WHO) to 140/90 mmHg (1993 JNC-V) and more recently to 130/85 mmHg (1997 JNC-VI)[2]. These new criteria have resulted in many patients who were previously classified as normotensive now being considered as hypertensive. For example, using JNC-V criteria (blood pressure > 140/90 mmHg) the proportion of Type 1 diabetic subjects with hypertension attending a Danish diabetes clinic was 42%, 52% and 79% in normo-, micro- and macroalbuminuric subjects, respectively [3]. In Type 2 diabetes, the corresponding proportions were 71%, 90% and 93% [3]. These prevalence rates are likely to be even higher once the stricter JNC-VI definition of hypertension in diabetes (>130/85 mmHg) has been taken into account. Indeed, in the JNC-VI guidelines, the presence of renal disease which is commonly observed in the hypertensive, diabetic patient requires the target for treatment to be further lowered to less than 125/75 mmHg [2].

Hypertension and subtype of diabetes

In Type 1 diabetes (insulin-dependent diabetes mellitus, IDDM), hypertension is usually a manifestation of diabetic nephropathy. Of the 35–40% of IDDM patients who ultimately develop nephropathy, the majority will be hypertensive during the phase of overt nephropathy. Longitudinal studies in this population have shown that as an individual subject progresses from normal urinary albumin excretion, to incipient nephropathy (microalbuminuria), to overt nephropathy, there is a gradual rise in systemic blood pressure [4]. By contrast, in the Type 2 (non-insulin-dependent diabetes mellitus, NIDDM) patient, hypertension is often present and may antedate the diagnosis of diabetes [5]. Hypertension is one of the major clinical features of the insulin resistance syndrome, also known as 'syndrome X', which includes glucose intolerance/diabetes [5].

The role of ambulatory blood pressure monitoring (ABPM)

In diabetic subjects ABPM is useful to identify a high-risk group of patients who require antihypertensive treatment. Progression from normo- to microalbuminuria is associated with a concomitant rise in blood pressure when assessed longitudinally by ABPM [4]. Previous work has shown that the nocturnal fall in blood pressure is less in normotensive, normoalbuminuric patients with Type 1 diabetes than in age-matched controls, thereby increasing the 24-hour blood pressure load [6]. Nocturnal blood pressure and heart rate are higher in hypertensive, normoalbuminuric patients with Type 2 diabetes and the nocturnal systolic dip in blood pressure is often absent. In patients with microalbuminuria and Type 1 diabetes the nocturnal dip in systolic blood pressure has been reported to correlate inversely with urinary albumin excretion [7]. In addition, reduced blood pressure variation was associated with increased prevalence of end-organ damage in these diabetic subjects [7].

Microalbuminuria

Studies evaluating the natural history of diabetic nephropathy identified a phase known as 'incipient nephropathy' in which there is an increase in urinary albumin excretion, not yet detectable by conventional Albustix methods (see Figure 8.4.1) [8]. This phase is also known as 'microalbuminuria' and is associated with an 80% risk of development of overt nephropathy with subsequent renal failure. It is now considered routine as part of the management of a diabetic patient to screen for the presence of microalbuminuria (Figure 8.4.2) [8]. If detected, optimization of glycemic control should initially be considered. However, if microalbuminuria persists, antihypertensive treatment is now considered to be appropriate, even in the absence of hypertension. ACE inhibitors are considered by many organizations to be the treatment of choice. The aim of treatment includes not only reduction in urinary albumin excretion but also reduction in blood pressure to relatively low targets. The target blood pressure remains controversial but is probably in the range of 125–130/75–85 mmHg [2,8].

Antihypertensive drugs and cardioprotection in diabetes

The choice of antihypertensive therapy in the diabetic population needs to be considered in the context of not only providing renoprotection but also the potential effects of these agents on atherosclerotic events. Indeed, diabetic patients with persistent microalbuminuria are at

Antihypertensive drugs
and cardioprotection in
diabetes

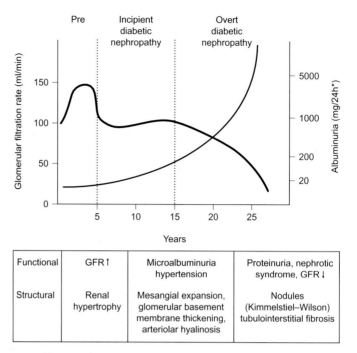

Functional	GFR↑	Microalbuminuria hypertension	Proteinuria, nephrotic syndrome, GFR↓
Structural	Renal hypertrophy	Mesangial expansion, glomerular basement membrane thickening, arteriolar hyalinosis	Nodules (Kimmelstiel–Wilson) tubulointerstitial fibrosis

Fig. 8.4.1 Natural history of Type 1 (IDDM) diabetes mellitus. (After Mogensen *et al.* [8].)

increased risk for all-cause mortality, especially from cardiovascular disease. Therefore, assessing other cardiovascular risk factors in these patients is critical (Figure 8.4.2). Several studies have suggested that ACE inhibitors may be superior to other classes of agents in conferring additional cardioprotection in hypertensive patients with either Type 1 or Type 2 diabetes. In the GISSI-3 trial, lisinopril treatment was associated with improved 30-day survival in diabetic patients after an acute myocardial infarct [9]. In the ABCD trial, in which cardiovascular endpoints were assessed, the hypertensive arm of the study was prematurely halted due to a possible superiority of the ACE inhibitor over the calcium-channel antagonist in terms of cardiovascular events [10]. In the FACET study involving 380 hypertensive Type 2 diabetic subjects, it was reported that the ACE inhibitor, fosinopril, was associated with less cardiovascular events than amlodipine [11]. In the CAPPP trial, an advantage of the ACE inhibitor over conventional therapy (diuretics, beta-blockers) was observed in the diabetic subgroup [12].

However, there is a number of other studies which have either failed to show a superiority of ACE inhibition or have demonstrated significant benefits on cardiovascular events with other antihypertensive agents. In the recent HOT study which involved calcium-channel antagonist based antihypertensive treatment, aggressive blood pressure reduction in the diabetic subgroup was associated with reduced cardiovascular mortality [13]. However, in that study the group with the lowest tertile of blood pressure had the highest prevalence of concomitant therapies including ACE inhibitors. Therefore, it remains to

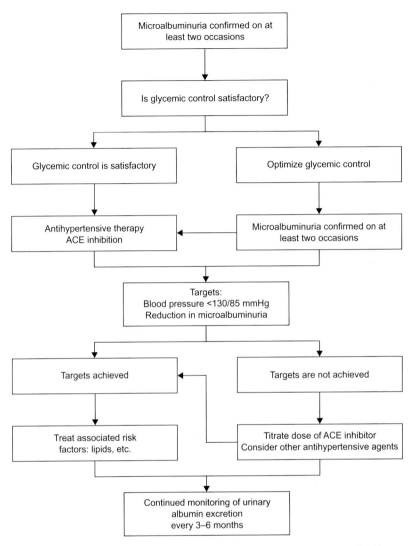

Fig. 8.4.2 Algorithm for screening microalbuminuria in diabetes (After Cooper [16].)

be determined if the improved cardiovascular outcome in the diabetic
population with the lowest blood pressure levels was due to effective
blood pressure reduction or to a specific vasoprotective effect of ACE
inhibition. In the United Kingdom Prospective Diabetes Study (UKPDS),
both captopril and atenolol were associated with reduced cardiovascular
events without evidence that one agent conferred a specific additional
benefit [14]. However, in that study a significant proportion of subjects
in each group were receiving additional antihypertensive agents making
it difficult to determine if the lack of difference between the two
treatment groups is real or is related to confounding effects of other
agents. In the recently published SYST-EUR subgroup analysis,
nitrendipine therapy was particularly effective in preventing vascular
events in diabetic subjects with isolated systolic hypertension [15].

However, this study was performed against placebo rather than an agent which interrupts the renin–angiotensin system. It is likely that over the next few years, results from other studies will become available which include even larger numbers of diabetic patients. In addition, several multicenter studies are currently examining the effects of AT_1-receptor antagonists on both renal and cardiovascular endpoints in Type 2 diabetic patients.

Diabetic renal disease

Experimental studies have clearly shown that hypertension is a major accelerating factor in both the functional and structural features of diabetic nephropathy. Epidemiological studies have reported a close association between systemic hypertension and the development of diabetic nephropathy. Over 15 years ago, two small Danish studies by Mogensen *et al.* [8] defined the importance of blood pressure reduction in retarding the decline in renal function in proteinuric Type 1 diabetic patients. Since then, a large number of studies have been completed exploring the role of antihypertensive treatment regimens in early and advanced diabetic nephropathy [16]. These studies have involved the use of hypotensive drugs in Type 1 and Type 2 diabetes, in the presence or absence of conventionally defined systemic hypertension and in various phases of diabetic renal disease as well as in normoalbuminuric subjects as part of a preventive approach [16]. These studies are summarized below.

Overt diabetic nephropathy

The initial studies, as described earlier, showed that conventional agents including beta-blockers, diuretics and vasodilators were effective at reducing proteinuria and preserving renal function. ACE inhibitors have been considered to be particularly useful in diabetic patients with overt proteinuria. These agents not only decrease proteinuria, but reduce the number of patients who will develop end-stage renal failure [17]. Over the last 15 years, the potential mechanisms of action of these drugs as renoprotective agents has been extensively investigated. These agents not only reduce systemic blood pressure but appear to reduce intraglomerular hypertension and reduce extracellular matrix accumulation by inhibiting angiotensin II-induced expression of prosclerotic cytokines within the kidney [16] (Table 8.4.1). Although ACE inhibition is clearly very useful in this population, in the Collaborative study there was clearly less benefit detected in those Type 1 diabetic subjects with serum creatinine less than 150 μmol/liter or normal blood pressure [17]. These findings are consistent with a meta-analysis, suggesting that the superiority of ACE inhibition over other antihypertensive agents is not as evident at maximum hypotensive doses [18]. A link between reduced rates of progression and improvement in prognosis in nephropathic Type 1 diabetic subjects has been noted by Parving's group using both ACE inhibitors and conventional agents [19], consistent with the view that the major focus is this population must remain aggressive blood pressure reduction.

Table 8.4.1 Postulated mode of action of ACE inhibitors as renoprotective agents

- Lowering of systemic blood pressure
- Lowering of intraglomerular pressure
- Reducing proteinuria (average of 40–50%)
- Affecting natriuresis
- Inhibiting non-hemodynamic effects of angiotensin II via reduced cytokine and growth factor expression, resulting in less proliferation, hypertrophy and matrix expansion
- Inhibiting macrophage activation, proliferation and migration

Even though ACE inhibitors may be antiproteinuric, many Type 1 diabetic subjects will still have inadequately controlled blood pressure. Indeed, a lack of strict blood pressure control may be a major factor in the continued rate of decline in renal function in the captopril treated group, albeit at a slower rate, in the Collaborative study [17]. Additional agents may need to be considered including the use of diuretics, the addition of other antihypertensive drugs such as calcium-channel blockers [20] or newer pharmacological agents such as the dual ACE/neutral endopeptidase inhibitors which are at present being investigated in heart failure and hypertension [21].

In Type 2 diabetic subjects with macroproteinuria, antihypertensive treatment has also been shown to be renoprotective (Table 8.4.2). The role of ACE inhibitors has not been as clearly defined in this population and this is an area of continued clinical investigation. For example, there are now several multicentered large-scale studies in progress which are evaluating the role of angiotensin II-receptor antagonists in this clinical

Table 8.4.2 The effect of antihypertensive agents on albuminuria, renal function and blood pressure in Type 2 diabetic subjects with proteinuria[31]

Agent	Duration	n	Albuminuria (%)*	Glomerular filtration rate	Blood pressure
Lisinopril	18 months	10	↓ (−42)	→	↓
Diltiazem		10	↓ (−45)	→	↓
Furosemide & atenolol		10	↓	↓	↓
Lisinopril	36 months	17	↓ (−55)	↓	↓
Atenolol		19	↓ (−15)	↓	↓
Enalapril	12 months	18	↓ (−87)	→	↓
Nifedipine		12	→	→	↓
Enalapril	52 weeks	7	↓ (−71)	→	↓
Nifedipine		10	→		↓
Captopril	18 months	24	↓(−27)	→	↓
Hydralazine		18	→		↓
Lisinopril	12 months	8	↓(−59)	↓	↓
Verapamil		8	↓(−50)	↓	↓
Lisinopril + Verapamil		8	↓(−78)	↓	↓
Guanfacine + hydrochlorothiazide		6	→	↓	
Verapamil	>4 years	18	↓(−60)	↓	↓
Atenolol		16	↓(−20)	↓↓	↓
Lisinopril	5 years	18	↓(−25)	↓	↓
Atenolol		16	→	↓↓	↓
Verapamil or diltiazem		16	↓(−18)	↓	↓

8

context. A number of recent studies have confirmed that ACE inhibitors are superior to other antihypertensive agents including the dihydropyridine calcium-channel blockers in reducing albuminuria in hypertensive Type 2 diabetic subjects with macroproteinuria (Table 8.4.2). Parving's group has reported a disparity in effects on albuminuria and renal function with different antihypertensive agents [22]. Whereas lisinopril was more effective than atenolol in reducing albuminuria, both agents were similar in efficacy in terms of rate of decline in glomular filtration rate. Bakris *et al.* have reported differences between the subclasses of calcium-channel blockers and have suggested that the dihydropyridine group (such as nifedipine), despite effectively reducing arterial pressure, do not confer the same degree of renoprotection as the non-dihydropyridines [23]. Nevertheless, the role of calcium-channel blockers as add-on therapy in the diabetic population must not be underestimated. The new targets for treatment of blood pressure in the diabetic population will require the use of multiple agents and dihydropyridine calcium-channel blockers are effective blood pressure lowering agents in these patients.

Antihypertensive treatment and microalbuminuria

Most Type 1 diabetic patients with microalbuminuria have normal blood pressure, even when considering the recent JNC-VI criteria [2]. However, experimental data indicate that ACE inhibitors could prevent the development of albuminuria and glomerular ultrastructural injury even in the absence of systemic hypertension. In the landmark studies by Marre *et al.*, enalapril was shown, over ten years ago, to reduce urinary albumin excretion in a cohort of predominantly Type 1 microalbuminuric diabetic patients without hypertension [24]. In a further study, this group compared ACE inhibition to an equally hypotensive dose of the diuretic, hydrochlorothiazide [25]. In that study, only the ACE inhibitor had a favorable effect on albuminuria. This was interpreted as indicating that ACE inhibitors have a renoprotective effect which is partly independent of systemic blood pressure. In a recent study, the Melbourne Diabetic Nephropathy Study Group has performed a placebo-controlled study in normotensive, microalbuminuric Type 1 diabetic subjects which involved a comparison between the ACE inhibitor, perindopril and the calcium-channel blocker nifedipine. After three years of treatment, despite similar (albeit modest) reductions in blood pressure, perindopril treatment was associated with a sustained 50% reduction in albuminuria whereas the calcium-channel blocker treated group had a progressive rise in albuminuria, indistinguishable from the placebo group.

Several other studies have confirmed the beneficial effect of ACE inhibition in this population (Table 8.4.3). The Microalbuminuria Captopril Study Group in a two-year study confirmed the ability of the ACE inhibitor, captopril to retard the rise in albuminuria. In a recent placebo-controlled study over eight years, captopril prevented the development of macroproteinuria and was associated with stabilization of renal function [26]. This study by Mathiesen and colleagues provides

Table 8.4.3 The effect of ACE inhibition in normotensive microalbuminuric subjects

Study	Type of diabetes	Agent	Duration of study	n	Change in albuminuria (%)	Change in glomerular filtration rate	Change in blood pressure
Mathiesen 1991 [32]	1	Captopril	4 years	21	↓(−32%)	→	↓
		Placebo		23	↑(+63%)	→	→
MDNSG 1991 [31]	2	Nifedipine	12 months	13	→	→	→
		Perindopril		11	→ %	→	→
O'Donnell 1993 [32]	1	Lisinopril	48 weeks	12	↓(−50%)	ND	↓
		Placebo		15	→	ND	→
Ravid 1993 [31]	2	Enalapril	5 years	49	→	→	→
		Placebo		45	↑(+152%)	↓	→
Viberti 1994 [33]	1	Captopril	2 years	46	↑	→	↓
		Placebo		46	↑	→	→
Sano 1994 [31]	2	Enalapril	48 months	12	↓(−47%)	→	↓
		Untreated		12	→	→	→
Laffel 1995 [33]	1	Captopril	2 years	67	↓(−36%)	→	↓
		Placebo		70	↑(+24%)	↓	→
Ahmad 1997 [31]	2	Enalapril	5 years	52	↓(−64%)	→	→
		Placebo		51	↓(+60%)	→	→
Marre *et al.* 1998 [24]	1	Enalapril	12 months	10	↓	→	↓
		Placebo		10	↑	↓	→
EUCLID 1997 [34]	1	Lisinopril	2 years	32	↓(−50%)	ND	↓
		Placebo		37	↑	ND	→
Crepaldi 1998 [31]	1	Lisinopril	3 years	32	↓(−47%)	ND	↓
		Nifedipine		26	↓(−18%)	ND	↓
		Placebo		34	↑(+35%)	ND	→
MDNSG 2001 [35]	1	Perindopril	>3 years	13	↓	→	↓
		Nifedipine		9	↑	↓	↓
		Placebo		14	↑	→	→

the first long-term evidence that appropriate timing of the commencement of ACE inhibitor therapy in this normotensive population postpones and possibly, in some patients, prevents the development of overt nephropathy. Since ACE inhibitors appear to be renoprotective in microalbuminuric Type 1 diabetic subjects and up to 40% are at risk of nephropathy, it has been suggested that ACE inhibition may be an appropriate preventative treatment in normoalbuminuric Type 1 diabetic subjects. However, in the EUCLID study, no evidence of a beneficial role for the ACE inhibitor, lisinopril, in normoalbuminuric Type 1 diabetic subjects was observed.

The use of antihypertensive therapy in Type 2 diabetic subjects with hypertension and microalbuminuria has been evaluated by an increasing number of investigators over the last decade (Table 8.4.4). In the largest of these studies which involved over 300 subjects, the ACE inhibitor, lisinopril, reduced albuminuria over 12 months whereas nifedipine failed to significantly influence urinary albumin excretion [27]. In normotensive microalbuminuric Type 2 diabetic subjects several placebo-controlled studies have reported the efficacy of ACE inhibition in either reducing or preventing a rise in albuminuria over at least four years (Table 8.4.3) [16]. In a recent study, Ravid *et al.* suggested a role for ACE inhibition in preventing the development of microalbuminuria in normotensive Type 2 diabetic patients [28]. In contrast to the relatively short duration of two years in the EUCLID study, in this study enalapril treatment was administered for six years.

Antihypertensive treatment and microalbuminuria

Table 8.4.4 The effect of antihypertensive agents on albuminuria, renal function and blood pressure in Type 2 diabetic subjects with hypertension and microalbuminuria

Agent	Duration of study	n	Change in albuminuria (%)	Change in glomerular filtration rate	Change in blood pressure
Captopril	36 months	9	↓ (–65%)	→	↓
Metoprolol or hydrochlorothiazide		12	→	→	↓
Enalapril	12 months	16	↓ (–70%)	→	↓
Nifedipine		15	→	→	↓
Enalapril	12 months	8	↓ (–28%)	↑	↓
Nitrendipine		8	↓ (–17%)	↑	↓
Lisinopril	12 months	156	↓ (–37%)	→	↓
Nifedipine		158	→	→	↓
Cilazipril	3 years	9	↓ (–27%)	↓	↓
Amlodipine		9	↓ (–31%)	↓	↓
Ramipril ± Felodipine	12 months	46	→	→	↓
Atenolol ± hydrochlorothiazide		45	↑	↓	↓
Enalapril + nifedipine	48 months	11	↓ (–42%)	→	↓
Nifedipine		13	↑ (+29%)	→	↓

Retinopathy

Hypertension has been shown epidemiologically to be closely associated with the development of retinopathy. Furthermore, in the recently published UKPDS, blood pressure reduction was associated with a reduction in microvascular complications including retinopathy. Angiotensin II has angiogenic properties and, therefore, it is possible that this hormone may play a role in mediating neovascularization in the diabetic retina. Indeed, the retina has all the components of the renin–angiotensin system (RAS). Although this possibility has not been extensively investigated, in the EUCLID study which evaluated the role of lisinopril in a population of predominantly normotensive, normoalbuminuric Type 1 diabetic subjects, ACE inhibition was associated with at least a 50% reduction in retinopathy including proliferative retinopathy [29]. This issue requires further investigation since this study provides preliminary evidence for a retinoprotective role for agents which interrupt the RAS.

Choice of antihypertensive agent in the metabolic syndrome

In Type 2 diabetes, hypertension is frequently associated with central obesity, insulin resistance, hyperuricemia, hypertriglyceridemia, low HDL-cholesterol levels and microalbuminuria [5]. The choice of antihypertensive agent needs to take into account the effect of drugs on lipid parameters and the clinical context [30]. Centrally acting agents, alpha-blockers, vasodilators, ACE inhibitors, angiotensin II-receptor antagonists and calcium-channel blockers have little effect on the lipid profile or glycemic status [30]. However, ACE inhibitors can induce hyperkalemia especially in those with Type 2 diabetes and hyporeninemic hypoaldosteronism and may precipitate renal failure in the context of undiagnosed bilateral renal artery stenosis. The prevalence of renal artery stenosis may be increased in the diabetic patient who has a high risk of atherosclerotic vascular disease. Nevertheless, careful introduction of the ACE inhibitor with early measurement of serum potassium and creatinine should result in early detection by the physician of functionally significant bilateral renal artery stenosis at a potentially reversible stage. Indeed, in the recent large studies of ACE inhibitors and angiotensin II-receptor antagonists in diabetic nephropathy, the precipitation of acute, renal failure has not been a major clinical problem.

References

1. Guidelines Subcommittee. World Health Organization – International Society of Hypertension guidelines for the management of hypertension. *J Hypertension* 1999;**17**:151–183.
2. Joint National Committee on Prevention, Detection, Evaluation, and Treatment of High Blood Pressure. The Sixth Report of the Joint National Committee on Prevention, Detection, Evaluation, and Treatment of High Blood Pressure. *Arch Intern Med* 1997;**157**:2413–2445.
3. Tarnow L, Rossing P, Gall M-A *et al*. Prevalence of arterial hypertension in diabetic patients before and after JNC-V. *Diabetes Care* 1994;**17**:1247–1251.
4. Poulsen PL, Hansen KW, Mogensen CE. Ambulatory blood pressure in the transition from normo- to microalbuminuria. A longitudinal study in IDDM patients. *Diabetes* 1994;**43**:1248–1253.
5. Williams B. Insulin resistance: the shape of things to come. *Lancet* 1994;**344**:521–524.
6. Gilbert R, Phillips P, Clarke C, Jerums G. Day–night blood pressure variation in normotensive, normoalbuminuric Type 1 diabetic subjects. Dippers and non-dippers. *Diabetes Care* 1994;**17**:824–827.
7. Lindsay RS, Stewart MJ, Nairn IM *et al*. Reduced diurnal variation of blood pressure in non-insulin dependent diabetic patients with microalbuminuria. *J Human Hypertension* 1995;**9**:223–227.
8. Mogensen CE, Keane WF, Bennett PH *et al*. Prevention of diabetic renal disease with special reference to microalbuminuria. *Lancet* 1995;**346**:1080–1084.
9. Zuanetti G, Latini R, Maggioni AP *et al*. Effect of the ACE inhibitor lisinopril on mortality in diabetic patients with acute myocardial infarction – data from the GISSI-3 study. *Circulation* 1997;**96**:4239–4245.
10. Estacio RO, Jeffers BW, Hiatt WR *et al*. The effect of nisoldipine as compared with enalapril on cardiovascular outcomes in patients with non-insulin-dependent diabetes and hypertension. *N Engl J Med* 1998;**338**:645–652.
11. Tatti P, Pahor M, Byington RP *et al*. Outcome results of the Fosinopril versus Amlodipine Cardiovascular Events randomised Trial (FACET) in patients with hypertension and non-insulin dependent diabetes mellitus. *Diabetes Care* 1998;**21**:597–603.
12. Hansson L, Lindholm LH, Niskanen L *et al*. Effect of angiotensin-converting-enzyme inhibition compared with conventional therapy on cardiovascular morbidity and mortality in hypertension: the Captopril Prevention Project (CAPPP) randomised trial. *Lancet* 1999;**353**:611–616.
13. Hansson L, Zanchetti A, Carruthers SG *et al*. for the HOT Study Group. Effects of intensive blood-pressure lowering and low-dose aspirin in patients with hypertension: principal results of the Hypertension Optimal treatment (HOT) randomised trial. *Lancet* 1998;**351**:1755–1762.
14. Stearne MR, Palmer SL, Hammersley MS *et al*. Efficacy of atenolol and captopril in reducing risk of macrovascular and microvascular complications in Type 2 diabetes – UKPDS 39. *Br Med J* 1998;**317**:713–720.

8

References

15. Tuomilehto J, Rastenyte D, Birkenhager WH *et al*. Effects of calcium-channel blockade in older patients with diabetes and systolic hypertension. *N Engl J Med* 1999;**340**:677–684.

16. Cooper ME. Pathogenesis, prevention and treatment of diabetic nephropathy. *Lancet* 1998;**352**:213–219.

17. Lewis EJ, Hunsicker LG, Bain RP, Rohde RD. The effect of angiotensin converting enzyme inhibition on diabetic nephropathy. *N Engl J Med* 1993;**329**:1456–1462.

18. Weidmann P, Schneider M, Bohlen L. Therapeutic efficacy of different antihypertensive drugs in human diabetic nephropathy: an updated meta-analysis. *Nephrol Dial Transpl* 1995;**10**(Suppl.):39–45.

19. Rossing P, Hommel E, Smidt UM, Parving HH. Reduction in albuminuria predicts a beneficial effect on diminishing the progression of human diabetic nephropathy during antihypertensive treatment. *Diabetologia* 1994;**37**:511–516.

20. Bakris GL, Weir MR, Dequattro V, McMahon FG. Effects of an ACE inhibitor calcium antagonist combination on proteinuria in diabetic nephropathy. *Kidney Int* 1998;**54**:1283–1289.

21. Tikkanen T, Tikkanen I, Rockell MD *et al*. Dual inhibition of neutral endopeptidase and angiotensin-converting enzyme in rats with hypertension and diabetes mellitus. *Hypertension* 1998;**32**:778–785.

22. Nielsen FS, Rossing P, Gall MA *et al*. Long-term effect of lisinopril and atenolol on kidney function in hypertensive NIDDM subjects with diabetic nephropathy. *Diabetes* 1997;**46**:1182–1188.

23. Bakris GL, Copley JB, Vicknair N *et al*. Calcium channel blockers versus other antihypertensive therapies on progression of NIDDM associated nephropathy. *Kidney Int* 1996;**50**:1641–1650.

24. Marre M, Chatelier G, Leblanc H *et al*. Prevention of diabetic nephropathy with enalapril in normotensive diabetics with microalbuminuria. *Br Med J* 1988;**297**:1092–1095.

25. Hallab M, Gallois Y, Chatellier G *et al*. Comparison of reduction in microalbuminuria by enalapril and hydrochlorothiazide in normotensive patients with insulin dependent diabetes. *Br Med J* 1993;**306**:175–182.

26. Mathiesen E, Hommel E, Smith U, Parving H-H. Efficacy of captopril in normotensive diabetic patients with microalbuminuria – 8 years follow up. *Diabetologia* 1995;**38**(Suppl. 1):A46.

27. Agardh CD, Garcia Puig J, Charbonnel B *et al*. Greater reduction of urinary albumin excretion in hypertensive Type 2 diabetic patients with incipient nephropathy by lisinopril than by nifedipine. *J Hum Hypertension* 1996;**10**:185–192.

28. Ravid M, Brosh D, Levi Z *et al*. Use of enalapril to attenuate decline in renal function in normotensive, normoalbuminuric patients with Type 2 diabetes mellitus – a randomized, controlled trial. *Ann Intern Med* 1998;**128**:982–988.

29. Chaturvedi N, Sjolie A-K, Stephenson JM *et al*. and the EUCLID study group. Effect of lisinopril on progression of retinopathy in people with Type 1 diabetes. *Lancet* 1998;**351**:28–31.

30. Stein P, Black H. Drug treatment of hypertension in patients with diabetes mellitus. *Diabetes Care* 1991;**14**:425–448.

31. Cooper ME, McNally PG. Antihypertensive treatment in NIDDM, with special reference to abnormal albuminuria. In: *The Kidney and Hypertension in Diabetes Mellitus* (ed. Mogensen CE), 4th edn., pp. 427–440. Kluwer Norwell, MA: 1998.

32. Cooper ME. Renal protection and ACE inhibition in microalbuminuric Type 1 and Type 2 diabetic patients. *J Hypertension* 1996;**14**(Suppl. 6):S11–S14.

33. The Microalbuminuria Captopril Study Group. Captopril reduces the risk of nephropathy in IDDM patients with microalbuminuria. *Diabetologia* 1996;**39**:587–593.

34. EUCLID study group. Randomised placebo-controlled trial of lisinopril in normotensive patients with insulin-dependent diabetes and normoalbuminuria or microalbuminuria. *Lancet* 1997;**349**:1787–1792.

35. Jerums G, Allen TJ, Campbell DJ *et al*. Long-term comparison between perindopril and nifedipine in normotensive patients with type 1 diabetes and microalbuminuria. *Am J Kidney Dis* 2001;**37**:890–899.

Further reading

Cooper ME, Gilbert RE, Epstein M. Pathophysiology of diabetic nephropathy. *Metab (Clin Exp)* 1998;**47**(Suppl. 1):3–6.

Cutler JA. Calcium channel blockers for hypertension. Uncertainty continues. *N Engl J Med* 1998;**338**:679–681.

Gilbert RE, Jerums G, Cooper ME. Diabetes and hypertension: prognostic and therapeutic considerations. *Blood Press* 1995;**4**:329–338.

Rodby RA. Antihypertensive treatment in nephropathy of Type 2 diabetes: role of the pharmacological blockade of the renin–angiotensin system. *Nephrol Dial Transplant* 1997;**12**:1095–1096.

8

8.5

Hypertension in pregnancy

MA Brown and GK Davis

8

8.5

Introduction

Hypertension affects 10–12% of all pregnancies and is, therefore, the most common medical disorder of pregnancy. It has a broad spectrum of importance during pregnancy, many cases not affecting the pregnancy significantly, whilst others may be fatal for mother or baby. As our current knowledge does not allow us to discriminate well at initial presentation between hypertensive women who will have a good pregnancy outcome and those who will not, all cases of hypertension in pregnancy should be treated with the utmost respect.

Managing hypertension during pregnancy is quite different from managing non-pregnant women with hypertension, the most striking difference being the speed at which the clinical condition may deteriorate during pregnancy. The detection of elevated blood pressure during pregnancy is one of the prime purposes of good antenatal care. This provides not only an opportunity to diagnose and treat the important condition of pre-eclampsia, but also to detect essential or secondary hypertension, which may otherwise have gone unnoticed for many years. This chapter will discuss the different types of hypertension during pregnancy, the differential diagnosis of these disorders, and their appropriate management.

Recording blood pressure in pregnant women

Unfortunately, a large number of methods have been employed to assess blood pressure during pregnancy. Such diversity means that, depending on the technique used, blood pressures as different as 20 mmHg can be recorded in the same woman [1]. This may have significant implications for a pregnant woman, leading to under- or overdiagnosis of hypertension.

Mercury sphygmomanometry remains the recommended technique for assessing BP in pregnancy (Table 8.5.1) because aneroid devices are unreliable in pregnant women and cannot, therefore, be recommended. It is likely that mercury will be banned in the future, for environmental reasons, necessitating an automated blood pressure recorder. To date, only a small number of ambulatory blood pressure monitors and an even smaller number of self-initiated automated blood pressure recorders have been validated for use in pregnancy [2]. Blood pressures taken in left lateral recumbency on the left arm do not differ substantially from those recorded sitting and the former is a reasonable alternative, particularly during labor.

The major controversy of sphygmomanometry in pregnancy has revolved around whether to measure the fourth (K4) or the fifth (K5)

Table 8.5.1 Recording blood pressure in pregnancy

- Use mercury sphygmomanometer
- Record blood pressure both arms, then right arm
- Pregnant woman seated
- Use 'large' cuff if mid upper arm circumference ⩾ 33 cm
- Record diastolic blood pressure as 5th Korotkoff sound

Hypertension in pregnancy

8.5

Recording blood pressure
in pregnant women

Recognizing hypertension
in pregnancy

Classification of
hypertension in pregnancy

Korotkoff sound to record the diastolic blood pressure. Recent research
has shown:

- K5 is nearly always present in pregnant women.
- The difference between K4 and K5 is generally only 5–6 mmHg,
  particularly in hypertensive pregnant women.
- K5 is detected more reliably than K4 during pregnancy [3].
- K5 is closer to intra-arterial diastolic pressure than K4 [4].
- Changing from use of K4 to K5 makes no difference to the clinical
  outcome for mother or baby [5].

For these reasons, the International Society for the Study of
Hypertension in Pregnancy now recommends recording the diastolic
blood pressure in pregnancy by K5.

Recognizing hypertension in pregnancy

Hypertension in pregnancy is defined as:

- An absolute blood pressure > 140 mmHg systolic and/or > 90 mmHg
  diastolic at any stage of pregnancy.
- Previous recommendations included a rise from 'booking' (first
  trimester) or pre-conception systolic blood pressure ⩾ 30 mmHg
  and/or diastolic blood pressure ⩾ 15 mmHg. The data for this
  method are less convincing [6]. A further diagnostic criterion has been
  suggested [7]: an initial blood pressure < 140/90 mmHg followed by a
  rise in diastolic blood pressure ⩾ 25 mmHg to reach a diastolic blood
  pressure ⩾ 90 mmHg.

However, in clinical practice any of these criteria are sufficient to
warrant increased antenatal monitoring to detect the emergence of pre-
eclampsia, as described below.

Classification of hypertension in pregnancy (Table 8.5.2)

Hypertension in pregnancy may arise *de novo* in the second half of
pregnancy, when a diagnosis of either gestational hypertension or pre-
eclampsia is made, or is present from the outset of the pregnancy, i.e.
chronic essential or secondary hypertension. Because pregnancy is often
the first time young women have repeated blood pressure recordings,
this affords the opportunity to diagnose chronic hypertension. In some
cases pre-eclampsia will develop in women with chronic hypertension
and, in a few cases, it is not possible to make a firm diagnosis of the
cause of the hypertension until after delivery, when blood pressure

Table 8.5.2 Classification of hypertension in pregnancy

• *De novo* hypertension
  Pre-eclampsia
  Gestational
	• Pre-eclampsia superimposed on chronic hypertension

• Chronic hypertension
  Essential
  Secondary
	• 'White coat' hypertension

8

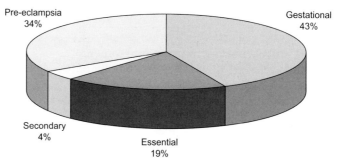

Fig. 8.5.1 Prevalence of different types of hypertension in pregnancy amongst 1183 hypertensive pregnant women. (Adapted from Brown and Buddle [16].)

returns to normal if it was solely due to the pregnancy. In our own unit gestational hypertension and pre-eclampsia are the most common causes of hypertension in pregnancy (Figure 8.5.1).

Initial assessment of the woman with hypertension in pregnancy

Is hypertension chronic or specifically caused by the pregnancy?

This is usually easily distinguished by observing whether the blood pressure was elevated in the first half of pregnancy, indicating chronic hypertension. On occasions, if the initial blood pressure was not recorded until towards the end of the first trimester or early in the second trimester, then it is possible that chronic hypertension was present but missed, as some chronic hypertensives still undergo the normal vasodilatation of pregnancy and their blood pressure falls early on.

Medical history, physical examination, urine microscopy and urinalysis and measurement of serum creatinine and potassium are generally sufficient to unearth clues to a secondary cause for hypertension. Investigations for a secondary cause during pregnancy are generally unrewarding in the absence of specific clues, e.g. elevated creatinine, abnormal urinalysis or symptoms of excess catecholamines, and we do not recommend an exhaustive search for a secondary cause during pregnancy.

Does the woman with *de novo* hypertension in the second half of pregnancy have gestational hypertension or pre-eclampsia?

Diagnosing pre-eclampsia requires the detection of something more than hypertension, such as abnormal renal, hepatic, cerebral or clotting functions or impaired fetal growth. These abnormalities can be detected from examination (Figure 8.5.2), and simple clinical investigations (Table 8.5.3). Gestational hypertension is diagnosed when there is *de novo* hypertension without any of the other features of pre-eclampsia.

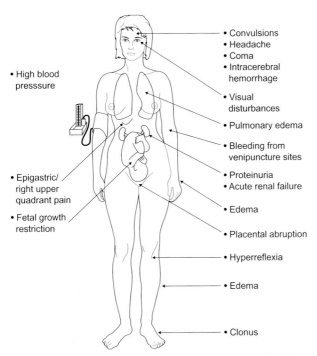

- High blood
  presssure

- Convulsions
- Headache
- Coma
- Intracerebral
  hemorrhage

- Visual
  disturbances

- Pulmonary edema

- Bleeding from
  venipuncture sites

- Epigastric/
  right upper
  quadrant pain

- Proteinuria
- Acute renal failure

- Fetal growth
  restriction

- Edema

- Placental abruption

- Hyperreflexia

- Edema

- Clonus

Fig. 8.5.2 The clinical features of pre-eclampsia. (Adapted from Brown [30].)

Table 8.5.3 Laboratory testing in hypertensive pregnancy

- Hemoglobin, hematocrit, platelet count
- Creatinine, uric acid, potassium
- Liver enzymes and bilirubin
- Urinalysis
- 'Spot' urine protein and creatinine if dipstick-positive proteinuria
- Coagulation studies*

*Only necessary if thrombocytopenia and/or abnormal liver function.

Management of gestational hypertension

Women whose pregnancy is complicated by gestational hypertension generally have a very good outcome; in our series none of 437 pregnancies resulted in maternal morbidity or fetal death and small for gestational age (SGA) rates were only 7–12% [8]. This contrasts with the more serious outcomes of pre-eclampsia, in which about half develop severe hypertension, one-third develop neurological problems, and one-quarter of babies are born SGA. Overall, perinatal mortality is around 30–40 per 1000 pre-eclamptic pregnancies. Therefore, the woman with gestational hypertension can be reassured she will have a good pregnancy outcome, provided her disorder does not progress to pre-eclampsia.

Thus, the two principles of managing gestational hypertension are:

- Control of hypertension, in order to reduce the likelihood of severe maternal hypertension and, therefore, the need for delivery.

8

Table 8.5.4 Day assessment unit (DAU) management of hypertensive pregnant women

Referrals
Hypertension without pre-eclampsia
Some essential hypertensives

Process
Four to six standardized blood pressures using sphygmomanometry.
Midstream urine – automated urinalysis for proteinuria.
    Accept nil/trace as negative.
Positive urinalysis: send for spot protein: creatinine ratio – >30 mg protein/mmol
creatinine is abnormal [34].
    No 24-hour urines collected.
CTG (cardiotocograph)
Blood
    Hemoglobin, platelets
    Creatinine
    Liver enzymes (aspartate transaminase, AST/alanine transferase, ALT)
    Uric acid
Review by obstetrician and physician

Criteria for admission to hospital from DAU
• Pre-eclampsia
• Blood pressure ⩾ 170/110 mmHg at any stage
• Impaired fetal growth
• 'Symptomatic' hypertension
• Planned delivery

• Constant surveillance to detect those women with gestational
  hypertension who will progress to develop pre-eclampsia.

Outpatient management

The first outpatient day care area for management of hypertensive
pregnant women was established at the Glasgow Royal Maternity
Hospital in 1981 and subsequent small randomized trials have shown
that good pregnancy outcomes can be achieved with this system [9,10].
Management in a day assessment unit generally involves a 4–5-hour
stay, with blood tests, urinalysis, clinical examination and four to six
blood pressures recorded over this time and averaged (Table 8.5.4). By
the end of the morning the woman with gestational hypertension has
been assessed for evidence of pre-eclampsia and the antihypertensive
regime altered as required. If pre-eclampsia is present, admission is
generally indicated.

Antihypertensives

Several antihypertensives have been used for the chronic management
of hypertension in pregnancy [11]. In general, first line treatment is with
beta-blockers retaining intrinsic sympathomimetic activity, e.g.
oxprenolol, or the centrally acting agent methyldopa. Additional
treatment usually entails hydralazine, prazosin or nifedipine in the
second half of pregnancy (Tables 8.5.5).

The aim is to maintain blood pressure around 110–140/80–90 mmHg
without inducing undue side effects. If a single episode of severe

8

Table 8.5.5 Drugs often used to lower blood pressure chronically during pregnancy (see text)

Choice	Usual doses (per day)	More common maternal side effects
First line		
Methyldopa	0.5–2 g	Sedation, dry mouth, nasal congestion, depression
Oxprenolol	80–480 mg	Insomnia, nightmares, bronchospasm
Labetalol	0.2–1.2 g	Fatigue; bronchospasm; sensation of 'tingling' over scalp and body
Second line		
Hydralazine	25–200 mg	Flushing; headaches; tachycardia; nausea; edema
Prazosin	1–15 mg	'First-dose' hypotension; edema
Nifedipine (slow release)	40–100 mg	Flushing; headache; tachycardia; nausea; edema
Drugs not recommended		
Atenolol		Associated with fetal growth restriction during long-term use
ACE inhibitors or angiotensin-receptor blockers		Oligohydramnios; fetal growth restriction; stillbirth; neonatal renal failure
Diuretics		Reduction in maternal blood volume; hyperuricemia

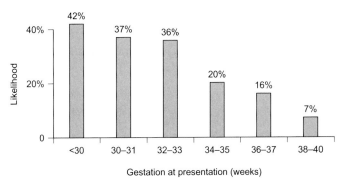

Fig. 8.5.3 Likelihood of a woman presenting with gestational hypertension progressing to develop pre-eclampsia according to gestation at presentation with gestational hypertension. The overall rate is 17%. (Adapted from Saudan *et al.* [8].)

Management of gestational hypertension

Antihypertensives

Risk factors for progression to pre-eclampsia

Pre-eclampsia

hypertension (≥ 170/110 mmHg) is present at any outpatient visit or the average blood pressure > 160/100 mmHg then admission to hospital is indicated for control of hypertension.

Risk factors for progression to pre-eclampsia

In a study of 773 women presenting with gestational hypertension we found that 15–25% developed pre-eclampsia, this being increasingly likely with earlier presentation (Figure 8.5.3) or if the woman had had a prior miscarriage. No single laboratory test or the change in blood pressure from the beginning of pregnancy were predictive of this development [8].

Pre-eclampsia

The causes of pre-eclampsia are outlined in Figure 8.5.4.

8

BOX 8.5.1 Etiology of pre-eclampsia

Placentation

As the only cure for pre-eclampsia is removal of the placenta and as this condition can occur in the absence of a fetus (with hydatidiform mole), the placenta is considered the root cause of this disorder. This is understandable in pre-eclampsia in otherwise healthy young primigravid women but it does not readily explain the increased risk of pre-eclampsia in women with underlying chronic hypertension. In the normal process of placentation the muscular coat of the spiral arteries is invaded by trophoblast, thereby converting them to capacitance vessels under low pressure, carrying a much higher blood flow. This process occurs initially in the first trimester and again at around 20 weeks' gestation. In pre-eclampsia trophoblast invasion is limited and the muscular coat is maintained, reducing blood flow through the placenta and presumably contributing to placental hypoxia. Because this process occurs equally in pre-eclamptic pregnancies with and without babies born small for gestational age, there must be other factors which limit fetal growth and lead to the final maternal expression of this disease [12].

Genetics

There is a genetic predisposition to pre-eclampsia, though the precise mode of inheritance remains unclear. The major histocompatibility complex does not appear to be substantially involved and although one molecular variant of the angiotensinogen gene (*T235*) has been observed, this has not yet been proven integral to the development of pre-eclampsia. Abnormalities of the gene for nitric oxide synthase and perhaps even maternal renin may be implicated. From a clinical perspective the importance is that pre-eclampsia does co-segregate in families, though it is not clear whether this is due to the maternal or fetal genotype.

Immunology

It has been postulated that the failure of normal trophoblast invasion is part of an abnormal immunological response during pregnancy. This has been supported epidemiologically by observations that the longer the sexual cohabitation before conception, the less likely pre-eclampsia will occur, implying maternal tolerance to paternal antigens on sperm [13]. Also, women who use barrier methods of contraception, thereby not being exposed to paternal antigens via sperm, have a higher incidence of pre-eclampsia [14]. Unfortunately these studies have not been reliably reproducible, though they remain intriguing possible clues to the etiology of pre-eclampsia.

Endothelium

A current hypothesis is that placental ischemia somehow leads to widespread maternal endothelial damage, perhaps through release of a cytokine or else production of oxygen-free radicals or lipid peroxides from the placenta. This endothelial cell injury creates a thrombogenic site, perhaps by secreting von Willebrand factor (a cofactor for platelet adhesion) and/or platelet-activating factor or thrombomodulin. At the same time altered production of vasoactive factors such as prostacyclin and other vasodilator prostaglandins, nitric oxide, thromboxane, kallikrein, serotonin and endothelin could all contribute to the enhanced vascular reactivity characteristic of this disorder. Unfortunately, only indirect measurements of these factors can be made, e.g. from blood or urine or else from endothelial tissue taken at delivery, and therefore this hypothesis remains difficult to prove.

8

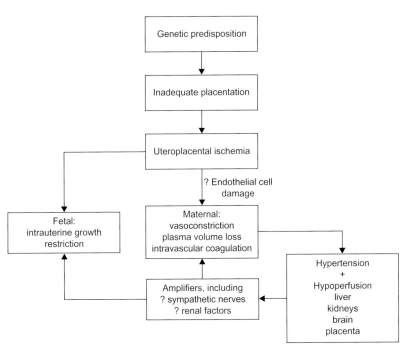

Fig. 8.5.4 Proposed mechanisms involved in the development of pre-eclampsia. (Adapted from Brown [31].)

Pathophysiology of pre-eclampsia

Pre-eclampsia is characterized by plasma volume reduction (with reduced cardiac output), systemic vasoconstriction and intravascular coagulation, processes which reduce organ perfusion, primarily affecting the maternal kidneys, liver and brain and compounding placental ischemia. Whilst these changes have been relatively well documented in established pre-eclampsia, it remains uncertain whether the pathophysiology is the same before pre-eclampsia can be recognized clinically. Cardiac output is actually increased prior to the clinical appearance of pre-eclampsia, but then falls [15], presumably related to preload reduction due to plasma volume loss (from the intravascular to the extravascular space) and to the increased afterload due to systemic vasoconstriction.

Intravascular thrombi occur commonly, either in the placenta, kidney or other organs, associated with platelet activation and thrombocytopenia. In some cases there are also abnormalities of the coagulation system, including decreased antithrombin III, inhibition of plasminogen activation and activated protein C resistance, but none of these processes occurs frequently enough to be the primary cause of pre-eclampsia.

Hypertension and reduced perfusion to the liver, kidneys, brain and placenta result in the clinical features of pre-eclampsia, discussed below, but the intriguing question remains as to why other maternal organ

8

Table 8.5.6 The woman 'at risk' of pre-eclampsia

- Primigravida
- Multipara with new partner
- Multiple pregnancy
- Pre-existing renal insufficiency
- Obesity
- Essential hypertension

- Diabetes
- Family history of pre-eclampsia
- Prior pre-eclampsia
- Autoimmune disorders, e.g. systemic lupus erythematosus
- Thrombophilic disorders, e.g. activated protein C resistance, antiphospholipid syndrome

- Male partner was the product of a pre-eclampsia pregnancy

systems (e.g. gut) are spared in this condition of intense vasospasm and reduced blood flow.

The woman 'at risk' of pre-eclampsia

There are several conditions which predispose to the emergence, or re-emergence, of pre-eclampsia (Table 8.5.6). Although more common in a first pregnancy, it is well recognized to occur in second or later pregnancies, particularly if there has been a change of partners for that pregnancy. Pre-eclampsia occurs more commonly in patients with essential hypertension, diabetes and impaired renal function but how this is mediated remains an area for further research. Conditions with large placentae (e.g. multiple pregnancy and diabetes) have a higher frequency of pre-eclampsia, possibly due to relative placental hypoxia due to increased oxygen demand. Finally, conditions increasing the risk of thrombosis such as activated protein C resistance and the presence of antiphospholipid antibodies also increase the pre-eclampsia risk, presumably by promoting placental thrombi.

Management of pre-eclampsia

Managing pre-eclampsia requires consistency (so that staff members know how to monitor the condition) and vigilance (because of the unpredictability of the condition and its propensity to change rapidly). Pre-eclampsia is most effectively managed in hospital using a team approach of obstetrician, physician, neonatalogist and midwife, monitoring all the while for the multisystem problems which may arise (Figure 8.5.2)

Treatment of hypertension

Acute severe hypertension requires treatment to prevent maternal cerebrovascular damage and possibly eclampsia and placental abruption. Blood pressures above 170 mmHg systolic and/or 110 mmHg diastolic require immediate intervention with a quick acting agent such as intravenous hydralazine or labetalol, or oral nifedipine (Table 8.5.7). To avoid rapid falls in blood pressure, which can reduce uterine artery flow and placental perfusion, culminating in fetal distress, volume replacement using 500 ml of colloid is safe and beneficial given with antihypertensives. These women need full assessment to exclude other signs of deteriorating disease and continuous fetal monitoring until blood pressure has stabilized (Table 8.5.8).

8

Table 8.5.7 Acute treatment of severe hypertension in pregnancy (protocol of St George Hospital Obstetrics Unit, Sydney, Australia)

Antepartum or early post-partum
NIFEDIPINE
Do not use during labor as may be tocolytic

10 mg orally immediately (tablet). Repeat up to *three* doses at 30–45-minute intervals. Check blood pressure every 10 minutes.
Commence Haemacel 500 ml over 4 hours.
Continuous CTG monitoring.

During labour or failure to respond to nifedipine
HYDRALAZINE
Side effects of hydralazine include flushing, tachycardia, headache and tremor
Give 5 mg i.v. infusion immediately. Check blood pressure every 10 minutes. Repeat up to *three* doses at 15-minute intervals.
Commence Haemacel 500 ml over 4 hours.
Continuous CTG monitoring.
If further escape of blood pressure control, use hydralazine *infusion* (80 mg hydralazine in 500 ml saline solution (1 mg/6.25 ml). Start at 30 ml/h (i.e. 5 mg/h).
Adjustments may be made by increasing or decreasing the infusion rate by 10 ml/h every 30 minutes.

For hypertension refractory to above treatments
SODIUM NITROPRUSSIDE
0.5–10 µg/kg/min i.v. infusion – only for women with severe hypertension refractory to above regimes and requiring immediate delivery. May be continued 24–48 h post-partum if required.

Table 8.5.8   Monitoring of women with severe hypertension in pregnancy*

Symptoms	Blood tests
headache	hematocrit, hemoglobin, platelets
visual disturbances	uric acid
epigastric pain	creatinine
decreased fetal movements	AST, ALT
Blood pressure	Signs
Urinalysis for proteinuria	hyperreflexia/clonus
	epigastric tenderness
	pulmonary edema

*Fetal monitoring: CTG and ultrasound scan.

When severe hypertension develops, oral antihypertensives should be commenced and/or the dose increased, except in labor when oral absorption is delayed and variable. During labor, if blood pressure does not stabilize after acute reduction, constant infusion of hydralazine, magnesium sulfate or labetalol have all been used safely and effectively. The most important requirement for the management of acute severe hypertension is the use of a standard protocol with which all staff in any one unit are familiar.

Indications for delivery

After 37 weeks' gestation, fetal outcome is likely to be excellent and the diagnosis of pre-eclampsia at this gestation is an indication for delivery. The decision on delivery becomes more difficult with increasing prematurity and should be made in consultation with obstetrician,

8

BOX 8.5.2 Maternal consequences of pre-eclampsia

Renal dysfunction (see Figure 8.5.5)

Proteinuria is a common renal manifestation of pre-eclampsia but not universal. Only about 50% of women who develop features consistent with pre-eclampsia have significant proteinuria [16] and only two-thirds of eclamptics have proteinuria prior to fitting [17]. Hypertensive pregnant women with significant proteinuria have worse maternal and fetal outcomes than those without proteinuria (see Figure 8.5.6) and in proteinuric pre-eclampsia, the indications for continuing pregnancy are for fetal reasons – to give steroids, to allow transfer or in the hope of reaching fetal viability in early onset cases.

Oliguria *and* rising creatinine are signs of deteriorating pre-eclampsia and if this does not respond to colloid infusion and vasodilatation is an indication for urgent delivery, to prevent acute renal failure and cortical necrosis. Persisting postpartum oliguria is one of the few indications for measurement of pulmonary capillary wedge pressure to assist further fluid management, usually in an intensive care setting.

Hematological disturbances

Progressive thrombocytopenia is a sign of worsening pre-eclampsia and may progress to disseminated intravascular coagulation (DIC) and is, therefore, an indication for delivery. The process may accelerate during labor and the first few days postpartum, and supportive therapy, including platelet and fresh frozen plasma transfusions, may be necessary. Coagulopathy is uncommon in the absence of significant thrombocytopenia, liver dysfunction or placental abruption. Intravascular hemolysis may accompany DIC or liver dysfunction in pre-eclampsia (so called 'HELLP' syndrome) and is another indication for delivery.

Liver dysfunction

Rising liver transaminases are another sign of progressive pre-eclampsia and an indication for delivery. These may rise slowly, allowing timely induction of labor, or acutely as part of fulminating pre-eclampsia necessitating immediate delivery. The latter process is often associated with thrombocytopenia and 'HELLP' syndrome.

The development of epigastric pain in a woman with hypertension in pregnancy is an ominous sign, usually due to subcapsular liver hemorrhages and almost invariably associated with deteriorating liver function. True liver failure is rare in developed countries but acute rupture of the liver is a possibility, with high maternal and neonatal mortality.

Cerebral dysfunction

Vasospasm in cerebral arteries can lead to cerebral irritability and, ultimately, convulsions (eclampsia). In the developed world eclampsia is now rare (0.05% of pregnancies) due to better attention to symptoms and signs of imminent fitting, viz. severe headaches and visual disturbances, hyperreflexia and clonus. However, 20% of convulsions occur in women without any elevation in blood pressure and 18% and 44% of eclamptic fits occur intra- and postpartum, respectively [17]. Intravenous diazepam is the drug of choice to terminate convulsions but considerable controversy exists on seizure prophylaxis. Intravenous magnesium sulfate reduces the risk of subsequent fitting and improves maternal and neonatal outcomes in women who have fitted [18]. The criteria for giving seizure prophylaxis are controversial and the subject of ongoing study; it is our practice to restrict this to women with symptoms and/or signs of imminent fitting and this has not resulted in adverse outcomes for those not receiving convulsion prophylaxis. Magnesium sulfate infusion requires close monitoring but this is not a major problem when appropriate protocols are followed (Table 8.5.9).

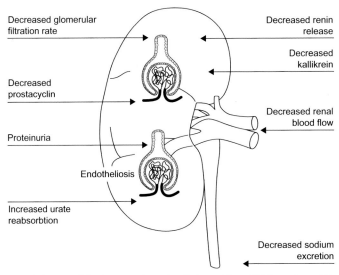

Fig. 8.5.5 Renal abnormalities in pre-eclampsia. (Adapted from Whitworth and Brown [32].)

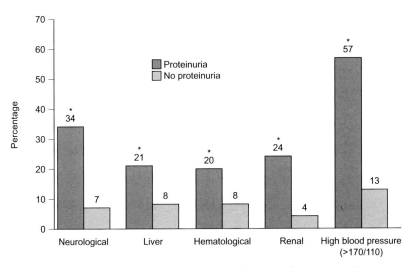

Fig. 8.5.6 Maternal and fetal outcomes in women with *de novo* hypertension in pregnancy according to the presence (*n* = 126) or absence of proteinuria (*n* = 614). *$P < 0.001$, proteinuria versus no proteinuria. (Adapted from Brown and Buddle [33].)

physician and neonatologist. In most cases, babies less than 34 weeks' gestation should have had the opportunity for maternal administration of steroids to improve fetal outcomes and, in particular, lung maturation In general, delivery is indicated when the risks of neonatal life are felt to be less than those of intrauterine life or at any time maternal safety is

Table 8.5.9 Protocol for convulsion prophylaxis using magnesium sulfate (protocol of St George Hospital Obstetrics Unit, Sydney, Australia)

Indications*
    After convulsion
    Hyperreflexia *with clonus* (three or more beats)
    Hyperreflexia *with severe headache*
    Repeated visual scotomata

Administration of magnesium sulfate**
Loading dose: 4 g $MgSO_4$ in 100 ml saline over 20 min i.v. infusion (peripheral line).
Warn patient she may experience flushing and to report pain at infusion site.
Maintenance dose: 1.5 g/h i.v. infusion until 24–48 h postdelivery.

Complications include:
hypotension, flushing, nausea, slurred speech, drowsiness;
absent reflexes;
respiratory paralysis;
cardiac conduction disturbances;
cardiac arrest.

Monitoring
Reflexes every 2 h – cease infusion if unable to elicit reflexes.
Respiratory rate + pulse oximetry every 30 min – cease infusion and review patient by doctor if respiratory rate < 10 per min or SaO_2 < 96%.
Hourly blood pressure – alert medical staff if < 110/70 or ⩾ 170/110 mmHg.
Urine output. Cease infusion if urine output <30 ml/hr for three consecutive hours and obtain medical review.
Continuous ECG monitoring.

For acute toxicity use
Calcium gluconate 10% – 10 ml i.v. infusion over 10 min (first take blood for magnesium level).

* For delivery.
** Magnesium sulfate is incompatible with calcium, chlorpromazine, potassium phosphates and sodium bicarbonate. Magnesium sulfate may also interfere with (anesthetic) paralyzing agents and paralysis may occur in women receiving aminoglycosides or lithium.

Table 8.5.10 Indications for delivery

Maternal	Fetal
Inability to control blood pressure	Fetal distress on CTG
Deteriorating liver or renal function	Failure to grow
Falling platelet count	Abnormal umbilical artery Doppler in
Symptoms and signs of imminent eclampsia	growth-restricted fetus

threatened. In practice, this means that evidence of progressive pre-eclampsia necessitates delivery, irrespective of gestation (Table 8.5.10).

Intrapartum management

During labor, blood pressure should be maintained in the range 110–160/80–100 mmHg. Higher blood pressures than this may lead to maternal cerebrovascular hemorrhage while lower pressures may cause acute fetal distress due to reduced uterine perfusion. Oral antihypertensive agents should not be given during labor because of variable absorption. If antihypertensives are required, intravenous hydralazine should be given with close supervision of blood pressure and fetal heart rate (Table 8.5.7). The hypotensive effect of epidural analgesia is useful in controlling blood pressure but should be preceded by a 500 ml colloid or crystalloid load 30 minutes prior to insertion of the epidural, in order to prevent sudden hypotension. Most anesthetists will not insert an epidural if the platelet count is less than 80–100 × 10^9/liter because of the risk of spinal cord hematoma.

Magnesium sulfate infusion has become the most widely used convulsion prophylaxis in the developed world though phenytoin, diazepam, barbiturates and numerous other agents are still used. Familiarity with the agent and its monitoring is possibly more important than the agent used (Table 8.5.9). We recommend seizure prophylaxis only in women with symptoms and/or signs of imminent eclampsia, which occurs in 10–12% of our hypertensive pregnant women.

A total fluid input of 80–120 ml/h is usually sufficient to maintain volume homeostasis; hourly urine output and regular clinical examination should be recorded.

Depending on the severity of the maternal condition, blood investigations (e.g. platelets, coagulation studies, potassium) may need to be performed frequently during labor, especially if the maternal condition is changing.

Management of chronic hypertension in pregnancy

Disorders such as renal artery stenosis, primary hyperaldosteronism, pheochromocytoma and Cushing's syndrome are uncommon during pregnancy. Renal disease is a more common secondary cause for hypertension in pregnancy, the prognosis depending upon the level of hypertension and renal impairment pre-conception. Women with serum creatinine < 130 μmol/liter generally have a good pregnancy outcome and their underlying renal disease does not progress. At least one-third of women with moderate renal impairment (creatinine 130–250 μmol/liter) will have some deterioration in renal function during pregnancy, often with progressive decline afterwards. Women with severe renal impairment (creatinine > 250 μmol/liter) have less than 50% chance of a successful pregnancy outcome with a high chance of deteriorating renal function and severe hypertension.

In most cases chronic hypertension in pregnancy is due to essential hypertension.

Pre-conception counseling

Older literature showed clearly that women whose initial pregnancy systolic blood pressures were > 140 mmHg and/or diastolic pressures > 90 mmHg had a higher risk of developing pre-eclampsia, accelerated maternal hypertension and increased perinatal loss. Careful review of this literature [19] shows that such women treated with antihypertensives have reduced prevalence of all these complications though even without the development of pre-eclampsia there is still an increased risk of fetal growth retardation.

8

There is debate about the level of blood pressure at which antihypertensives should be commenced in these women. Ideally, women should begin pregnancy with blood pressure less than 140/90 mmHg. If not, current recommendations of the Australasian Society for the Study of Hypertension in Pregnancy (ASSHP) are to commence antihypertensives for systolic blood pressures ⩾ 160 mmHg and/or diastolic blood pressures ⩾ 90 mmHg [20], while the (USA) National High Blood Pressure Education Program (NHBPEP) working group recommends antihypertensives when diastolic blood pressure is ⩾ 100 mmHg [21].

Antihypertensives

The same antihypertensives as discussed for gestational hypertension and pre-eclampsia are used for management of chronic hypertension in pregnancy. ACE inhibitors and angiotensin II-receptor blockers should be avoided due to the risks of fetal growth restriction, neonatal renal failure, oligohydramnios and fetal death. Likewise, diuretics are best avoided due to their propensity to reduce plasma volume further than already occurs in hypertensive pregnancies. Nifedipine has not been recommended in the first half of pregnancy, though recent studies suggest that this may indeed be safe [22]. Blood pressures should be controlled to around 110–140/80–90 mmHg where possible.

Maternal and fetal monitoring

Initial investigations of the woman with chronic hypertension should include baseline tests which may be relevant later in the pregnancy, i.e. hemoglobin, platelet count, liver function, creatinine, uric acid and urinalysis. Further investigations are indicated only if there is a clinical suspicion of a secondary cause.

Early pregnancy ultrasound is of great value in such pregnancies, in order to estimate gestation as accurately as possible. Thereafter, ultrasound is indicated if there is suspicion of diminished fetal growth. In general, hypertensive pregnant women should be seen every second week (alternately by obstetrician and physician) until 34 weeks, then weekly. Management is optimally done as an outpatient and there is no indication that bed rest is of any benefit, in the absence of fetal growth restriction. In the absence of superimposed pre-eclampsia, the only indications for delivery are failure of fetal growth or inability to control maternal hypertension.

It is common for essential hypertension to worsen during pregnancy and increasing doses of antihypertensives are needed particularly in the last trimester, followed by a reduction in the requirement for antihypertensives postpartum. It is wise to reduce medications fairly slowly postpartum as sudden rises in blood pressure may occur. Most importantly, the pregnant woman with essential hypertension should be reviewed three months postpartum to plan her long-term management.

8

White coat hypertension in pregnancy

Very little is known about the impact on pregnancy of 'white coat hypertension'. We have found that this is present in < 5% of women presenting with *de novo* hypertension in the second half of pregnancy, particularly when they are screened in a day assessment unit or with repeated inpatient blood pressure measurements.

A much more demanding situation is the woman presenting early in pregnancy with apparent essential hypertension, about 25% of whom prove to have 'white coat hypertension'. Our early studies suggest that this is not an entirely benign condition, with at least half this group developing ambulatory hypertension (gestational hypertension) and a small percentage also developing pre-eclampsia. To date, fetal outcomes have been very good in this group but the data are preliminary. On the basis of this limited information, we currently recommend withholding antihypertensives in women documented by ambulatory blood pressure monitoring (ABPM) to have 'white coat hypertension' early in their pregnancy, but repeated 24-hour ABPM (monthly) or home blood pressure monitoring is mandatory to detect any change from 'white coat' to true gestational hypertension or pre-eclampsia. It is imperative that these women be reassessed at least three months postpartum to determine whether they still have 'white coat hypertension' or have developed true ambulatory hypertension.

Postpartum management of hypertension in pregnancy

Early postpartum period

Women with pre-eclampsia should be treated with the same degree of caution for the first five days postpartum as during pregnancy because all the complications, including eclampsia, can develop or worsen during this period. Blood tests should be repeated during this time only if there were antenatal abnormalities, e.g. thrombocytopenia, abnormal liver or renal function, to ensure that they return rapidly to normal. Likewise, urinalysis should be checked to ensure the disappearance of proteinuria, which in some cases can take up to 12 months. Antihypertensives can generally be tapered and about 80% of pre-eclamptic or gestational hypertensive women will leave hospital without the need for antihypertensives. In the remainder these can be slowly withdrawn over the next few weeks and certainly within three months.

Women with gestational hypertension or essential hypertension alone can be discharged from hospital earlier as their immediate postpartum risks are minimal.

The late postpartum period

Follow up of all women with hypertension in pregnancy three months postpartum is mandatory. At this visit, it is important to be sure that the resting blood pressure and urinalysis are normal. This visit offers the

8

opportunity to discuss the long-term cardiovascular outcome and the likelihood of subsequent hypertension in pregnancy. Data on both these issues are inadequate. General advice is that a single episode of pre-eclampsia or eclampsia is not likely to increase long-term cardiovascular risk but ongoing (unpublished) work from Glasgow questions this point; women with recurrent gestational hypertension or recurrent pre-eclampsia seem to be at increased risk of hypertension in later life. Women who have had recurrent hypertension in pregnancy are likely to do so again whilst women with a first episode of pre-eclampsia have only about a 5–10% risk of recurrence, unless this occurred at an early gestation (less than 28 weeks) in which case the likelihood of recurrence is as high as 25%.

Advice about prevention of pre-eclampsia

Aspirin

Initial non-randomized trials reported that aspirin reduced the incidence of pre-eclampsia and improved fetal outcome in 'at risk' women but large randomized, controlled trials failed to confirm these findings [23,24]. Despite this, there is reason to believe that aspirin used from early pregnancy only in specific high risk women may be of benefit [25]. At present, the best *general* advice to patients is that aspirin is not effective in reducing the risk of pre-eclampsia. A recent systematic review has shown a statistically significant benefit of aspirin in preventing pre-eclampsia, but approximately 90 women need to be treated to benefit one[26].

Calcium

Reports from South America in the 1980s suggested that calcium supplementation reduced the incidence of both pre-eclampsia and preterm labor. Subsequent trials have refuted this [27] and suggested that calcium may have a role only in regions where calcium deficiency is common.

Ketanserin

Ketanserin, a selective serotonin-receptor blocker, given in combination with low dose aspirin to women with raised blood pressure in the second trimester of pregnancy, resulted in significantly fewer cases of pre-eclampsia and severe hypertension [28]. There was also a trend towards reduced perinatal mortality although the trial was not large enough to demonstrate this statistically.

Glyceryl trinitrate

The nitric oxide donor, glyceryl trinitrate, has theoretical benefits in pregnancy and, although appearing to have minimal hypotensive action, has been shown in small, non-randomized studies to improve uterine blood flow and amniotic fluid volume in growth restricted fetuses of pre-eclamptic women. Trials are underway to determine whether this reduces the incidence of pre-eclampsia or improves pregnancy outcome.

Vitamin C and E

One study has demonstrated a reduced incidence of pre-eclampsia in women already considered high risk of developing this disorder if they took vitamins C and E, as antioxidants, from early in pregnancy[29]. These data are yet to be confirmed in other populations and the safety of these vitamin supplements in pregnancy has yet to be established. Nevertheless, this may offer a future opportunity to prevent pre-eclampsia in some women who have had prior pre-eclampsia.

Acknowledgements

The authors wish to thank Ms Teresa Baldassarre and Mrs Jodie Hendley for their expert help in preparing the manuscript.

References

1. Brown MA, Simpson JM. Diversity of blood pressure recording during pregnancy: implications for the hypertensive disorders. *Med J Australia* 1992;**156**:306–308.
2. Halligan A, Shennan A, Thurston H *et al*. Ambulatory blood pressure measurement in pregnancy: the current state of the art. *Hypertension Pregnancy* 1995;**14**:1–16.
3. Shennan A, Gupta M, Halligan A *et al*. Lack of reproducibility in pregnancy of Korotkoff phase IV as measured by mercury sphygmomanometry. *Lancet* 1996;**347**:139–142.
4. Brown MA, Reiter L, Smith B *et al*. Measuring blood pressure in pregnant women: a comparison of direct and indirect methods. *Am J Obstetr Gynaecol* 1994;**171**:661–667.
5. Brown MA, Buddle ML, Farrell TJ *et al*. Randomised trial of management of hypertensive pregnancies by Korotkoff phase IV or phase V. *Lancet* 1998;**352**:777–781.
6. Levine RJ, Ewell MG, Hauth JC *et al*. Should the definition of preeclampsia include a rise in distolic blood pressure of > 15 mmHg to a level of < 90mmHg in association with proteinuria? *Am J Obstet Gynecol* 2000;**183**:787–792.
7. Redman CW, Jefferies M. Revised definition of pre-eclampsia. *Lancet* 1988;809–812.
8. Saudan P, Brown MA, Buddle ML, Jones M. Does gestational hypertension become pre-eclampsia? *Br J Obstetr Gynaecol* 1998;**105**:1177–1184.
9. Crowther CA, Bouwmeester AM, Ashurst HM. Does admission to hospital for bed rest prevent disease progression or improve fetal outcome in pregnancy complicated by non-proteinuric hypertension? *Br J Obstet Gynaecol* 1992;**99**:13–17.
10. Tuffnell DJ, Lilford RJ, Buchan PC *et al*. Randomised controlled trial of day care for hypertension in pregnancy. *Lancet* 1992;**339**:224–227.
11. Brown MA, Whitworth JA. Pregnancy. In: *Contemporary Issues in Nephrology*, Vol. 28. *Pharmacology and Management of Hypertension* (eds Bennett WM, McCarron DA), pp. 89–116. Churchill Livingstone: New York, 1994.
12. Salas SP. What causes pre-eclampsia? *Baillière's Clin Obstetr Gynaecol* 1999;**13**:41–57.
13. Robillard PY, Hulsey TC, Perianin J *et al*. Association of pregnancy-induced hypertension with duration of sexual cohabitation before conception. *Lancet* 1994;**344**:973–975.
14. Klonoff-Cohen HS, Savitz DA, Cefalo RC, McCann MF. An epidemiologic study of contraception and pre-eclampsia. *J Am Med Ass* 1989;**262**:3143–3147.
15. Bosio PM, McKenna P, O'Herlihy C *et al*. Maternal cardiovascular haemodynamic adaptation in pre-eclampsia and gestational hypertension – a process unravelled. (Abstract.) *11th World Congress of the International Society for the Study of Hypertension in Pregnancy*, Kobe, Japan, p. 97. 1998.

8

References

16. Brown MA, Buddle ML. What's in a name? Problems with the classification of hypertension in pregnancy. *J Hypertension* 1997;**15**:1049–1054.

17. Douglas KA, Redman CWG. Eclampsia in the United Kingdom. *Br Med J* 1994;**309**:1395–1400.

18. Eclampsia Trial Collaborative Group. Which anticonvulsant for women with eclampsia? Evidence from the Collaborative Eclampsia Trial. *Lancet* 1995;**345**:1455–1463.

19. Gallery EDM. Chronic essential and secondary hypertension in pregnancy. *Baillière's Clin Obstetr Gynaecol* 1999;**13**:115–130.

20. Brown MA, Hague WM, Higgins J *et al.* The detection, investigation and management of hypertension in pregnancy. *Aust NZ J Obstet Gynecol* 2000;**40**:133–135.

21. Report of the National High Blood Pressure Education Program working group on high blood pressure in pregnancy. *Am J Obstet Gynecol* 2000;**183**:1–22.

22. Magee L, Schikk B, Donnenfeld A *et al.* The safety of calcium channel blockers in human pregnancy: a prospective, multicenter cohort study. *Am J Obstetr Gynaecol* 1996;**174**:823–828.

23. CLASP Collaborative Group. CLASP: a randomised trial of low-dose aspirin for the prevention and treatment of pre-eclampsia among 9364 pregnant woman. *Lancet* 1994;**343**:619–629.

24. Caritis S, Sibai B, Hauth J *et al.* Low-dose aspirin to prevent pre-eclampsia in women at high risk. *N Engl J Med* 1998;**338**:701–705.

25. Visser W, Wallenburg HCS. Prediction and prevention of pregnancy-induced hypertensive disorders. *Baillière's Clin Obstetr Gynaecol* 1999;**13**:131–156.

26. Duley L, Henderson-Smart D, Knight M, King J. Antiplatelet drugs for prevention of pre-eclampsia and its consequences: systematic review. *BMJ* 2001;**322**:392–393.

27. Levine RJ, Hauth JC, Curet LB *et al.* Trial of calcium to prevent pre-eclampsia. *N Engl J Med* 1997;**337**:69–76.

28. Steyn DW, Odendaal HJ. Randomised controlled trial of ketanserin and aspirin in prevention of pre-eclampsia. *Lancet* 1997;**350**:1267–1271.

29. Chappell LC, Seed PT, Briley AL *et al.* Effect of antioxidants on the occurence of pre-eclampsia in women at increased risk: a randomised trial. *Lancet* 1999;**354**:810–816.

30. Brown MA. Pregnancy-induced hypertension: pathogenesis and management. *Aust NZ J Med* 1991;**21**:257–273.

31. Brown MA. Pre-eclampsia: a case of nerves? *Lancet* 1997;**349**:297–298.

32. Whitworth JA, Brown MA. Hypertension and the kidney. *Kidney Int.* 1993;**44**(Suppl. 42):552–558.

33. Brown MA, Buddle ML. The importance of non-proteinuric hypertension in pregnancy. *Hypertension Pregnancy* 1995;**14**:57–65.

34. Saudan PJ, Brown MA, Farrell T, Shaw L. Improved methods of assessing proteinuria in hypertensive pregnancy. *Br J Obstetr Gynaecol* 1997;**104**:1159–1164.

8

Hypertension in the transplant patient

G Mourad, J Ribstein and A Mimran

Introduction

Arterial hypertension was a common complication of transplantation under conventional immunosuppressive therapy (i.e. azathioprine and steroids). The incidence of *de novo* post-transplant hypertension sharply increased in the 1980s when cyclosporine (CsA) was introduced, with a prevalence of hypertension ranging from a low 30% after liver transplantation to a high 90% after cardiac transplantation, and varying between 60 and 80% after renal transplantion. Although less common than under CsA therapy, hypertension is also a side-effect of FK506 (tacrolimus), another calcineurin inhibitor used in liver transplantation in the early 1990s and in renal transplantation thereafter.

In the transplant patient as well as in the general population, hypertension contributes to the accelerated vascular disease and mortality [1]. Similar to most parenchymal renal diseases, it is also a significant risk factor for the progression of chronic renal allograft nephropathy (CAN)[2]. For all these reasons, post-transplant hypertension should be identified and arterial blood pressure should be optimally controlled in such patients.

What is 'special' in a transplant patient?

More often than in the general population, post-transplant hypertension may result from a specific cause, such as renal dysfunction or the prohypertensive properties of drugs used in this setting. When persistent hypertension is observed in a transplant patient, a number of factors potentially contributing to hypertension should be analyzed and a search for a curable cause should be undertaken.

Transplant patients generally receive a combination of immunosuppressive drugs, usually a calcineurin inhibitor with or without azathioprine or mycophenolate mofetil and steroids. Antihypertensive medications, particularly some calcium antagonists, may competitively inhibit the hepatic cytosolic cytochrome P4503A, and induce a sudden increase in blood levels of calcineurin inhibitors resulting in acute nephrotoxicity. Angiotensin-converting enzyme (ACE) inhibitors may also result in deterioration of renal function in renal graft recipients with transplant renal artery stenosis (TRAS) or CAN, as well as in non-renal transplant patients with chronic CsA nephrotoxicity. When prescribing an antihypertensive drug, the clinician should be aware of these interactions in order to make appropriate modifications and prevent undesirable side effects.

Overall, renal dysfunction is a common problem in renal as well as non-renal transplantation, and it certainly participates to the higher incidence of hypertension. The renal allograft is often the target of immunologic and non-immunologic insults, resulting in suboptimal function. In heart and liver transplants, the kidneys suffer from the nephrotoxicity of immunosuppressive drugs as well as the consequences of cardiac or hepatic failure.

8

What are the prominent features and the main mechanisms?

Kidney graft recipients

Post-transplant hypertension is multifactorial (Table 8.6.1), and the diagnosis workup of every patient must be structured in order to assess a variety of possible mechanisms (Figure 8.6.1).

Renovascular hypertension

The incidence of TRAS ranges between 2 and 12%, depending on the definition of 'significant stenosis' and the reference population undergoing angiography. A stenosis proximal to the arterial anastomotic site – sometimes due to peripheral vascular disease involving the iliac system, i.e. a pseudoTRAS, usually results from atherosclerosis in an old recipient with pretransplant hypertension [3]. Anastomotic lesions may be related to faulty surgical technique or fibrosis, and distal stenosis to mechanical or immunological damage. Stenosis was more frequent when the donor was cadaveric or pediatric; following improvement in harvesting techniques and the generalized use of aortic arterial patchs, the incidence of anastomotic lesions sharply decreased.

TRAS often occurs within six months after grafting. Arterial murmur is neither a constant finding nor a specific sign for TRAS. Hypertension may be severe, yet a number of patients are normotensive in the presence of more than 50% narrowing of the renal artery. Renal function may be altered by TRAS, usually when the stenosis exceeds 80%, and improve following correction [4]. An increase in plasma creatinine concentration upon initiation of antihypertensive therapy is suggestive (especially when blood pressure does not decrease), but not specific of TRAS.

Table 8.6.1 Causes of hypertension after renal transplantation

- Allograft
    Transplant renal artery stenosis (TRAS)
    Chronic allograft nephropathy (CAN)
    Recurrence of original disease

- Native kidneys (inappropriate renin secretion)

- Drugs
    Steroids
    Calcineurin inhibitors (cyclosporine, tacrolimus)

- Others causes
    Obesity (pre- or post-transplantation)
    Hypertension transmitted by donor
    Genetic predisposition to hypertension of the recipient
    Hypercalcemia

8

What are the prominent
features and the main
mechanisms?

Kidney graft recipients

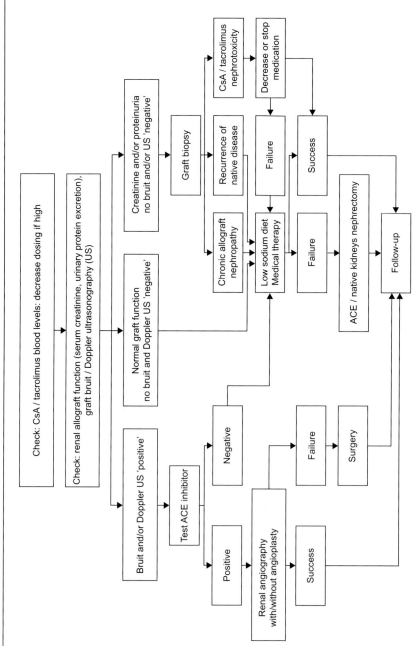

Fig. 8.6.1 General recommendations for the work-up of hypertension in the transplant patient.

What are the prominent
features and the main
mechanisms?

Kidney graft recipients

BOX 8.6.1 Investigating renal artery stenosis

Doppler ultrasonography is routinely used in the surveillance of the renal allograft. Prospective studies documented that an increased peak velocity in the graft artery yielded a sensitivity of 100% and a specificity of 75–95% in the detection of TRAS. However, the reference values are exceedingly variable in transplant recipients [5], with threshold values varying between 100 and 250 cm/s. In practice, the accuracy of the procedure is highly dependent upon the ultrasonographer, which is not the case with magnetic resonance angiography. Small series based on technical improvements such as gadolinium-enhancement and three-dimensional phase contrast analysis led to the claim of a sensitivity and specificity of 100% with the latter method. Depending on local availability, Doppler ultrasonography or magnetic resonance angiography have become the preferred screening modality for TRAS in different centers.

Arteriography is the definitive method for diagnosing TRAS, and the first step of revascularization. However, the procedure entails some risk and gives poor information about the functional significance of the stenosis (beyond the visual appearance, i.e. more than 50% narrowing of the vessel, and/or the presence of a pressure gradient).

Functional assessment of a stenosis remains an unresolved issue. TRAS resembles the one-clip, one-kidney Goldblatt model; hemodynamic studies usually showed a significant decrease in glomerular filtration rate (especially in the absence of a significant fall in blood pressure) with no change or a slight decrease in renal plasma flow in patients with TRAS studied after acute (see Table 8.6.2) or chronic ACE inhibitor treatment prior to the CsA era [6]. In our experience, acute administration of captopril is associated with a fall in glomerular filtration rate of more than 20% in CsA-treated patients with TRAS only when receiving diuretics. Radioisotope renography combined with ACE inhibitor, or the captopril test based on the response of blood pressure and renin, are neither sensitive nor specific enough in the transplant patient to be used at face value [7]. Decision upon revascularization is thus best given by a combination of angiographic/Doppler data, some sort of ACE inhibitor challenge, and clinical judgment.

Chronic allograft nephropathy

Chronic allograft nephropathy, the most common cause of late kidney graft loss (5% annual attrition rate after the first post-transplant year), is usually manifested by a gradual increase in serum creatinine, appearance or worsening of proteinuria, and the development of hypertension over months to years [8]. As in parenchymal renal diseases, there is a decrease in renal blood flow and glomerular filtration rate, and an increase in renal vascular resistance. The renin–angiotensin system is usually activated, yet ACE inhibitors are not regularly effective in lowering blood pressure because some degree of hypervolemia is often present, due to the fall in glomerular filtration rate.

Hypertension associated with CAN may be mild, but it often worsens in parallel with the loss of renal function. In practice, patients with CAN may become severely hypertensive during the three to six months period preceding reinstitution of dialysis.

8

What are the prominent
features and the main
mechanisms?

Kidney graft recipients

It is reasonable to suggest that optimal lowering of blood pressure may slow deterioration of renal function in CAN as it does in parenchymal renal disease. However, progression of renal failure in this setting is due to a number of immunologic and non-immunologic factors and well-controlled studies demonstrating the nephroprotective effect of antihypertensive drugs in CAN are lacking.

Recurrence of original renal disease

Recurrence of glomerular and vascular diseases of the kidney is frequent after transplantation. Recurrence of IgA nephropathy is often clinically asymptomatic. Recurrence of focal and segmental glomerulosclerosis is observed in 20–40% of patients within one month post-transplant and rarely after one year. Recurrence of membranoproliferative glomerulonephritis occurs in 20–30% in Type 1, and up to 80% in Type II [9]. Recurrence of glomerular diseases is usually manifested by heavy proteinuria or nephrotic syndrome, decreased renal function, and hypertension. Optimal control of blood pressure is difficult to obtain, particularly in some severe cases in which rapid deterioration of renal function results in graft loss and reinstitution of dialysis.

Recurrence of the hemolytic uremic syndrome (HUS) is observed in 10–50% of patients whose original disease was HUS. In addition, CsA and tacrolimus may also insult vascular endothelium and result in *de novo* HUS. Clinically, both *de novo* and recurrent HUS may be associated with renal failure and severe hypertension [10]. The degree of elevated blood pressure observed in recurrent diseases often parallels the progressive loss in renal function.

Hypertension due to native kidneys

Because of continued secretion of vasoconstrictive substances (mainly activation of the renin system) and decreased production of vasodilating agents, native diseased kidneys may be a major cause of post-transplant hypertension. This type of hypertension resembles the one-clip, two-kidney Goldblatt model. Usually, hypertension is already a problem during the dialysis period, then persists after a successful renal transplantation. In such patients, dialysis-associated hypertension is typically resistant to volume extraction and sensitive to ACE inhibition; following transplantion, administration of an ACE inhibitor results in normotension as well as improvement in overall renal function (Table 8.6.2) [11]

Genetic determination of hypertension

As shown by cross-transplantation studies in experimental models, inherited tendency to hypertension may be transmitted by the kidney allograft. In humans, it was reported that hypertension and increased need of antihypertensive therapy occurred more frequently in recipients from 'normotensive' familes who received a kidney from a donor with a 'hypertensive' family [12].

Table 8.6.2 Acute hemodynamic effects of angiotensin-converting enzyme inhibitors in renal transplant patients

Patient group	Glomerular filtration rate	Renal plasma flow	Renal vascular resistance	Filtration fraction
Transplant renal artery stenosis*	↓	↔ or ↓	↔	↓
Native kidneys	↑	↑	↓	↔
Chronic allograft nephropathy	↔ or ↓	↔ or ↓	↔	↔

* This pattern, observed mostly in patients receiving azathioprine and steroids, may still be disclosed under cyclosporine therapy following short-term diuretic or chronic administration of angiotensin-converting enzyme inhibitors.

What are the prominent features and the main mechanisms?

Non-renal transplantations

Non-renal transplantations

Heart transplantation

Virtually all CsA-treated heart transplant patients develop hypertension, independent of renal failure and irrespective of classical risk factors such as age, body weight and family history of hypertension. In fact, the incidence of hypertension rose from less than 20% in patients receiving azathioprine and steroids to more than 90% after the introduction of CsA [13]. The deleterious role of CsA is due to vasoconstriction (at the systemic as well as the renal, preglomerular level) and nephrotoxicity. Post-cardiac transplant hypertension is associated with normal cardiac output, elevated systemic vascular resistance, increased sympathetic stimulation of the renin system, and some impairment of renal function. Post-cardiac transplant hypertension is often severe and inadequately controlled, despite the use of multiple classes of potent antihypertensive medications, including diuretics, calcium antagonists, and sympatholytic drugs. Some success has been reported with the use of minoxidil [14], or combined enalapril, frusemide and verapamil [15].

Liver transplantation

About half of long-term (i.e. over two years) survivors after liver transplantation are hypertensive under CsA, essentially due to the vasoconstrictive and nephrotoxic effects of the drug. The incidence of hypertension dramatically decreases when liver transplant recipients are treated with tacrolimus, a more potent immunosuppressive drug. Hypertension is observed in 78 and 28% of patients receiving CsA and tacrolimus respectively [16]. It was reported from this series that tacrolimus resulted in similar renal vasoconstriction, but less systemic vasoconstriction, when compared to CsA [16]. Antihypertensive treatment is based on the same drugs as those used in other organ transplantation.

Bone-marrow transplantation

Prior to the availability of CsA, the incidence of hypertension was less than 10% in bone-marrow transplant patients. CsA conferred a 30-fold increase in the risk of hypertension, and 60% of graft recipients are

8

What are the prominent
features and the main
mechanisms?

Non-renal transplantations
Iatrogenic hypertension

hypertensive shortly after starting CsA [17]. In addition, CsA may result in severe HUS in some patients. Children appear to be very susceptible to the hypertensinogenic effect of CsA, as 86% developed hypertension and 28% seizures [18].

Iatrogenic hypertension

Steroids

The use of steroids may contribute to post-transplant hypertension, probably via enhanced vascular reactivity. Steroid dosage was inversely correlated with night-time decrease in blood pressure. Withdrawal of steroids in stable transplant recipients was followed by a modest reduction in arterial pressure and the requirement in antihypertensive drugs [19].

Cyclosporine

The hypertensinogenic role of CsA is less clear-cut in renal compared to non-renal transplantation because of the high incidence of hypertension under standard immunosuppression, the relatively low dose of CsA used, and possibly renal denervation. Hypertension prior to transplant and the presence of native diseased kidneys, but not age, sex, source of donor, number of acute rejection episodes, are usually correlated with the incidence of hypertension in such patients.

The exact participation of renal dysfunction to the development of CsA-induced hypertension is still a matter of debate [20]. In healthy volunteers, acute administration of CsA was associated with changes in arterial pressure independently from renal resistance or sodium balance. In renal transplant recipients on chronic CsA, each administration of the drug was associated with a transient episode of renal hypoperfusion and a slight increase in arterial pressure [21], thus suggesting that repeated episodes of hypoperfusion may play a role in the development of hypertension and nephrotoxicity. In most series of patients on CsA, the incidence of hypertension or the increase in arterial pressure was directly correlated with serum creatinine levels.

Both clinical and experimental data suggest that CsA results in vascular dysfunction (first at the endothelium level) with systemic vasoconstriction/impaired vasodilatation, and that early changes in renal function are the consequence of a predominant afferent vasoconstriction (Table 8.6.3). In addition, chronic CsA may decrease the glomerular ultrafiltration coefficient in humans as it does in rats. That sodium retention plays a major role in CsA-induced hypertension, is a well-accepted concept based on controversial evidences [20]. In non-transplant patients on CsA, a progressive increase in arterial pressure was associated to increased sodium intake and enhanced natriuretic response to salt loading, thus suggesting that circulating volume was expanded or that exaggerated natriuresis resulted from increased renal perfusion pressure as in essential hypertension. Of note, low-to-normal circulating levels of renin and aldosterone were regularly found in such patients.

Table 8.6.3 Arguments in favor of the use of calcium antagonists or ACE inhibitors in patients on immunosuppression with the calcineurin inhibitors cyclosporine (CsA) and tacrolimus

	Calcium antagonists	ACE inhibitors
PRO	Efficacy	Efficacy
	Immunomodulation	
	Favorable outcome on graft function	
	Decreased need for CsA/tacrolimus	No effect on Cs/tacrolimus level or need
	Renal vasodilation: afferent arteriole	Renal vasodilation: efferent arteriole
		Decrease in filtration fraction and possibly glomerular pressure
	Effect on endothelial function?	Inhibition of angiotensin-stimulated cell growth
	Influence on vasoactive mediators of cell growth?	
CON	Side effects	Poor effect of acute administration
	Pharmacologic interaction with CsA/tacrolimus	Hyperkalemia
		Renal failure (TRAS, diuretics)

The effective role of the renin–angiotensin system in CsA-associated hypertension and renal dysfunction is not clearly elucidated. The association of low–normal plasma renin activity, increased inactive renin, and hyperplasia of juxtaglomerular cells is suggestive of impaired processing of prorenin or altered mechanisms of renin secretion. Chronic, but not acute, administration of an ACE inhibitor is beneficial to arterial pressure and renal hemodynamics [22]. As depicted on Table 8.6.3, a prominent role in renal and systemic vasoconstriction may be played by excess adrenergic nerve activity and profound alteration in vasoactive substances, including eicosanoids, kinins, nitric oxide, and endothelin. The vascular and tubulointerstitial impact of chronic CsA therapy may occur independently.

Tacrolimus

Tacrolimus is increasingly used in transplant patients, as it effectively reduces incidence of acute rejection and may reverse steroid-resistant rejection. The incidence of *de novo* hypertension seems lower after tacrolimus than after CsA in liver [16] and renal transplant patients. Although tacrolimus and CsA share a number of mechanisms of action as well as side effects, the benefits of treatment with tacrolimus have included a decreased need for antihypertensive drugs, possibly because of a reduction in episodes of acute rejection, and presumably CAN, as well as a reduction in steroid dose [23]. Of note, tacrolimus may also induce less renal vasoconstriction, as measured by Doppler ultrasound at the level of interlobar arteries in renal grafts [24].

How to manage the hypertensive transplant recipient?

What is the rationale for lowering blood pressure?

In transplantation patients, as in the non-transplant population, hypertension leads to significant chronic morbidity and mortality through stroke and myocardial dysfunction [25]. Hypertension may also induce or amplify graft injury. During the follow up of 30 000 patients, a progressive increase in systolic and diastolic blood pressure following transplant was associated with a graded incidence of subsequent graft failure [2]. In a smaller cohort, blood pressure at one-year post-transplant strongly predicted graft survival adjusted for baseline renal function [26]. Thus, post-transplant hypertension should be treated in order to protect against both cardiovascular disease in the recipient and hypertensive injury to the graft. However, despite experimental evidence showing that antihypertensive therapy improved graft survival and function [27], there are no prospective studies demonstrating that aggressive lowering of blood pressure improves long-term transplant outcome. On the contrary, the retrospective analysis of 144 kidney graft recipients followed up for 3–13 years suggested that hypertension was a strong risk indicator for renal graft survival, but that control of blood pressure alone did not alter the risk, since 10-year graft survival was 81%, 58% and 50% in normotensive, controlled hypertensive and uncontrolled hypertensive patients, respectively [28].

Change in lifestyle

General recommandations are of the utmost importance in the transplant patient:

- stop smoking,
- exercise regularly,
- avoid obesity and
- quit alcohol.

In addition, glucose intolerance and hyperlipemia, which contribute to the vascular risk, must be treated with dietary measures and appropriate medications.

Immunosuppressive drugs

Corticosteroid dosage should be decreased to the lowest maintenance level. Similarly, an attempt to reduce CsA or tacrolimus dosage should be made. Some authors have reported that it may be possible to withdraw steroids [19] or CsA [29], thus resulting in improved metabolic profile and better control of hypertension. However, steroid or CsA withdrawal may be associated with an unacceptably high rate of rejection and a decreased long-term graft survival.

Prevention of CsA-associated hypertension has been studied in heart transplant recipients: compared to corn oil as a placebo, ω-3 fatty acids prevented the development of hypertension [30]. However, ω-3 fatty acids have also been tried without success in renal transplant recipients [31].

Antihypertensive drugs

All antihypertensive agents may be used in the transplant patient, inasmuch as one is aware of their specific benefits and limitations in this special setting. The choice of a drug depends on the main mechanism of hypertension (i.e. diseased native kidneys, CAN, recurrence of original disease, calcineurin inhibitors) and the presence of associated comorbid conditions. Since it is often difficult to identify a single predominant factor responsible for post-transplant hypertension, it is important to systematically address all the possibilities in every individual.

Specific conditions in transplant patients

Hypertension due to native kidneys

This type of hypertension is usually due to increased renin secretion by the diseased kidneys. ACE inhibitors are the treatment of choice, because they usually result in good control of hypertension and improvement in renal function [11]. In very exceptional cases with severe hypertension, native kidney nephrectomy may be performed. Alternatively, a favorable outcome has been reported by the Oxford group after embolization of both native kidneys.

Cyclosporine

In patients with hypertension, normal renal function, and no signs of chronic rejection or recurrence, one can assume that CsA plays a prominent role. As CsA-associated hypertension is mainly due to systemic and renal vasoconstriction, potent vasodilators such as calcium antagonists have been advocated as first-line therapy. Calcium antagonists are commonly used because they alleviate the renal effect of CsA: they preferentially vasodilate the afferent, preglomerular arteriole, and increase natriuresis. Whether these beneficial effects observed in short-term follow up translate into long-term nephroprotection is still unproven. In addition, a few anecdotal reports suggested that calcium antagonists may decrease nephrotoxicity as well as the incidence of acute rejection episode an observation that was not confirmed by more recent studies [32]. When using calcium antagonists, it is important to remember that they may interact with CsA metabolism: some dihydropyridine derivatives (such as nitrendipine or lacidipine) as well as diltiazem and verapamil may increase CsA blood levels by 40–50%, whereas other dihydropyridines (such as nifedipine or amlodipine) do not interfere significantly with the metabolism of CsA. Some physicians have taken advantage of these interactions, and use CA in all patients in order to decrease CsA doses, thereby decreasing the cost of treatment. In our practice, we consider that this approach may complicate the management of immunosuppression, and we continue to avoid medications which interfere with CsA.

ACE inhibitors are an alternative for the treatment of CsA-associated hypertension (Table 8.6.3). We previously demonstrated that renal transplant patients treated by the ACE inhibitor lisinopril had similar blood pressure and renal function over a three-year period when compared to those treated by nifedipine [22]. Also isinopril had a good antihypertensive and antiproteinuric effect in renal transplant patients

8

[33]. As ACE inhibitors have renoprotective effects in diabetic and non-diabetic glomerular diseases as well as cardioprotective effects in patients with pre-existing cardiovascular disease [34], we consider that these drugs may be used as a first-line treatment in the transplant population. ACE inhibitors may result in some side effects, like reversible renal failure, hyperkalemia, or anemia. However, we do not know whether angiotensin II-receptor antagonists have any advantage over ACE inhibitors in transplant patients. Preliminary data suggest that they share with ACE inhibitors both efficacy and side effects.

Chronic rejection and recurrent nephropathy

These conditions resemble parenchymal renal diseases in which extracellular volume excess is the prominent feature of hypertension. Sodium restriction and diuretics are the first-line treatment. ACE inhibitors and, if needed, calcium antagonists or beta-blockers may be added. Side effects of ACE inhibitors, including reversible acute renal failure, hyperkalemia or anemia have been reported in these patients in the absence of TRAS; thus monitoring of renal function and electrolytes is advised within one week following introduction of ACE inhibitors.

Hypertension and post-transplantation

Polycythemia
Post-transplant polycythemia occurs in 10–15% of renal transplant recipients with well-functioning grafts [35], and it is associated with increased morbidity. When these patients are hypertensive, ACE inhibitors are the best choice because they are very effective in reducing erythrocytosis as well as controlling hypertension. Recently, it was reported that the angiotensin receptor antagonist losartan was safe and effective in treating such patients [36].

Transplant patients with cardiovascular diseases

Since cardiovascular diseases, including ischemic heart disease and peripheral arterial disease, are common in dialysis and renal transplant patients, antihypertensive drugs with cardioprotective effects or associated cardiovascular beneficial effects will be preferentially used. Thus, ACE inhibitors are indicated in patients with heart failure and prior myocardial infarction, and beta-blockers in those with coronary heart disease and arrythmias.

Transplant renal artery stenosis (TRAS)

This results in a correctable form of hypertension, and sometimes in renal functional degradation, thus revascularization of a significant narrowing is warranted. Medical management may be an option in patients with moderate degree of stenosis (i.e. debatable hemodynamic significance) and/or high risk associated with treatment. In addition, the extent of parenchymal injury (i.e. chronic rejection or recurrent nephropathy) should be considered before embarking on complex revascularization procedures.

Percutaneous balloon angioplasty is technically feasible in most patients, although it may be difficult due to arterial geometry and fibrosis of the stenosis. The procedure is not free of complications, including arterial injury and distal embolus or renal artery thrombosis leading to transplantation nephrectomy. The rate of recurrence is about 10–20%. Stent placement was proposed in such cases, since repeat angioplasty is usually unsuccessful. In small series, the patency of stented arteries has been documented at three-year follow up, but no prospective, formal evaluation of this procedure has been performed in comparison to alternative approaches.

The indication of surgical revascularization is currently restricted to failure of endoluminal procedures, including recurrence and proximal atheromatous stenosis when associated with severe hypertension and renal functional deterioration. Surgical repair may be hampered by the extent of fibrosis and scarring as well as the complex medical condition of many patients. In the absence of well-controlled studies in centers with similar experience of both techniques, it is not possible to compare the rate of graft loss following surgical versus endoluminal procedures.

References

1. Hill MN, Grossman RA, Feldman HI *et al*. Changes in causes of death after renal transplantation, 1966 to 1987. *Am J Kidney Dis* 1991;**17**:512–518.
2. Opelz G, Wujciak T, Ritz E, for the Collaborative Transplant Study. Association of chronic kidney graft failure with recipient blood pressure. *Kidney Int* 1998;**53**:217–222.
3. Becker BN, Odorico JS, Becker YT *et al*. Peripheral vascular disease and transplant renal artery stenosis: a reappraisal of transplant renovascular disease. *Clin Transplant* 1999;**13**:349–355.
4. Mourad G, Ribstein J, Argiles A *et al*. Contrasting effects of acute angiotensin-converting enzyme inhibitors and calcium antagonists in transplant renal artery stenosis. *Nephrol Dial Transplant* 1989;**4**:66–70.
5. Loubeyre P, Abidi H, Cahen R, Van Tran Minh A. Transplanted renal artery: Detection of stenosis with color Doppler US. *Radiology* 1997;**203**:661–665.
6. Mimran A, Mourad G, Ribstein J. The renin–angiotensin system and renal function in kidney transplantation. *Kidney Int* 1990;**38**(Suppl. 30);S114–117.
7. Erley CM, Duda SH, Wakat JP *et al*. Non-invasive procedures for diagnosis of renovascular hypertension in renal transplant recipients: a prospective analysis. *Transplantation* 1992;**54**:863–867.
8. Remuzzi G, Perico N. Protecting single-kidney allografts from long-term functional deterioration. *J Am Soc Nephrol* 1998;**9**:1321–1332.
9. Charpentier B, Hiesse C, Marchand S *et al*. De novo and recurrent diseases: recurrent glomerulopathies. *Transplant Proc* 1999;**31**:264–266.
10. Ducloux D, Rebibou JM, Semhorn-Ducloux D *et al*. *De novo* hemolytic uremic syndrome in renal transplant recipients: a meta-analysis. *Transplantation* 1998;**65**:1405–1407.
11. Ribstein J, Mourad G, Mion C, Mimran A. Chronic angiotensin-converting enzyme inhibition as an alternative to native kidneys removal in post-transplant hypertension. *J Hypertension* 1986;**4**:(Suppl. 5):S255–S257.
12. Guidi E, Minghetti D, Milani S *et al*. Hypertension may be transplanted with the kidney in humans: a long-term historical prospective follow-up of recipients grafted with kidneys coming from donors with or without hypertension in their families. *J Am Soc Nephrol* 1996;**7**:1131–1138.

8

13. Thompson ME, Shapiro AP, Johnsen AM *et al*. New onset of hypertension following cardiac transplantation: a preliminary report and analysis. *Transplant Proc* 1983;**15**:2573–2577.

14. Starling RC, Cody RJ. Cardiac transplant hypertension. *Am J Cardiol* 1990;**65**: 106–111.

15. Angermann CE, Spes CH, Willems S *et al*. Regression of left ventricular hypertrophy in hypertensive heart transplant recipients treated with enalapril, frusemide and verapamil. *Circulation* 1991;**84**:583–593.

16. Textor SC, Wiesner R, Wilson DJ. Systemic and renal hemodynamics differs between FK506 and cyclosporine in liver transplant recipients. *Transplantation* 1995;**55**:1332–1339.

17. Loughran TP Jr, Deeg HJ, Dahlberg S *et al*. Incidence of hypertension after bone marrow transplantation among 112 patients randomized to either cyclosporine or methotrexate as graft-versus-host disease prophylaxis. *Br J Dermatol* 1985;**59**:547–553.

18. Joss DV, Barrett AJ, Kendra JR *et al*. Hypertension and convulsions in children receiving cyclosporin A. *Lancet* 1982;**i**:906.

19. Hricik DE, Lautman J, Bartucci MR *et al*. Variable effects of steroid withdrawal on blood pressure reduction in cyclosporine treated renal transplant patients. *Transplantation* 1992;**53**:1232–1235.

20. Mimran A, Mourad G, Ribstein J, Halimi JM. In: *Cyclosporine-associated Hypertension in Hypertension: Pathophysiology, Diagnosis, and Management* (eds Laragh JH, Brenner BM), pp. 2459–2469. Raven Press: New York, 1994.

21. Kiberd BA. Cyclosporine-induced renal dysfunction in human renal allograft recipients. *Transplantation* 1989;**48**:965–969.

22. Mourad G, Ribstein J, Mimran A. Converting-enzyme inhibitor versus calcium antagonist in cyclosporine-treated renal transplant recipients. *Kidney Int* 1993;**43**:419–425.

23. Knoll GA, Bell RC. Tacrolimus versus cyclosporin for immunosuppression in renal transplantation: meta-analysis of randomised trials. *Br Med J* 1999;**318**:1104–1107.

24. Radermacher J, Meiners M, Bramlage C *et al*. Pronounced renal vasoconstriction and systemic hypertension in renal transplant patients treated with cyclosporin A versus FK506. *Transplant Int* 1998;**11**:3–10.

25. Kasiske BL, Guijarro C, Massy Z *et al*. Cardiovascular disease after renal transplantation. *J Am Soc Nephrol* 1996;**7**:158–165.

26. Mange KC, Cizman B, Joffe M, Feldman HI. Arterial hypertension and renal allograft survival. *J Am Med Ass* 2000;**283**:633–638.

27. Paul LC, Benediktsson H. Post-transplant hypertension and chronic renal allograft failure. *Kidney Int* 1995;Suppl.**52**:S34–S37.

28. Cheigh JS, Haschemeyer RH, Wang JC *et al*. Hypertension in kidney transplant recipients. Effect on long-term renal allograft survival. *Am J Hypertension*, 1989;**2**:341–348.

29. Kasiske BL, Heim-Duthoy KL, Ma JZ. Elective cyclosporine withdrawal after renal transplantation. A meta-analysis. *J Am Med Ass* 1993;**269**:395–400.

30. Andreassen AK, Hartmann A, Offstadt J *et al*. Hypertension prophylaxis with omega-3 fatty acids in heart transplant recipients. *J Am Coll Cardiol* 1997;**29**:1324–1331.

31. Kooijmans-Coutinho MF, Rischen-Vos J, Hermans J *et al*. Dietary fish oil in renal transplant recipients treated with cyclosorin-A: no beneficial effects shown. *J Am Soc Nephrol* 1996;**7**:513–518.

32. Ladefoged SD, Andersen CB. Calcium channel blockers in kidney transplantation. *Clin Transplant* 1994;**8**:128.

33. Traindl O, Falger S, Reading S *et al*. The effects of lisinopril on renal function in proteinuric renal transplant recipients. *Transplantation* 1993;**55**:1309–1313.

34. The Heart Outcomes Prevention Evaluation study. Effects of an angiotensin-converting enzyme inhibitor, ramipril, on cardiovascular events in high-risk patients. *N Engl J Med* 2000;**342**:145–153.

35. Gaston RS, Julian BA, Curtis JJ. Post-transplant erythrocytosis: an enigma revisited. *Am J Kidney Dis* 1994;**24**:1.

36. Klaassen RJ, Van Gelder T, Rischen-Vos J *et al*. Losartan, an angiotensin II receptor antagonist, reduces hematocrits in kidney transplant recipients with posttransplant erythrocytosis. *Transplantation* 1997;**64**:780–782.

8

Resistant hypertension

M Barenbrock and KH Rahn

Introduction

Definition

A substantial percentage of patients with hypertension still have elevated blood pressure levels despite receiving antihypertensive therapy. Hypertension resistant to drug therapy has been defined in the recent International Society of Hypertension Guidelines for the Management of Hypertension [1]: hypertension should be considered resistant if blood pressure cannot be reduced to below 140/90 mmHg in patients who are adhering to an adequate and appropriate triple-drug regimen that includes a diuretic, with all three drugs prescribed in near maximal doses. For patients with isolated systolic hypertension, resistance is defined as failure of an adequate triple-drug regimen to reduce systolic blood pressure to below 140 mmHg. Resistant hypertension can be considered primary if desired blood pressure control is never achieved or secondary if blood pressure appearing after adequate control had been accomplished.

Prevalence of resistant hypertension

The prevalence of resistant hypertension is difficult to estimate and it depends on criteria used to define the phenomenon and characteristics of the study population. The percentage of patients with resistant hypertension is likely to be higher in patients with more severe degrees of hypertension and in secondary causes. In tertiary centers designed to handle patients with hypertension it has been estimated that the prevalence of resistant hypertension is anywhere from less than 5% to 18% [2]. However, in 1781 patients with mild hypertension, who were studied at work, Alderman *et al.* found that 2.9% of subjects had primary resistant hypertension [3].

Causes and management

Pseudoresistance

A number of patients who appear to have resistant hypertension in the usual office setting are actually well controlled when blood pressure is assessed out of office [4–6]. It has been shown that 20% of patients with diastolic readings between 90 and 104 mmHg have normal readings during 24-hour blood pressure monitoring. Self-measurements of blood pressure at home may distinguish sustained hypertension from office hypertension. Continuous 24-hour ambulatory blood pressure measurement is most helpful to exclude 'office hypertension'.

It is not uncommon that elderly patients and those with diabetes mellitus or with advanced renal failure have pseudohypertension from rigid, calcified arteries that do not collapse beneath the sphygmomanometer even when the balloon pressure is above the true intraarterial pressure [7,8]. Pseudohypertension can be suspected when radiologic evidence of pipe-stem calcification is found in brachial arteries. It has been suggested that patients who have pseudohypertension can be distinguished from others because their arteries remain palpable when the cuff is inflated above the systolic pressure, a so-called positive Osler's maneuver [8]. Since Osler's maneuver does not appear to be very reliable, the only method to rule out pseudohypertension is a direct intra-arterial blood pressure recording.

Pseudoresistance should be suspected in patients whose pressures do not respond to increasing therapy. Missing pseudoresistance can result in hazardous overmedication. When antihypertensive therapy produces symptoms consistent with hypotension in the absence of an excessive reduction in blood pressure, pseudoresistance has to be excluded. It should also be ruled out in patients whose blood pressure levels seem out of proportion to the extent of organ damage.

Non-adherence to therapy

Poor adherence to antihypertensive therapy is one of the most important factors contributing to resistant hypertension [9,10]. Non-adherence should, therefore, be suspected in all patients with resistant hypertension. Studies have shown that patients must take 80% or more of their prescribed antihypertensive therapy each month before a significant change in blood pressure can be observed [11]. Guidelines to improve patient adherence to therapy have been published in the Joint National Committee's Sixth Report on Detection, Evaluation, and Treatment of High Blood Pressure [12] (Table 8.7.1). The responsibilities of physicians include:

- convincing the patient of their intent and interest in treating hypertension,
- educating the patient,
- selecting and individualizing therapy, and
- responding quickly and effectively to adverse effects caused by antihypertensive therapy.

Table 8.7.1 Guidelines* to improve patients' adherence to antihypertensive therapy

Be aware of signs of patients' non-adherence to antihypertensive therapy
Establish the goal of therapy: to reduce blood pressure to target levels with minimal or no adverse effects
Educate patients about the disease, and involve them and their families in its treatment
Have them measure blood pressure at home
Maintain contact with patients; consider telecommunication
Keep care inexpensive and simple
Encourage lifestyle modification
Integrate pill-taking into routine activities of daily living
Prescribe medications according to pharmacologic principles, favoring long-acting formulations
Be willing to stop unsuccessful therapy and try a different approach
Anticipate adverse effects and adjust therapy to prevent, minimize or ameliorate side effects
Continue to add effective and tolerated drugs, stepwise, in sufficient doses to achieve the goal of therapy
Encourage a positive attitude about achieving therapeutic goals

* Joint National Committee. Sixth Report of the Joint National Committee on Detection, Evaluation, and Treatment of High Blood Pressure [12].

8

Of the many variables in the doctor–patient relationship that influence compliance, good communication appears to be particularly important. The best way to assess whether patients are non-adherent is to simply ask them if they take their medication regularly. A frank and non-judgmental discussion is the best way to elicit the patient's assessment of adherence to the treatment schedule. Patients who claim steadfast adherence to a regimen are not always truthful. Indirect evidence of non-adherence includes failure to keep appointments regularly, failure to renew prescriptions on time, failure to know what medications they are taking and at what intervals, frequent complaints about side effects or cost of medication. Pill counting or monitoring the changes in response to the medication may provide clues about patient's compliance. This may also involve assessing their pharmacological effects such as lowering serum potassium or raising serum urate levels in case of diuretic or decreasing heart rate in case of beta-blocker therapy. Multiple drugs and frequent daily dosing have adverse effects on medication adherence. Reducing complexity will decrease non-adherence, extending the duration of action of medication helps to bridge the gap between errors in frequency of dosing [13]. Once-a-day formulation of every class of antihypertensive drugs are available and it is possible to control the majority of patients with resistant hypertension with multiple drugs all given once daily [13,14].

Drug-related causes

It has been shown that nearly half of patients with resistant hypertension are treated with suboptimal regimens [15]. When referred to a tertiary center, blood pressure levels of most patients with refractory hypertension can be substantially improved if antihypertensive therapy is modified [15]. The combination of antihypertensive drugs can also increase the fraction of hypertensive patients having their blood pressure controlled [16]. The four classes of antihypertensive drugs, which have been advocated as suitable for first-line antihypertensive treatment can be combined with each other. However, it is obvious that not all combinations are equally effective or logical from a pharmacodynamic viewpoint. Combining drugs that lower blood pressure by different mechanisms can increase the fraction of hypertensive patients adequally controlled [1]. The enhanced antihypertensive efficacy is related to the simultaneous attack on several regulatory systems involved in the abnormal blood pressure elevation. Indeed combinations, such as beta-blockers and dihydropyridine-derived calcium antagonists or ACE inhibitors and diuretics, are more effective in lowering blood pressure than ACE inhibitors and beta-blockers or calcium antagonists and diuretics [17]. It is important to point out that hypertension can only be considered resistant in patients with an antihypertensive triple-drug regimen that includes a diuretic. There are several causes of poor response to antihypertensive drugs (Table 8.7.2). Non-diuretic antihypertensive drugs can lose their effectiveness by a stimulation of renal sodium retention due to

Table 8.7.2 Causes of resistant hypertension

- Pseudoresistance
  White coat or office hypertension
  Pseudohypertension
- Nonadherence to therapy
  Side effects of medication
  Instructions unclear and/or not given to the patient in writing
  Lack of involvement of the patient in the treatment plan
  Inconvenient dosing
  Cost of medication
  Organic brain syndrome (e.g. memory deficit)
- Drug-related causes
  Doses too low
  Inappropriate combinations
  Medication or substances that may interfere with blood pressure control (adrenal corticosteroids, antidepressants, nasal decongestants, NSAIDs, sympathomimetics, cyclosporine, erythropoietin, cholestyramine, licorice, cocaine, amphetamine)
- Associated conditions
  Obesity
  Sleep apnea
  Excess alcohol intake
  Smoking
- Secondary hypertension
  Renal failure
  Renovascular hypertension
  Pheochromocytoma
  Primary aldosteronism
- Volume overload
  Inadequate diuretic therapy
  Fluid retention from reduction of blood pressure
  Excessive sodium intake
  Progressive renal failure

Modified from Joint National Committee. Fifth report of the Joint National Committee on Detection, Evaluation, and Treatment of High Blood Pressure [12].

stimulation of a variety of hormonal mechanisms. Sodium and water retention can be frequently observed in patients treated with centrally acting alpha-adrenergic agonists and direct vasodilators. With refilling of the vascular bed that has been dilated by these antihypertensive drugs, blood pressure remains as high as when therapy was started [18]. This phenomenon can even be observed in patients treated with furosemide once daily. Since furosemide is a short-acting drug, sodium and volume retention occurs during the time when the drug is not working. In these patients diuretic therapy with longer-acting diuretic agents or with two or three doses of furosemide can result in effective blood pressure control.

Resistant hypertension can be caused by interactions with other drugs or substances [19,20]. The elimination of such agents can obviate the need for unnecessary, costly and potentially dangerous evaluations or treatments. Non-steroidal anti-inflammatory drugs can nullify the effectiveness of thiazide diuretics due to retention of salt and water and to the loss of the vasodilatory effects of prostaglandins [20]. Oral contraceptives or other steroids and tricyclic antidepressants may also antagonize the effectiveness of certain antihypertensive drugs. Cyclosporine or erythropoietin is often responsible for the development

8

of hypertension that may be very resistant to therapy. The consumption of licorice, cocaine, amphetamines or anabolic steroids may also be responsible for the development of hypertension resistant to therapy.

Associated conditions

Obese patients are more likely to be resistant to antihypertensive therapy. Several studies have shown that obesity, glucose intolerance and hyperinsulinemia can lead to high blood pressure and can lower the effectiveness of antihypertensive treatment [21,22]. In patients with glucose intolerance and hyperinsulinemia, higher doses of antihypertensive drugs are necessary irrespective of the body mass index suggesting that refractory hypertension is closely related to insulin resistance. The role of dietary factors has to be explained by the physician. All patients with resistant hypertension who are over their desirable weight should be prescribed an individualized, monitored weight reduction program involving caloric restriction and increased physical activity.

Excessive alcohol use has clearly been shown to elevate blood pressure and to increase resistance to appropriate antihypertensive therapy [19,23]. The blood pressure effects of alcohol are independent of obesity, salt intake, cigarette smoking and potassium intake. However, the mechanism of alcohol-related hypertension remains unclear. Patients should be counselled to limit their daily intake to no more than 30 g ethanol in males and 15 g ethanol in females.

It has to be pointed out that smoking can also contribute to resistant hypertension. It has been shown that hypertension resistant to therapy is more frequent in smokers than in hypertensive patients who do not smoke [24].

Hypertension resistant to treatment can also be related to obstructive sleep apnea. Clinicians have to ask hypertensive patients for symptoms suggesting sleep apnea such as snoring, disrupted breathing during sleep and daytime somnolence. Studies have shown that treatment of sleep apnea is associated with an improvement of blood pressure elevation [25].

Secondary hypertension

It has been estimated that about 10% of patients with resistant hypertension have an identifiable secondary cause [26]. Secondary hypertension must, therefore, be excluded in every patient resistant to therapy. Common causes are renoparenchymal disease, renal artery stenosis [27], pheochromocytoma [28] and primary aldosteronism.

Salt and water retention is the major cause of resistant hypertension in patients with renal failure setting off a vicious cycle. Blood pressure elevation leads to a progressive deterioration of renal function, the subsequent decrease of glomerular filtration rate is associated with an increase of salt and water retention further accentuating hypertension. Careful control of plasma volume is therefore necessary in hypertensive patients with renal failure. Often it is possible to control blood pressure simply by adding a diuretic to the regimen, increasing the dose of the diuretic, or changing to a diuretic appropriate to the individual patient's renal function.

Renovascular hypertension is difficult to identify by clinical observation. Renal artery stenosis has to be particularly considered in patients whose renal function deteriorates when treated with ACE inhibitors and in subjects with extensive atherosclerotic disease in other parts of the body. Renal artery stenosis should be excluded in refractory hypertension. Atherosclerotic renovascular hypertension is often diagnosed when previously easily managed hypertension becomes resistant to antihypertensive therapy [21]. Hypertension accompanied by headache, palpitations, pallor and perspiration can indicate pheochromocytoma [22]. Primary aldosteronism is often seen with severe or resistant hypertension. Unprovoked hypokalemia gives the clinical clue to detect this endocrine cause of hypertension.

Volume overload

Volume overload is an important cause of resistant hypertension, often related to excessive sodium intake, reactive sodium retention, inadequate diuretic therapy and deterioration of renal function [27,28]. Excessive consumption of dietary sodium will reduce the effectiveness of antihypertensive drugs in general as well as that of diuretic agents. Measurements of 24-hour urinary sodium excretion are helpful to evaluate daily sodium intake. Reactive salt retention often comes into play when blood pressure is lowered with non-diuretic antihypertensive drugs. The lower pressure leads to reduced renal sodium excretion which can be enhanced by an activated renin–angiotensin and sympathetic system. The role of salt and water retention points out clearly the need for adequate diuretic therapy in resistant hypertension. Unfortunately, diuretic therapy is often inadequate due to the widespread use of once daily furosemide and the increasing avoidance of diuretics because of concerns about their metabolic mischiefs [29]. Because of the important role of sodium and water retention for resistant hypertension, antihypertensive action provided by a diuretic given in adequate dosage is mandatory to maintain a slightly contracted plasma volume in hypertensive patients refractory to therapy [29].

References

1. Guidelines Subcommittee: World Health Organization–International Society of Hypertension Guidelines for the Management of Hypertension. *J Hypertension* 1999;**17**:151–183.
2. Setaro JF, Black HR. Refractory hypertension. *N Engl J Med* 1992;**327**:543–547.
3. Alderman MH, Budner N, Cohen H *et al*. Prevalence of drug resistant hypertension. Hypertension 1988;**11**(suppl. II):II-71–75.
4. Pickering TG, James GD, Boddie C *et al*. How common is white coat hypertension? *J Am Med Ass* 1988;**259**:225–228.
5. Waeber B, Petrillo A, Nussberger J. Are some hypertensive patients overtreated? A prospective study of ambulatory blood pressure recording. *Lancet* 1987;**ii**:732–734.

8

6. Mejia AD, Egan BM, Schork NJ, Zweifler AJ. Artefacts in measurement of blood pressure and lack of target organ involvement in the assessment of patients with treatment resistant hypertension. *Ann Intern Med* 1990;**112**:270–277.

7. Zweifler AJ, Shahab ST. Pseudohypertension: A new assessment. *J Hypertension* 1993;**11**:1–6.

8. Messerli FH, Ventura HO, Amodeo C. Osler's maneuver and pseudohypertension. *N Engl J Med* 1985;**312**:1548–1551.

9. Sharkness CM, Snow DA. The patient's view of hypertension and compliance. *Am J Prev Med* 1992;**8**:141–146.

10. Shea S, Misra D, Ehrlich MH *et al*. Predisposing factors for severe, uncontrolled hypertension in an inner-city minority population. *N Eng J Med* 1992;**327**:776–781.

11. Luscher TF, Vetter H, Siegenthaler W, Vetter W. Compliance in hypertension: facts and concepts. *J Hypertension* 1985;**3**(Suppl. 1):3–9.

12. The Sixth Report of the Joint National Committee on Prevention, Detection, Evaluation, and Treatment of High Blood Pressure. *Arch Intern Med* 1997;**157**:2413–2443.

13. Rudd P, Ahmed S, Zachary V *et al*. Issues in patient compliance: the search for therapeutic sufficiency. *Cardiology* 1992;**80**(Suppl. 1):2–10.

14. Spitalewitz S, Porush JG, Reiser IW. Minoxidil, nadolol, and a diuretic. Once-a-day therapy for resistant hypertension. *Arch Intern Med* 1986;**146**:882–887.

15. Yakovlevitch M, Black HR. Resistant hypertension in a tertiary care clinic. *Arch Intern Med* 1991;**151**:1786–1792.

16. Chalmers J. The place of combination therapy in the treatment of hypertension in 1993. *Clin Exp Hypertension* 1993;**15**:1299–1313.

17. Waeber B, Brunner HR. Combination antihypertensive therapy: does it have a role in rational therapy? *Am J Hypertension* 1997;**10**:131S–137S.

18. Dustan HP. Causes of inadequate response to antihypertensive drugs: volume factors. *Hypertension* 1983;**5**:SIII26–30.

19. Clyburn EB, DiPette DJ. Hypertension induced by drugs and other substances. *Semin Nephrol* 1995;**15**:72–86.

20. Pope JE, Anderson JJ, Felson DT. A meta-analysis of the effects of nonsteroidal anti-inflammatory drugs on blood pressure. *Arch Intern Med* 1993;**153**:477–484.

21. Modan M, Almog S, Fuchs Z *et al*. Obesity, glucose intolerance, hyperinsulinemia, and response to antihypertensive therapy. *Hypertension* 1991;**17**:565–573.

22. Reaven GM. Insulin resistance and compensatory hyperinsulinemia: role in hypertension, dyslipidemia, and coronary heart disease. *Am Heart J* 1991;**121**:1283–1288.

23. Puddey IB, Beilin LJ, Vandongen R. Regular alcohol use raises blood pressure in treated hypertensive subjects. A randomized controlled trial. *Lancet* 1987;**i**:647–651.

24. Toner JM, Close CF, Ramsay L. Factors related to treatment resistance in hypertension. *Q J Med* 1990;**77**:1195–1204.

25. He J, Kryger MH, Zorick FJ *et al*. Mortality and apnea index in obstructive sleep apnea: experience in 385 male patients. *Chest* 1988;**94**:9–14.

26. Andersson O. Management of hypertension: clinical and hemodynamic studies with special reference to patients refractory to treatment. *Acta Med Scand* 1977;**617**(Suppl.):1–62.

27. Tarazi RC, Dustan HP, Frohlich ED *et al*. Plasma volume and chronic hypertension: relationship to arterial pressures in different hypertensive diseases. *Arch Intern Med* 1970;**125**:836–842.

28. Graves JW, Bloomfield RL, Buckalew VM. Plasma volume in resistant hypertension: guide to pathophysiology and therapy. *Am J Med Sci* 1989;**298**:361–365.

29. Kaplan N. Southwestern Internal Medicine Conference: difficult-to-treat hypertension. *Am J Med Sci* 1995;**309**:339–346.

8

Section

9

Changing aspects of hypertension

9

9.1

Malignant-accelerated hypertension

YK Seedat

9

Introduction

Volhard and Fahr first described malignant hypertension as a disease entity in 1914. Untreated it carries a high mortality, with 99% risk of death by 5 years. However, with the advent of new and effective antihypertensive agents and the increasing availability of renal dialysis and transplantation, the mortality has been reduced to <26% by 5 years.

Hypertension should be severe with bilateral retinal hemorrhages and exudates. Papilledema may or may not be present and is not absolutely necessary for the diagnosis. Other features like microangiopathic hemolytic anemia or renal failure need not be present.

Diastolic blood pressure is usually greater than 130 mmHg but there is no absolute level above which malignant hypertension always develops and below which it never develops. Lower blood pressure is recognized as occurring in patients with renal failure or in patients with eclampsia and acute glomerulonephritis.

Epidemiology of malignant-associated hypertension

In the elderly, the diastolic blood pressure is lower than the younger group although there is no significant difference in the systolic blood pressures [1]. Malignant hypertension is more common in lower social class groups. Insufficient sleep, overwork and/or mental burden of long duration are factors noticed within one year before the occurrence of malignant hypertension [2].

Malignant hypertension can occur at any age but is less common in those over 70 years. It is more common in males compared to females and seems commoner in Blacks compared to Whites. Whilst it is considered to be uncommon in the developed world, it remains a common problem in developing countries.

Pathogenesis of malignant-associated hypertension

The generally accepted view is that increased arterial pressure is the primary event, and that the rate of rise is more important than the actual level present. Another hypothesis is that increased arterial pressure is not the only factor but that other factors like immunological changes, intravascular coagulation, renal failure, cigarette smoking, the oral contraceptive pill and vasoactive agents are also important. Angiotensin II may play a role both in fibrin deposition and subintimal cellular proliferation which is characteristic of malignant hypertension. Deposition of more fibrin, not only in the vessel wall but also within the microcirculation causes microangiopathic hemolytic anaemia. Peptides and endothelial factors including endothelin, endothelial-derived relaxing factor, cytokines and platelet-derived growth factor may also contribute to malignant hypertension [3]. Decreased urinary kallikrein could indicate depressed activity in the renal kallikrein–kinin system, which may be associated with the initiation of essential malignant hypertension [4].

Underlying causes

Different series have reported a considerable variation in the number of patients in whom an underlying cause for this malignant hypertension can be identified, which is probably a reflection of the extent to which they were investigated [3]. However, any cause of secondary hypertension including primary hypertension may result in malignant hypertension. The most frequent renal parenchymal cause is probably IgA nephropathy[5].

Patients with malignant hypertension are more likely to have an underlying cause than patients with non-malignant hypertension. Renal and renovascular diseases are those most commonly identified. In the investigation of patients for an underlying cause, it should be emphasized that whilst most patients have irreversible disease with renal impairment, only a few can be cured of their hypertension by specific intervention.

Thus it is just as important to control the hypertension and associated risk factors of coronary heart disease, such as cigarette smoking, as to investigate patients for underlying pathologies.

Cigarette smoking

Smoking does not cause essential hypertension with the exception of malignant hypertension. Malignant hypertension has been documented from workers in Glasgow to be five times more common in those who smoked compared to those who did not smoke [3]. The possibility remains that smoking could act as a trigger in susceptible patients and that it exerts its effect by promoting intravascular coagulation. In some patients the combination of smoking and caffeine use is additive and may reflect an extreme pressure effect [6].

The oral contraceptive pill

A causal relation between the oral contraceptive pill and malignant hypertension seems likely when patients develop malignant hypertension within a few weeks or months of starting the oral contraceptive pill [7]. It has also been stated that oral contraceptives are not an important cause of malignant hypertension. Among a sample of malignant hypertensive patients of childbearing age, a past history of hypertension in pregnancy was important. Such patients also had a longer duration of hypertension and poorer function at follow up, and their blood pressure did not fall to normal when the pill was stopped. The oral contraceptive pill may cause activation of the coagulation system, and *in situ* thrombosis. If the pill is stopped and underlying renal disease excluded, the long-term prognosis for such patients is excellent.

Immunology

The frequency of T-lymphocytes and their baseline thymidine incorporation have been shown to be significantly depressed in patients with previously malignant hypertension compared with control subjects. Patients with antiphospholipid syndrome, primary or secondary to systemic lupus erythematosus may develop malignant hypertension with renal involvement [8].

9

625

9.1

Clinical features

In contrast to patients with non-malignant hypertension, which is essentially a symptomless disease, patients with malignant hypertension nearly always present with symptoms. Headaches and visual symptoms are the commonest. The headaches of malignant hypertension are typically worse in the mornings.

Renal failure is the most serious complication of malignant hypertension. Despite investigation, it is often difficult to know whether the hypertension preceded the renal failure or whether the underlying renal disorder caused the hypertension. Exclusion of renovascular hypertension is important, because surgical intervention may improve the blood pressure and renal function. However, in the majority of cases, the value of distinguishing primary hypertension and primary renal disease is mainly for prognostic reasons and does not need any change in management.

BOX 9.1.1 Pathogenesis of acute renal failure

The pathogenesis of the acute renal failure in malignant hypertension is ischemic tubular necrosis secondary to the occlusive vasculopathy. This has been confirmed on histology. In the kidney it is the arteriole which is most severely affected. Musculomucoid hyperplasia results in partial or complete occlusion of the arteriolar lumen. Fibrinoid necrosis also contributes to the vascular lumen and the presence of fibrin in the lumen and blood vessel wall further aggravates the occlusive vasculopathy. Additional reduction in renal perfusion may follow severe hypertensive heart failure or dehydration. Rapid lowering of the blood pressure may follow severe hypertensive heart failure or dehydration. Hypotension results in preferential cortical perfusion at the expense of medullary blood flow and tubular ischemia ensues. Musculomucoid hyperplasia and fibrinoid necrosis have been reported to be partially reversible with control of the hypertension [3].

Cardiac features

The heart is involved frequently in malignant hypertension. The commonest symptom is dyspnea. In contrast, ischemic heart disease is rare. Left ventricular hypertrophy is prominent and when absent suggests that the malignant hypertension is recent and not preceded by a long period of non-malignant hypertension.

Neurological features

Neurologic manifestations consist of hypertensive encephalopathy, acute cerebral infarction, uremic encephalopathy, multi-infarct dementia, and chronic paranoid schizophrenia [9].

Gastrointestinal features

Gastrointestinal manifestations consisting of anorexia, nausea, vomiting, abdominal pain and weight loss may occur. The weight loss is

9

unexplained and is not as a result of the severity of renal impairment. Abdominal pain due to acute pancreatitis or small bowel infarction may occur.

Other features

These include microangiopathic hemolytic anemia which is due to red cell fragmentation by fibrin strands within the microcirculation. It is associated with a low hemoglobin, low platelets and raised reticulocyte count. The hematuria in malignant hypertension may be a presenting manifestation. Red cells in the urine in malignant hypertension are usually isomorphic and not dysmorphic, particularly in the presence of glomerular fibrinoid necrosis. With control of blood pressure, the hematuria and proteinuria due to malignant hypertension secondary to glomerular disease persists, whereas it is usually absent in malignant hypertension due to essential hypertension.

Secondary hypertension leading to hypokalemia, raised plasma renin levels is common. The renin–angiotensin system may be activated by renal ischemic or sodium depletion. The raised plasma renin levels are of no value in determining the cause of the hypertension or of prognostic significance.

Malignant hypertension in developing countries

Whilst malignant hypertension seems rare amongst Whites, it remains a common problem in developing countries. The exception to the rarity of malignant hypertension in Whites is the experience of Lip *et al.* [10] who found that the incidence has failed to decline in Birmingham, England, over a survey period of 24 years. Data from the South African Dialysis and Transplantation Registry has shown that hypertension was responsible for 35% of end-stage renal failure in Blacks. Malignant hypertension was the diagnosis in 57% of essential hypertensives [11]. The poor outlook for Black patients could be explained by their late presentation and the higher prevalence of renal impairment. Moreover, the follow up and control of blood pressure in Black patients is poor because of poor education and inability to understand the severity of their illness or facilities may be wanting or to understand the existing facilities. Fibrinoid necrosis was found in 92% of the autopsy sections of the South African Blacks with malignant hypertension in contrast to African Americans in whom fibrinoid necrosis is rare and the renal changes in malignant hypertension consisted of myxoid internal thickening of small arteries consisting predominantly of smooth-muscle cells [12].

Prognosis in malignant hypertension

In 1939, the five-year survival of untreated patients with malignant hypertension was as low as 1% [15]. This has been confirmed in the UK [16]. With the advent of new and effective antihypertensive agents and the increasing availability of renal dialysis and transplantation, the prognosis of malignant hypertension has dramatically improved and a

9

BOX 9.1.2 Special features of malignant hypertension in the Blacks of South Africa and India

The majority of South African Blacks have essential hypertension and not secondary hypertension. This has epidemiological and therapeutic implications. There is a striking absence of cardiovascular and hypertensive risk factors, smoking, alcohol consumption and obesity.

   Renal failure remains the most important factor regarding prognosis. Approximately 20% of patients with malignant hypertension recover some renal function over time [13]. Before considering renal transplantation or bilateral nephrectomy for blood pressure control, a waiting period of six months is suggested in anticipation of recovery. Where chronic dialysis and renal transplantation facilities are scarce, as is the case in most developing countries, all malignant hypertension renal failures should be treated as acute renal failures for as long as possible under the prevailing local conditions. The clinical and laboratory predictors could assist in the selection of patients most likely to recover.

Malignant hypertension in India is commonly due to aortoarteritis. These patients are treated with steroids and antihypertensive agents and in selected cases renal angioplasty or surgical correction and repair [14].

---

five-year survival of 74% occurs [17]. Renal impairment at initial presentation is regarded as the most important predictor of survival in malignant hypertension. Patients with malignant essential hypertension and malignant hypertension due to renovascular disease may have a higher mortality than those of malignant hypertension due to chronic glomerulonephritis, because of more widespread vascular disease. It has been suggested by Lip *et al.* [18] that renal function continues to deteriorate in some patients with malignant hypertension despite a good degree of control of their blood pressure having been achieved at follow up. However, the renal function of 16 of the 33 patients with severe renal impairment either remained invariant or was found to have improved in some patients at follow up. There was no evidence that those patients whose renal function remained invariant was confined to those who had presented with less renal impairment. The severity of malignant hypertension and the amount of renal impairment did not predict the outcome. This is contrary to an acceptable viewpoint[18]. The quality of control of the blood pressure that had been obtained at follow up did predict the outcome and that careful monitoring of renal function and effective control of the blood pressure is mandatory in patients with malignant hypertension [18].

Renal outcome

With long-term therapy Woods and Blythe [19] were the first to show that control of blood pressure did not result in deterioration of renal function. When vigorous antihypertensive therapy has begun, renal function often worsens transiently, but those who will eventually improve will begin to do so within two weeks. There has been greater knowledge in the syndrome of malignant hypertension with acute renal failure. The typical features include oliguria, normal-sized kidneys on ultrasonography, and marked vascular changes with normal glomeruli. The renal function of patients with an underlying renal disease like glomerulonephritis or interstitial nephritis on long-term follow up, irrespective of the control of blood pressure, invariably developed end-stage renal failure. The deterioration in renal function in these patients probably reflects the natural history of progression of the disease. The renal function in malignant hypertension with renovascular disease does not usually deteriorate in patients whose blood pressure is well controlled. Overall survival in these patients is no better than the renal parenchymal disease group because they have widespread atheromatous disease affecting the coronary and cerebral vessels.

BOX 9.1.3 The renal outcome of malignant hypertension, due to underlying essential hypertension [3]

- Patients with a serum creatinine <300 µmol/liter on presentation generally do well with effective antihypertensive therapy.
- Patients who present with chronic renal failure not requiring dialysis are less likely to maintain or show improvement of renal function and progression to chronic renal failure is almost inevitable.
- A small group may present with acute renal failure. The diagnosis can only be made by renal biopsy.
- Thus in malignant essential hypertension, irreversible renal damage will usually have occurred in a patient with a serum creatinine of 300 µmol/liters unless acute renal failure is superimposed.

Hypertensive encephalopathy

Hypertensive encephalopathy is due to progressively higher blood pressure with or without structural defects of accelerated malignant hypertension. With changes in blood pressure, cerebral vessels dilate or constrict to maintain a constant level of cerebral blood flow. This process of autoregulation is controlled by the sympathetic nervous system.

Chronic hypertensives are able to handle high pressures without obvious trouble and the blood vessels adapt to the chronically elevated blood pressure with structural changes, probably mediated by sympathetic nerves. The entire curve of autoregulation is shifted to the right. Even with this shift, vasodilation occurs if pressures are raised beyond a mean arterial pressure of 180 mmHg [20]. However, normotensives who become hypertensive suddenly may develop encephalopathy at relatively low levels of hypertension which is beyond their level of autoregulation. This occurs in children with acute glomerulonephritis, eclampsia in young females or sympathomimetic drug abuse.

Rapid reduction of blood pressure in chronic hypertensives is not tolerated and cerebral hypoperfusion with features of weakness and dizziness may develop. These symptoms occur at levels of blood pressure within the normal range of autoregulation and within the normotensive range. This fall-off of cerebral blood flow occurs at levels of mean arterial pressure of 100–120 mmHg. Chronic hypertensives may also lose their ability to autoregulate, increasing their risk of brain damage when blood pressure is lowered acutely.

BOX 9.1.4 Hypertensive encephalopathic patients

These have the same laboratory findings as seen in malignant hypertension, but they have more central nervous system manifestations. The cerebrospinal fluid rarely shows pleocytosis, but is usually under pressure. The EEG may show transient, variable, focal or bilateral disturbances. Computed tomography scan or MRI may show white-matter edema, mostly in the posterior part of the brain.

Management of hypertensive encephalopathy

The initial management of hypertensive encephalopathy does not require a knowledge of the cause of the hypertension, but a reduction of blood pressure to a lower level is most important. The choice of therapy may however, differ with the diagnosis. A less aggressive approach is indicated in patients with neurologic features that suggest cerebrovascular accidents when a rapid reduction in blood pressure may extend the lesion. The presentation of cerebrovascular accidents is usually gradual and progressive over hours, whereas hypertensive encephalopathy is usually abrupt.

Patients must be treated quickly in order to prevent further deterioration of cerebral edema. Further increases in the volume of the ischemic tissue as a result of lack of autoregulation may cause acute herniation or more gradual compression of normal brain. Moreover, with increased intracranial pressure, the Cushing reflex may cause the systemic pressure to rise further in an attempt to maintain cerebral blood flow. A shift to the right of the curve of autoregulation leads to the hazards of a fall in cerebral blood flow when systemic pressure is lowered by more than 25% even though these are levels not truly hypotensive.

Table 9.1.1 and Figure 9.1.1 outlines the management of hypertensive encephalopathy. Patients with hypertensive encephalopathy should be admitted to an intensive care unit, and intravenous access and frequent

Table 9.1.1 Management of hypertensive encephalopathy (see also Figure 9.1.1)

- Sodium nitroprusside
  Starting dose is 0.25 μg/kg/min. The dose is 0.25–10 μg/kg/min as i.v. infusion. If cyanide toxicity is suspected, nitroprusside should be discontinued, and 4–6 mg of 3% sodium nitrate should be given intravenously over 2–4 min, followed by an infusion of 50 ml of 25% sodium thiosulphate. Cyanide toxicity has been prevented by concomitant administration of hydroxycobalamin.
- Labetalol
  Dosage is 20–80 mg i.v. bolus every 10 min or 2 mg/min i.v. infusion.
- Nicardipine
  Dose is 5–15 mg/h i.v.

Malignant-accelerated hypertension

Hypertensive
encephalopathy

Management of
hypertensive
encephalopathy

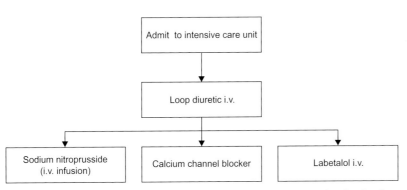

Fig. 9.1.1 Management of hypertensive encephalopathy (see Table 9.1.1 for details of administration).

monitoring of blood pressure should begin. Thereafter, antihypertensive therapy should start. Abrupt falls in blood pressure should be avoided and the goal of immediate therapy should be a diastolic blood pressure of 110 mmHg. Caution should be taken in elderly patients and in those with known cerebrovascular disease. If the neurologic status worsens as treatment continues, intracranial pressure may be elevated, most likely from cerebral edema associated with hypertensive encephalopathy. In such an instance hypotensive agents should be stopped.

The choice of a parenteral drug depends on the experience of clinicians and their knowledge of a particular antihypertensive agent. All antihypertensives are capable of causing profound hypotension, a risk that mandates careful monitoring of blood pressure.

A potent diuretic, usually a loop diuretic, furosemide or bumetanide is usually given intravenously together with a parenteral antihypertensive agent.

Sodium nitroprusside is a valuable antihypertensive agent **and the blood pressure always falls**. The onset is immediate and the duration of action is 1–2 min. Sodium nitroprusside is an exogenous nitrate and is an arteriolar and venous dilator. By dilating cerebral vessels, sodium nitroprusside may increase cerebral blood flow and increase intracranial pressure. However, the fall in systemic pressure moderates the rise in cerebral blood flow and most patients with encephalopathy respond well. It should be used in patients with very high intracranial pressure or azotemia. Sodium nitroprusside is metabolized to cyanide by the sulfydryl group in red cells and the cyanide is rapidly metabolized to thiocyanate in the liver. High levels of thiocyanate may cause fatigue, nausea, disorientation and psychosis.

Labetalol, a combined alpha- and beta-blocker, is given either intravenously or by continuous infusion. It starts acting within 5 min and lasts for 3–6 h. Labetalol should be used in patients with left ventricular dysfunction as it could be worsened by predominant beta blockade. The main side effects are vomiting, scalp tingling, burning in the throat, dizziness, nausea, heart block and orthostatic hypotension.

Nicardipine and other calcium-channel blockers produce a steady progressive fall in blood pressure with little change in heart rate. The

9

onset of action is 5–10 min and the duration of action is 1–4 h. Side effects are few and include headache, nausea, flushing, tachycardia, and local phlebitis. It should be used with caution with left ventricular dysfunction as acute left ventricular failure may occur.

Oral or sublingual agents should not be used in hypertensive encephalopathy as they are more likely to cause precipitous falls in blood pressure because the medications cannot be titrated. Only under the very unlikely event of a patient with rapidly advancing target organ damage, or when intensive care management is not freely available as in developing countries should oral or sublingual therapy be considered.

Therapy for hypertensive urgency

Patients with malignant accelerated hypertension can usually be managed by oral therapy. Patients who are seen in a nursing home or a clinic, whose blood pressure is found to be above some arbitrary danger level like a blood pressure of 180/120 mmHg *should not have a rapid reduction in blood pressure. Do not use sublingual nifedipine.*

Figure 9.1.2 outlines the management of hypertensive urgency. The oral agents are effective in patients with severe uncontrolled hypertension, few having true hypertensive urgencies. There is no ideal antihypertensive agent for hypertensive urgency.

BOX 9.1.5 Nifedipine

Nifedipine has been widely used for the treatment of hypertensive emergency. Liquid nifedipine 5–10 mg sublingually or when chewed and the contents swallowed will rapidly lower pressure within minutes. The problem with sublingual or oral nifedipine is that it is often too effective too rapidly and no way to titrate or overcome the response *Do not use sublingual or oral short-acting nifedipine.* Grossman *et al.* [21] state:

In true hypertensive emergencies, nifedipine capsules are contraindicated because of the unpredictability of the fall in arterial pressure. Given the seriousness of the adverse effects and the complete lack of outcome data, the routine use of short-acting nifedipine in hypertensive emergencies should be abandoned. Other slower and therefore probably safer long-acting calcium-channel blockers can be used.

Captopril is the fastest acting of the oral angiotensin-converting enzyme inhibitors. It can also be used sublingually in patients who cannot swallow. Captopril shifts the entire curve of cerebral autoregulation to the left, so cerebral blood flow should be maintained as the systemic pressure falls. Caution is needed in patients with significant renal insufficiency or who are volume depleted. Abrupt and marked first-dose hypotension after captopril is uncommon and occurs in patients with high renin status. Despite the small potential for hypotension, oral captopril may be the safest of non-parenteral agents for urgent hypertension [22]. Moreover, if renovascular hypertension is suspected, a blood sample for plasma renin activity can be obtained

Malignant-accelerated hypertension

Hypertensive
encephalopathy

Therapy for hypertensive
urgency

References

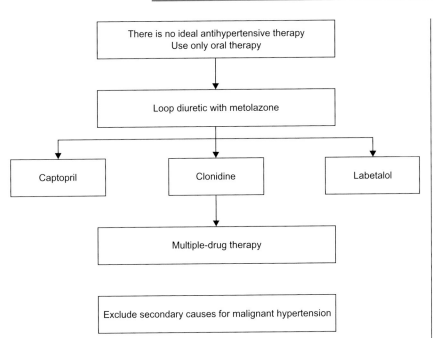

Fig. 9.1.2 Management of hypertensive urgency (see text for details of administration).

before and 1 hour after the 25 mg dose as a reasonably accurate screening test.

Clonidine a central alpha-agonist has been widely used in a dosage of 0.3 mg t.i.d to reduce very high blood pressures. It works more slowly than nifedipine and brings down the blood pressure more safely and effectively. Its main disadvantage is sedation and rebound hypertension if the drug is stopped suddenly. It should not be given in patients who have been shown to be poor compliers.

Labetalol, an alpha- and beta-blocker has been used in hourly doses of 100–200 mg. It has reduced blood pressure as effectively as oral nifedipine and acts more slowly and effectively.

Diuretics specifically furosemide or bumetanide (loop diuretics) combined with metolazone are needed in hypertensive urgencies both to lower blood pressure by removing excess volume and to prevent loss of potency from tendency to cause fluid retension. Volume depletion should be watched in patients on diuretics.

After the patient is out of danger a careful search should be done to exclude a secondary cause for the malignant hypertension. The patient should then be put on the regime of multiple-drug therapy.

References

1. Lip GYH, Beevers M, Potter JF, Beevers DG. Malignant hypertension in the elderly. *Q J Med* 1995;**88**(9):641–647.
2. Sesoko S, Akema N, Matsukawa T, Kaneko Y. Predisposing factors for the development of malignant essential hypertension. *Arch Intern Med* 1987;**147**(10):1721–1724.

9

3. Isles CG. Hypertensive emergencies. In: *Textbook of Hypertension* (ed. Swales JD), pp. 1234–1235. Blackwell Scientific Publications: Oxford, 1994.
4. Hilme E, Herlitz H, Gyzander E, Hansson L. Urinary kallikrein excretion is low in malignant essential hypertension. *J Hypertension* 1992;**10**(8):869–874.
5. Subias R, Botey A, Darnell A, Montoliv J, Revert L. Malignant or accelerated hypertension IgA nephropathy. *Clin Nephol* 1987;**27**:1–7
6. Freestone S, Yeo WW, Ramsay LE. Effects of coffee and cigarette smoking on the blood pressure of patients with accelerated (malignant) hypertension. *J Hum Hypertens* 1995;**9**(2):89–91.
7. Lim KG, Isles CG, Hodsman GP *et al*. Malignant hypertension in women of childbearing age and its relation to the contraceptive pill. *Br Med J* 1987; **294**(6579):1057–1059.
8. Cacoub P, Wechsler B, Piette JC *et al*. Malignant hypertension in antiphospholipid syndrome without overt lupus nephritis. *Clin Exp Rheumatol* 1993;**11**(5):479–485.
9. Healton EB, Brust JC, Feinfeld DA, Thomson GE. Hypertensive encephalopathy and the neurologic manifestations of malignant hypertension. *Neurology* 1982; **32**(2):127–132.
10. Lip GYH, Beevers M, Beevers DG. The failure of malignant hypertension to decline: a survey of 24 years experience in a multiracial population in England. *J Hypertension* 1994;**12**:1297–1305.
11. Veriava Y, Du Toit E, Lawley CG, Milne FJ, Reinach SG. Hypertension as a cause of endstage renal failure in South Africa. *J Hum Hypertens* 1990;**4**:379–383.
12. Isaacson C, Milne FJ, van Niekerk I *et al*. The renal histopathology of essential malignant hypertension in Black South Africans. *South African Med J* 1991;**80**(4):173–176.
13. James SH, Meyers AM, Milne FJ, Reinach SG. Partial recovery of renal function in Black patients with apparent end-stage renal failure due to primary malignant hypertension. *Nephron* 1995;**71**(1):29–34.
14. Sharma BK, Singh G, Sagar S. Malignant hypertension in north west India. A hospital based study. *Jpn Heart J* 1994;**35**(5):601–609.
15. Keith NM, Wagener HP, Barker NW. Some different types of essential hypertension: their course and prognosis. *Am J Med Sci* 1939;**197**:332–343.
16. Breckenridge A, Dollery CT, Parry EHO. Prognosis of treated hypertension. Changes in life expectancy and causes of death between 1952 and 1967. *Q J Med* 1970;**39**(155):411–429.
17. Lip GYH, Beevers M, Beevers DG. Complications and survival of 315 patients with malignant-phase hypertension. *J Hypertension* 1995;**13**(8):915–924.
18. Lip GYH, Beevers M, Beevers DG. Does renal function improve after diagnosis of malignant phase hypertension? *J Hypertension* 1997;**15**(11):1309–1315.
19. Woods JW, Blythe WB. Management of malignant hypertension complicated by renal insufficiency. *N Engl J Med* 1967;**277**:57–61.
20. Strandgaard S, Olesen J, Skinhof E, Lassen NA. Autoregulation of brain circulation in severe arterial hypertension. *Br Med J* 1973;**i**(852):507–510.
21. Grossman E, Messerli FH, Grodzicki T, Kowey P. Should a moratorium be placed on sublingual nifedipine capsules given for hypertensive emergencies and pseudoemergencies? *J Am Med Ass* 1996;**276**(16):1328–1331.
22. Kaplan NM. *Clinical Hypertension*, 8th edn., pp. 265–280. Williams & Wilkins: Baltimore, MD, 1998.

9

9.2

Impact of guidelines for management of hypertension

J Chalmers

9

9.2

Why so many guidelines?

Guidelines are multiplying rapidly in the health sector and this is reflected in the field of hypertension. The pressure for their production stems from many factors. One is the needs of doctors faced by an explosion of knowledge and literature, yet expected to remain abreast of current opinion and modern technology. Another is the wide diversity amongst nations, in terms of culture, of resources, and of the nature of medical practice, making it highly desirable to develop locally or regionally relevant guidelines. Scientific societies and professional bodies too, like to put their imprimatur on the fields in which they operate. Governments and funding agencies such as health maintenance organizations also wish to provide doctors with independent, authoritative advice, not influenced by commercial considerations or by the pharmaceutical industry. Informed consumers too, increasingly seek to ensure that health professionals practice within well-defined and well-informed guidelines.

All of these influences are represented in the growing emphasis on 'evidence-based medicine' which have given guidelines a more focused role. Where it was once sufficient to produce an authoritative summary, guidelines are now expected to lead the way towards 'best practice', or at least better practice! It has become apparent that this requires a well-orchestrated and comprehensive educational program in which guidelines are only one element, albeit a central one. While guidelines alone may have a limited influence on clinical practice, their potential impact on government policy and on the allocation of scarce resources makes it essential that they be rigorous and based on the best available evidence.

The need for improvement in the management of hypertension

The original 'rule of halves' described the situation in the 1970s, when only half the people with hypertension were aware they had it, only half of these (25% of the total) were on treatment, and only half of those (12% of the total) had their hypertension well controlled. While this has improved in some countries such as the USA [1,2] where the hypertension is well controlled in about one-quarter of the hypertensive population, it still holds in many developing countries [3] and in some advanced countries – such as the UK – where the latest survey in 1988, reported that hypertension may only be well controlled in as few as 6% [4]. In general, there is a wide gap around the world, between the diagnosis of hypertension and its effective control (Table 9.2.1) [1–9].

The importance of 'achieved blood pressure' in determining the benefits of treatment in hypertensive patients [10,11] and the continuing difficulties in lowering the incidence of coronary heart disease events [12,13] serve to emphasize the importance of achieving real improvements in clinician behavior and in health outcomes in relation to this group of patients.

9

Table 9.2.1 Effectiveness of hypertension control in the 1990s [1–9]

Country	Blood pressure < 140/90 mmHg
Australia	19%
Belgium	43%
China	11%
France	27%
Italy	23%
Spain	20%
UK	6%
USA	24%

Criteria for evaluating the impact of guidelines

The impact that guidelines have exerted on the practicing doctor can be assessed at different levels of sophistication (Table 9.2.2). At the simplest level, an investigation of the impact achieved might examine the level of awareness of the guidelines on the level of knowledge of guideline recommendations, among the target group of physicians or other health professionals. It is now recognized that this bears little relationship to real changes in physician behavior [14,15].

A more useful measure requires assessment of the extent to which physicians' clinical decisions and practice have been altered by publication of the guidelines or consensus statements. Two main methods have been used for this purpose, and both must be applied before and after dissemination of the guidelines. The most used, but least reliable, tool is the self-report questionnaire, which is simple and cheap but often gives an artificially favorable view of the extent of change in physician behavior. The most reliable method is to carry out analysis of practice data from the same group of clinicians, before and after publication of the guidelines, using trained and independent evaluators. This is expensive and requires thorough planning from the very beginning of the process of producing a set of guidelines.

Available reports in the literature indicate that the mere production and dissemination of Guidelines produces little change in medical practice. For example, Hill *et al.* [16] investigated the impact of the Third Report of the Joint National Committee in the USA (JNC III) on a group of Maryland physicians and found high levels of awareness (62%) but low levels of change in practice (18%). Lomas *et al.* investigated the impact of a Canadian Consensus Conference on the use of cesarean section and found a negligible change in practice, using on site evaluation of clinical data, despite suggestions of extensive compliance with the consensus recommendations, using self-report questionnaire [15]. Lomas *et al.* concluded that substantial change in practice requires a comprehensive program of actions implemented at the local level, accompanied by economic incentives [14,15].

Table 9.2.2 Methods for evaluating the impact of guidelines

- Assessment of physician awareness
- Assessment of physician performance
- Assessment of health outcomes

9

Criteria for evaluating the
impact of guidelines

Qualities that influence
the use of guidelines in
clinical practice

The final test and the main objective, of course, is to produce better health outcomes in the population with the disorders targeted by the Guidelines. It is absolutely clear from more recent investigations reported below that favorable changes in health outcomes require that guidelines be accompanied by a comprehensive package of actions reaching deep into the practice site, and involving active participation of the responsible clinicians.

Qualities that influence the use of guidelines in clinical practice

A recent Dutch study examined the influence of 47 recommendations from 10 sets of national clinical guidelines, published in a national scientific journal for general practice, on the clinical practice of 61 general practitioners in The Netherlands [17]. Included were guidelines on hypertension, Type 2 diabetes, urinary tract infection, and acute otitis media. Each general practitioner recorded his or her decisions on specially designed forms, after each consultation pertaining to one of the 10 guidelines being surveyed.

On average, the recommendations from the guidelines were followed in 61% of the 12 880 decisions monitored. The frequency of compliance was correlated with a set of 16 attributes used as descriptions for each of the 47 recommendations evaluated (Table 9.2.3). Controversial recommendations were only followed in 35% of decisions, compared to non-controversial ones which were observed in 68%. Vague and non-specific recommendations were followed in 36% of cases compared to clear recommendations in 67%. Those that required a significant change in existing practice routines were only followed in 44% of decisions compared with those that did not in 67%. Evidence-based recommendations were also observed more frequently (71%) than those not based on evidence from research (57%) [17]. The messages for authors of guidelines, summarized in Table 9.2.3 are clear – 'Make your recommendations clear and simple, and base them squarely on reliable evidence'. Other conclusions derived by the authors are less helpful, in that guidelines are often most needed in relation to controversial issues, and the whole purpose may well be to change the ingrained habits of clinical practice. The authors stress the importance of testing the feasibility and acceptance of clinical guidelines in the target groups of clinicians, to improve their implementation [17].

Table 9.2.3 Qualities that influence the use of clinical guidelines

- Positive qualities (favoring compliance)
  Clear and precise
  Based on good evidence
  Not controversial
- Negative qualities (favoring non-compliance)
  Vague and non-specific
  Not evidence-based
  Controversial
  Requiring change in practice routines

Table 9.2.4 Effectiveness of CME: evidence from 50 randomized controlled trials (after Davis *et al.* [19])

- Predisposing interventions
  Predisposing interventions based on communication and dissemination alone have little effect on physician performance and no effect on health outcomes.
  Practice guidelines alone are not effective.
- Enabling interventions
  Facilitating change in practice site.
- Reinforcing interventions
  Using reminders and feedback.
- Multifaceted interventions (combinations of the above)
  Enabling, re-inforcing and multifaceted interventions using practice-based strategies at the practice site, consistently improve physician performance and in some instances health outcomes.

Influence of continuing medical education (CME) on physician performance and health outcomes

Doctors are often cynical about the value of formal CME programs in improving the quality of their clinical care. However, as recently reviewed in relation to hypertension guidelines [18] there is now a substantial body of evidence to assess the influence and effectiveness of a large variety of modes of intervention. The McMaster Group reviewed 50 randomised controlled trials, evaluating the efficacy of CME interventions [19]. These 50 studies were selected from over 700 in the literature, as they fulfilled four basic criteria [19]:

- that they be randomized controlled trials,
- that at least 50% of the clinicians were doctors,
- that at least 70% of participants be followed up, and
- that they examine objective measures of physicians' performance on health outcome.

They found that intervention based mainly on the production and dissemination of reports and educational materials, which they called 'predisposing' interventions, had little influence on physician behavior and none on health outcomes [19] confirming Lomas' groups' opinion [14,15]. Indeed, the authors make the categoric statement that 'Practice Guidelines alone were not effective' [19]. However, their analysis revealed that interventions which reached deep into the clinicians' practice site, 'enabling' or 're-enforcing' interventions, consistently improved physician performance and occasionally achieved the ultimate objective – that of improving health outcomes! (Table 9.2.4). The same positive outcome was found for multifaceted interventions using all three types of intervention 'predisposing', 'enabling', and 're-enforcing' [19].

Effectiveness of interventions to improve clinical practice

Physicians would like to think that their clinical practice was squarely based on evidence from medical literature. In fact, medical practice will often diverge considerably from recommendations based on the best

9

Effectiveness of
interventions to improve
clinical practice

Conclusions: place of
guidelines in management
of hypertension

Table 9.2.5 Effectiveness of interventions to promote professional behavioral change (from Bero *et al.* [21])

- Consistently effective
  Educational outreach visits
  Reminders – manual or computerized
  Multifaceted interventions
  Interactive educational meetings
- Mixed effectiveness
  Audit and feedback.
  Local opinion leaders
  Local consensus process
  Patient-mediated interventions
- Little or no effect
  Educational materials
  Printed recommendations
  Published clinical practice guidelines
  Didactic lectures

available evidence [20]. This is certainly true of hypertension, where around three-quarters of hypertensive subjects do not have their blood pressure lowered to recommended levels [1–9].

A careful review of 102 controlled trials differentiated clearly between interventions that were effective in influencing practices, and those that were not [20]. All the studies reviewed fulfilled strict criteria that ensured reliability, including the use of objective measures of clinician performance and of health outcomes [20]. The authors conclude:

> There are no magic bullets for improving the quality of health care, but there are a wide range of interventions that, if used appropriately, could lead to important improvements in professional practice and patient outcomes.

A critical analysis of the methods of intervention used within the studies reviewed indicated once again that the mere production, publication and distribution of guidelines and other educational materials had little or no discernible influence on professional behavior [20,21]. On the other hand, interventions that included interactive discussions with health professionals, particularly in their own practice settings, were consistently effective in improving clinician performance and often effective in improving health outcomes (Table 9.2.5) [4,20].

Conclusions: place of guidelines in management of hypertension

Guidelines alone will not alter physician behavior, nor improve health outcomes, however well written and valid they may be. Change in practice and improved control of hypertension plainly require a comprehensive set of actions embedded in a well-conceived program that reaches into the doctor's practice location in an interactive manner. This does not mean that Guidelines have no value; they do. Their value is at least twofold. Firstly, they help codify 'best practice' and provide a reference point for practitioners, for opinion leaders, and for health authorities. Secondly, they serve as one critical component of a well-constructed program designed to improve professional practice and health outcomes.

References

1. Burt VL, Whelton P, Rocella EJ *et al*. Prevalence of hypertension in the US adult population. Results from the Third National Health and Nutrition Examination Survey 1988–1991. *Hypertension* 1995;**25**:305–313.
2. Burt VL, Cutler JA, Higgins M *et al*. Trends in the prevalence, awareness, treatment and control of hypertension in the US adult population: data from the health examination surveys 1960 to 1991. *Hypertension* 1995;**26**:60–69.
3. Marques-Vidal P, Tuomilehto J. Hypertension awareness, treatment and control in the community: is the rule of halves still valid? *J Human Hypertension* 1997;**11**:213–220.
4. Colhoun HM, Dong W, Poulter NR. Blood pressure screening, management and control in England: results from the Health Survey for England 1994. *J Hypertension* 1998;**16**:747–752.
5. Mancia G, Sega R, Milesi C *et al*. Blood pressure control in the hypertensive population. *Lancet* 1997;**349**:454–457.
6. De Henauw S, De Bacquer D, Fonteyne W *et al*. Trends in the prevalence, selection, treatment and control of arterial hypertension in the Belgian adult population. *J Hypertension* 1998;**16**:277–284.
7. Jamrozik K, Hockey R. Trends in risk factors for vascular disease in Australia. *Med J Australia* 1989;**150**:14–18.
8. Plans P, Pardell H, Salleras L. Epidemiology and cardiovascular disease risk factors in Catalonia (Spain). *Eur J Epidemiol* 1993;**9**:381–389.
9. Tao SQ *et al*. Hypertension prevalence and status of awareness, treatment and control China. *Chinese Med J* 1995;**108**:483–489.
10. Lindholm L, Ejlertsson G, Schersten B High risk of cerebrocardiovascular morbidity in well treated male hypertensives: a retrospective study of 40–59 year old hypertensives in a Swedish primary care district. *Acta Med Scand* 1984;**216**:251–259.
11. Isles CG, Walker LM, Beevers GD *et al*. Mortality in patients of the Glasgow Blood Pressure Clinic. *J Hypertension* 1986;**4**:141–156.
12. Collins R, Peto R, MacMahon S *et al*. Blood pressure, stroke and coronary heart disease – part 2, short-term reductions in blood pressure: overview of randomised drug trials in their epidemiological context. *Lancet* 1990;**335**:827–838.
13. Collins R, MacMahon S. Blood pressure, antihypertensive drug treatment and the risks of stroke and coronary heart disease. *Br Med Bull* 1994;**50**:272–298.
14. Lomas J. Words without action? The production, dissemination and impact of consensus recommendations. *Ann Rev Public Health* 1991;**12**:41–65.
15. Lomas J, Anderson GM, Pierre KD *et al*. Do practice guidelines guide practice? The effect of a consensus statement on the practice of physicians. *N Engl J Med* 1989;**321**:1306–1311.
16. Hill MN, Levine DM, Whelton PK. Awareness, use and impact of the 1984 Joint National Committee Consensus Report on High Blood Pressure. *Am J Public Health* 1988;**78**:1190–1194.
17. Dalhuison J, Thomas S, Cees in't Veld *et al*. Attributes of Clinical Guidelines that influence use of guidelines in general practice: observational study. *Br Med J* 1998;**317**:858–861.
18. Chalmers J. Implementation of Guidelines for the management of hypertension. *Clin Exp Hypertension* 1999;**21**:647–657.
19. Davis DA, Thomson MA, Oxman AD, Haynes RB. Evidence for the effectiveness of CME. A review of 50 randomised controlled trials. *J Am Med Ass* 1992;**268**:1111–1117.
20. Oxman AD, Thomson MA, Davis DA, Haynes RB. No magic bullets: a systematic review of 102 trials of interventions to improve professional practice. *Canad Med Ass J* 1995;**153**:1423–1431.

9

9.2

References

21. Bero L, Guilli R, Grimshaw J *et al*. Closing the gap between research and practice: An overview of systematic reviews of intervention to promote implementation of research findings by health care professionals. On behalf of the Cochrane Collaboration on Effective Professional Practice.

Failure of antihypertensive treatment in the population

SA Gregory, SE Bakir and S Oparil

Introduction

Advances in the understanding of a disease and improved techniques for its management have little impact if they do not reach the population. Progress in the field of hypertension has led to many important discoveries and therapeutic developments over the last fifty years. It is known that hypertension is an important risk factor for the development of myocardial infarction, stroke, heart failure, end-stage renal disease, and peripheral vascular disease. This knowledge has been accompanied by both non-pharmacological and medical therapies which effectively lower blood pressure. Further, pharmacologic treatment of hypertension has been shown to prevent target-organ damage and cardiovascular disease morbidity and mortality. Despite these advances, failure to adequately treat those who suffer from hypertension remains a major worldwide health problem.

In 1972, Wilber and Barrow described a 'rule of halves' for the detection, treatment, and control of high blood pressure in the population. This rule stated that of those with hypertension, one-half are aware of having the disorder, one-half of those receive treatment, and of those treated only one-half are at or below their target blood pressure [1]. Awareness of this problem spurred international efforts to detect and control high blood pressure in the population. Programs throughout the world improved antihypertensive treatment in many industrialized nations. In recent years, however, this trend has slowed and even worsened, prompting a reexamination of our strategies for detecting and controlling high blood pressure.

Time trends

The implementation of educational programs and guidelines for healthcare providers, screening and awareness programs for patients, new management strategies and knowledge, and an expanding number of antihypertensive therapies have improved the treatment of hypertension. In the 1970s and 1980s, awareness, treatment, and control of hypertension improved in those populations exposed to these advances. In the past decade, there has been a decline in this progress. The National Health and Nutrition Examination Survey (NHANES) studies illustrate the pattern in the United States (Figure 9.3.1). Data from the 1975–80 period revealed that 51% of those with hypertension were aware of their diagnosis; 31% were receiving treatment, and 10% had control to a blood pressure <140/90 mmHg. Improvement was recorded in the 1988–91 period, when 73% were aware, 55% receiving therapy, and 29% under control [2]. These initial improvements were accompanied by a 60% reduction in the age-adjusted death rate for stroke and a 53% reduction in the age-adjusted death rate for coronary heart disease. Since the publication of the fifth report of the Joint National Committee on Prevention, Detection, Evaluation, and Treatment of High Blood Pressure (JNC V) in 1993, which noted these improvements, there has been a slowing in the decline of cardiovascular

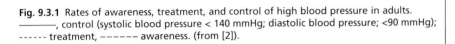

Fig. 9.3.1 Rates of awareness, treatment, and control of high blood pressure in adults. ———, control (systolic blood pressure < 140 mmHg; diastolic blood pressure; <90 mmHg); ------ treatment, – – – – – awareness. (from [2]).

disease morbidity and mortality and increasing rates of end-stage renal disease and heart failure [3] (Figures 9.3.2–9.3.5). These unfavorable trends in cardiovascular disease morbidity and mortality may, in part, be accounted for by deterioration in hypertension management on a population basis. Data from phase 2 of the third National Health and Nutrition Examination Survey (NHANES III) covering the years 1991–4 showed that awareness of hypertension decreased to 68%, treatment to 53%, and control of blood pressure to 27% [2].

BOX 9.3.1 Minnesota Heart Survey

The trend observed in NHANES is supported by studies in Minnesota. The Minnesota Heart Survey showed that, in the 10-year period between 1980–2 and 1990–2, control of hypertension in men fell from 66% to 61%, while awareness decreased from 86% to 83%. Results for women showed an increase in control from 71% to 77% from 1980–2 to 1985–7, followed by a decrease to 73% in 1990–2. This was accompanied by an initial increase in awareness from 90% to 94%, followed by a decrease to 91%. These changes were accompanied by a decrease in the rate of decline in strokes in the study population from 6–7% per year to 1–2% per year. Another study carried out in Minnesota showed worsening of blood pressure control in the decade from 1986 to 1996, using home blood pressure monitoring. A 1996 survey, of a random sample of those in the population over age 45, showed increases in mean systolic blood pressure of 6.6 mmHg (4.9%) and in diastolic blood pressure of 3.6 mmHg (5%) compared to 1986 levels. When adjusted for other variables affecting blood pressure, the increases were still statistically significant, with an estimated increase of 2% in systolic and 4% in diastolic blood pressure. The study also reported a decrease in control rates from 28% in 1986 to 14% in 1996 [3].

Data from the United States show major differences in hypertension prevalence according to gender and ethnicity (Figures 9.3.6 and 9.3.7). The NHANES III shows the overall prevalence of hypertension in the

9

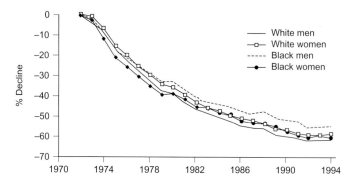

Fig. 9.3.2 Decline in age-adjusted mortality rates for stroke by gender and race in the USA (from [3]).

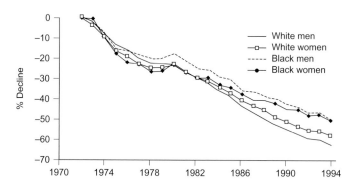

Fig. 9.3.3 Decline in age-adjusted mortality rates for coronary heart disease by gender and race in the USA (from [3]).

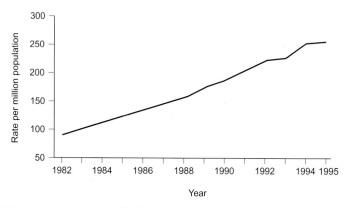

Fig. 9.3.4 Increase in the reported incidence rates of end stage renal disease therapy per million in the US population, adjusted for age, gender, and race (from [3]).

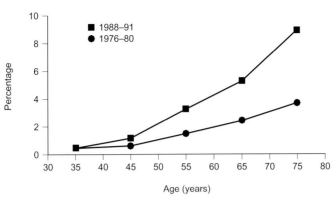

Fig. 9.3.5 Increase in the age-adjusted prevalence of congestive heart failure in the US population from 1976–80 to 1988–91 (from [3]).

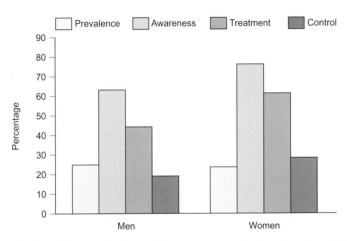

Fig. 9.3.6 Gender differences in the prevalence, awareness, treatment, and control of high blood pressure (from [2]).

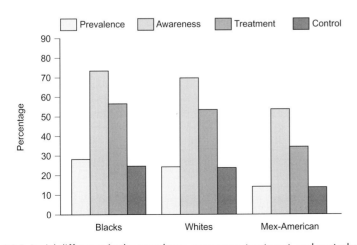

Fig. 9.3.7 Racial difference in the prevalence, awareness, treatment, and control of high blood pressure (from [2]).

US population to be 24% (~43 186 000 individuals). The highest age-adjusted prevalence is in non-Hispanic Blacks (32.4%), followed by non-Hispanic Whites (23.3%), and then Mexican-Americans (22.6%). Men have a slightly higher prevalence than women up to age 59 in all racial groups. However, non-Hispanic blacks 60 years and older with hypertension are more likely to be female, as are non-Hispanic White hypertensives over 70. Increasing age is associated with increasing systolic blood pressure, pulse pressure, and prevalence and severity of hypertension regardless of gender or race. The rate of rise of the systolic blood pressure with age is higher in women than in men. However, men, as a group, have mean systolic and diastolic blood pressures 6–7 mmHg and 3–5 mmHg higher than women [2]. Interestingly, the blood pressures of females following menopause or ovariectomy are similar to males. Females with functioning ovaries have lower blood pressures than females without ovarian function and males. In laboratory animals, hypertensive males and hypertensive females without functional ovaries tend to have salt-sensitive blood pressure, while females with functioning ovaries have salt-resistant hypertension. Synthetic estrogens and progestins, such as those found in oral contraceptive pills tend to elevate blood pressure, while naturally-occurring estrogens, such as those used in hormone replacement therapy, tend to lower, or have no effect on, blood pressure [4].

Gender and racial differences are also observed in hypertension awareness, treatment, and blood pressure control rates (Figures 9.3.6 and 9.3.7). Women are more likely to be aware of having hypertension (76% versus 63%), to be receiving antihypertensive therapy (61% versus 44%), and to have their blood pressures under control (28% versus 19%) than are men. Non-Hispanic Blacks and Whites have higher awareness (74% and 70%), treatment (57% and 54%), and control rates (25% and 24%) than do Mexican-Americans (54%, 35%, and 14% respectively). Of note, the blood pressures of Mexican-American men respond better than those of White men when treatment is given. White men had a mean reduction in blood pressure of 6/4 mmHg with therapy versus 17/9 mmHg in Mexican-American men [2].

Similar patterns but more alarming values for cardiovascular disease morbidity and mortality and for hypertension awareness, treatment, and control rates are apparent worldwide (Figure 9.3.8). The World Health Organization (WHO) notes decreasing cardiovascular mortality with improved control of hypertension in the industrialized nations of North America, Western Europe, and Australasia over the last fifty years. Some parts of Asia, Africa, and Latin America are largely unstudied, while other parts of the world which have been examined show disturbing data. The WHO warns against a 'second wave' epidemic of cardiovascular disease in developing countries and predicts that coronary heart disease will be the number one killer and cerebrovascular disease number four worldwide by 2020 [5].

Marques-Vidal and Tuomilehto reviewed studies on the prevalence, awareness, and treatment of hypertension in various populations. Their review showed that the percent aware varied from 23% in one study of

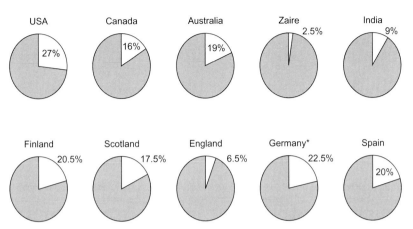

Fig. 9.3.8 Blood pressure control in ten nations. The percentage of hypertensive patients achieving blood pressure reduction to <140/90 mmHg in the US and England, and < 160/95 mmHg in the other nations *Age > 65 years; blood pressure < 140/90 mmHg USA and England, <160/95 mmHg in all other countries. (from [3,6,7]).

men from the People's Republic of China to 97% in a cohort of women from the United States. Those receiving treatment ranged from a low of 5% in Chinese men to 97% in a study of US women. Control was achieved in no female patients in a study from Zaire, while a US study showed 97% control in a group of women. The review noted that women generally fare better than men worldwide. However, in contrast to the US, men in other parts of the world are more likely than women to be aware of having hypertension. The data, not surprisingly, show that developing countries perform worse than industrialized ones. The authors concluded that the developing countries are 20 years behind more developed nations with respect to hypertension management [6].

A study by Colhoun *et al.* compared awareness, treatment, and control of high blood pressure in England to the US. The prevalence of hypertension in England, as defined by blood pressures >160/95 mmHg, was 19.5%, rising to 38% if 140/90 mmHg was used as the cutoff. In 1994, with hypertension defined as blood pressure >160/95 mmHg, 63% of English hypertensives were aware of their diagnosis, 50% were receiving treatment and 30% were under control. Using the more contemporary definition of >140/90 mmHg, 40% were aware, 26% treated, and only 6% under control. After comparing their data with those obtained from the US population a few years prior, the authors concluded that hypertension is more effectively managed in the US, with England lagging approximately 15 years behind [7].

Screening programs

Hypertension education and screening programs have contributed to an improvement in hypertension treatment in those countries employing them over the last 50 years. The greatest impact, as expected, has been in awareness. However, recent trends suggest that further efforts are needed in this area. The screening test for hypertension, blood pressure

Table 9.3.1 Blood pressure measurement (from [3] and [5])

- Patients should be seated with back supported and arm bared and supported.
- The cuff should be at the level of the patient's heart.
- Patients should refrain from smoking or ingesting caffeine for 30 minutes prior to measurement.
- The patient should be allowed to rest in a quiet room for 5 minutes prior to measurement.
- Appropriate cuff size (the bladder within the cuff should encircle at least 80% of the patient's arm) and calibrated equipment should be used.
- Record both systolic and diastolic blood pressures.
- Two or more readings separated by at least 2 minutes should be averaged.
- Measure the blood pressure in both arms on the first visit if there is evidence of peripheral vascular disease.
- Measure blood pressure in the standing and seated positions in elderly individuals, diabetics, and others in whom orthostatic hypotension is common.

measurement, has the ideal characteristics of being safe, easy to perform, inexpensive, and widely available (Table 9.3.1). The WHO recommends that multiple blood pressure measurements be recorded on several separate occasions in order to make an accurate diagnosis of hypertension. JNC VI guidelines call for blood pressure measurement at each patient encounter. However, this is not being done. In a study performed at Veterans Administration hospitals in the US, patients had a mean of 6.4 clinic visits per year but only 5.1 blood pressure measurements [8]. In England, Colhoun *et al.* found that 49% of those discovered to have hypertension had not had their blood pressures measured for at least one year [7].

Screening programs must involve regular blood pressure measurements of the population. This can be accomplished through both community programs and efforts by healthcare providers. The latter appear to be much more important. The National Heart, Lung, and Blood Institute (NHLBI) notes that community screening programs reach an estimated 25% of the population, while roughly 70% of people will have a healthcare visit within a given year [9]. Therefore, the most fruitful screening program will consist of healthcare providers measuring blood pressure during each patient encounter. Equally important as blood pressure measurement is the recording of values over time in order to confirm the diagnosis of hypertension and guide referral and, if appropriate, therapy. For those who are not reached by encounters with healthcare providers, community-based programs offer another opportunity for hypertension screening. These take the form of job-related health screens and health fairs at gathering places such as shopping centers, entertainment events, places of worship, and schools.

Appropriate follow-up of those found to have elevated blood pressures in a screening program is crucial for future blood pressure control. Healthcare providers and those involved with community programs must be able and willing to educate hypertensives about the importance of seeking further evaluation and controlling blood pressure. The impact of elevated blood pressure on cardiovascular and cerebrovascular disease and the importance of treatment should be emphasized, and arrangements facilitated for timely follow-up.

9

Guidelines for the intervals between healthcare visits are provided in the JNC VI report [3]. Close attention to those with intermittent or labile hypertension and borderline or high normal blood pressure values is warranted due to their future risk of developing hypertension and increased likelihood of cardiovascular events. This is particularly true for persons with other cardiovascular risk factors or comorbid conditions such as diabetes. The WHO has provided a strategy for risk stratification in their most recent guidelines (Table 9.3.2 and 9.3.3) [5].

Improved follow-up is fostered by home blood pressure monitoring. This is useful in differentiating 'white coat' hypertension from sustained hypertension as the measurement is taken in a comfortable environment by the patient's friend, relative, or partner. Repeated measurements in such a setting are helpful in establishing the patient's true mean blood pressure by accounting for fluctuations during the day. Home

Table 9.3.2 WHO: Risk stratification for cardiovascular events (from [5])

Other risk factors and disease history	Blood Pressure (mmHg)		
	Grade 1 (mild hypertension) SBP 140–159 or DBP 90–99	Grade 2 (moderate hypertension) SBP 160–179 or DBP 100–109	Grade 3 (severe hypertension) SBP ⩾ 180 or DBP ⩾ 110
I. No Other Risk Factors	Low risk	Medium risk	High risk
II. One or two risk factors	Medium risk	Medium risk	Very high risk
III. Three or more risk factors, target organ damage, or diabetes	High risk	High risk	Very high risk
IV. Associated clinical conditions	Very high risk	Very high risk	Very high risk

SBP = sysolic blood pressure; DBP = diastolic blood pressure.

Table 9.3.3 WHO: Factors affecting risk stratification (from [5])

Risk factors for cardiovascular disease	Target-organ damage	Associated clinical conditions
• Levels of systolic and diastolic blood pressures (grades 1–3) • Men > 55 years old • Women > 65 years old • Smoking • Total cholesterol > 6.5 mmol/l (250 mg/dl) • Diabetes • Family history of premature cardiovascular disease	• Left ventricular hypertrophy (by electrocardiogram, echocardiogram, or radiogram) • Proteinuria and/or elevation of plasma creatinine concentration (1.2–2.0 mg/dl) • Ultrasound or radiological evidence of atherosclerotic plaque (carotid, iliac and femoral arteries, aorta) • Generalized or focal narrowing of the retinal arteries	• Cerebrovascular disease Ischemic stroke Cerebral hemorrhage Transient ischemic attack • Heart disease Myocardial infarction Angina Coronary revascularization Congestive heart failure • Renal Disease Diabetic nephropathy Renal failure (plasma creatinine concentration > 2.0 mg/dl) • Vascular disease Dissecting aneurysm Symptomatic arterial disease • Advanced hypertensive retinopathy Hemorrhages or exudates Papilledema

9

monitoring also improves adherence to care by actively involving patients in the management of their disorder, giving them results to show progress and promote goals, and providing frequent reminders of the presence of their hypertension. The WHO cites data from Mancia *et al.* that suggest blood pressures taken at home are generally lower than those observed at office visits. They assert that a home reading of 125/80 mmHg is equivalent to a measurement of 140/90 mmHg in a healthcare provider's office [10]. JNC VI recommends using a cut-off of 135/85 mmHg as the upper limit of normal for home blood pressure measurements [3].

Prevention of hypertension

International guidelines, such as those of the WHO Expert Committee, National High Blood Pressure Education Program (NHBPEP), and the JNC, have stressed the importance of primary prevention of hypertension. The goals of such an intervention would include preventing the blood pressure rise observed with aging, lowering overall blood pressure levels in the population, and addressing other modifiable risk factors in an effort to decrease cardiovascular morbidity and mortality. The NHBPEP estimates that a population-based program to slightly lower overall blood pressure levels and prevent the rise of blood pressure associated with aging would have an effect on cardiovascular disease equal to or greater than that of treating patients with established hypertension [11].

Published guidelines for primary prevention of hypertension include lifestyle modifications such as weight reduction, increased physical activity, moderation of alcohol intake, and dietary salt restriction (Table 9.3.4). Obesity, a sedentary lifestyle, and intake of alcohol and salt have all been associated with increased risk of developing hypertension. Data from the Framingham Heart Study suggest that 78% of hypertension in men and 65% in women is attributable to obesity as defined by a subscapular skinfold thickness of at least one centimeter. Sedentary individuals with normal blood pressures were found to have a 20–50% increased risk of developing hypertension, and alcohol intake was shown to be a risk factor in another study. Sodium intake has been associated with increased blood pressure, and reducing dietary sodium to less than 75–100 mmol per day has been effective in lowering blood pressure in some studies. Programs involving weight reduction, exercise, and salt reduction decreased the incidence of hypertension in patients with risk factors such as obesity, high normal blood pressures,

Table 9.3.4 Recommendations for lifestyle modification (from [16])

- Reduce dietary sodium and fat
- Increase calcium, potassium, magnesium, vitamins, and fiber from food sources
- Weight loss if overweight
- Regular physical activity
- Moderation of alcohol intake
- Smoking cessation

and family histories of hypertension [12,13]. The NHBPEP estimates that such interventions could decrease the prevalence of hypertension in the US population by 20–50% [11]. The INTERSALT [14] Study, Smith *et al* [15] and Opril [16] illustrate the controversy over the effectiveness of dietary measures.

Recent data have caused controversy over the recommendation of salt restriction to lower blood pressure in the population. The INTERSALT study, which involved approximately 11 000 subjects from 52 centers in 39 countries, set out to examine the relationship between 24-hour sodium excretion in the urine (and thus salt intake) and blood pressure [14]. The data from this study showed no significant relationship between the two in 48 of the participating centers. Inclusion of the other four study centers, which had populations with very low salt intake, alcohol use, body weight, and blood pressure, resulted in a weak but statistically significant positive relationship between sodium excretion and blood pressure. Reanalysis of the data has shown a stronger relationship, but has been criticized for its statistical methods. A similar study in Scotland examined over 11 000 subjects to find a relationship between sodium excretion and blood pressure [15]. After correcting for other variables such as alcohol intake and body mass, no correlation was found.

A review of the literature on dietary sodium restriction and blood pressure shows that studies on the subject have been limited by numerous factors [16]. These include: the fact that restricting sodium frequently alters the intake of other nutrients, which may affect outcomes, that noncompliance with low salt diets is often seen, but infrequently accounted for in data analyses, and that quantitating salt intake is very difficult and prone to error. The review asserts that the published studies on the subject are often not blinded and/or placebo controlled, and generally lack statistical power due to insufficient study periods and too few subjects. This has prompted several meta-anaylses, which have been complicated by significant heterogeneity among the studies examined. Also, it should be noted that sodium restriction may not be free of adverse consequences. Several studies have shown sustained increases in study subject plasma renin and aldosterone proportional to the level of sodium restriction achieved [17]. This is concerning due to observations of increases target organ damage and coronary events in the setting of increased plasma renin activity and hypertension [18, 19].

A recent trial by the Dietary Approaches to Stop Hypertension (DASH) Collaborative Research Group suggests that total diet is more important than altering individual micronutrients such as sodium [20]. The study examined the effects of a diet high in fruits, vegetables, and low-fat dairy products, and lowe in saturated and total fat (combination diet) on blood pressure. The study enrolled 459 individuals with systolic blood pressure < 160 mmHg and diastolic blood pressures of 80–95mmHg and randomized them to one of three diets: the combination diet, a diet rich in fruits and vegetables, or a control diet low in fruits, vegetables, and low-fat dairy products with a fat content

9

approximating that of the average American diet. The subjects' sodium intake and body weights were held constant during the study period. Eight weeks following initiation of these diets, blood pressure reductions were observed in those on the combination diet and the diet rich in fruits and vegetables (Figure 9.3.9). The combination diet lowered blood pressure by 3.5/2.1 mmHg more than the control diet in normotensive individuals and by 11.4/5.5 mmHg more in those with hypertension. The authors of the study have noted that the effects of the DASH combination diet cannot be attributed to micronutrients alone, and advise that their diet can be approximated better by taking four servings of fruit, four servings of vegetables, and three of low-fat dairy products per day rather than attempting to ingest specific amounts of micronutrients. Although patients may desire a 'hypertensive supplement', the current data suggest they would be better served by eating a well-balanced diet low in fat and rich in calcium, potassium, magnesium, and vitamins. This is supported by the fact that in many studies attempting to find a role for various nutrients in blood pressure

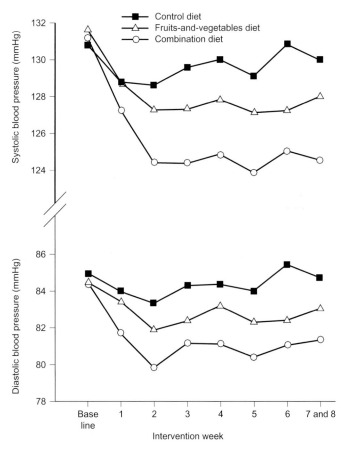

Fig. 9.3.9 Mean systolic and diastolic blood pressures of participants in the DASH study based on diet. Blood pressures were recorded at baseline and then weekly following institution of the diets (from [20]).

control, effects are most pronounced for individuals with deficiencies of the nutrient in question. The DASH study suggests that preventing these deficiencies and others with a balanced, healthy diet can be helpful in preventing hypertension.

Despite the dissemination of guidelines and data on the effectiveness and importance of primary prevention, two million new cases of hypertension are diagnosed each year in the US alone. In 1996, Kannel [13] cited data from the Framingham Heart Study suggesting that, if those on therapy who have achieved normal blood pressures are excluded, there has been no decline in the prevalence of hypertension. In the Framingham cohort, there has been no consistent change in the age-adjusted blood pressure in those not receiving therapy over the three decades of the study. In addition, two-thirds of those who started the study with normal blood pressures subsequently developed hypertension. Kannel suggests that this indicates an urgent need for primary prevention. He also notes that the measures used to prevent hypertension are also beneficial in reducing other cardiovascular risk factors – which are found in 80% of hypertensives [13].

Healthcare providers should assess the need for preventive measures in all of their patients. Those with high normal blood pressures (>130/85 but <140/90 mmHg) are at higher risk of developing hypertension and cardiovascular disease than those with normal or optimal blood pressures [21], and are, therefore, excellent targets for primary prevention. African-Americans, those with a family history of hypertension, and those with a predisposition to developing obesity or diabetes are also excellent candidates for programs to decrease weight, salt intake, alcohol use, and improve dietary habits while increasing exercise due to their increased risk of developing high blood pressure [13]. These recommendations help promote health in all, but are especially important in those persons with other risk factors for hypertension-associated conditions such as coronary heart disease, stroke, renal disease, and peripheral vascular disease.

Studies concerning awareness, treatment, and control of high blood pressure, as well as the continued high prevalence of hypertension, suggest that primary prevention is not being effectively practiced. In 1997, the American Heart Association (AHA) addressed problems with preventative strategies in their statement on compliance [22]. As in the larger issue of compliance with or adherence to therapeutic recommendations, they saw the lack of effectiveness of preventative strategies to be due to problems with patients, providers, and healthcare systems. The AHA statement noted that patients and providers overestimate compliance with lifestyle behaviors, and that these and other recommendations for health promoting and disease preventing behaviors will not be heeded without a multilevel approach to the issue.

The AHA asserts that one of the key areas in need of improvement is provider and patient communication (Table 9.3.5). The lifestyle changes used to help prevent hypertension are very difficult for many people, especially those at highest risk, who often must give up many long-term habits. Recommendations for dietary and activity changes by a provider

9

Table 9.3.5 Suggestions to increase patient adherence/compliance with prevention recommendations (from [22])

- Educate patients about risk factors
- Stress the importance and potential benefits of lifestyle modifications
- Improve patient skills in lifestyle modification
- Set goals for the patient, monitor progress, and provide feedback
- Improve the counseling skills and knowledge of providers
- Involve other healthcare providers (nurses, nutritionists, psychologists, etc.) in prevention strategies
- Healthcare organizations should develop systems to incorporate prevention strategies into medical practice

have little chance of being followed if their importance and potential benefits are not communicated to the patient. The AHA Expert Panel states that such communication is dependent on the provider's confidence in his or her ability to teach patients the necessary skills to follow recommendations, and the amount of time available for preventative services. Studies cited in the AHA recommendations maintain that physicians lack such skills and time. Another problem is that physicians feel that peers are not providing such counseling and, therefore, it is not the standard of care. There is also a lack of reimbursement for patient education. The panel suggests that healthcare organizations help remedy this problem by providing training, personnel, and support to address patient education and counseling [22].

Treatment of hypertension

The lifestyle modifications recommended as helpful for the prevention of hypertension are also beneficial in the treatment of high blood pressure. The WHO and JNC guidelines cite numerous studies which support the use of weight reduction, moderation of alcohol consumption, decreased dietary sodium, and increased exercise to reduce blood pressure. Both guidelines note that the blood pressure lowering effects of these measures can reduce or obviate the need for drug therapy with its associated costs and side effects. The DASH study supports an increased emphasis on a well-balanced diet in treating hypertension. In addition, such dietary modifications help reduce other risk factors for cardiovascular disease.

Lifestyle modifications should be used in all patients with high blood pressure as either the definitive treatment or an adjunct to drug therapy. However, data from the NHANES suggest that this is not being done (Figure 9.3.1). In a survey of those patients reporting a diagnosis of hypertension, 24% had received no prior prescription of any of the following: weight loss, sodium restriction, increased physical activity, or moderation of alcohol intake. Of those patients with blood pressures >140/90 mmHg on medical therapy, 14% had never been prescribed any of the non-pharmacological therapies and 24% reported no current use of any one of them [2]. These data suggest that at least some of the problems with blood pressure control in the population are due to providers not prescribing lifestyle modification to all of their patients.

9

Another study has also provided evidence that many physicians are not aggressive enough in their medical treatment of hypertension. This study included 800 hypertensive men with a mean age of approximately 65 years who received medical care at Veterans Administration Medical Centers. Despite averaging six hypertension-related visits to these centers per year, 40% of the subjects had blood pressures of at least 160/90 mmHg. Medications were increased in only 6.7% of hypertension-related visits and 11.2% of such visits with recorded blood pressure measurements. Using a model to assess the intensity of therapy, the investigators found that those patients in the most intensive treatment category had a mean decline of 6.3 mmHg in systolic blood pressure while those in the least intensive treatment group had a mean increase of 4.8 mmHg in systolic pressure over the two-year study period [8].

Data from the Hypertension Optimal Treatment study (HOT) also suggest that most hypertensive patients are not receiving enough medication. At the beginning of the study, the subjects had a mean blood pressure of 161/98 mmHg. Approximately 60% of these patients were receiving single-drug therapy, while 30% took two medications for their hypertension. By the end of the study period, the mean blood pressure had fallen to 142/83 mmHg, and 52% of the study patients required at least two drugs to achieve this level of blood pressure control [23]. Taken together, data from HOT and other studies support the concept that undertreatment can take the form of too few drugs and/or inadequate doses of drugs, as well as a lack of nonpharmacological augmentation.

BOX 9.3.2 Framingham Heart Study

Data from the Framingham Heart Study highlight the potential benefit of increases in drug therapy to hypertensive patients on a population basis. The study involves over 10 000 participants who have been followed for approximately 40 years. The authors noted that from 1950 to 1989, the rate of use of antihypertensive drugs increased from 2.3% to 24.6% in men, and from 5.7% to 27.7% in women. This improvement was accompanied by declines in the age-adjusted prevalence of blood pressures $\geqslant 160/100$ mmHg from 18.5% to 9.2% in men, and from 28% to 7.7% in women. Target-organ damage, in the form of left ventricular hypertrophy, also declined, from 4.5% to 2.5% in men, and from 3.6% to 1.1% in women [24].

When combining two or more antihypertensive drugs, agents with additive or synergistic effects should be used. WHO and JNC guidelines note that it is often more helpful to add a small dose of a second drug rather than to increase the dose of the original medication. A diuretic is an excellent choice as a second drug because diuretics potentiate the effects of most other antihypertensive agents. Potentiation can be achieved with low doses of diuretic, thus avoiding many of the side effects associated with diuretic therapy. Effective combinations take advantage of differing mechanisms of action of their component drugs. The WHO and JNC recommendations include combinations of:

- diuretic and beta-blocker,
- diuretic and ACE inhibitor or angiotensin-receptor blocker,
- dihydropyridine calcium-channel blocker and beta-blocker, and
- calcium-channel blocker and ACE inhibitor.

The WHO guidelines also list combining an alpha-blocker with a beta-blocker. However, this approach may not be ideal, as the antihypertensive effects of the two drugs are not additive and there is a risk of rebound hypertension if the agents are withdrawn [21]. Fixed-dose combination pills are available which offer convenience and many other advantages, such as improved compliance, as will be discussed later (Table 9.3.6).

Hypertension is a condition with a heterogeneous pathophysiology. This provides a rationale for using combination therapy with agents which have differing mechanisms of action, and for a new strategy of treatment that involves rotating different classes of drugs in order to find the best choice for an individual. This strategy was examined by Dickerson *et al.* who took 56 young, untreated hypertensives with a mean blood pressure of 161/98 mmHg and rotated them through monotherapy with an agent from each of four major classes of

Table 9.3.6 Fixed-dose antihypertensive combinations (modified from [32])

- Calcium-channel blockers and angiotensin-converting enzyme (ACE) inhibitors
    Amlodipine/benazepril (Lotrel)
        Diltiazem/enalapril (Teczem)
        Felodipine/enalapril (Lexxel)
    Verapamil/trandolapril (Tarka)
- ACE inhibitors and diuretics
        Benazepril/hydrochlorothiazide (Lotensin HCT)
            Captopril/hydrochlorothiazide (Capozide)
            Enalapril/hydrochlorothiazide (Vaseretic)
    Lisinopril/hydrochlorothiazide (Prinzide, Zestoretic)
        Moexipril/hydrocholorothiazide (Uniretic)
- Angiotension II-receptor antagonists and diuretics
        Losartan/hydrochlorothiazide (Hyzaar)
        Valsatan/hydrochlorothiazide (Diovan HCT)
            Irbesartan/hydrochlorothiazide (Avalide)
- Beta-blockers and diuretics
        Atenolol/chlorathalidone (Tenoretic)
        Bisprolol/hydrochlorothiazide (Ziac)
        Metoprolol/hydrochlorothiazide (Lopressor HCT)
            Nadolol/bendlumethiazide (Corzide)
        Propranolol/hydrochlorothiazide (Inderide)
    Propranolol extended release/hydrochlorothiazide (Inderide LA)
            Timolol/hydrochlorothiazide (Timolide)
- Other combinations
            Amiloride/hydrochlorothiazide (Moduretic)
        Spironolactone/hydrochlorothiazide (Aldactazide)
    Triamterene/hydrochlorothiazide (Dyazide, Maxzide)
            Clonidine/chlorthalidone (Combipres)
        Hydralazine/hydrochlorothiazide (Apresazide)
            Methydopa/chlorothiazide (Aldochlor)
            Prazosin/polythiazide (Minizide)

9

antihypertensive medication in a systematic manner [25]. The four classes were (1) ACE inhibitors (A), (2) beta-blockers (B), (3) calcium-channel blockers (C) and (4) diuretics (D). They noted a large amount of variablility in the responses of their patients to the various agents. By using their rotational strategy, however, they were able to improve blood pressure control rates (goal <140/90 mmHg) on monotherapy from 39% to 73%. The authors put forth an AB/CD rule in which one agent from either the AB group or the CD group was selected first and, if that agent failed to control the patient's blood pressure, an agent from the other group was chosen next. This strategy is based upon the strong correlations in response observed between A and B agents ($r = 0.5$), and between C and D agents ($r = 0.6$). For combination therapy, the study recommends using an agent from the AB group with one from the CD group. It should be noted that the difficulty in practicing the rotational strategy, which requires multiple clinic visits and medication/dosage adjustments, is ameliorated by using the AB/CD rule.

The choice of the best initial medical therapy for hypertensive patients has been hotly debated among experts/consensus committees. JNC VI recommends that, in the absence of contraindications or specific indications for the use of another agent, a diuretic or beta-blocker should be chosen. This is based on data from randomized controlled clinical trials showing decreased morbidity and mortality from hypertension-related endpoints in patients receiving one of these agents. The WHO guidelines do not make this direct recommendation, but they do mention diuretics and beta-blockers first in their discussion of drug selection. Other guidelines, such as those of the Hypertension Guidelines Committee of Australia in 1991, do not recommend these agents as first choice, and the expert committee of the British Hypertension Society was divided on the issue in 1993 [26]. Actual prescribing practices reinforce these differences of opinion.

Caro and Speckman reviewed prescribing practices for high blood pressure during the period between 1988 and 1998 (Figure 9.3.10) [27]. They found a great deal of variation between countries in the choice of initial therapy of hypertension. In the US, Canada, and Sweden an ACE inhibitor or calcium-channel blocker was used most often. A diuretic or beta-blocker was used more often in Germany and the United Kingdom. Variation was also observed within countries and between practitioners. The authors suggested that this lack of adherence to the recommendations of groups such as the JNC may reflect practice patterns that are actually beneficial because they take into account the issue of persistence with therapy.

Problems with adherence/compliance

Adherence/compliance with hypertension management is a major obstacle to achieving adequate control of high blood pressure in the population. Each step in management is associated with significant numbers of patients being lost from medical care. In the US, approximately 50% of individuals do not follow through with referral

9

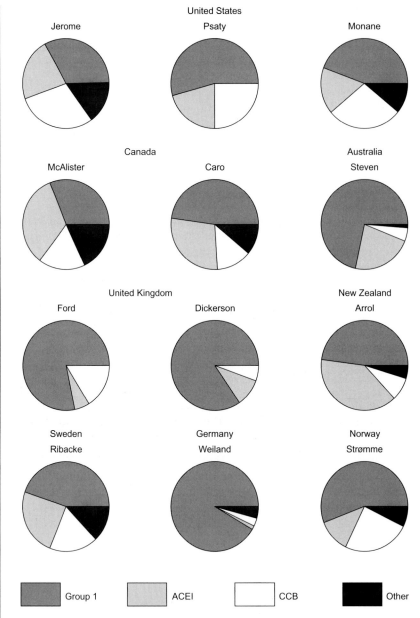

Fig. 9.3.10 Medications prescribed to newly-diagnosed hypertensive patients by country. Differences are observed in the use of four major classes of antihypertensive agents (from [27]).

advice; approximately 40% do not take their medications as directed, and over 50% of those who begin treatment are not in care one year later [9]. In the UK, 50–70% of new medications are changed or discontinued within six months of their initiation [28].

Caro and colleagues suggest that persistence with medical therapy is related to the choice of initial antihypertensive agent (Figure 9.3.11) [29]. They analyzed data obtained from the Saskatchewan Health system

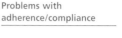

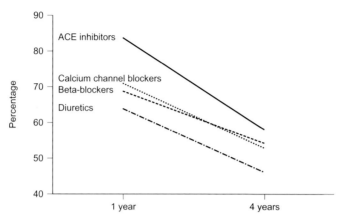

Fig. 9.3.11 Adherence to therapy based on class of antihypertensive agent used. ———,
ACE inhibitor; ·········· calcium-channel blocker; − − − − − beta-blocker; ·−·−·−·, diuretic
(from [34]).

from 1989 to 1994, and found that only 78% of those diagnosed with
hypertension and prescribed medication persisted with therapy at one
year, and 46% persisted with therapy four years after its initiation. The
rate of persistence varied with the initial choice of medication. ACE
inhibitors performed best, with persistence of 84% at one year, and 58%
at four years; they were followed by calcium-channel blockers (71% and
53%), beta-blockers (69% and 54%), and diuretics (64% and 46%). The
authors noted that the difference in persistence between ACE inhibitors
and the agents recommended as initial therapy by JNC VI (beta-blockers
and diuretics) remained significant after controling for age, gender, and
utilization of healthcare resources. Caro suggests that this might explain,
and justify, many providers choosing agents other than diuretics and
beta-blockers as initial therapy for hypertension.

Initial choice of medication was also important in determining
adherence to treatment in a study of patients in California (Figure 9.3.12)
[30]. The population studied received healthcare support from Medicaid

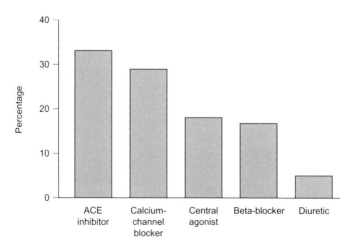

Fig. 9.3.12 Adherence to therapy based on initial medication choice (from [30]).

due to poverty or disability. In this group, only 14.3% maintained continuous antihypertensive drug therapy over one year, and only 16.6% of those who interrupted therapy restarted it later that year. Again, those whose initial drug was an ACE inhibitor were most likely to adhere to treatment (33%). The rates of continuous therapy for the other agents were: calcium-channel blockers 29%, central adrenergic agonists 18%, beta-blockers 16.8%, and diuretics 4.9%. Of the significant number of patients who stopped therapy within the first month, 65.5% were prescribed diuretics and 29.7% ACE inhibitors. The performance of the ACE inhibitors has been attributed to their tolerability [18].

Another factor affecting persistence with therapy is the number of times a patient has his/her medical regimen changed. In the Saskatchewan population, patients who had their therapy changed two or more times within any six-month period were 25% less likely to persist with medication over the ensuing six months. A single change in therapy decreased persistence by 7% for the next six-month period [27]. Changes in therapy are often associated with patient frustration, as the patient may feel as if he/she is making little progress against his/her high blood pressure. Patients may see little benefit in enduring the costs and possible/actual side effects of medical therapy, and may even doubt the provider's ability to manage their blood pressure. Since many changes of medication are due to lack of tolerability, patients may anticipate and dread such adverse effects from their next prescription.

The Losartan Effectiveness and Tolerability Study (LET) supports the use of angiotensin-receptor blockers as antihypertensive agents with excellent tolerability [31]. These newer agents, which were not included in the previous studies of adherence/compliance, show promise in improving persistence with therapy. LET compared a losartan/hydrochlorothiazide regimen with a usual care regimen over a 16-week period. Participants were all in need of a change in their antihypertensive therapy at the start of the study due to uncontrolled blood pressure (82%) or intolerable side effects (18%). Blood pressure control was the same in each group, but the patients on losartan had a lower incidence of side effects and fewer medication switches (9%) than the usual care group (23%). The authors asserted that this improved tolerability may translate into better adherence and, therefore, better control of high blood pressure.

The promising results of LET also highlight the potential of fixed-dose combination therapy in improving adherence to treatment (Table 9.3.7). A fixed-dose combination agent obviously reduces the number of pills that the patient on two or more drugs must take. In addition, these agents offer improved tolerability as the individual components can be given in lower doses in combination than as monotherapy. Combinations of antihypertensive drugs have been produced in which one component decreases or attenuates the side effects of the other. For example, adding an ACE inhibitor to a calcium-channel blocker can help with the peripheral edema associated with the latter. Many of the combinations take advantage of synergistic or additive blood pressure-lowering effects. Fixed-dose combination agents are often cheaper than their individual

9

Table 9.3.7 Advantages of fixed-dose combination therapy (adapted from [32])

Convenience for patient and physician
Improved compliance/adherence
Often cost less than individual components
Potentiation of antihypertensive effects through the additive or synergistic effect of combining the individual components
Reduction in adverse events through lower dosages of individual components
Attenuation of adverse effects through interaction of individual components
Improved overall antihypertensive effect if the ratio of components is superior to what is available in the absence of a fixed-dose combination

components due to insurance reimbursement policies and, most likely, improved tolerability and effectiveness [32].

In addition to the discomfort of side effects, poor tolerability of an agent may contribute to non-adherence through increased costs. Side effects often lead to more clinic visits and laboratory testing, additional medications, and changes in therapy. The choice of antihypertensive medication is important to the overall cost of care, with diuretics and beta-blockers proving more expensive than other agents in some studies. For example, in a tertiary care hypertension clinic, diuretic or beta-blocker therapy had to be switched to another agent in 122/357 patients, while only 44/270 patients receiving other agents required a change in therapy over a four-year period. The cost of the switch from a diuretic or beta-blocker to another drug was $1333 per patient, while that of changing from one of the other agents to a different drug was $1017. The additional cost was attributed to the need for more clinic visits and laboratory testing. This analysis did not include the additional costs of poorly controled blood pressure occurring as a consequence of intolerance and/or non-adherence to therapy [21].

Data from the California Medicaid population suggest that lack of persistence with therapy significantly raises healthcare costs [30]. Patients whose therapy was not continuous over one year accounted for $873 ($637 of which were hospitalization costs) more in costs than those who adhered to therapy. The effect was more pronounced in subjects previously hospitalized ($1840) than those with no such history ($673). The additional costs accrued by those not adherent to therapy were offset by savings in drug costs of only $281. It should be noted that continued lack of therapy would most likely result in additional healthcare costs as the patient's hypertension-related diseases progressed.

Strategies to improve adherence and, therefore, blood pressure control must involve the patient, provider, and health care system (Table 9.3.8). The AHA notes that the most beneficial approach combines several interventions: patient and provider education, treatment contracts, self-monitoring of blood pressure, social support, telephone follow-up, tailoring of therapy, and involvement of other healthcare professionals such as pharmacists [22]. Healthcare systems should provide time, training, personnel, educational material, and tracking technology to make all of this possible.

The physician can make it easier for the patient to adhere to therapy by designing a treatment regimen with patient convenience, tolerability,

9

Problems with
adherence/compliance

Table 9.3.8 Suggestions for increasing patient adherence to antihypertensive therapy (from [22])

Educate the patient about hypertension and the importance of treatment
Describe the potential complications of uncontrolled hypertension
Schedule a follow-up appointment during the office visit and reconfirm by telephone
Prescribe the drug regimen least likely to result in adverse effects
Choose the least costly regimen likely to be effective
Prescribe a once-a-day regimen, if feasible
Simplify drug regimen by using a fixed-dose combination product
Track attendance
Set a blood pressure goal for the patient
Provide feedback about progress toward the goal
Have patients monitor their blood pressure at home
Inquire about difficulties with the prescribed regimen
Discuss new treatment strategies with the patient, and involve him/her in the decision process

and understanding in mind. If feasible, the physician should utilize long-acting, once-a-day drugs to minimize the number of pills the patient must take and provide consistent blood pressure control. Fixed-dose combination pills are also useful in this regard. Pill boxes or special packaging measures, such as blister packaging, should be used to help the patient keep track of his/her medicine. The taking of medication should be incorporated into the patient's daily routine and associated with a regular activity such as brushing teeth, going to bed, or eating a particular meal. The treatment regimen must include education of the patient on the importance of adhering to therapy, and on the consequences of poorly controlled blood pressure. Family members and friends should be involved in the process if possible.

Patients have great difficulty adhering to lifestyle modifications prescribed for hypertension. The measures recommended are often very difficult for a patient and his/her family to accept. Dietary and activity habits must often undergo dramatic changes. The AHA Expert Panel on Compliance points out that these changes require the development of new skills such as reading food labels, knowledge of healthy cooking methods, time management, and making appropriate food choices outside of the home [22].

Lifestyle modifications involve more than just the patient. Family members and those who live with the patient will be affected by changes in the patient's diet and physical activity. Success in making these changes depends, at least in part, on the assistance, understanding, encouragement, and approval of the patient's loved ones. This is particularly true when someone other than the patient usually prepares meals or schedules outings. Such a person will also need to develop new skills and strategies. For all of these reasons, the changes engendered by lifestyle modifications are difficult to achieve and sustain even when extensive counseling and support are provided.

The second phase of the Trials of Hypertension Prevention (TOHP II) Collaborative Research Group was undertaken to evaluate the feasibility of maintaining lifestyle modification in individuals with high normal blood pressures in order to prevent the development of hypertension

[33]. The study subjects received intensive counseling on lifestyle modifications, but still had difficulty in adhering to prescribed measures. The study enrolled 2382 individuals who were moderately overweight, had high normal blood pressures, and were not receiving any antihypertensive medication. These participants were randomized to weight loss with a goal decrease of 4.5 kg, sodium reduction with goal intake of 80 mmol/day or less, a combination of weight loss and sodium reduction, or usual care. The sodium reduction and combination groups achieved mean daily sodium intakes of 104 and 124 mmol/day six months after initiation of the study, and both had increases in intake throughout the next 30 months. Weight loss was also difficult to achieve and maintain. Although the weight loss and combination groups came close to achieving their weight loss goal of 4.5 kg at six months (with mean losses of 4.4 kg and 4.1 kg respectively), they showed significant accumulation of weight over the rest of the study period.

The Treatment of Mild Hypertension Study (TOMHS) also shows a lack of sustainability in weight loss, sodium reduction, and increased physical activity in hypertensive subjects [34] (Figure 9.3.13). Participants in the study were hypertensive subjects (diastolic blood pressures <100 mmHg) who received what the authors described as 'intensive nutritional-hygenic intervention' with or without conventional antihypertensive drug treatment. At the end of the four-year study period, the mean weight loss achieved was 2.6 kg – approximately one-half of that achieved one year into the study. Sodium reduction, as measured by urinary sodium excretion, at four years was approximately one-third of that achieved at the end of the first year of study. Measurements of physical activity also declined from an initial

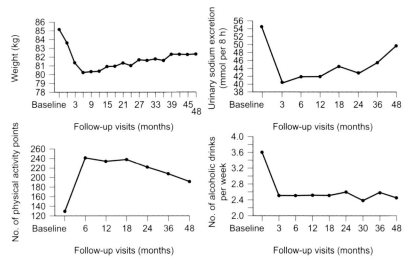

Fig. 9.3.13 Adherence to lifestyle modifications in TOMHS participants. The top left shows average weight over four years. Bottom left, average number of physical activity points (with one activity point defined as 16.8 joules) expended. Top right, average urinary sodium excretion (used to estimate salt intake). Bottom right, average number of alcoholic drinks consumed per week (from [34]).

improvement over baseline. In contrast, decreased alcohol consumption was maintained over four years.

As mentioned previously, physicians generally do not have the time or skills to effectively counsel their patients on lifestyle modification. Further, patients and their families usually lack the skills and knowledge necessary to put prescribed modifications into practice. Thus, healthcare providers such as nurses, nutritionists, educators, and psychologists are needed to improve patient adherence to lifestyle interventions as well as treatment recommendations. Patients also need motivation, support, and follow-up as they attempt to learn new skills and change their daily habits. The resources to make all of these measures possible require commitment by healthcare organizations and systems, as well as patients and providers [22].

Refractory hypertension

Refractory or resistant hypertension may be defined as blood pressure $\geq 140/90$ mmHg despite an optimal two-drug regimen that has been given adequate time to take effect (at least one month since the last dosage adjustment or addition of a drug) [35]. Studies evaluating the prevalence of refractory hypertension in the general hypertensive population have resulted in estimates of 2.9–18% [36]. There are many causes of refractory hypertension, including secondary hypertension, problems with blood pressure treatment, patient-related factors, and inappropriate therapy (Table 9.3.9).

Secondary hypertension is high blood pressure due to a specific, potentially curable disorder (Table 9.3.10). Approximately 10% of patients with refractory hypertension have an identifiable disorder such as chronic renal disease, renovascular disease, pheochromocytoma, or primary aldosteronism, as its cause [36]. These patients often fail to respond to typical antihypertensive regimens, and manifest symptoms and signs of their primary disorder. Further, the patient's history and screening laboratory data often give clues to the diagnosis. Although secondary hypertension is far less common than essential hypertension, it should always be considered as a cause of high blood pressure in any

Table 9.3.9 Causes of refractory hypertension (from [3])

Non-adherence to therapy
White coat hypertension
Spurious hypertension (pseudohypertension)
Antihypertensive drug dose too low
Too few antihypertensive agents
Inappropriate combinations of agents
Use of drugs with short half-lives
Interaction of antihypertensive drug(s) with other agents
Weight gain or obesity
Excessive alcohol intake
Sedentary lifestyle
Obstructive sleep apnea
Volume overload
Secondary hypertension

9

Table 9.3.10 Causes of secondary hypertension (modified from [3])

Renal parenchymal disease
Renal vascular disease
Organ transplantaion with use of immunosuppressive agents
Renin-secreting tumors
Primary aldosteronism
Overproduction of mineralocorticoids
Congenital adrenal hyperplasia
Cushing's syndrome
Pheochromocytoma
Extra-adrenal chromaffin tumors
Hyperparathyroidism/hypercalcemia
Acromegaly
Pregnancy-induced hypertension
Obstructive sleep apnea
Coarctation of the aorta
Dysautonomia
Increased intracranial pressure
Quadriplegia
Lead poisoning
Guillan–Barré syndrome
Postoperative hypertension
Thyrotoxicosis
Anemia
Aortic insufficiency
Arteriovenous shunts
Paget's disease of bone
Beriberi
Carcinoid syndrome

given patient, especially in those resistant to therapy. Interventions directed at the primary disorder can be effective in lowering blood pressure, and have great potential benefit to the patient.

Inadequate therapy is a common cause of uncontrolled blood pressure, whether or not the high blood pressure is truly treatment resistant. Among patients referred to a tertiary care hypertension clinic for resistant hypertension, 43% were receiving a suboptimal regimen according to the hypertension specialists staffing the clinic. The specialists noted that there was inadequate use of diuretic therapy in several of these patients [37]. Patients with renal insufficiency (serum creatinine >3 mg/dl and/or glomerular filtration rate <30 ml/min) should receive a loop diuretic to help control blood pressure and volume. However, patients with normal renal function should receive a thiazide diuretic instead of a loop diuretic, as the former is more effective in controlling blood pressure in that population. These points are very important in that volume overload is the most common cause of resistant hypertension in those patients who adhere to therapy [21]. The hypertension specialists were able to control blood pressure in 50% of those patients whose regimens had been considered suboptimal by adding a diuretic, increasing the dose of diuretic, or changing the diuretic to the proper class for the patient's renal function [37].

Non-adherence to prescribed therapy is another important cause of refractory hypertension. In a tertiary care hypertension clinic, 19% of cases of refractory hypertension were, at least partially, due to a lack of adherence to treatment [37]. Other studies have estimated that up to

9

50% of refractory hypertension is caused by non-adherence. There are measures for detecting non-adherence to antihypertensive treatment in the population. Non-adherence should be suspected in all patients with resistant hypertension due to its frequent occurrence in that setting. Additional clues include missed appointments, failure to manifest expected biological effects of medication such as a decreased heart rate with beta-blocker treatment, and substance abuse [38]. Strategies to enhance adherence have been discussed previously.

Refractory hypertension has been associated with the use of various substances, including decongestants, bronchodilators, corticosteroids, non-steroidal anti-inflammatory drugs (NSAIDs), and others (Table 9.3.11). These agents can act by directly raising the blood pressure, interfering with the actions of antihypertensive medications, or both. For example, NSAIDs can directly raise blood pressure by inhibiting natriuresis and causing volume expansion. They can also elevate blood pressure by indirect mechanisms, such as interfering with the actions of agents such as ACE inhibitors. Heavy alcohol use can increase blood pressure and make it more difficult to control, as can illicit drugs, e.g. cocaine and amphetamines. Abuse of alcohol and other substances also contributes to non-compliance with therapy. Caffeine and nicotine can cause transient refractory hypertension by their ability to temporarily raise blood pressure after their ingestion [35,36].

Other patient-related factors such as obesity, hyperinsulinemia, and sleep apnea are associated with refractory hypertension. Modan *et al.* showed that obese patients (body mass index (BMI) of >27.8 in men and 27.3 in women) required more antihypertensive medication to achieve blood pressure control than leaner patients, and that the requirement increased in proportion to increasing BMI. Glucose intolerance and hyperinsulinemia, even in non-obese patients, were associated with increased medication requirements as well [38]. Sleep apnea increases blood pressure through the stimulation of the sympathetic nervous system that occurs in response to upper airway closure. It should be considered in patients with resistant hypertension and other findings such as: obesity, large neck size (17 inches or more in men and 16 inches or more in women), a history of loud snoring and interrupted sleep, daytime somnolence, polycythemia, and carbon dioxide retention [35]. It is often useful to interview the patient's sleeping partner, as most patients are unaware of having this disorder.

Inappropriate therapy resulting in a diagnosis of refractory hypertension may be due to 'white coat' hypertension (office

Table 9.3.11 Substances that raise blood pressure (adapted from [36])

Anabolic steroids	Chlorpromazine
Caffeine	Corticosteroids
Cocaine	Cyclosporine
Ethanol	Erythropoietin
Nicotine	Monoamine oxidase inhibitors
Sympathomimetic agents	Oral contraceptives
NSAIDs	Tricyclic antidepressants

9

hypertension) or spurious hypertension (pseudohypertension). 'White coat' hypertension is elevated blood pressure found in health care offices and clinics, but not outside of such settings. However, it may not be benign [35]. 'White coat' hypertension should be suspected in those resistant to therapy, but without target-organ damage. These patients often exhibit symptoms of overmedication such as orthostasis, and report home blood pressure values lower than those obtained by the healthcare provider. This cause of refractory hypertension can be screened for with home blood pressure monitoring. The upper limit of normal for home blood pressure is usually set at 135/85 mmHg. Treatment should be based on the values obtained at home; and patients should have careful monitoring for evidence of target-organ damage, combined with preventative strategies and risk factor modification.

Spurious hypertension (pseudohypertension) is artefactually elevated blood pressure obtained by indirect cuff measurement secondary to reduced arterial compliance [35]. This most often occurs in the elderly and is caused by atherosclerotic disease. The Systolic Hypertension in the Elderly Program (SHEP) found that 7% of elderly patients screened had spurious hypertension [39]. This should be suspected in patients with refractory hypertension, no target-organ damage, and/or symptoms of overmedication. The diagnosis is difficult to make as the classic physical diagnosis test, the Osler maneuver, which consists of palpating a pulse in the radial or brachial artery despite the blood pressure cuff being inflated above the auscultated systolic blood pressure, has questionable accuracy and usefulness [39]. The diagnosis can be made by intra-arterial blood pressure measurement or, less invasively and less dangerously, with an infrasonic or plethysmographic device [35].

References

1. Wilber JA, Barrow JG. Hypertension – a community problem. *Am J Med* 1972;**52**:653–663.
2. Burt VL, Whelton P, Rocella EJ *et al.* Prevalence of hypertension in the U.S. adult population. Results from the Third National Health and Nutrition Examination Survey, 1988–1991. *Hypertension* 1995;**25**:305–313.
3. Joint National Committee on Detection, Evaluation, and Treatment of High Blood Pressure. The Sixth Report of the Joint National Committee on the Detection, Evaluation, and Treatment of High Blood Pressure. *Arch Intern Med* 1997;**157**:2413–2446.
4. Calhoun DA, Oparil S. High blood pressure in women. *Int J Fertil* 1997;**42**:198–205.
5. World Health Organization–International Society of Hypertension Guidelines Subcommittee. 1999 World Health Organization–International Society of Hypertension Guidelines for the Management of Hypertension. *J Hypertension* 1999;**17**:151–183.
6. Marques-Vidal P, Tuomilehto J. Hypertension awareness, treatment and control in the community: is the 'rule of halves' still valid? *J Hum Hypertension* 1997;**11**:213–220.
7. Colhoun HM, Dong W, Poulter NR. Blood pressure screening, management and control in England: results from the health survey for England 1994. *J Hypertension* 1998;**16**:747–752.
8. Berlowitz DR, Ash AS, Hickey EC *et al.* Inadequate management of blood pressure in a hypertensive population. *N Engl J Med* 1998;**339**:1957–1963.

9

References

9. National Heart, Lung, and Blood Institute Working Group, United States Department of Health and Human Services. Management of patient compliance in the treatment of hypertension. *Hypertension* 1982;**4**:415–423.

10. Mancia G, Sega R, Bravi D *et al*. Ambulatory blood pressure normality: results from the PAMELA Study. *J Hypertension* 1995;**13**:1377–1390.

11. Working Group on Primary Prevention of Hypertension. Report of the National High Blood Pressure Education Program Working Group on Primary Prevention of Hypertension. *Arch Intern Med* 1993;**153**:186–208.

12. Trials of Hypertension Prevention Collaborative Research Group. The effects of nonpharmacologic interventions on blood pressure of persons with high normal levels: results of the Trials of Hypertension Prevention, phase I. *JAMA* 1992;**267**:1213–1220.

13. Kannel WB. Blood pressure as a cardiovascular risk factor: prevention and treatment. *JAMA* 1996;**275**:1571–1576.

14. INTERSALT Cooperative Research Group. INTERSALT: An international study of electrolyte excretion and blood pressure. Results for 24-hour urinary sodium and potassium excretion. *Br Med J* 1988;**297**:319–328.

15. Smith WCS, Crombie IK, Tarendale RT *et al*. Urinary electrolyte excretion, alcohol consumption, and blood pressure in the Scottish Heart Health Study. *Br Med J* 1988;**297**:329–330.

16. Oparil S. Diet – micronutrients – special foods. In: (eds, Oparil S, Weber MA). *Hypertension: Companion to Brenner and Rector's The Kidney*. WB Saunders: Philadelphia, PA, 1999.

17. Gradual NA, Galloe AM, Gamed P. Effects of sodium restriction on blood pressure, renin, aldosterone, catecholamines, cholesterols, and triglycerides. *JAMA* 1998;**279**:1381–1391.

18. Brunner HR, Laragh JH, Baer L *et al*. Essential hypertension: renin and aldosterone, heart attack and stroke. *N Engl J Med* 1972;**286**:441–449.

19. Alderman MH, Madhavan S, Ooi WL *et al*. Association of the renin–sodium profile with the risk of myocardial infarction in patients with hypertension. *N Engl J Med* 1991;**324**:1098–1104.

20. Appel LJ, Moore TJ, Obarzanek E *et al*. The effect of dietary patterns on blood pressure: results from the Dietary Approaches to Stop Hypertension (DASH) clinical trial. *N Engl J Med* 1997;**336**:1117–1124.

21. Calhoun DA, Oparil S. The National Health and Nutrition Examination Survey (NHANES) III: how are we doing with blood pressure control? In: *The Practice of Hypertension* (ed. Weber MA). The Humana Press: Totowa, NJ, 1999.

22. AHA Expert Panel on Compliance. The multilevel compliance challenge: recommendations for a call to action. *Circulation* 1997;**95**:1085–1090.

23. Hansson L, Zanchetti A, Carruthers SG *et al*. for the HOT Study Group. Effects of intensive blood pressure lowering and low-dose aspirin in patients with hypertension: principal results of the Hypertension Optimal Treatment (HOT) randomized trial. *Lancet* 1998;**351**:1755–1762.

24. Mostard A, D'Agostino RB, Silbershatz H *et al*. Trends in the prevalence of hypertension, antihypertensive therapy, and left ventricular hypertrophy from 1950–1989. *N Engl J Med* 1999;**340**:1221–1227.

25. Dickerson JEC, Hingorani AD, Ashby MJ *et al*. Optimisation of antihypertensive treatment by crossover rotation of four major classes. *Lancet* 1999;**353**:2008–2013.

26. Kaplan NM, Gifford RW Jr. Choice of initial therapy for hypertension. *JAMA* 1996;**275**:1577–1580.

27. Caro JJ, Speckman JL. Current prescribing practices. In: (eds, Oparil S, Weber MA). *Hypertension: Companion to Brenner and Rector's The Kidney*. WB Saunders: Philadelphia, PA, 1999.

28. Jones JK, Garkin L, Lian JF *et al*. Discontinuation of and changes in treatment after start of new courses of antihypertensive drugs: a study of a United Kingdom population. *Br Med J* 1995;**311**:293–295.

29. Caro JJ, Salas M, Speckman JL *et al*. Persistence with treatment for hypertension in actual practice. *Canadian Med Assoc J* 1999;**160**:31–37.

9

30. McCombs JS, Nichol MB, Newman CM, Sclar DA. The costs of interrupting antihypertensive drug therapy in a Medicaid population. *Med Care* 1994;**32**:214–226.
31. Moore MA, Gazdick LP, Edelman JM *et al.* Losartan effectiveness and tolerability (LET) study. *Am J Hypertension* 1998;**11**:104A.
32. Sica DA. Fixed-dose combination antihypertensive drugs. Do they have a role in rational therapy? *Drugs* 1994;**48**:16–24.
33. The Trials of Hypertension Prevention Collaborative Research Group. Effects of weight loss and sodium reduction intervention on blood pressure and hypertension incidence in overweight people with high-normal blood pressure. The Trials of Hypertension Prevention, phase II (TOHPII). *Arch Intern Med* 1997;**157**:657–667.
34. Neaton JD, Grimm RH Jr., Prineas RJ *et al.* Treatment of Mild Hypetension Study (TOMHS). Final results. *JAMA* 1993;**270**:713–724.
35. Oparil S, Calhoun DA. Managing the patient with hard-to-control hypertension. *Am Fam Phys* 1998;**57**:1007–1014.
36. Setaro JF, Black HR. Refractory hypertension. *N Engl J Med* 1992;**327**:543–547.
37. Yakovlevitch M, Black HR. Resistant hypertension in a tertiary care clinic. *Arch Intern Med* 1991;**151**:1786–1792.
38. Modan M, Almog S, Fuchs Z *et al.* Obesity, glucose intolerance hyperinsulinemia, and response to antihypertensive drugs. *Hypertension* 1991;**17**:565–573.
39. Wright JC, Looney SW. Prevalence of positive Osler's manoeuver in 3387 persons screened for the Systolic Hypertension in the Elderly Program (SHEP). *J Hum Hypertension* 1997;**11**:285–289.

References

9

Assessment of cost-benefit in antihypertensive treatment

FV Costa and E Ambrosioni

9

Introduction

The great benefits of reducing cardiovascular events using antihypertensive treatment have been clearly demonstrated in a large number of controlled clinical trials. However, as shown by recent reports [1] a large proportion of patients are either untreated or fail to achieve 'normal' blood pressure. Since the severity and the frequency of cardiovascular complications, due to hypertension, are related to blood pressure, it is reasonable that better blood pressure control in the population could produce greater benefits in terms of reductions in cardiovascular complications. However, since hypertension is a very common disease, needing life-long therapy, an increase in the number of treated subjects along with more aggressive treatment, will produce a proportional increase in social costs. This could increase healthcare expenses. Projected healthcare spending will show a steep increase in the next thirty years. Indeed, in the USA by the year 2030, health spending will represent 30% of gross domestic product [2].

Until recently, only a minority of physicians were aware of the economic impact of therapeutic choices but all physicians must also consider now the economic aspects of their practice.

In the USA, with a population of around 250 million people, the acquisition cost of antihypertensive drugs is about $8 billion per year. In Italy, the costs are similar since, with a population of about 60 million, the yearly direct cost of antihypertensive drugs is about $1.5 billion. However, these costs have been calculated in countries where blood pressure control in the population has greatly improved in the last three decades, but where a large proportion of patients are untreated or undertreated. Therefore, any strategy to improve hypertension control should increase the costs but also the benefit.

The necessity of correct therapeutic choices in a field like hypertension, where treatment options are very large and, apparently, widely different in costs, creates the need for physicians to critically evaluate their practice patterns in order to maximize cost-benefit ratios for their patients. Physicians must play a primary role in the processes of pharmacoeconomic evaluations. If not, they risk being excluded from the process and if cost-containing strategies are planned without an adequate clinical input, the effects may be very deleterious, both for patient health and future medical progress. The result would e a situation in which politicians and health managers put costs first and consider health as they would any other commodity. On the other hand, excessive reductions in pharmaceutical-company profits will cause a fall in investments for research into new drugs.

Only physicians have the scientific and clinical outlook to be responsible for the management of a patient's health and only physicians can accurately evaluate the costs and benefits of treatment. The first goal of a physician must be towards the health of patients and not how much it will cost.

Methods for economic evaluations of antihypertensive treatment

The cost-benefit of treatment in hypertension depends on the magnitude of the pretreatment cardiovascular risk which, in turn, is related to blood pressure levels, on the success of treatment of blood pressure reduction and in reducing total risk as well as on the net cost of this. Net costs depend on the balance between the expenses for treatment and the savings linked to prevention of complications. However, in the case of hypertension, both cost and benefit determinations are not easy to obtain since there are many confounding variables.

Appropriate approach to the economic evaluation of alternative treatments can be performed on the basis of four different kinds of economic models [3]:

- cost minimization,
- cost-effectiveness,
- cost-utility and
- cost-benefit analysis.

The approach to cost evaluation is similar in all these analyses whereas the evaluation of outcomes is quite different.

BOX 9.4.1 Approaches to the economic evaluation of treatments

- *Cost-minimization* is the most limited type of economic analysis. This approach to evaluation compares only the costs, and not the effects, of alternative treatments. Using this kind of analysis, cheaper drugs are considered cost-effective because differences in effects are not taken into account. Furthermore, this kind of analysis frequently considers only the wholesale price of different drugs and does not include associate costs of treatment which can represent a great proportion of the final (real) costs. This kind of analysis indicates which treatment has the lowest cost, but does not take into account possible different (quantitative and qualitative) results in terms of blood pressure control and prevention of complications. Therefore, cost-minimization analysis has a place only in situations in which economic resources are very poor.
- *Cost-effectiveness analysis* evaluates effects of treatment which are qualitatively similar but, possibly, quantitatively different. Using this analysis, we can evaluate which drug gives the highest proportion of responders, the greatest blood pressure reduction, the greatest reduction in cardiovascular events or the greatest gain in years of survival.
- *Cost-utility analysis*, is more complex, and also takes into account parameters which are strictly patient-related (e.g. quality of life) but which are very important. In a disease such as hypertension, where symptoms are absent or minimal and where side effects of drugs, complex treatment schedules, need for frequent clinical visits or laboratory evaluations can interfere with everyday life, an evaluation of its quality is very important. The most adequate evaluation should be the cost per quality-adjusted life-year (QALY) which considers not only how much the survival of that patient would be increased by that therapy, but also what will be the quality of his or her life. However, the methodology for QALY measurements is still in its infancy and needs to be refined to become widely used.

9

> **BOX 9.4.1** *Continued*
>
> ● *Cost-benefit analysis* is the most difficult form of economic analysis and requires that all costs and effects of treatment are valued in dollars. This kind of analysis takes into account the effects of alternative treatment which can differ from one drug to another, both qualitatively and quantitatively. With cost-benefit evaluation, not only can survival or prevention of major complications be considered, but also the effects on intermediate endpoints. For example, it is known that different drugs producing a similar blood pressure reduction can have differing effects on other parameters like left ventricular hypertrophy: it has been shown that even if ACE inhibitors have a higher acquisition cost than diuretics or beta-blockers, their greater impact on left ventricular mass results in a better cost : benefit ratio [4]. However, for clinicians it is very hard to decide the dollar value of a year of life and thus this kind of analysis is not frequently used.

Determination of costs of treatment

An accurate evaluation of costs should first take into account costs which produce no benefit (Table 9.4.1).

A *correct diagnosis* is the first step for best utilization of resources. However, the diagnosis of hypertension is frequently made on a few (or even a single) casual blood pressure measurement and thus treatment can be prescribed to patients not needing it. Accurate, repeated blood pressure measurements are needed to avoid a false diagnosis of patients and to prevent unnecessary therapy in subjects who would not benefit from treatment and where medications could increase the risk. Diagnosing a patient who is not as hypertensive increases costs not only because of the pharmacological treatment but also because it has been shown that after a diagnosis hypertension, the number of absences from work increases as do clinical visits and laboratory tests.

Inadequate blood pressure control, due to ineffective or partially effective treatments (both pharmacological and non-pharmacological), is a certain expense with little or no benefit. In treated hypertensive patients, the probability of having a stroke is related to blood pressure, the risk being fivefold higher in patients whose diastolic blood pressure is 95 mmHg or more, in comparison with those having a diastolic blood pressure below 90 mmHg [5]. Lifestyle intervention programs are generally cheaper than drug treatment but when they are ineffective, their costs may be high. Unsuccessful long-term attempts to reduce body weight can produce frustration and may not reduce blood pressure. This may also be costly in terms of long-term complications. Since *low compliance*

Table 9.4.1 Causes of costs without benefits in the management of hypertension

- Wrong diagnosis
- Inadequate blood pressure control
- Ineffective lifestyle changes
- Poor compliance

is the most frequent cause of unsuccessful therapies, its economic impact is great. Finally, it should always be remembered that other cardiovascular risk factors should be controlled to maximize the benefits of antihypertensive treatment.

Factors affecting costs of treatment

Cost of treatment is only a part of the total costs in hypertension. In the USA, costs of hypertension are mainly due to clinical visits and hospitalization, while medication costs are only about 20% of total costs [6]. Frequently, when physicians compare the costs of alternative treatments, they think that the cost of treatment is simply the acquisition cost of the drugs. This is only part of the problem since other parameters contribute in a significant way to the final, cumulative, cost of therapy, and each must be considered for a correct evaluation (Table 9.4.2).

The acquisition cost of drugs represents only a part of the cumulative costs of treatment. In the Emilia Romagna region of Italy we observed (Figure 9.4.1) that the acquisition cost of drugs is only about 50% of the total cost of hypertension treatment even if these data are calculated over a short period of time (three months) during which the relative weight of hospitalization was insignificant [7]. Drugs with low

Table 9.4.2 Factors determining the total costs of treatment

- Acquisition of drugs
- Medical visits
- Laboratory investigations
- Hospitalization
- Side effects of drugs
- Level of compliance to treatment
- Changes in treatment
- Patient transportation
- Loss of work

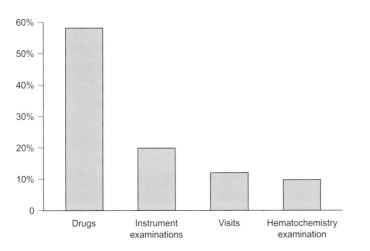

Fig. 9.4.1 Costs of hypertension in Italy evaluated in 460 patients followed for three months by family doctors and specialists (the GREAT study). The acquisition cost of drugs represents only 52% of the total costs. (From Ambrosioni *et al.* [7]).

9

acquisition costs but needing more frequent laboratory controls, clinical visits, or causing side effects (thus reducing compliance) have cumulative costs which can become much higher than their acquisition price. In spite of a strikingly different acquisition price, between the cheapest diuretics and the most expensive calcium antagonists, taking into account the other parameters generating costs (clinical visits, side effects, laboratory studies and the need of other medications) a large prospective study has shown that no significant differences in cost of treatment were detectable during one year of therapy (Table 9.4.3) [8]. The same study has also shown that within each class of drugs, the more recent ones, even at a higher price, owing to their better kinetic profile and compliance, are not usually more expensive than older drugs.

The newer drugs, such as ACE inhibitors, angiotensin II-antagonists and calcium-channel blockers have a yearly cost which is about $200–300 greater than that of diuretics and beta-blockers. However, they are generally better tolerated than the older drugs. Their antihypertensive efficacy is at least comparable to that of the older drugs, and it has been shown that ACE inhibitors and angiotensin II-antagonists are highly effective in diabetic nephropathy and in heart failure. Long-acting calcium antagonists are effective in preventing stroke in older patients whereas diltiazem and verapamil can reduce reinfarction rate. No data are available at present about the effects of these drugs on coronary artery disease. Ongoing trials may show their superiority to diuretics and beta-blockers and this would further improve their cost : benefit ratio.

The economic role of compliance

The role of compliance is crucial since only compliant patients achieve reasonable blood pressure control, and thus obtain the benefits of treatment. About 50% of prescription medications dispensed each year in the USA are not taken correctly and non-compliance tends to increase with the frequency of adverse reactions, the number of medications

Table 9.4.3 Mean costs per drug per cost category

Drug class	Acquisition cost($)	Supplemental drug cost ($)	Laboratory cost ($)	Clinic Visit cost ($)	Side effect cost ($)	Total cost ($)
Diuretics	133±107*	232±203	117±32†	298±102†	263±480	1043±667
Beta-blockers	334±170	115±192	56±32	187±87	203±418	895±545
α-blockers	401±151	290±290	114±30	227±69	256±485	1288±697
Centrally acting α-agonists	285±224	295±338	125±52	267±114	193±390	1165±658
ACE inhibitors	444±301	291±315	95±33	218±87	195±400	1243±800
Calcium-channel blockers	540±219	278±398	87±29	214±84	306±642	1425±962

It can be observed that while the acquisition costs vary up to 400% the differences in the total costs are much less evident.
Values are expressed as mean ± SD (after [8]).
ACE = angiotensin-converting enzyme.
*P<0.05, versus any other class of drugs.
†P<0.05, versus all other classes of drugs except centrally acting α-agonists.

taken and the complexity of the regimen. Low compliance, however, affects not only the benefits, but also the costs of treatment. When a treated patient has an uncontrolled blood pressure, rarely does the physician look to non-compliance. Usually, other drugs are added to the already prescribed therapy. Since compliance is inversely related to the number of pills to be taken daily, the result will be an increase cost of drugs with even lower compliance. The physician, when deciding which drug to prescribe, should always consider the tolerability profile and the costs associated with side effects.

Discontinuing and switching prescriptions also has an impact on costs. Discontinuation of treatment is very frequent, especially in everyday practice, and it has been calculated that discontinuation rate in the first six months of therapy is about 60% for the most prescribed classes of drugs [9]. However, discontinuation is not always due to inefficacy or side effects of treatment, but sometimes simply because there is a new drug to try. Frequently patients ask the doctor to prescribe them the latest 'miracle drug'. Physicians should resist the temptation of changing drugs with no real clinical need to do so. The economic importance of simple treatment schemes has been underlined by a study in which several drugs administered in a transdermal formulation were compared with traditional ones. The transdermal formulation, even if its acquisition costs were higher, were cheaper owing to the higher levels of compliance and tolerability [10].

Controlled clinical trials have shown that the probability of good compliance increases with drug toleration and is maximal with angiotensin II-antagonists, whereas poorest compliance is observed with diuretics [11,12]. A recent study performed by family doctors showed that patients needing a change in treatment and receiving a treatment based on the angiotensin II-antagonist losartan, in comparison with subjects receiving traditional therapies, achieved a similar level of blood pressure control but had less side effects and a less need of changing treatment [13].

In another recent study, it was shown that, over 26 months, patients followed by general practitioners who switched from initial therapy had a 20% increase in yearly costs in comparison with patients who continued on the original therapy. The main reasons for the switch from initial therapy were either lack of antihypertensive efficacy or unacceptable side effects [14]. Since both the efficacy in terms of blood pressure reduction, or in the percentage of responders does not greatly differ from one drug to another, the most important variable in determining differences between drugs is tolerability and thus compliance.

All these data suggest that physicians should choose (especially in drug-naïve patients) the drug which, in that patient, guarantees best compliance.

Benefits of treatment

Evaluation of the benefits obtained with antihypertensive treatment is usually based on the results of controlled clinical trials. In economic analyses, benefit is generally calculated from meta-analysis of trials which result in an average fall in diastolic blood pressure of only 5–6 mmHg. This cannot be considered as *the* benefit of treatment since it is clear that much greater blood pressure reduction and a much higher proportion of well-controlled patients can be achieved with an appropriate and intensive use of all the drugs at present available. Thus, it is highly probable that the results of some trials underestimate the favorable effects of treatment. [15,16]:

- First, the duration of some studies usually does not exceed four or five years and this is a too short time to evaluate the impact of therapy especially in patients with mild hypertension. This trial duration could be adequate in older patients in whom life expectancy is not significantly greater than the duration of the study, but not in young or middle-aged subjects. This kind of approach could lead to the paradox of calculating that the cost per year of life gained is by far smaller for elderly patients in whom prolongation of life can be only minimal or modest whereas in younger subjects life can be prolonged by several decades.
- Second, in many intervention studies, patients on placebo progressing from less severe to more severe hypertension were switched to active treatment and this must have an impact on the final evaluation.
- Third, the evaluation of benefits of treatment should not be limited to the reduction in deaths, events or hospitalizations. Other important intermediate (but clinically relevant) endpoints should be included (Table 9.4.4).
- Fourth, recruitment of patients in clinical trials usually excludes subjects at high risk such as recent stroke or myocardial infarction, renal failure, severe diabetes or obesity. These are the patients in whom short-term treatment could produce best results.
- Finally, many studies often lacked the statistical power to detect significant benefits from therapy.

These then are some of the reasons why pharmacoeconomic models tend to underestimate the benefits of therapy. Some studies [17] have suggested that treatment of hypertension should be maximally cost-effective in high-risk patients (elderly males with high blood pressure) and that only in very high-risk subjects therapy can money be saved in the long term. However, basing results on short-term intervention trials does not take into account the natural history of hypertension which, especially in its milder forms, needs decades to manifest clinically relevant complications.

The analysis of actuarial data [18] on untreated patients has suggested that the costs of antihypertensive treatment per expected additional year of life gained is much lower than that calculated when considering the results of clinical trials and has shown that cost differences between low-risk and higher risk patients are not so great and that the absolute cost of a year of life gained is low (Figure 9.4.2). Calculations based on the actuarial approach are made on logical but unproven assumptions but the same could well be said about

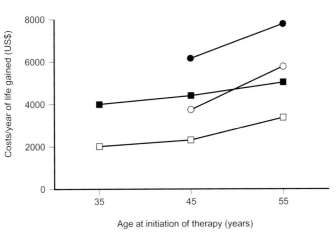

Fig. 9.4.2 Calculated costs of antihypertensive treatment per additional year of life gained as calculated by Zanchetti and Mancia [18] on the basis of actuarial data. Values are blood pressure (mmHg) at initiation of treatment. □ = males 150/100; ■ = males 145/95; ○ = females 150/100; ● = females 145/95 mmHg.

calculations based on the results of clinical trials. Furthermore, the actuarial approach, is supported by observational data over a very long period of time (1950–1990) showing that long-term therapy of hypertension patients leads to a 60% reduction in the 10-year cardiovascular mortality rate [19].

Over the next few years, several large prospective intervention trials will be published and should help us to get information about any significant benefits (at least in the short term) which can be obtained with antihypertensive treatment based on these new drugs.

How to improve the cost-benefit of antihypertensive treatment

An improvement in the cost : benefit ratio can obviously be obtained by reducing the costs, by increasing the benefits, or both.

A reduction in costs can be obtained in several ways. Correct diagnosis is the first step. Secondly, it is important to limit laboratory examinations to those really necessary, and to limit the number of clinical visits, especially those in hypertension clinics, to two or three per year. A reduction in the price of antihypertensive drugs is another effective way but this could have detrimental effects on research investment. Investment is proportional to the profits of a pharmaceutical company. With some patients, the use of generic drugs could cut the costs. The use of drugs with lower acquisition costs seems not to be an effective way, since cheaper drugs usually have higher accessory costs and are usually associated with poor compliance.

It should always be remembered that arbitrary cost-cutting in the pharmaceutical sector can have detrimental consequences on other health areas, e.g. by increasing costs due to hospitalization. Lifestyle changes can be useful in reducing the drug dosage necessary to

9

maintain blood pressure within the normal limits even if compliance to lifestyle changes is very hard to assess.

Another important step is to increase compliance. Most important is good doctor–patient communication. If the patient is clearly informed about the risks of the disease, the advantages of treatment and how to conduct it, it will minimize potential problems and compliance can be greatly improved. Self-measurement of blood pressure is yet another very useful tool to improve compliance. For those patients in whom non-compliance is due to memory problems, reminding systems can be tried.

An improvement of benefits can be obtained firstly by increasing the proportion of treated patients with good blood pressure control. This can be achieved by improving compliance, minimizing the risk of side effects and simplifying treatment schedules by using, where possible, once-a-day drugs and fixed-dose combination treatments. Additional benefits can be obtained by non-pharmacological measures.

Advantages can be also obtained by prescribing drugs effective in correcting possible associated diseases. Examples include ACE inhibitors and AT-II antagonists in diabetic patients with nephropathy, or alpha-blockers in subjects with prostate disorders, and clonidine or beta-blockers in patients suffering from headache. Benefits which cannot be clearly demonstrated by short-term clinical trials but which can be of great importance in the long term (see Table 9.4.4) should also be considered.

Conclusions

The cost-benefit profile of a given treatment depends on the different points of view of those involved in treatment decisions. It is clear that physicians, healthcare providers, patients, employers, the pharmaceutical industry and government, can have different perspectives and their opinions can be conflicting. However, physicians should clearly know the factors that generate costs and the issues necessary to make cost-effective therapeutic decisions. The main goal is to find the best outcome for patients. In hypertension treatment, this is efficacy in reducing complications at a reasonable cost [20]. The benefits for patients both in terms of a reduction in morbidity and mortality require many strategies and should not focus only on cost-containment measures.

Table 9.4.4 Factors besides costs which should be considered in the economic evaluation of antihypertensive treatment

- Prevention/regression of atherosclerosis
- Prevention/regression of myocardial ischemia
- Prevention/regression of renal damage
- Prevention/regression of left ventricular hypertrophy
- Improvement of endothelial function
- Prevention of heart failure
- Effects on lipid metabolism
- Effects on glucose metabolism
- Effects on blood coagulation

Over the next few years, further information about the clinical and prognostic importance of the effects of drugs on other parameters (Table 9.4.4) will become available. However, it should always be remembered that full benefits of treatment can only be obtained if patients achieve normal blood pressure and maintain it in the long term. Thus, the winning strategy in terms of cost-benefit will be that of prescribing a treatment which, in the individual patient, gives the best probability of continuing it in the long term. Such a strategy should also be beneficial from the point of view of economics.

References

1. The Sixth Report of the Joint National Committee on Prevention, Detection, Evaluation, and Treatment of High Blood Pressure. NIH Publication, pp. 98–4080, National Institutes of Health: Bethesda, MD, 1997.
2. Burner ST, Waldo DR, McCusick DR. National health expenditures projections through 2030. *Health Care Financing Rev* 1992;**14**:1–30.
3. Maynard A. The economics of hypertension control: some basic issues. *J Human Hypertension* 1992;**6**:417–420.
4. Eagle KA, Blank DJ, Aguiar F, Firth LM. Economic impact of regression of left ventricular hypertrophy by antihypertensive drugs. *J Human Hypertension* 1993;**7**:341–344.
5. Du X, Cruikshank K, McNamee R *et al*. Case–control study of stroke and the quality of hypertension control in north-west England. *Br Med J* 1997;**314**:272–276.
6. Moser M. The cost of treating hypertension. Can we keep it under control without compromising the level of care? *Am J Hypertension* 1998;**11**:120s–127s.
7. Ambrosioni E, Beluci A, Bustacchini S *et al*. and the GREAT investigators. The cost of hypertension and its correlates in Emilia Romagna region (Italy): results from the GREAT study. *Proceedings of the European Conference of the International Society of Pharmacoeconomics and Outcome Research, Edinburgh*, 1999;302.
8. Hilleman DE, Mohiuddin SM, Lucas BD *et al*. Cost-minimization analysis of initial antihypertensive therapy in patients with mild-to-moderate essential diastolic hypertension *Clin Ther* 1994;**16**:88–102.
9. Jones JK, Gorkin L, Lian JF *et al*. Discontinuation of and changes in treatment after start of new courses of antihypertensive drugs: a study of United Kingdom population. *Br Med J* 1996;**311**:293–295.
10. Cramer MP, Saks SR. Translating safety, efficacy, compliance and economic value for controlled release dosage forms. *Pharmacoeconomics* 1994;**5**:482–504.
11. Gregoire JP. Choice of initial antihypertensive medication and continuation of use. *Can J Cardiol* 1999;**15**(Suppl F):39–41.
12. Bloom BS. Continuation of initial antihypertensive medication after 1 year of therapy. *Clin Ther* 1998;**20**:671–681.
13. Moore MA, Edelman JM, Gadzdick LP *et al*. for the LET investigators. Choice of initial antihypertensive medication may influence the extent to which patients stay on therapy: a community-based study of losartan-based regimen vs. usual care. *High Blood Press* 1998;**7**:156–167.
14. Hughes D, McGuire A. The direct costs to the NHS of discontinuing and switching prescriptions for hypertension. *J Human Hypertension* 1998;**12**:533–537.
15. Ambrosioni E, Costa FV. Cost-effectiveness calculations from trials. *J Hypertension* 1996 (Suppl 2):s47–s52.
16. Simpson FO. Fallacies in the interpretations of the large scale trials of treatment of mild to moderate hypertension. *J Cardiovasc Pharmacol* 1990;**16** (Suppl. 7):92s–95s.
17. Johannesson M. The cost-effectiveness of hypertension treatment in Sweden. *Pharmacoeconomics* 1995;**7**:242–250.
18. Zanchetti A, Mancia G. Editor's corner: benefits and cost-effectiveness of antihypertensive therapy. The actuarial versus the intervention trial approach. *J Hypertension* 1996;**14**:809–811.

9

References

19. Sytkowski PA, D'Agostino RB, Belanger AJ, Kannel WB. Secular trends in long-term sustained hypertension, long-term treatment and cardiovascular mortality: the Framingham Heart Study 1950–1990. *Circulation* 1996;**93**:697–703.

20. McMurray J. The health economics of the treatment of hyperlipidemia and hypertension. *Am J Hypertension* 1999;**12**:99s–104s.

9

Isolated office hypertension

G Mancia and G Parati

Introduction

Isolated office hypertension is the condition in which systolic and/or diastolic blood pressure are elevated (i.e. equal to or above 140 mmHg and/or 90 mmHg, respectively) when repeatedly measured in the clinic environment by a doctor or a nurse, but normal when self-measured at home or assessed through automatic or semiautomatic ambulatory blood pressure monitoring techniques [1]. Critical for the diagnosis of isolated office hypertension is the persisting presence of elevated blood pressure at the time of consultation and of extraoffice 'normotension' over time. Isolated office blood pressure elevations that can be found only at the initial or at the first few visits, and that later disappear, should be regarded as temporary blood pressure abnormalities with no obvious adverse prognostic significance [2], and should not lead to the diagnosis of isolated office hypertension.

Prevalence of isolated office hypertension

The prevalence of isolated office hypertension in various countries has not been conclusively determined [3]. The reported figures range from more than 60% to less than 10% of the overall hypertensive population. However, the highest figures reported are likely to largely overestimate this phenomenon, either because of the inclusion of subjects with a temporary rather than a persistent office hypertension (see above), and/or because of the inclusion in this category of all subjects in whom office blood pressure values above 140 mmHg systolic (and/or 90 mmHg diastolic) corresponded to home, daytime average or 24-hour average values just below 140/90 mmHg. It is now clear that the upper limit of normality for home and daytime or 24-hour average blood pressure is much lower than 140/90 mmHg [4–9], the values reported in a large population study performed in Italy being lower than 132/81, 132/85 and 126/80 mmHg, respectively [9]. This means that a subject having an office blood pressure equal to or greater than 140/90 mmHg together with a home or a daytime blood pressure of, for example, 136/88 mmHg should be regarded as hypertensive both inside and outside the doctor's office. Isolated office hypertension should only be diagnosed where persistent office hypertension is accompanied by blood pressure values below 130/85 mmHg when measured at home or over the daytime and below 126/80 mmHg when measured over 24 hours. Under these conditions the prevalence is not greater than 10–15% of the hypertensive population.

Mechanisms of isolated office hypertension

The mechanisms responsible for isolated office hypertension have not yet been completely clarified [3]. However, it is believed that an emotional reaction to the measurement of blood pressure in the clinic environment is involved, which is the reason for this condition to be widely known also as 'white coat hypertension' [10]. This is justified by several findings:

9

- Blood pressure can indeed increase acutely when measured by a doctor and to a lesser extent by a nurse (Figures 9.5.1 and 9.5.2) [11,12].
- Blood pressure values can have widely different magnitudes in different subjects with no relationship with baseline values and age [11], and no consistent attenuation when the patient is repeatedly visited by the same doctor, over a relatively narrow time span (Figure 9.5.3) [12].

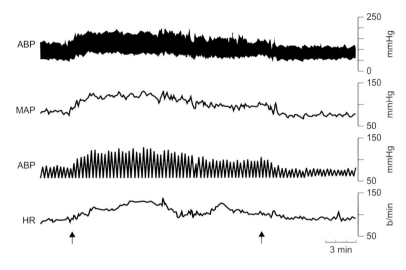

Fig. 9.5.1 Original intra-arterial blood pressure and heart rate tracing showing the pressor and tachycardic effect of the physician's visit in a representative subject. Arrows at the bottom refer to the beginning and the end of the visit. ABP: pulsatile blood pressure; MAP: mean arterial pressure; ∫ABP, blood pressure integrated every 10 s, HR: heart rate. (Reproduced with permission[11].)

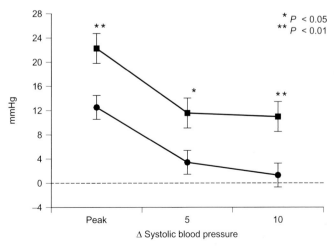

Fig. 9.5.2 Intra-arterial systolic (S) blood pressure changes induced during the visit by a doctor and a nurse. Data are shown as average values ± SE from 35 patients. Values obtained at the time of maximal changes (peak), after 5 and 10 min since the beginning of the visit are separately shown. (Reproduced with permission[12].)

Mechanisms of isolated
office hypertension

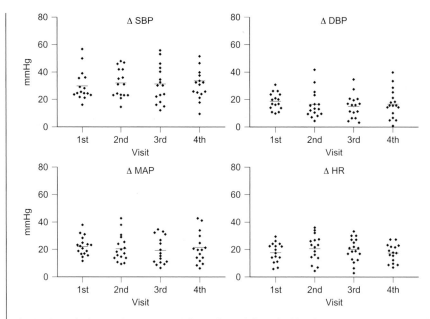

Fig. 9.5.3 Peak changes in intra-arterial systolic and diastolic blood pressures, mean arterial pressure and heart rate values during a physician's visit in 46 hypertensive patients. Data are separately shown for four consecutive visits by the same physician performed over a 48 hour period. (Reproduced with permission[12].)

- In contrast, no blood pressure increase characterizes semiautomatic or automatic blood pressure measurements during the day (Figures 9.5.4 and 9.5.5) except perhaps for the first few measurements only [13].

  Nevertheless, several findings also suggest that a pressor response to the emotion elicited by a doctor's or nurse's blood pressure measurement is not the only mechanism involved:

- While the white coat effect is characterized not only by a pressor but also by a tachycardic response (see Figures 9.5.1–9.5.3), office heart rate values have not been shown to be systematically greater than the home or ambulatory ones (Figure 9.5.6) [9–14].
- The clinic-daytime or clinic-home blood pressure differences increase with clinic hypertension and ageing (Figure 9.5.6) while the white coat effect is independent of the baseline blood pressure value or whether the subject is young, middle-aged or elderly.
- No significant relationship has been found between white coat effect when measured directly (beat-to-beat blood pressure monitoring before, during and after a doctor's visit) and indirectly quantified from the clinic-daytime blood pressure difference [15].
- This difference has been shown to correlate directly with baseline clinic blood pressure, but inversely with baseline ambulatory blood pressure [14]. This suggests that factors modulating blood pressure values in daily life, such as for example the degree of physical activity [16,17] and of environmental stimuli to blood pressure [18] participate together with the white coat effect in the determination of this phenomenon.

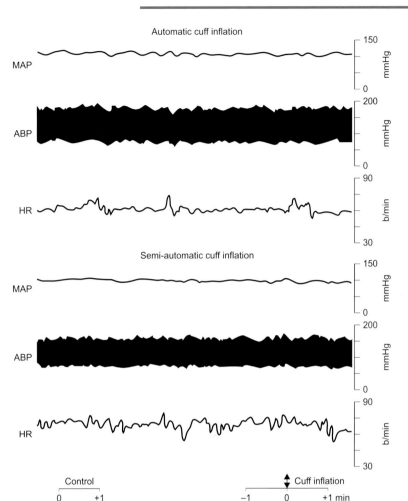

Fig. 9.5.4 Original intra-arterial blood pressure recordings performed in a representative subject at the time of non-invasive blood pressure measurements in which cuff inflation was started automatically (upper panel) or was self-triggered by the patient (semi-automatic measurement, lower panel). Arrows refer to the time of cuff inflation. (Reproduced with permission[13].)

Clinical significance

The clinical significance of isolated office hypertension is also uncertain [3]. This is because while a number of cross-sectional studies have reported this condition to be associated with metabolic abnormalities typical of hypertension (dyslipidemia and insulin resistance) [19] or with damage in various organs targeted by hypertension [20–25], other studies have shown it to have organ structures and functions indistinguishable from those of normotensive individuals [26–29]. Furthermore, longitudinal studies on the outcome of subjects with isolated office hypertension are limited and controversial [30–32]. This is exemplified by a study which showed that over an average of 3.2 years,

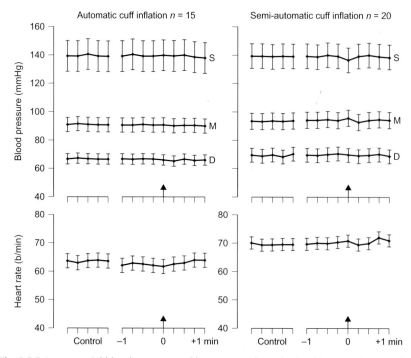

Fig. 9.5.5 Intra-arterial blood pressure and heart rate values obtained in 15 patients at the time of automatic blood pressure measurements and in 20 patients when the cuff inflation was triggered by the patient himself. Data are shown as average values ± SEM for 10-s segments of the intra-arterial tracing taken 5 min before cuff inflation, and during the 1-min period immediately preceding and following cuff inflation. Arrows refer to the time of cuff inflation. S: systolic blood pressure; D: diastolic blood pressure; M: mean arterial pressure. (Reproduced with permission[13].)

normotensive subjects and subjects with isolated office hypertension had a similarly low number of cardiovascular events as compared to patients with both clinic and ambulatory hypertension (Figure 9.5.7) [30]. However, this study did not provide comprehensive information on the extent of treatment, the type of treatment and the blood pressure values achieved by treatment in the hypertensive groups. Moreover, because of the low number of events occurring in the normotensives and isolated office hypertensives, it could not determine statistically whether isolated office hypertension is entirely innocent or carries a risk that is greater than that of the normotensive condition.

This is also exemplified by a study which showed that subjects with isolated office hypertension frequently progress, over a few years, to ambulatory hypertension [31]. However, no comparison was made with a normotensive group regarding clinical outcomes.

Information is limited and controversial with regard to the clinical significance of a phenomenon related to isolated office hypertension, i.e. the absolute difference between office and ambulatory blood pressure, regardless of whether the former shows hypertensive or normotensive values. Again, there are studies which show this difference to be related to target-organ damage [24,33] and suggest it to

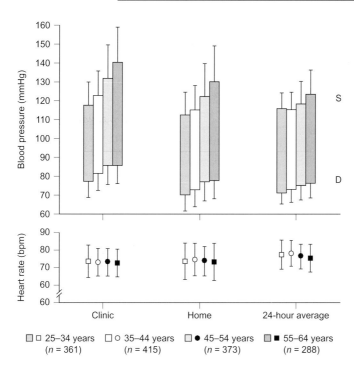

Fig. 9.5.6 Clinic, home and 24-hour average blood pressure and heart rate values in normotensive and untreated hypertensive subjects included in the PAMELA study. Data are shown as average values ± SEM separately for different age decades. S: systolic blood pressure, D: diastolic blood pressure. (Reproduced with permission[9].)

be due to its reflection of the white coat effect and, more generally, of the blood pressure tendency to increase as a result of stressful stimuli [34]. However, other studies show subjects with large office-ambulatory blood pressure differences to have cardiovascular structures and functions similar to those with small office-ambulatory blood pressure differences, thereby leading to the conclusion that this phenomenon is non-pathological [35–37]. In a recent study performed by our group on hypertensive patients with echocardiographic left ventricular hypertrophy [38], the office-daytime blood pressure difference was attenuated during a one-year antihypertensive treatment. The degree of the attenuation, however, did not bear any relationship with the reduction of left ventricular mass index which depended on the treatment-induced change in ambulatory blood pressure alone (Figure 9.5.8) [39].

Treatment of isolated office hypertension

Because its clinical significance is uncertain, the decision whether to start drug treatment in patients with isolated office hypertension is difficult. However, there can be little doubt that lifestyle changes aimed at reducing overall cardiovascular risk should be implemented and antihypertensive drug treatment should be considered if these patients

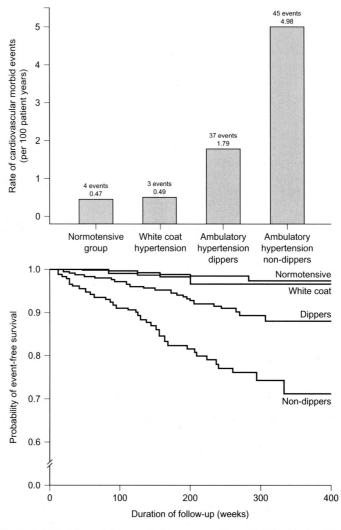

Fig. 9.5.7 Probability of event-free survival in a population of 1187 subjects with essential hypertension and 205 healthy control subjects with clinic normotension included in the PIUMA study. Hypertensive patients are further subdivided into 'white coat' hypertensives and ambulatory hypertensives with (dippers) or without (non-dippers) a nocturnal blood pressure fall >10% of daytime blood pressure. Comparison between survival curves was highly significant ($P < 0.02$). (Reproduced with permission[30].)

belong to the very high- or high-risk categories as defined by the WHO/ISH 1999 Guidelines [1], namely if they have:

- cardiovascular diseases related to hypertension (e.g. myocardial infarction, cerebrovascular disease, etc.),
- signs of organ damage (left ventricular hypertrophy, large artery plaques, silent myocardial ischemia, renal damage, etc.) and
- diabetes and/or multiple risk factors of a metabolic (e.g. dyslipidemia) or non-metabolic (e.g. smoking) nature.

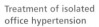
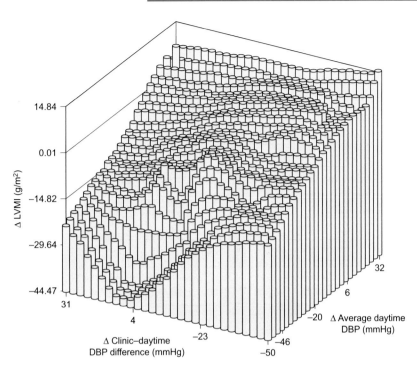

Clinical relevance of 'surrogate' estimates of white coat effect (Δ with treatment)

Fig. 9.5.8 Three-dimensional plots simultaneously illustrating the relationship between treatment-induced changes in left ventricular mass index (Δ-LVMI), in average daytime or home blood pressure (Δ-BP) and in clinic-daytime or clinic-home blood pressure differences (Δ-differences). Data refer to 206 essential hypertensive patients with left ventricular hypertrophy included in the Study on Ambulatory Monitoring And Lisinopril Evaluation (SAMPLE) and treated for 12 months with the ACE inhibitor lisinopril associated with a diuretic if needed.

Under these circumstances, drugs should be started at low doses and titrated upwards cautiously, to avoid possible excessive falls in ambulatory blood pressure, and underperfusion of vital organs.

If, on the other hand, patients with isolated office hypertension belong to the low- or medium-risk category [1] drug treatment might be avoided. However, in this case, lifestyle changes should always be implemented both to pursue some reduction of the elevated office blood pressure values and to keep the overall risk profile low. In addition, patients should be monitored frequently to initiate antihypertensive drug administration if ambulatory or home blood pressure becomes abnormal (and thus patients no longer fit the definition of 'isolated office hypertension') or organ damage becomes manifest. It should be emphasized, however, that the above recommendations (see Table 9.5.1) are based on common sense rather than on conclusive scientific evidence and that thus careful judgment of any individual situation by physicians is required. Physicians should also be aware that, because of the large body of evidence that patient's outcome depends on office blood pressure [40] and improves with its reduction [41], avoiding or delaying treatment when its value is persistently elevated carries a legal

9

9.5

Table 9.5.1 Clinical management of patients with isolated office hypertension

- High-or very high-risk categories (WHO/ISH Guidelines 1999) [1]
    Antihypertensive drug treatment
    Lifestyle changes
- Low- or medium-risk categories (WHO/ISH Guidelines 1999) [1]
    Drug treatment may be avoided
    Lifestyle changes to be implemented
    Close follow up over time by monitoring ambulatory or home blood pressure and
    appearance of organ damage

responsibility and should thus be done only after the patient has been given information and has approved it.

References

1. 1999 World Health Organization–International Society of Hypertension Guidelines for the Management of Hypertension. *J Hypertension* 1999;**17**:151–183.
2. Neaton JD, Grimm RH, Prineas RJ *et al.* for the Treatment of Mild Hypertension Study Research group. Treatment of Mild Hypertension Study: final results. *J Am Med Ass* 1993;**270**:713–724.
3. Mancia G, Zanchetti A. White-coat hypertension: misnomers, misconceptions and misunderstandings: what should we do next? *J Hypertension* 1996;**14**:1049–1052.
4. O'Brien E, Murphy J, Tyndal A *et al.* Twenty-four hour ambulatory blood pressure in men and women aged 17 to 80 years: the Allied Irish Bank Study. *J Hypertension* 1991;**9**:355–360.
5. Staessen JA, Fagard R, Lijnen P *et al.* Ambulatory blood pressure and blood pressure measured at home: progress report on a population study. *J Cardiovasc Pharmacol* 1994;**23** (Suppl. 5):S5–S11.
6. Staessen JA, Fagard R, Lijnen P *et al.* Mean and range of ambulatory blood pressure in normotensive subjects from a meta-analysis of 23 studies. *Am J Cardiol* 1991;**67**:723–727.
7. Imai Y, Nagai K, Sakuma M *et al.* Ambulatory blood pressure of adults in Ohasama, Japan. *Hypertension* 1993;**22**:900–912.
8. Rasmussen SL, Torp-Pedersen C, Borch-Johnsen K, Ibsen H. Normal values for ambulatory blood pressure and differences between casual blood pressure and ambulatory blood pressure: results from a Danish population survey. *J Hypertension* 1998;**10**:1415–1424.
9. Mancia G, Sega R, Bravi C *et al.* Ambulatory blood pressure normality: results from the PAMELA study. *J Hypertension* 1995;**13**:1377–1390.
10. Pickering TG, James GD, Harshfield GA *et al.* How common is white-coat hypertension? *J Am Med Ass* 1988;**259**:225–228.
11. Mancia G, Bertinieri G, Grassi G *et al.* Effects of blood pressure measurement by the doctor on patients' blood pressure and heart rate. *Lancet* 1983;**ii**:695–698.
12. Mancia G, Parati G, Pomidossi G *et al.* Alerting reaction and rise in blood pressure during measurement by physician and nurse. *Hypertension* 1987;**9**:209–215.
13. Parati G, Pomidossi G, Casadei R, Mancia G. Lack of alerting reactions to intermittent cuff inflation during non-invasive blood pressure monitoring. *Hypertension* 1985;**7**:597–601.
14. Parati G, Omboni S, Staessen J *et al.* On behalf of the SYST-EUR investigators. Limitations of the difference between clinic and daytime blood pressure as a surrogate measure of the 'white-coat' effect. *J Hypertension* 1998;**16**(1):23–29.
15. Parati G, Ulian L, Santucciu C *et al.* Difference between clinic and day-time blood pressure is not a measure of the white-coat effect. *Hypertension* 1998;**31**:1185–1189.
16. Shimizu M, Kitazumi H, Kawabe T *et al.* Exercise performance in essential hypertension with special preference to blood pressure response and left ventricular hypertrophy. *Am J Hypertension* 1992;**5**:92–94.

9

17. Fagard R, Staessen J, Thijs L, Amery A. Prognostic significant of exercise versus resting blood pressure in hypertensive men. *Hypertension* 1991;**17**:574–578.

18. Mancia G, Parati G, Di Rienzo M, Zanchetti A. Blood pressure variability. In: *Handbook of Hypertension*, Vol. 17: *Pathophysiology of Hypertension* (eds Zanchetti A, Mancia G), pp. 117–169. Elsevier: Amsterdam, 1997.

19. Julius S, Mejia A, Jones K *et al*. White-coat versus sustained borderline hypertension in Tecumseh, Michigan. *Hypertension* 1990;**16**:617–623.

20. Hoegholm A, Kristensen KS, Madsen NH, Svendsen TL. White-coat hypertension diagnosed by 24-hour ambulatory monitoring. Examination of 159 newly diagnosed hypertensive patients. *Am J Hypertension* 1992;**5**:64–70.

21. Kuwajima I, Suzuki Y, Fujisawa A, Kuramoto K. Is white-coat hypertension innocent? Structure and function of the heart in the elderly. *Hypertension* 1993;**22**:826–831.

22. Cardillo C, De Felice F, Campia U, Folli G. Psychological reactivity and cardiac end-organ changes in white-coat hypertension. *Hypertension* 1993;**21**:836–844.

23. Burnier M, Biollaz J, Magnin JL *et al*. Renal sodium handling in patients with untreated hypertension and white-coat hypertension. *Hypertension* 1994;**23**:496–502.

24. Palatini P, Penzo M, Canali C *et al*. Interactive action of the white-coat effect and the blood pressure levels on cardiovascular complications in hypertension. *Excerpta Medica* 1997;**103**:208–216.

25. Chang NC, Lai ZY, Chan P, Wang TC. Left ventricular filling properties in young white-coat hypertensive patients without hypertrophy. *Hypertension* 1997;**30** (part 2):746–752.

26. Verdecchia P, Schillaci G, Bodrini F *et al*. Variability between current definitions of 'normal' ambulatory blood pressure. *Hypertension* 1992;**20**:555–562.

27. Gosse P, Promax H, Durandet P, Clementy J. White-coat hypertension. No harm for the heart. *Hypertension* 1993;**22**:766–770.

28. White W, Schulman P, McCabe EJ, Dey H. Average daily blood pressure, not office blood pressure, determines cardiac function in patients with hypertension. *J Am Med Ass* 1989;**261**:873–877.

29. Sokolow M, Perloff D, Cowan R. Contribution of ambulatory blood pressure to the assessment of patients with mild to moderate elevations of office blood pressure. Cardiovasc. *Rev Rep* 1980;**1**:295–303.

30. Verdecchia P, Porcellati C, Schillaci G *et al*. Ambulatory blood pressure. An independent predictor of prognosis in essential hypertension. *Hypertension* 1994;**24**:793–801.

31. Waeber B, Burnier M, Heynen G, Brunner HR. Clinical utility of ambulatory blood pressure monitoring in the evaluation of patients with borderline hypertension. *J Cardiovasc Risk* 1994;**2**:120–126.

32. Waeber B, Scherrer U, Petrillo A *et al*. Are some hypertensive patients overtreated? *Lancet* 1987;**ii**:732–733.

33. Cerasola G, Cottone S, Nardi E, D'lgnoto D *et al*. White-coat hypertension and cardiovascular risk. *J Cardiovasc Risk* **2**(6):545–549.

34. Mancia G, Parati G. Reactivity to physical and behavioural stress and blood pressure variability in hypertension. In: *Handbook of Hypertension, Behavioural Factors in Hypertension* (eds Julius S, Basset DR), Vol. 9, pp. 104–122. Elsevier: Amsterdam, 1987.

35. Verdecchia P, Schillaci G, Borgioni C *et al*. White-coat hypertension and white-coat effect: similarities and differences. *Am J Hypertension* 1995;**8**:790–798.

36. Verdecchia P, Schillaci G, Borgioni C *et al*. Prognostic significance of the white-coat effect. *Hypertension* 1997;**29**:1218–1224.

37. Cavallini MC, Roman MJ, Pickering TG *et al*. Is white-coat hypertension associated with arterial disease or left ventricular hypertophy? *Hypertension* 1995;**26**(3):413–419.

38. Mancia G, Zanchetti A, Agabiti-Rosei E *et al*. the Sample Study Group. Ambulatory blood pressure is superior to clinic blood pressure in predicting treatment-induced regression of left ventricular hypertrophy. *Circulation* 1997;**95**:1464–1470.

39. Parati G, Ulian L, Sampieri L *et al*. on behalf of the SAMPLE Study Group. Attenuation of the 'white-coat' effect by antihypertensive treatment and regression of target organ damage. *Hypertension* 2000;**35**:614–620.

9

References

40. Collins R, Peto R, MacMahon S *et al.* Blood pressure, stroke and coronary heart disease. Part 2. Short-term reductions in blood pressure: overview of randomised drug trials in their epidemiological context. *Lancet* 1990;**335**:827–839.
41. MacMahon S, Peto R, Cutler J *et al.* Blood pressure, stroke, and coronary heart disease. Part 1. Prolonged differences in blood pressure: prospective observational studies corrected for the regression dilution bias. *Lancet* 1990;**335**:765–774.

9

Index